MATERNAL AND CHILD HEALTH NURSING

MATERNAL & CHILD HEALTH NURSING

A. JOY INGALLS, R.N., M.S.

Instructor, Maternal and Child Health Nursing,
Grossmont Vocational Nursing School,
La Mesa, California

M. CONSTANCE SALERNO, R.N., M.S.

Professor of Pediatric Nursing,
San Diego State University,
San Diego University,

Special contributions:

CHAPTER 18 *Intensive care of the newborn*

LINDA JEAN CRAMER, R.N., B.S.

Senior Staff Nurse, Neonatal Special Care Unit,
University Hospital, University of California,
San Diego, California

JOHN E. WIMMER, Jr., M.D.

Perinatal Research Fellow, University Hospital,
University of California, San Diego, California

CHAPTER 23 *Rehabilitation of the long-term pediatric patient*

LARRY D. CHRISTENSON, R.N.

Assistant Director of Nursing Service; former Coordinator
of Rehabilitation, Children's Hospital,
San Diego, California

THIRD EDITION

with 627 illustrations

The C. V. Mosby Company

SAINT LOUIS   1975

Conversion chart on back endpaper from
Chinn, P. L.: Child health maintenance:
concepts in family-centered care, St. Louis, 1974,
The C. V. Mosby Co.

THIRD EDITION

Printed in the United States of America

Distributed in Great Britain by Henry Kimpton, London

Library of Congress Cataloging in Publication Data

Ingalls, A. Joy.
    Maternal and child health nursing.

    "Special contributions: chapter 18: Intensive care of
the newborn, Linda Jean Cramer and John E. Wimmer, Jr. . . .
chapter 23: Rehabilitation of the long-term pediatric patient,
Larry D. Christenson."
    Bibliography: p.
    Includes index.
    1. Obstetrical nursing. 2. Pediatric nursing.
I. Salerno, M. Constance, joint author. II. Title.
[DNLM: 1. Obstetrical nursing. 2. Pediatric nursing.
WY157 I44m]
RG951.I5 1975   610.73′62   75-2480
ISBN 0-8016-2330-8

VH/VH/VH   9 8 7 6 5 4 3 2 1

To

THE BEDSIDE NURSE

whatever her title

Preface

The third edition of *Maternal and Child Health Nursing* reflects the vast changes in medical technology, specialization of services, expansion of roles, and continuing challenges, opportunities, and frustrations of nursing in the mid-seventies. Hardly a page remains as it was in the previous revision. New developments of each day outdate publications of the day before. One puzzles over priorities, roles, and systems, as the "future shock" of modern technology, worldwide dilemmas, and deeply personal problems merge in the experience of the contemporary nurse.

One of the newer specialties in pediatrics, which nurses may encounter with varying levels of involvement, is the pediatric intensive care unit or special care nursery. They should be aware of the types of therapy and nursing intervention offered in these intensive care units and the progression of care that pediatric patients may have experienced. As a graduate, the pediatric nurse may wish to pursue this interest further. We are indebted to John E. Wimmer Jr., M.D., and Linda Cramer, R.N., who contributed Chapter 18, Intensive Care of the Newborn.

We also welcome as a contributor representing another recently defined pediatric specialty, Larry D. Christenson, R.N. Mr. Christenson shares his considerable experience and knowledge in Chapter 23, Reha-bilitation of the Long-Term Pediatric Patient.

In an attempt to combine the best of two worlds, the problems concerning the body systems (unit eleven) have been arranged according to the age groups primarily affected: infant, toddler, preschool and school-age child, and adolescent. This rearrangement was made with the realization that just as childhood illnesses do not always fit neatly into an anatomical category, they often refuse to be confined to one age group.

Considerable material has been added and much deleted in an effort to maintain a volume of approximately the same size. Among special areas of addition are: an expanded treatment of nutrition in prenatal care; an introduction of fetal monitoring; a reevaluation of the problem of toxemia of pregnancy; more material concerning methods of assessing fetal health and premature labor; characteristics of the immature infant; methods of infant feeding and the development of maternal attachment. The discussion of pediatric abnormalities has been enhanced by an increased explanation of genetics, congenital hip dislocation, tracheoesophageal fistula, hydrocephalus, scoliosis, asthma, and pneumonia. Recent progress in the treatment of leukemia, osteogenic sarcoma, and congenital heart disease has also been included. Students and teachers may also be interested to know that a separate Student Study Guide based on the text is now available.

Artistically, the text has been enhanced by the retention of many of Martha Lackey's original line drawings and the addition of the sensitive work of Mary Fritchoff and Kalman Erdeky. Karla Barber, who again offered her exceptional talent, and a very competent Ron Ray were responsible for many of the new photographs.

Again, our deep-felt appreciation must be extended to Anne Blythe, our main typist and consistent support in both calm and crisis, and to the Director of Health Occupations of the Grossmont Union High School District, Adult Education, Ellen M. Abbott, who has offered continuous, generous encouragement and help throughout this extended endeavor. We must also acknowledge the long period of altered lifestyle that this modest but time-consuming project necessitated for our respective families and thank them for all their understanding and assistance.

One may not know the shape of tomorrow, but nurses today seek to prepare themselves to function in a variety of settings and at many levels to meet the needs of people of all ages. It is our hope that this new edition will make the task a little easier as nurses face the challenges of maternal and child health care.

A. Joy Ingalls
M. Constance Salerno

Contents

Contents

MATERNAL AND CHILD HEALTH NURSING

unit one
Introduction

1

Current perspectives in maternal-child care

Nurses working in hospital maternity and pediatric departments and clinics need to know about the development of these specialties and the current goals of these services not only locally but also from a national perspective. This brief introductory chapter contains some definitions and important statistics and a short historical review designed to increase the student's appreciation of the progress that has been made and the problems that still remain.

That progress has been made cannot be denied. Great reductions have been realized in the amount of illness and death involving both mothers and children. The overlapping disciplines of *obstetrics,* the art and science of maternal-fetal and newborn care, and *pediatrics,* the art and science of the care of children and youth, have made tremendous, almost miraculous advances in the last 50 years.

To help the student understand the extent of the improvement that has been made in the field, it will be necessary to introduce some statistics; however, they need not be complicated or lengthy to tell an important story.

Maternal mortality

Among health statistics we often encounter the term "mortality," which means the number of persons per given population who died in a given period of time. Maternal mortality refers to the number of mothers who die per 100,000 live births for a certain period. In 1915 maternal mortality in the United States equaled 608 per 100,-000. By 1973 maternal mortality for this country had fallen to 15.2 per 100,000 (provisional figure).*

Although this figure represents a splendid reduction in the maternal death rate, it should be much lower. The national statistics for 1973 continue to demonstrate a great but narrowing difference between the maternal death rate among nonwhite mothers (34.6 per 100,000) and white mothers (10.7 per 100,000), reflecting a significant inequality in the availability or use of maternity services. Shifting centers of population, lack of education, strained, understaffed public facilities, and ineffectual health delivery systems all help contribute to a higher maternal death rate than should be recorded by the United States.

Leading causes. Statistically, as of 1973 the most common causes of maternal death (when abortions with various complications were computed separately) were the toxemias, 23%; infections, 20.5%; hemorrhage, 12.5%; and abortions, 7.5% (provisional figure).*

The toxemias of pregnancy include several associated signs and symptoms such as elevated blood pressure (hypertension), albumin in the urine (albuminuria), and an abnormal amount of fluid in the tissues (edema). Edema reveals itself by swelling

*U. S. Department of Health, Education, and Welfare, Public Health Service, Health Resources Administration, Monthly Vital Statistics Report, vol. 23, Suppl. 2, Feb. 10, 1975, pp. 2, 18.

1

and rapid weight gain, headache, and, in extreme cases, even convulsions. At this time there is no agreement among clinicians regarding its cause.

Hemorrhage is by far the most common major obstetrical complication. It should be appreciated that many times hemorrhage may predispose a mother to fall victim to other difficulties, such as infection. The greatest progress in the overall reduction of maternal mortality through the years has been in the prevention of infection.

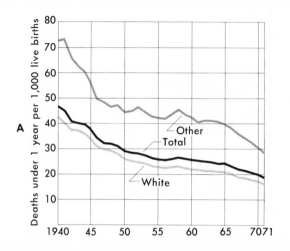

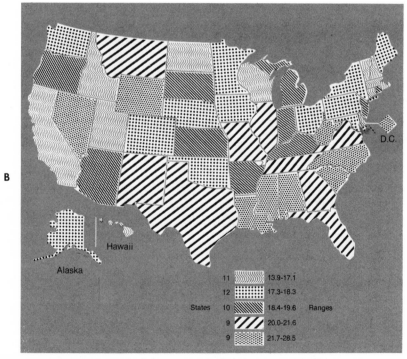

Fig. 1-1. **A,** U. S. infant mortality trends: 1940-1971 (1970-71 figures are provisional). **B,** Infant mortality in each state, 1971. U. S. provisional rate: 19.1 deaths under 1 year per 1,000 live births. Source: Maternal and Child Health Project, George Washington University. (From Maternal and child health service reports on: Promoting the health of mothers and children, Washington, D. C., FY 1973, Department of Health, Education, and Welfare.)

Fetal mortality

Another type of statistic that is often cited is fetal mortality, a combination of words that may mean different things to different people. The usual definition is the number of fetuses of 20 weeks' gestational development or more that die before birth. However, in 1950 the World Health Organization (WHO) recommended that the definition be based on death of a fetus, regardless of age, before its complete removal from its mother. We have no accurate way to determine the extent of fetal death as defined by WHO, but we know that the waste of life is very significant. The loss of a pregnancy before the fetus is *viable* (sufficiently developed to live independently outside his mother), regardless of the cause, is termed an abortion by professional personnel. Viability has become a legal consideration. Communities differ in their definitions. Some regard the 20-week-old gestation as viable; others use the term only after 24 weeks of fetal development. "Legal viability" may not agree with the survival rate statistics, however. The survival of a child of appropriate weight who completes 25 weeks of gestation is at best tenuous.

Infant mortality

Infant mortality statistics concern the number of children per 1,000 live births who die before their first birthday. In 1900 the average rate in those states reporting was 200 per 1,000; in 1973 the rate had dropped to 17.7 per 1,000 live births.* But lest we become too self-congratulatory, we should be aware that this figure is not consistent throughout the United States and still ranks approximately sixteenth among the nations recording such statistics. Reduced to more shocking proportions, our infant mortality statistics means that 1 out of every 56 babies born dies before his first

birthday. Our national lag in lowering infant mortality is related to the reasons cited for the rate of maternal mortality. It is no doubt caused by the many different economic, cultural, and educational backgrounds and levels found in the United States and our failure to meet the needs of these diversified groups. Our international standing may also be influenced slightly by the different ways in which statistics are formulated in various countries, despite attempts at standardization. However, the fact remains that, comparatively speaking, our performance leaves much to be desired.

About 70% of infant deaths occur in the first 28 days of life, the *neonatal* period. The leading causes of infant death are immaturity, asphyxiation (improper ventilation), congenital malformations, influenza and pneumonia, and birth injury. Prematurity is the leading cause of neonatal death. It will readily be seen that any

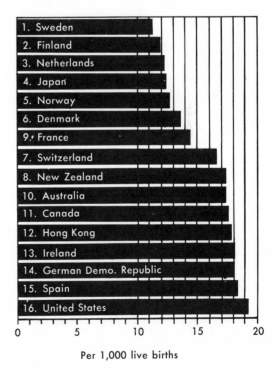

Fig. 1-2. International infant mortality statistics, 1971: deaths per 1,000 live births. (Data from Demographic yearbook 1972, United Nations, New York, pp. 503-523.)

---

*U. S. Department of Health, Education, and Welfare, Public Health Service, Health Resources Administration, Monthly Vital Statistics Report, vol. 23, Feb. 10, 1975, p. 2.

method decreasing the incidence of prematurity or improving medical-nursing management of premature infants would profoundly affect infant mortality statistics. The most commonly used definition of prematurity has been a birth weight of less than 5½ pounds (2,500 grams), although it is recognized that not all infants of low birth weight are born before term. Infants born before the end of 37 weeks' intra-uterine development is perhaps a better definition but not always verifiable.

Another statistical category is that of *perinatal mortality*. This figure includes recorded deaths of fetuses of more than 20 weeks' gestation added to those of the first 4 weeks of life (the neonatal period).

PROGRESS IN OBSTETRICS

Although we have a great deal of room for improvement in our maternity care, it is clear that conditions have changed radically for the better. It would be worthwhile for us to discuss the major reasons for this great progress.

Acceptance of the germ theory

First, the acceptance of the germ theory led to a greater understanding of the causes of infection. Less than a hundred years ago, infection was such a common companion of childbirth in some communities, notably among poor hospital patients, that its symptoms were termed childbed, or puerperal, fever (referring to the puerperium, the approximate 6-week period after delivery). Standards of cleanliness in most nineteenth century hospitals were nonexistent, and the suggestion that illness might be spread by the contaminated hands of physicians and medical students met with much opposition and scorn. Nevertheless, despite much difficulty and even persecution, certain individuals began to persuade the medical world that puerperal fever was really a contagion borne by many hands and common objects.

Chief among these medical pioneers was a Hungarian, Ignaz Philipp Semmelweis (1818-1865), whose sad and fascinating bi-

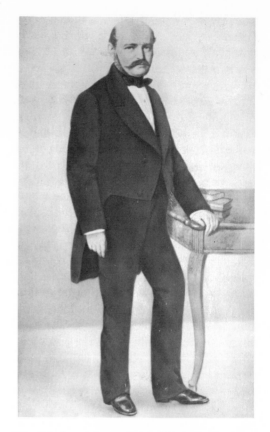

Fig. 1-3. Ignaz Semmelweis (1818-1865), a pioneer in the struggle against puerperal fever. Modern obstetricians and mothers are greatly indebted to him. (From Bettmann, O. L.: A pictorial history of medicine, Springfield, Ill., 1956, Charles C Thomas, Publisher; courtesy The Bettmann Archive, Inc.)

ography should be read by every obstetrical nurse. The American poet-physician, Oliver Wendell Holmes (1809-1894), is probably more remembered for his "Chambered Nautilus," but medical historians record his concern with maternal mortality and his widely criticized paper entitled "The Contagiousness of Puerperal Fever." The famed French chemist, Louis Pasteur, confirmed that childbed fever was indeed caused by bacteria and was contagious in character.

Improvement of techniques and teaching

Second, there has been a vast improvement in obstetrical techniques and teaching. With the acceptance of the germ theory, new concepts of care were evolved. Britain's Joseph Lister, the Father of Antisepsis, began to combat infection by chemical means and new wound-dressing techniques. Students of obstetrics were given more clinical instruction at the bedside, and their "experience" was not so confined to the printed page or the dissecting table. New tools, such as improved obstetrical forceps, sutures, and syringes, and antibiotic medications, laboratory clinical tests, transfusions, and anesthesia were developed. Hospitalization of the laboring or delivered mother and her child became an asset.

More recently there has been the development of new laboratory methods of assessing fetal maturity and health, the wider use of ultrasonic and electronic fetal monitoring, and more aggressive techniques in treating the immature or sick newborn. There has also been greater technological aid available to the mother facing high-risk pregnancy and labor. These advances along with the beginning of regional maternal and infant intensive care centers have made possible a further reduction in mortality and morbidity.

Development and extension of prenatal care

Third, and probably most significant, has been the development of *prenatal care* and extended obstetrical services by private and governmental public health facilities. It is with pride that nurses relate that prenatal care began as a nursing contribution instigated by the Instructive Nursing Association of the Boston Lying-In Hospital in 1901. From one visit prior to delivery, prenatal care has now developed into the close supervision of the expectant mother considered necessary today. Prenatal care has been extended to more and more Americans through the services of public health departments, visiting nurses, and nurse midwives, as well as private clinics and individual doctors. However, despite these efforts, many women in the United States still do not obtain adequate prenatal care.

Much analysis of health delivery systems, funding, promotional expertise, and education are still needed in this area.

CHANGE AND PROGRESS IN CHILD CARE

Naturally, the same factors that improved maternity care have helped to enhance the lives of children of all ages. However, pediatrics is a more recent speciality than obstetrics. Until the 1800's there was little formalized recognition of the special needs of children, the medical and surgical problems peculiar to childhood, or the different ways in which infants and children, in contrast to adults, respond to the presence of disease.

Development of pediatrics

In 1802 the first children's hospital was founded in Paris, France. In 1855 the first children's hospital in the United States was established in Philadelphia. But in most regions sick hospitalized children were often quartered with ill adults, sometimes in the same bed! Gradually, the consideration of pediatrics as a separate study was initiated, and as medical schools recognized the unique qualities of the childhood period, nursing schools followed their lead and offered special classes in pediatric nursing, general hospitals established pediatric departments, and more separate treatment centers for children were inaugurated. An early leader in the recognition of the special needs of children was Abraham Jacobi, first president of the American Pediatric Society and founder of the first clinic operated exclusively for children.

Responses of a changing society to children's needs

Change in itself does not automatically guarantee progress, and certainly the vast technological changes of the late nineteenth and early twentieth centuries did little to improve the immediate outlook of a great number of the world's growing children. The new demands of the rapidly accelerating industrial revolution, often untempered by regard for the individual, child or adult, caused sudden urban congestion, and while standards of living rose for some, many times the industrial laborer suffered from deprivation and exploitation. Some of those laborers working in the mills, factories, and mines were children. Two early major events, the inauguration of the White House Conferences and the establishment of the Children's Bureau, reflected a definite improvement and promotion of a better life for all children.

White House Conferences. Since 1909, at the beginning of each decade the very important national White House Conferences have been held. These have focused attention on the current prominent needs of children and youth. Delegates of private and governmental agencies at local, state, and federal levels concerned with maternal and child care as well as selected youth representatives meet for serious evaluation of these needs and ways in which they can be met. One of the most significant documents in the history of child care was prepared at the 1930 White House Conference on Child Health and Protection. Entitled "The Rights of the Child as an Individual in the State," it has been called the "Children's Charter." The 1970-71 White House Conference focused on children and youth in the changing social scene. For the first time youth delegates participated in the formal deliberations of the Conference.

Children's Bureau. It is principally because of the problem of child labor that the Children's Bureau, founded in 1912 as a result of the support of the first White House Conference on Children and Youth, was initially placed under the jurisdiction of the Department of Labor. Later when the Department of Health, Education, and Welfare was created in 1953, it became part of the responsibility of this cabinet post. In its founding legislation, as amended, the Children's Bureau is charged with the responsibility "to investigate and report on all matters pertaining to the welfare of children and child life among all classes of our people . . ."; to carry out research, demon-

stration, and training functions; to help coordinate the programs for children and parents throughout the Department of Health, Education, and Welfare; to promote programs for youth; and to identify areas requiring the development of new projects.

Social security legislation. The Social Security Act, passed in 1935, has been amended twice recently (1965 and 1967). It established the principle that all people in the United States, through the federal government, share responsibility with the state and local governments for helping to provide essential community services for children. To back up this principle, the Social Security Act authorizes Congress to appropriate funds each year to be given to the states to help them extend and improve their maternal and child health, crippled children's, and child welfare services. Whether a child is eligible for such aid depends on his problem or diagnosis and the financial position of his family. In 1973 an extension of Title XIX of the Social Security Act provided that "early and periodic screening, diagnosis, and treatment" be made available to all Medicaid recipients *under 21,* and each state is now in the process of determining the content and procedures for such a program. The implications of this legislation are far reaching for our pediatric population and health care services.

Project Head Start. Continued organized public concern for the health and welfare of children has resulted in great progress in society's efforts to protect their rights and promote their well-being. One of the most recent advances has been the establishment of Project Head Start.

Project Head Start is a comprehensive program launched by the Office of Economic Opportunity in the summer of 1965 and delegated to the Department of Health, Education, and Welfare in July, 1969. It is designed particularly for preschool children from disadvantaged backgrounds to help them develop their full potential and promote individual social competence. It provides a daily program of learning activities, nutritious meals, medical and dental care, and psychological, social, and economic services for these children and their families. Parental participation is a vital requirement of the program.

The Parent and Child Center Program (part of Head Start) is a demonstration project providing a full range of services to disadvantaged families having at least one child under 3 years of age. It is planned to provide practical encouragement and assistance to parents in overcoming economic and personal problems and learning the importance of their role in child development. Head Start has been considered helpful in preparing culturally disadvantaged children for their public school experience. Its effectiveness is prolonged and enhanced by continuing educational enrichment by parents and elementary school programs. It has excelled in its detection and treatment of health problems in the preschooler. But, since a relatively small number of children are involved, it has been an extremely expensive program to implement.*

Office of Child Development. In July, 1969, the Office of Child Development was established within the Department of Health, Education, and Welfare. It administers the activities and programs of the Children's Bureau and Project Head Start. It also coordinates and serves as an advocate for all children's programs throughout the federal government in an attempt to improve the wide range of services for children, youth, and their families.

Also in 1969 the Report of the Joint Commission on Mental Health of Children, "Crisis in Child Mental Health: Challenge for the 1970's," was published. It contained another statement of children's rights expressed from a broad psychosocial perspective. These rights included: the right to be wanted, the right to be healthy and to live in a healthy environment, the right to pro-

vision of basic needs and consistent loving care, and the right to acquire the intellectual and emotional skills necessary to fulfill individual aspirations.* As a reflection of some of the attempts to secure these rights, the Family Planning Services and Population Research Act was passed in 1970.

Private volunteer programs. Numerous private voluntary organizations are interested in certain specific diseases or conditions and provide considerable funds for research, diagnosis, and treatment. The National Foundation is now particularly interested in birth defects. The Cystic Fibrosis Research Foundation, the American Cancer Society, the Muscular Dystrophy Association, The American Heart Association, the Epilepsy Association of America, and the National Association for Retarded Children are all examples of such private voluntary groups. Other private social agencies help by providing essential community services, such as adoption, care of the unwed mother, counseling and psychiatric services, homemaking and recreational facilities.

International organizations. On an international scale two organizations under the auspices of the United Nations immediately come to mind. Perhaps the first is the United Nations International Children's Emergency Fund, called the United Nations Children's Fund since 1950, although the former initials, UNICEF, have been retained. This worthy organization, supported entirely by voluntary contributions, was established in 1946 primarily to meet the distress of children caused by war. It has now greatly expanded its scope. It currently includes not only the distribution of food, clothing, and medicine but also the provision for education and training of needed national workers in the health field. It is the world's largest international agency devoted to children and has received the Nobel Peace Prize for its efforts in behalf of children. In 1973 it approved new com-

---

*Zigler, E. F.: Project Head Start: success or failure? Children Today **2**:2-7+, Nov.-Dec., 1973.

*Crisis in child mental health: challenge for the 1970's, report of the Joint Commission on Mental Health of Children, Washington, D. C., 1969.

mitments totaling more than 76 million dollars.

The second United Nations–sponsored agency is the World Health Organization (WHO) formed in 1948. It helps coordinate efforts for disease control, provides a method of sharing new information in the fight against disease, and cooperates with UNICEF in promoting maternal and child health.

In 1956 the General Assembly of the United Nations, showing international concern for a popular topic, approved another important statement in the history of child care, "The Declaration of the Rights of the Child."

The continuing challenge

In spite of significant progress made during the past decade, much remains to be done. Although our nation is ranked as the most affluent, more than 30 million Americans continue to be burdened with poverty, hunger, illness, and despair. Our concentrated urbanized and dispersed rural poor, changing population patterns, increasing health costs, and unevenly distributed medical care have necessitated alterations in health care delivery. More extended nursing roles, involving advanced preparation, are now being defined. These include those of the pediatric and school nurse practitioners and the nurse-midwife. To meet the desires of consumers for more control over health care decisions and more emphasis on the promotion of health rather than the treatment of disease, new types of health insurance and prepaid medical care are being formulated. Nursing in the combined maternal-child or family care settings of the future may change in form, but its basic intent, to promote health and to cope with the threat and discomfort of disease, remains constant.

These are some of the many challenges still to be met in our society that profoundly affect the quality of our basic unit, the family and the child it produces. Continued effort must be exerted to strengthen this unit and lend stability, depth, and purpose to our daily lives so that individually and collectively we and coming generations may enjoy creatively the best that life can offer.

The present day obstetrical or pediatric nurse finds herself working in an area that demands increasing knowledge, skill, and appreciation. Her responsibilities embrace an understanding of the reproductive process, its possible complications, care of the mother and her growing child in health and illness, ability in health teaching, an appreciation of the role of the family, and a knowledge of community resources. Each patient is an individual with particular needs. For the alert nurse there is abundant opportunity for real challenge and achievement.

unit one
Suggested selected readings and references

Carlucci, F. C.: The future outlook for delivery of human services, Health Services Reports **88:**891-893, Dec., 1973.

Close, K.: Selecting priorities at the White House Conference on Children, Children **18:**42-48, March-April, 1971.

Dunlop, R.: Abraham Jacobi, the children's physician, Today's Health **48:**58+, April, 1970.

Eiduson, B. T.: Looking at children in emergent family styles, Children Today **3:**2-6, July-Aug., 1974.

Eliot, M. M.: Six decades of action for children, Children Today **1:**2-6, March-April, 1972.

Falkner, F.: Infant mortality: an urgent national problem, Children **17:**82-87, May-June, 1970.

Ferro, F.: Addressing children's needs, Children Today **2:**12-13+, Nov.-Dec., 1973.

Fitzpatrick, E., Eastman, N. J., and Reeder, S. R.: Maternity Nurs., ed. 12, Philadelphia, 1971, J. B. Lippincott Co.

Gaylin, W.: The patient's bill of rights, Nurs. Digest **1**:89-91, Nov., 1973; reprinted from Saturday Review **1**:22, March, 1973.

Hasselmeyer, E. G.: The infant mortality problem in the United States, J. Prac. Nurs. **19**:26-29, Jan., 1969.

Hunt, E.: Infant mortality trends and maternal and infant care, Children **17**:88-90, May-June, 1970.

Ledney, D. M.: Nurse-midwives: can they fill the OB gap? RN **33**:38-45, Jan., 1970.

Lerch, C.: Maternity nursing, ed. 2, St. Louis, 1974, The C. V. Mosby Co.

Lesser, A. J.: Progress in maternal and child health, Children Today **1**:7-12, March-April, 1972.

Lubic, R. W.: What the lay person expects of maternity care: are we meeting these expectations? J. Obstet. Gynecol. Neonatal Nurs. **1**: 25-31, June, 1972.

Marlow, D. R.: Textbook of pediatric nursing, ed. 4, Philadelphia, 1973, W. B. Saunders Co.

The maternal and child health service report on: promoting the health of mothers and children, U. S. Department of Health, Education, and Welfare, FY 1973.

Midwife: coming of age, Medical World News **14**: 114-115, Oct. 12, 1973.

NAACOG statement on the role of the OB-GYN nurse practitioner, J. Obstet. Gynecol. Neonatal Nurs. **1**:56, June, 1972.

Quinn, N. K., and Somers, A. R.: The patient's bill of rights: a significant aspect of the consumer revolution, Nurs. Outlook **22**:240-244, April, 1974.

Reid, J. H., and Phillips, M.: Child welfare since 1912, Children Today **1**:13-18, March-April, 1972.

Sato, I. S.: The culturally different child—the dawning of his day? Exceptional Children **40**: 572-577, May, 1974.

Scelsi, M. N.: UNICEF at work around the world, Children Today **1**:19-23, March-April, 1972.

Schulkind, M. L., and Morton, H. G.: Neonatal health insurance, Clin. Pediatr. **13**:209-210, March, 1974.

Valdes-Dapena, M. A.: Prognosis for neonates: what do the data show, Contemp. OB/GYN **5**: 17-20, Jan., 1975.

Wallace, H., Gold, E., and Lis, E., editors: Maternal-child health practice, problems, resources and methods of delivery, Springfield, Ill., 1973, Charles C Thomas Publisher, pp. 5-83.

Work, H.: Advocacy for children: challenge for the 1970's, Children **18**:31-32, Jan.-Feb., 1971.

unit two
Reproductive anatomy and physiology

2
Female reproductive anatomy

THE PELVIS, THE BONY PASSAGEWAY

To understand the events of labor and delivery we must be acquainted with the first journey the fetus takes—the all-important journey of a few inches through the mother's birth canal. Since this canal is shaped largely by the bones of the pelvis, we will begin with a discussion of its formation and contours.

The word pelvis means basin. We encounter the word at least twice when we study human anatomy. It is used in describing the cavity in the kidneys into which the urine drains before flowing down the ureter. It is also used to describe the bony ring located between the trunk and thighs, joining the spine above and the femurs below. This is the pelvis to which we refer now.

Anatomy

The pelvis is formed by the two innominate bones and the sacrum and coccyx. Each innominate bone, however, is the end result of the fusion of three once-upon-a-time distinct bones: ilium, ischium, and pubis.

Landmarks and joints

The names of these three bones often recur as we describe the following interesting pelvic landmarks:

anterosuperior iliac spines the lower front end of the iliac crest line.
iliac crests the hip bones. Convenient for book or baby balancing.
iliopectineal line (linea terminalis, brim) divides the upper, or false, pelvis and the lower, or true, pelvis.
ischial spines two important landmarks in determining the depth of the fetus in the passageway. The location of the presenting part of the fetus in the pelvic canal in relation to the ischial spines is termed its "station." If the presenting part is at the level of the ischial spines, its station is said to be 0, or zero. If it is above the ischial spines, it is termed minus so many centimeters (for example, −1 or −2 cm.). If the presenting part is below the ischial spines, its location is termed plus so many centimeters (for example, +1 or +2 cm.). Naturally, it is important for the nurse to be able to interpret this information. When a patient in labor nears full cervical dilatation and has a station of +2 cm., the nurse must realize that if the mechanism of labor is normal, it will probably be only a relatively short time before the infant will be born.
ischial tuberosities major bony sitting support; important in measuring a transverse diameter of the pelvis.
pubic arch formed by the lower border of the symphysis pubis and the ischial bones.
sacral promontory the internal junction of the last lumbar vertebra and the sacrum; important in obtaining an internal obstetrical measurement, known as the true conjugate, conjugata vera, or C.V.
sacrococcygeal joint located between the sacrum and coccyx, retains limited mobility, which may offer additional room for the passage of the fetus by bending the coccyx slightly backward. Some authorities say that as much as 1 inch is occasionally gained in this way at the outlet.
sacroiliac joints found at either side of the sacrum joining with the iliac bones.
symphysis pubis junction of the pubic bones.

True and false pelvis

The *false pelvis,* formed chiefly by flaring wings of the iliac portions of the innomi-

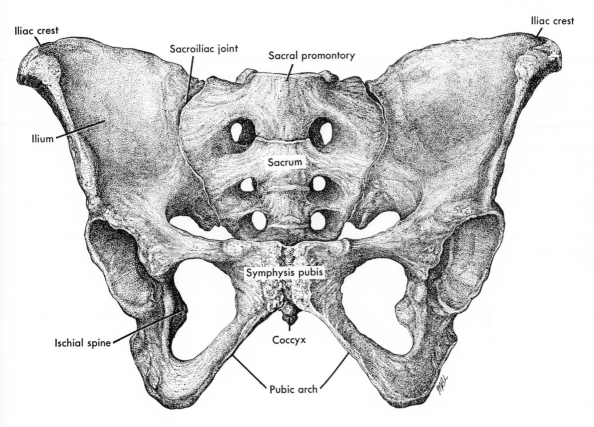

Iliac crest

Iliac crest

Sacroiliac joint

Sacral promontory

Ilium

Sacrum

Symphysis pubis

Ischial spine

Coccyx

Pubic arch

Fig. 2-1. Female pelvis, anterior view.

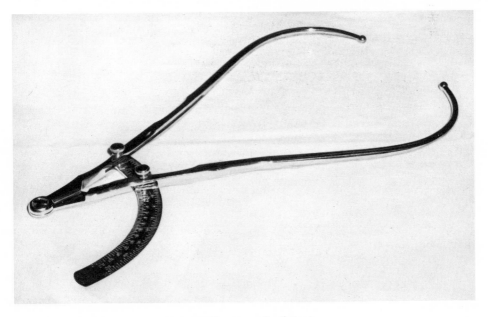

Fig. 2-2. One type of pelvimeter.

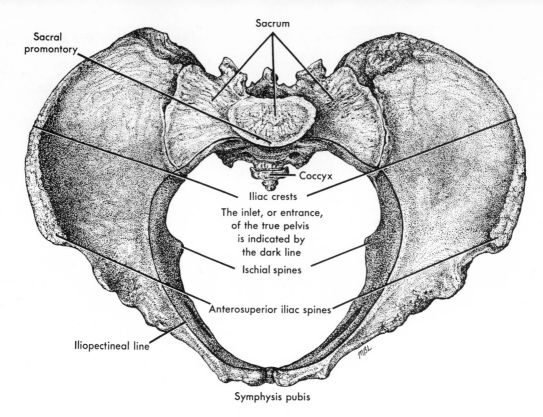

Sacrum

Sacral
promontory

Coccyx

Iliac crests

The inlet, or entrance,
of the true pelvis
is indicated by
the dark line

Ischial spines

Anterosuperior iliac spines

Iliopectineal line

Symphysis pubis

Fig. 2-3. The inlet.

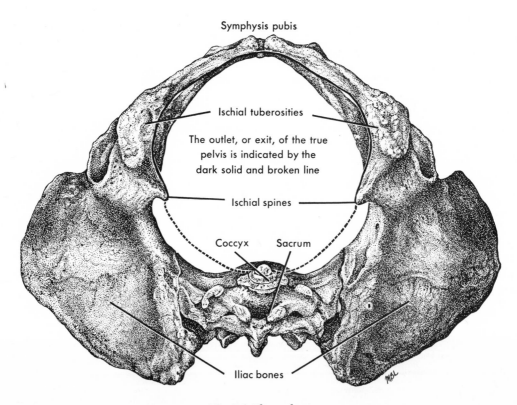

Symphysis pubis

Ischial tuberosities

The outlet, or exit, of the true
pelvis is indicated by the
dark solid and broken line

Ischial spines

Coccyx   Sacrum

Iliac bones

Fig. 2-4. The outlet.

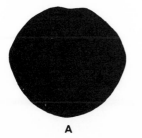 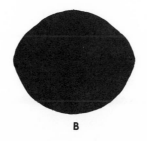 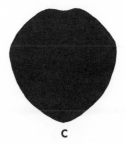

| A | B | C |

Fig. 2-5. Types of pelves. *A,* Normal female pelvic inlet (gynecoid); *B,* flattened female pelvic inlet (platypelloid); *C,* typical male pelvic inlet (android).

nate bones, helps guide the fetus into the true obstetrical canal. Its measurements may indicate possible difficulties in the structure of the true pelvis just below. The *true pelvis* is of real concern to the obstetrician. In its journey the fetus must adapt to its different diameters and shapes to successfully reach the outside world.

Inlet and outlet

The entrance to the true pelvis is termed the "inlet." Its shape is traced, in part, by the iliopectineal line. It is wider from side to side than from front to back. Therefore the head usually enters the true pelvis with its longest diameter (which is from front to back) pointed from side to side or in transverse position. Mechanically, it is either easier or absolutely necessary.

The exit of the true pelvis is termed the "outlet." The outlet is wider from front to back than from side to side. To pass through the outlet, the head, in most cases, must turn to accommodate its longest diameter to the longest diameter of the exit. This turning is called *internal rotation.* The canal formed by the true pelvis forms a slight curve near the outlet and has been likened in shape to the letter J.

Pelvic differences

Classifications. No two pelves are exactly alike although they may be classified according to their measurements. The most common classification concerns the shape and dimensions of the inlet. The typical female pelvic inlet is labeled "gynecoid." The typical male inlet is "android." Unfortunately, some women have android-type pelves. A look at a male pelvis should tell you at least one reason why the masculine member of the family would not bear children. The inlet is heart shaped and angular. The whole pelvic structure is heavier and more confining than that of the female. The pubic arch, under which every fetus should pass, is steep and narrow. In contrast, a typical woman's pelvis is relatively light and commodious, and the pubic arch is shallow and wide. Occasionally, a woman's pelvic inlet will be abnormally flat or platypelloid, with a decreased anteroposterior diameter or other abnormalities. These problems may necessitate a cesarean section, or abdominal delivery. But whether a birth will terminate abdominally or vaginally will depend on several factors: the type of passageway, the size and position of the fetus, the strength of the uterine contractions, and the condition of the laboring mother.

Causes of abnormalities. A history of certain conditions may alert the physician to expect trouble because of pelvic abnormalities. The five main causes of abnormal pelvic measurements are (1) heredity (characteristic familial problems, dwarfism), (2) infections (poliomyelitis, osteomyelitis, tuberculosis of the bone), (3) poor nutrition (rickets), (4) accidents (fractured pelves), and (5) poor posture and exercise habits.

Four methods of pelvic measurement

The pelvis may be measured by:
1. *External palpation* with instruments

13

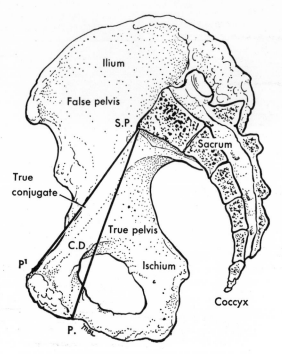

Fig. 2-6. Female pelvis, sagittal section. *C.D.*, Diagonal conjugate; P^1, inner superior border of the pubis; *P.*, outer inferior border of the pubis; *S.P.*, sacral promontory.

3. X-ray pelvimetry generally involving two views, one made with the patient in a semirecumbent position, her pelvic inlet parallel with the x-ray plate, and another with the patient upright and sideways to secure a lateral view of the pelvis. This method is the most accurate and allows evaluation of additional crucial obstetrical diameters as well as the relationship of the size and posture of the fetus to the passageway. But it should be scheduled only near term or during labor, for significant reasons: to reduce the exposure of the young developing fetus to radiation and to avoid possible damage to fetal structures during early gestation, the most vulnerable period.

4. Ultrasonography, the use of ultrasound to detect differences in tissue density, is now of clinical importance in obstetrics. Although it has seemingly not been used to determine relative pelvic and fetal size as has x-ray, with perfection of technique and experience, it probably will be. It offers no known hazards to the mother or fetus. It has been employed to detect single or multiple pregnancy and abnormal fetal or placental positions. It also supplies helpful estimates of the fetal size and growth through the determination of the biparietal diameter of the infant skull.

There has been a growing trend for physicians working in areas well supplied with adequate hospital facilities to discontinue the determination of external pelvic measurements except perhaps an evaluation of the pubic arch. In fact, some believe that if cephalopelvic disproportion becomes a practical problem it can be evaluated and faced best at the time of labor using the more refined diagnostic and treatment facilities available in the hospital.

A knowledge of the structure of the obstetrical passageway is basic to an understanding of the mechanism of labor and the problems faced by the physician. So far, we have only discussed the bony pelvis. We shall continue now with a consideration of the soft structures involved—the muscles of the pelvic floor and the organs they support.

called pelvimeters. The most important external measurement that may be determined is the distance between the ischial tuberosities (Bi. Isch. or T.I., averaging 10 to 11 cm.). This measurement may indicate the distance between the ischial spines, a critical transverse measurement that is possible only with x-ray pelvimetry.

2. *Internal palpation* with a lubricated gloved finger. The distance between the sacral promontory and the outer inferior border of the pubis known as the *diagonal conjugate* (C.D., averaging 12.5 cm.) may be sought. From this measurement a closer estimate of the anteroposterior diameter of the inlet, referred to as the *true conjugate,* conjugata vera, or C.V., may be made. To do this, one subtracts 1.5 to 2 cm. from the diagonal conjugate to compensate for the thickness and tilt of the pubic bone. The true conjugate usually averages 11 cm. (Fig. 2-6).

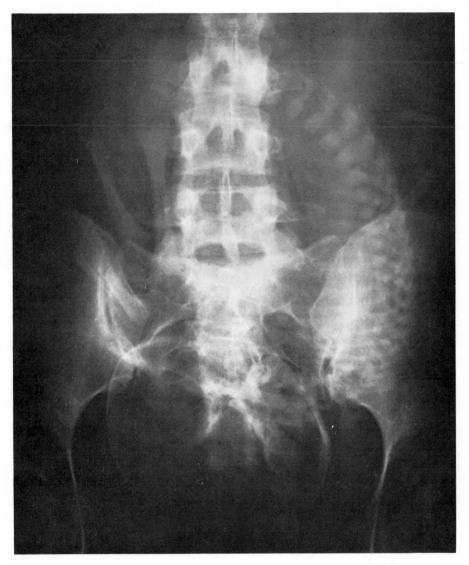

Fig. 2-7. Photograph of x-ray film. Pelvimetry showing a cephalic presentation. (Courtesy Grossmont Hospital, La Mesa, Calif.)

THE PELVIC CONTENTS AND SUPPORT

The pelvis, through which the fetus must pass, contains many soft tissue structures vital to normal body function. These structures are supported by layers of muscle, fibrous coverings called *fasciae*, and various ligaments and tendons. They help to cushion the passage of the fetus through the hard, bony canal, help direct its descent, occasionally impede its progress, and may sustain damage at the time of birth.

Soft tissues of the vulva

Looking at the external female genitalia as they are observed when the patient is on her back with her knees flexed, we discover the superficial relationships of many of these vital soft tissue organs. The vulva, or external genital area, includes the following structures:

1. *Mons veneris* (Mount of Venus—mons pubis). A fatty pad over the symphysis pubis, which after puberty becomes covered

15

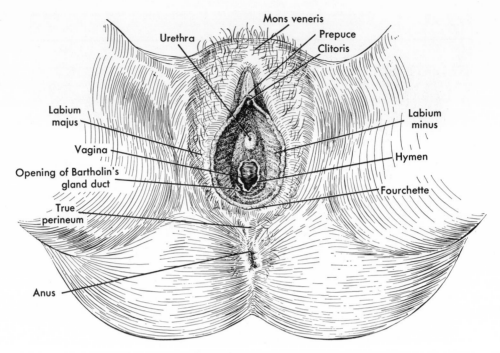

Fig. 2-8. Female external genitalia.

with curly hair in the form of an inverted triangle extending between the legs.

2. *Labia majora* (larger lips.) Two fleshy, hair-covered folds, extending on each side of the midline from the mons veneris almost to the anus. In a child or a woman who has not borne a child, these folds almost completely cover the structures between. They correspond to the two halves of the scrotum in the male. Their inner surfaces are rich in oil and sweat glands.

3. *Labia minora* (small lips). Two smaller, more delicate folds of tissue, located just under the labia majora. These small folds are somewhat erectile and are also supplied with oil and sweat glands.

4. *Clitoris.* A small, sensitive, erectile structure located at the anterior junction of the labia minora. Actually, folds of the small labia surround the clitoris; the top fold forms a fleshy hood, or *prepuce*, and the lower fold, the *frenulum*. The clitoris corresponds to the penis in the male as the primary anatomical center of sexual arousal.

5. *Vestibule.* The triangular space be-

tween the labia minora in which we find the openings of the urethra, the vagina, and the *Bartholin glands.*

6. *Urethral opening.* The urethra, a tissue tube leading from the urinary bladder to the exterior, opens in the midline between the clitoris and vagina. This opening usually appears as a dimple or slit and after delivery may be slightly displaced or more difficult to locate because of local swelling. On the floor of the urethra open two ducts that lead to *Skene's glands*, structures that have no known purpose but unfortunately may become infected rather easily.

7. *Vaginal opening.* The vagina, a large distensible tube or sheath, leads down and back to the uterine cervix. It serves as the exit point for menstrual flow, the female organ of intercourse, or coitus, and the soft tissue birth canal in labor and delivery. In virgins, it usually is partially covered by a membrane called the *hymen,* or maidenhead. However, absence of a hymenal membrane does not preclude virginity, since this tissue may be accidentally torn during

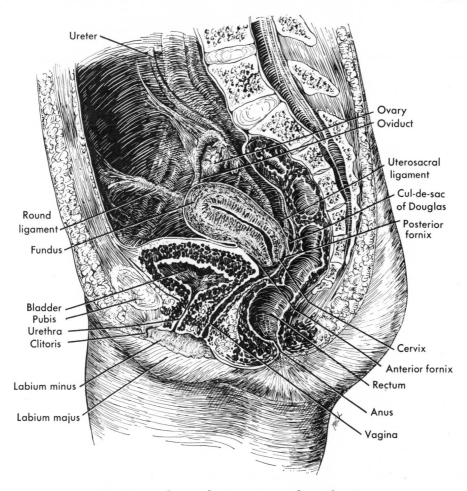

Ureter

Ovary
Oviduct

Uterosacral
ligament

Cul-de-sac
of Douglas

Posterior
fornix

Round
ligament

Fundus

Bladder
Pubis
Urethra
Clitoris

Cervix

Anterior fornix

Rectum

Anus

Vagina

Labium minus

Labium majus

Fig. 2-9. Female reproductive system, midsagittal section.

childhood. On the other hand, the presence of the hymen is no proof of virginity, since it may be very elastic and fail to tear during intercourse. Rarely, the hymen completely covers the vaginal opening. This condition is termed "imperforate hymen" and is relieved by a hymenectomy.

8. *Bartholin's glands.* Two in number, the Bartholin glands produce a mucoid substance, which drains into the vestibule on either side of the vagina via two ducts during sexual stimulation. This drainage in addition to mucoid secretion from the vaginal walls themselves provides lubrication for intercourse. Occasionally, these glands become infected, and painful abscesses may form.

9. *Fourchette.* A tissue fold below the

vaginal opening, formed by the fusion of the posterior edges of the labia minora, often lacerated by childbirth.

10. *Perineum.* Sometimes considered to be the entire body area between the patient's legs. However, when we speak of the *true perineum,* we mean that tissue block found between the posterior edge of the vagina and the anus or rectal opening. It contains the *perineal body,* a mass of connective tissue that forms the point of attachment for the muscles and fascia of the pelvic floor. It is this area that is most frequently injured during delivery. The true perineum is a critical area of pelvic support. Such pelvic organs as the vagina, uterus, bladder, and rectum may be affected by its injury or inadequate repair.

A look at Fig. 2-9, which shows these internal pelvic organs, will clarify their relationships and need for support.

Uterus and adnexa
Uterus and fallopian tubes

An adult, nonpregnant *uterus,* or womb, is a pear-shaped, hollow muscular organ about 3 inches long, 2 inches wide, and 1 inch thick. It serves as a protector and nourisher of the developing baby and aids in his

birth. Attached to either side of the uterus are the *fallopian tubes,* also called the oviducts or uterine tubes, which help conduct the female sex cell to the uterus.

The uterus is composed of three layers. The vascular mucus-producing endometrium, or inner lining, alters periodically in depth and character, demonstrating the uterine changes of the menstrual cycle. The middle layer, or myometrium, made up of muscular fibers that run in circular, length-

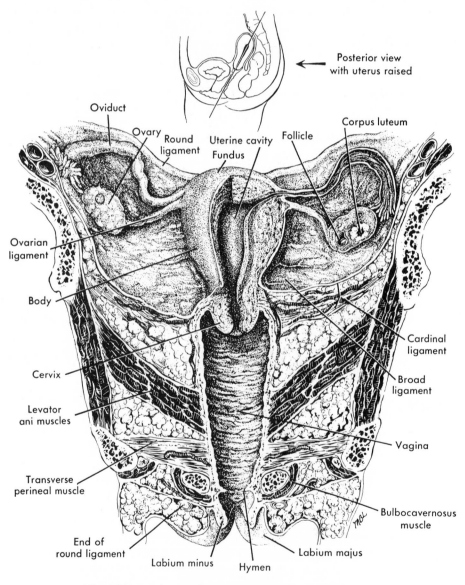

Fig. 2-10. Female reproductive system, inclined posterior view.

wise, and figure-8 patterns, provides forceful, efficient contraction of the uterine wall during and after delivery. The outermost covering layer of the uterus is formed by the enfolding pelvic peritoneum and the parametrium, both strong connective tissues.

The uterus may also be divided into three main parts: the neck portion, or cervix; the main or central portion called the body, or corpus; and the area above the oviducts, the fundus. Normally, the uterus is tipped toward the front of the body, resting on the urinary bladder just below. The cervix dips down into the posterior portion of the vagina from above. Vaginal and cervical tissue ultimately join, forming two pouches, referred to as the anterior and posterior fornices (singular fornix). The posterior fornix is adjacent to a fold in the peritoneal lining of the pelvic cavity, termed the pouch, or cul-de-sac, of Douglas. Occasionally, be-

cause of infection of the pelvis or abdomen, pus may drain into this cul-de-sac and is aspirated vaginally or rectally by the physician.

Uterine support

Ligaments. The uterus is not only indirectly supported by the true perineum but also, along with portions of the oviducts and ovaries, is infolded in layers of the so-called *broad ligaments*, portions of the abdominal peritoneal lining. The lower portions of the broad ligaments are thicker and are sometimes called the *cardinal ligaments*. They connect the upper portion of the cervix to the lateral pelvic walls. The uterus is also positioned and stabilized by other fibrous attachments, such as the *round ligaments* leading from the uterine walls toward the front, just below the fallopian tubes, down the inguinal canals, and to the labia majora. The round ligaments hold the

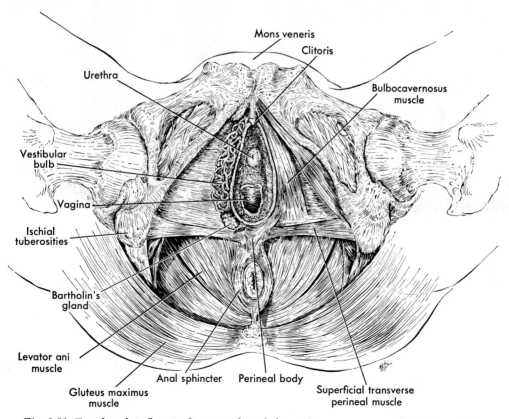

Fig. 2-11. Female pelvic floor in dissection from below. The coccygeus muscle is obscured by the gluteus maximus muscle.

uterus in its forward position. The *uterosacral ligaments* connect the posterior cervival portion of the uterus to the sacrum. The oviducts and ovaries and such soft tissue attachments are often referred to as the *adnexa,* or adjacent parts. The ovaries, two almond-shaped glands that produce female hormones and the female sex cells, or ova, are held one on each side of the uterus principally by the ovarian and broad ligaments.

Muscles. The deep muscles of the pelvic floor are arranged in such a way that they form a type of hammock pierced only by the urethra, vagina, and rectum. This muscle grouping, often termed the pelvic diaphragm, is formed by the branches of the large *levator ani* muscles and the *coccygeus* muscles. More muscles converge at the point of the previously described true perineum, reinforcing the levator ani. These are the *bulbocavernosus* muscles, the *transverse* muscles, and the *anal sphincter.*

Protection of the perineum

Various attempts are made to preserve or protect the muscles of the true perineum from tears (lacerations) at the time of delivery. The head of the infant is slowly extended by external, manual pressure to force the presentation of the smallest cephalic diameter. It is delivered slowly between contractions. Because the tissues of women bearing their first babies are not so easily stretched, many physicians, particularly in the United States, will perform a prophylactic perineal incision called an *episiotomy* to avoid an uncontrolled, jagged tear, reduce possible prolonged pressure on the baby's head, and speed delivery. Episiotomies may be performed in several ways. The midline, or median, episiotomy extends from the vagina straight down to the anus. It is said to be easier to repair and more comfortable for the mother in the healing period, but one difficulty is that it may extend into the anal sphincter. Many physicians now use a combination episiotomy known as a mediolateral, which starts at the midline but then angles off, missing the sphincter. Because of its angle, it is more difficult to repair and more painful during the postpartum period, since the suturing is done "on the bias." Episiotomies are so common now that most delivery room setups routinely include the instruments and supplies needed for their execution and repair. Low or outlet forceps are frequently used to speed delivery and lessen the pounding of the presenting part on the perineum. Obvious damage to the perineal floor does not always occur as a result of childbirth. Perineal lacerations and other problems related to possible delivery trauma are discussed in greater detail in the chapters on labor and delivery and obstetrical complications.

It is well to note, however, that despite the difficulties that can occur during this first journey taken by all human beings through the pelvic passageway, with proper care and management relatively few major problems actually materialize. Probably our first journey from internal to external space, though demanding for mother and child, is far less dangerous than the freeway trip we negotiate every afternoon going home from work.

3

The menstrual cycle

We have reviewed the anatomy of the pelvis. However, in order to study the physiology or function of the pelvic organs, we must discuss more than the contents of the pelvis itself.

ROLE OF THE PITUITARY GLAND

The proper functioning of the ovaries and uterus also depends on a gland located a considerable distance from the pelvic cavity but which empties its powerful products directly into the bloodstream, exerting influence on the body far beyond that expected, considering their gland's size and position. Remember, glands that empty their manufactured products directly into the blood circulation are called *endocrine* glands. Their products are termed "hormones." The gland outside the pelvis that is so important in ovarian and uterine function is the *pituitary,* located at the base of the brain. It, in part, is regulated by that portion of the brain called the hypothalamus. Some of the pituitary hormones help to regulate one of the events universal among women, *menstruation.*

MENSTRUATION

Menstruation may be defined as the monthly elimination, through a bloody vaginal discharge, of a portion of the lining of the uterus that had been prepared to protect and nurture the fertilized egg in the event of pregnancy. Menstruation is also properly called menses, catamenia, or, more commonly, a period, or monthly flow. Terminology that implies an undesirable condition or illness should be avoided because menstruation is not an illness but an expected and necessary part of healthy mature womanhood. It may at times be individually inconvenient and troublesome, but

it is the way all normal women function, and it declares the possibility for a type of growth unmatched in meaning and wonder by that provided by any other form of life.

Menarche

The advent of menstruation in a girl is a signal of impending physical maturity. This first menses is called *menarche.* It is one of the signs of "growing up." Menstruation occurs periodically throughout the childbearing years, except during periods of pregnancy and lactation, or breast feeding. The age of onset and termination differs from person to person but seems to be affected by heredity, racial background, nutrition, and perhaps climate. On the average, menarche occurs between 10 and 14 years of age. It is preceded by other body changes, such as the development of breasts, a rounding off of the many angles characteristic of the body of the preadolescent, and the appearance of axillary and pubic hair. Psychologically, a girl's interest turns toward members of the opposite sex.

The cycle

Menstruation occurs approximately every 28 days in most women and lasts about 5 days. The time between the beginning of one period and the beginning of the next is called the menstrual cycle. It generally repeats itself about every 4 weeks (Fig. 3-1), though variations of several days in the cycles of different women or even in the cycles of the same woman are quite normal. Day 1 is distinguished by the appearance of the menstrual flow.

ANATOMY AND PHYSIOLOGY

The physiology of menstruation is complex. However, a basic understanding of

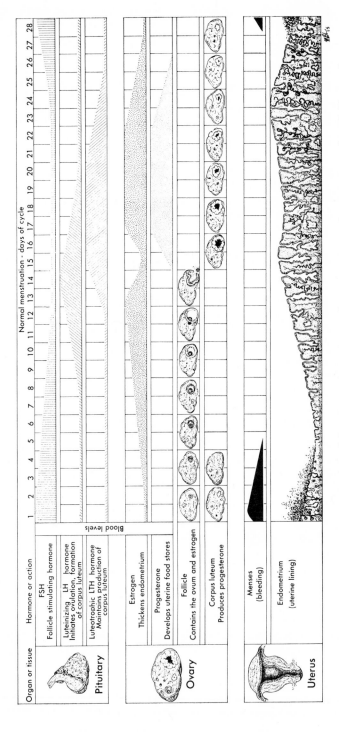

Fig. 3-1. Normal menstrual cycle. (Adapted from Physiology of normal menstruation, Schering Corp., Bloomfield, N. J.)

some of the relationships involved will increase our appreciation of the human body and its potential. Three organs are primarily involved: the pituitary gland, the ovaries, and the uterus. We will begin our explanation with a description of the ovaries.

The ovaries

The ovaries have two basic functions—first, the production of hormones (*estrogen* and *progesterone*), which help regulate the activities of the uterus and pituitary gland and thus bring about the obvious changes that make a little girl a woman, and, second, the formation of the microscopic eggs that carry the hereditary possibilities of her family heritage. United with a male sex cell, or sperm, the fertilized egg grows to become a new human being. These eggs are stored in varying degrees of immaturity in the underlying tissues of the ovary. Each month one egg develops to maturity within a protective tissue envelope called a follicle. This follicle and other ovarian tissue are filled with estrogenic fluid, which is secreted in large amounts into the blood to thicken the lining of the uterus. As the follicle develops, it pushes to the surface of the ovary to create a blisterlike bulge that may be clearly seen if the ovary is observed directly (for example, during surgery). The growth of the follicle in the ovary and the development of the egg, or ovum, it contains are not primarily the results of activity carried on by the ovary but of that faraway master gland, the pituitary, which directs ovarian activity.

The pituitary gland

The anterior portion of the pituitary manufactures three hormones that govern the ovarian and, more indirectly, the uterine cycles. During the first and last days of the cycle, the pituitary secretes particularly large amounts of the *follicle-stimulating hormone* (FSH), which triggers and helps sustain the development of the follicle and ovum. Toward the middle of the cycle, a second potent pituitary product is released,

the *luteinizing hormone* (LH), which furthers the development of the follicle and causes it to gently break open to expel the mature or ripe egg and begin its manufacture of progesterone. The rupture of the follicle on the surface of the ovary and the expulsion of the ovum is called *ovulation*. It occurs about the fourteenth day. After ovulation the mature egg is normally swept up into the fallopian tube to begin its journey to the uterus. After ovulation the empty follicle changes its name and alters its function. The walls of the follicle begin to thicken and form a yellow deposit about the size of a lima bean. This deposit is called the *corpus luteum* (yellow body). The name "follicle" is no longer used. The corpus luteum continues to produce estrogen but, in addition, manufactures another hormone, *progesterone*, initiated by LH and possibly maintained by a third pituitary secretion the *luteotrophic hormone* (LTH). The role of LTH in the regulation of progesterone production during the menstrual cycle appears somewhat debatable, but it is clear that LTH, or prolactin, as it is also called, is involved in the formation of breast milk after delivery.

Progesterone helps in the storage of foodstuffs in the wall of the uterus, built up and thickened by the action of estrogen. Progesterone, which means "a hormone designed to promote pregnancy," helps maintain the soft nutritious wall long enough to receive any fertilized egg and to nourish it until the developing fetus is able to establish its more elaborate lifeline of placenta and umbilical cord. Progesterone is sometimes given therapeutically to mothers who are having difficulty keeping their pregnancies and face the possibility of miscarriage. About the twenty-sixth day of the menstrual cycle, if no pregnancy has developed, the corpus luteum, lacking continued hormonal support from the pituitary, begins to degenerate. Approximately 2 days later the thickened lining of the uterus starts to disintegrate, having lost its progesterone and estrogen support.

CYCLE CONTROL
Pregnancy

If pregnancy does occur, hormones released by the developing fertilized egg interrupt the normal menstrual cycle by maintaining the level of estrogen and progesterone and inhibiting ovulation. Secreted early in the pregnancy is *chorionic gonadotropic hormone* (CGTH). Identification of this substance in the urine of the patient forms the basis of some pregnancy tests.

Artificial hormonal control

In recent years oral estrogen- and progesterone-like compounds, which simulate to some degree the changes in the uterine lining and the regulation of ovarian and pituitary activity occurring during pregnancy, have been used to control ovulation and aid in planned parenthood. (See discussion of contraception, Chapter 14.)

Ovulation and menses

The menstrual flow consists of less than 60 ml. of cellular debris, mucus, and blood. Its appearance signals the advent of another cycle. It is interesting to note that ovulation may not occur each time the menstrual cycle repeats and is not dependent on menstruation. The occurrence of ovulation can be detected by the careful recording of rectal temperatures taken before arising in the absence of a temperature-causing disease. Just before ovulation, the temperature drops to the lowest level found in the first half of the cycle. This drop is followed by an abrupt rise of perhaps one half of a degree Fahrenheit, indicating ovulation has occurred. This information has also been used in trying to plan pregnancies, since the most fertile period is during this temperature change (see Fig. 14-2).

PROBLEMS
Dysmenorrhea

The most common menstrual disturbance is dysmenorrhea, or painful menstruation. Although most women observe some discomfort (for example, pelvic congestion, fatigue, or irritability), severe cramping and incapacitation should not be the rule. Repeated experiences of dysmenorrhea should be evaluated by a physican. Occasionally, a physical cause may be found, such as an abnormal narrowing of the cervical opening, poor uterine positioning, the presence of pelvic tumors, or possible glandular imbalance. Dysmenorrhea may be caused or aggravated by constipation. Its possibility is also greatly increased by fatigue and emotional upset. The maintenance of meticulous hygiene, proper diet, and good mental health is of prime importance to the body's total response during menstruation. Excellent teaching aids dealing with the anatomy, physiology, and hygiene of menstruation are now available through public health departments and private commercial outlets.

Treatment of dysmenorrhea, of course, depends on the cause, but moderate exercise, fresh air, a serene philosophy, prevention or relief of constipation, possible application of heat to the pelvis, and mild sedatives or muscle relaxants usually help greatly. Because it has been found that many times dysmenorrhea is not experienced if a menstrual cycle does not include ovulation, contraceptive preparations containing estrogen or estrogen-progesterone combinations are occasionally prescribed with good effect. However, if the contraceptive action of the medication or possible side effects present problems, this method of treatment may not be appropriate.

Disturbances in flow

Other types of menstrual disorders should at least be defined. *Amenorrhea* means the abnormal absence of menses. *Menorrhagia* refers to abnormally excessive flow. *Metrorrhagia* identifies the presence of bloody vaginal discharge between periods. All these conditions should be investigated by a physician.

4

The male parent: his contribution

The role of the mother in the creation of new life has often been emphasized, but the role of the responsible male parent is also very important. Truly for an emotionally, socially, and physically healthy child both marriage partners must make considerable contributions of time and effort. This does not mean that if these contributions are absent the child will never achieve a happy, productive life, but if he does, he does so "in spite of" instead of "because of" his early family life. For the mature parent, capable of giving as well as receiving, parenthood is a demanding responsibility but one that gives a deserved sense of fulfillment and pride.

The male role in the initial physical creation of his offspring is relatively brief but no less miraculous because of its brevity. The male reproductive system is an intricate mechanism worthy of study.

ANATOMY AND PHYSIOLOGY
Puberty

Puberty, or the maturation of the reproductive system, usually occurs late in the male when compared with the female. The development of the male sex organs and secondary sex characteristics takes place, on the average, two years later. It involves such changes as the enlargement of the larynx and the deepening of the voice, the appearance of axillary, pubic, and facial hair, the development of increased musculature, the production of semen, and the normal occurrence of nocturnal emissions, or "wet dreams." Finally, there is a psychological change, and the boy who could not stand girls rather suddenly finds them quite attractive.

Genetic considerations

Perhaps a brief digression concerning genetics, the study of inheritance, is now in order. All cells that compose living things, animal or plant, have within their nuclei the potential of inheritance not only for the species but also for the individualized representatives of that species. Each living thing has a certain number of threadlike strands (chromosomes) of transmittable characteristics (genes) within the nuclei of its tissue cells. This number is constant for each species. For example, human beings have forty-six chromosomes in each body tissue cell. However, because the child necessarily inherits qualities from both parents and the body tissue chromosome count must be unaltered for the species, the sex cells of the male and female are different from the rest of the cells found in the body. Through a special process called meiosis, the chromosome count in these cells is reduced by half. When male and female sex cells unite, fertilization, or conception, takes place, and the species' chromosome count is restored in the new developing representative of the race.

Male organs of reproduction
(Figs. 4-1 and 4-2)

The male sex cells, or spermatozoa, are manufactured in two oval endocrine glands called *testes* (singular testis), or *testicles,* located in a fleshy pouch suspended from the abdomen called the *scrotum.* In addition to the manufacture of sperm, the testes also manufacture a hormone called *testosterone,* which is responsible for the appearance of male characteristics as estrogen in the female is responsible for feminine qual-

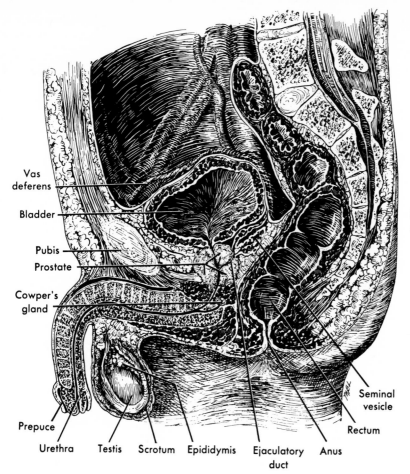

Vas
deferens

Bladder

Pubis

Prostate

Cowper's
gland

Fig. 4-1. Male reproductive
system, midsagittal view.

Seminal
vesicle

Rectum

Prepuce

Urethra   Testis   Scrotum   Epididymis   Ejaculatory   Anus
                                               duct

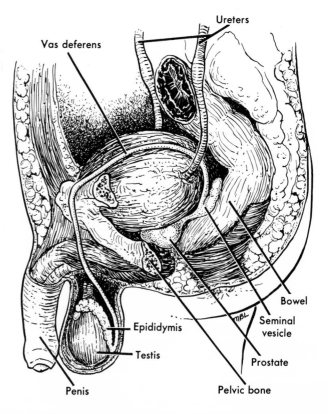

Ureters

Vas deferens

Fig. 4-2. Male reproductive system,
sagittal view with partial
dissection.

Bowel

Seminal
vesicle

Epididymis

Testis

Prostate

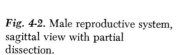

Penis

Pelvic bone

ities. The testes are found in the abdominal cavity proper during part of fetal development, but before birth they usually migrate to the scrotal sac via the inguinal canal. Occasionally, this migration does not occur, and a condition known as undescended testicles, or cryptorchidism, may exist. If this persists, sterility may occur, since the higher temperature of the abdominal cavity seems to interfere with the manufacture of sperm. If the condition continues, malignant changes are occasionally diagnosed.

Attached to the top of each testis is a coiled structure called an *epididymis,* which is actually an extension of the tubules of the testis where sperm are formed. In the epididymides (plural of epididymis) the male sex cells mature. Each epididymis is in turn attached to a long tube called the *ductus deferens,* or *vas deferens,* which with associated nerves and blood vessels travels up the inguinal canal as the *spermatic cord.* The ductus deferens eventually loops downward in back of the urinary bladder. Attached to the ductus in this area is the *seminal vesicle.* This small pouch secretes a product that is added to the spermatozoa and aids the motility of the sex cell. The tube leading forward from the point of attachment of the seminal vesicle is called the *ejaculatory duct.* It joins the long urethra after passing through tissue of the *prostate gland.* Three paired glands add secretions to the spermatozoa traveling from the testes to the exterior to form *semen,* or *seminal fluid:* the seminal vesicle, the prostate (already mentioned), and the bulbourethral, or Cowper's, gland, which opens into the urethra proper. These secretions regulate the acidity of the semen and influence the sperm's motility and life-span. As a result of sexual excitement and subsequent ejaculation of 2 to 6 ml. of semen, approximately 250 to 500 million sperm are released at a time from the penis, the male organ of intercourse, through the urethral meatus.

When not sexually stimulated, the penis serves as the excretory organ of the male urinary system. The urethra opens at the tip of the penis in a sensitive portion called the *glans.* The glans is hooded by a fold of skin called the *prepuce,* or *foreskin,* which is slit or at least partially removed if a circumcision is performed.

SEX DETERMINATION

Because there has been considerable consternation in the past concerning the sex of certain heirs, perhaps it should be pointed out that the potential sex of the child is determined by the type of sex cell contributed by the male that penetrates the ovum, or egg. Only the male sex cells, the spermatozoa, may carry the Y chromosome, which dictates the conception of a boy. When the sperm that unites with an ovum carries the Y chromosome, a boy will result; but if the sperm that fertilizes the egg carries an X chromosome, a girl will result. There is some evidence that suggests that the acidity or alkalinity of the vagina and the timing and techniques of intercourse may influence the type of sex cell that survives to penetrate the ovum. However, this has been disputed.[*]

"OUR HUMANITY"

Although few people would deny that a baby is a human being, it must be agreed that the true process of reproduction of the human race does not end at conception or at birth. It only enters another phase. Just how "human," in the best sense of the word, the child becomes depends on the humanity he observes and feels about him within his own family circle—what he finds within the lives of his mother and father that he values as true and lasting.

---

[*]Shettles, L. B., and Vande Wiele, R. L.: Can parents choose the sex of their baby? Birth and Fam. J. 1:3-5, Spring, 1974.

unit two
Suggested selected readings and references

Anthony, C. P.: Textbook of anatomy and physiology, ed. 8, St. Louis, 1971, The C. V. Mosby Co.
Anthony, C. P.: Structure and function of the

body, ed. 4, St. Louis, 1972, The C. V. Mosby Co.

Crouch, J. E.: Functional human anatomy, ed. 2, Philadelphia, 1972, Lea & Febiger.

Fitzpatrick, E., Reeder, S. R., and Mastroianni, L., Jr.: Maternity nursing, ed. 12, Philadelphia, 1971, J. B. Lippincott Co.

Guyton, A. C.: Basic human physiology: normal function and mechanisms of disease, Philadelphia, 1971, W. B. Saunders Co.

King, B. G., and Showers, M. J.: Human anatomy and physiology, ed. 6, Philadelphia, 1969, W. B. Saunders Co.

Laros, R. K., Work, B. A., Jr., and Witting, W. C.: Prostaglandins, Am. J. Nurs. **73:**1001-1003, June, 1973.

Memmler, R. L., and Rada, R. B.: The human body in health and disease, ed. 3, Philadelphia, 1970, J. B. Lippincott Co.

Netter, F. H., and Oppenheimer, E., editors: The Ciba collection of medical illustrations, vol. 2, The reproductive system, Summit, N. J., 1954, Ciba Pharmaceutical Products, Inc.

Rorvik, D. M., and Shettles, L. B.: You can choose your baby's sex, Look **34:**88-98, April 21, 1970.

Rothberg, L.: A new sound in obstetrics, RN **34:** 38-40, Dec., 1971.

Shettles, L. B., and Vande Weile, R. L.: Can parents choose the sex of their baby? Birth and Fam. J. **1:**3-5, Spring, 1974.

5

Embryology and fetal development

The event of *conception* (Fig. 5-1), the union of the male sex cell (sperm) and the female sex cell (ovum) within the mother, sets into motion a period of growth unequaled at any other time in the life of the individual.

Just after *fertilization*, or conception, the ovum is not quite as large as the dot used to complete a sentence, but within approximately 9 calendar months, or 266 days, that particle of life will increase in size approximately 200 billion times and become the highly complex structure and personality known as a baby.

EMBRYOLOGY
Early beginnings

Fertilization normally takes place in the fallopian, or uterine, tube. The single cell soon becomes two, then four, then eight, multiplying until keeping count would be impossible. The egg assumes the bumpy appearance of a mulberry and for that reason is called a *morula* as it journeys down the tube in search of a warm, safe place to grow. The journey from ovary to uterine cavity, where nesting, or *implantation*, takes place, involves about 7 days. At the end of this time the fertilized egg burrows into the soft uterine lining. The outer surface of the egg is covered by fingerlike tissue projections called *chorionic villi*, which aid in the process of implantation. These villi also manufacture the chorionic gonadotropic hormone that initially signals the corpus luteum in the ovary to continue to manu-

facture progesterone and estrogen to prevent menstruation and additional ovulation. The aggregation of cells begins to form a definite pattern. A hollow develops in its center, and the microscopic embryo forms, suspended within this hollow by a slender stalk that later becomes the umbilical cord.

Placental development and role

Fairly soon a "supply and disposal system" across the uterine wall is initiated through a special intermediary organ called the *placenta*, or *afterbirth*. The placenta, a miraculous structure, forms from part of the chorionic villi that extended from the outside of the egg. Attached to the uterine wall, it manufactures estrogen, progesterone, chorionic gonadotropin, and various other hormones and enzymes, which apparently influence the growth and maintenance of the pregnancy and maternal preparation for delivery and lactation. It also obtains the food and oxygen necessary for the growth of the fetus from the mother's blood. In addition, through the process of osmosis, hormones and protective substances called antibodies cross over the placental link to the fetus via the umbilical cord. Then, too, the placenta handles waste products brought to its tissue from the fetus: it allows the carbon dioxide and other metabolic wastes to pass over from the fetal circulation to the maternal bloodstream. The mother and fetus do not share a common bloodstream. The fetus manufactures its own blood. Normally, the whole blood

THE MENSTRUAL CYCLE

• Menstruation

• Ovulation

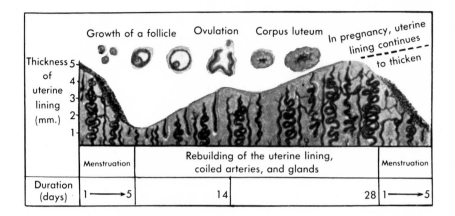

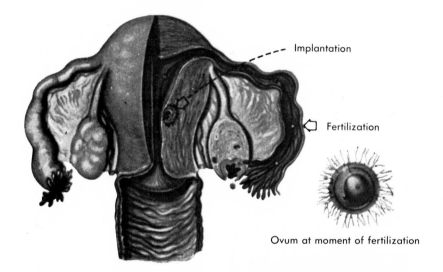

Implantation

Fertilization

Ovum at moment of fertilization

Fig. 5-1. The event of pregnancy. (Courtesy Carnation Co., Los Angeles, Calif.)

of the mother and that of the fetus stay within their own designated though closely related channels. Blood flows from the placenta to the fetus via a large umbilical vein in the cord. The two arteries in the cord, wound about the umbilical vein, carry the waste to the placenta.

"Bag of waters"

As the embryo develops, the chorionic villi that face the interior of the uterus and

are not involved in the formation of the placenta fall off the spherical covering, leaving a transparent sac made up of two membranous layers called the *chorion* and *amnion*. The inner layer, the amnion, secretes a salty liquid known as amniotic fluid in which the fetus may be said to float. It helps to control the environmental temperature of the fetus as well as shield it from bumps and pressure. Perhaps weightlessness is not such an extraordinary condition for mankind

THE FIRST THREE MONTHS

Actual size, ³/₁₄ inch

At end of four weeks

Heart pulsating and pumping blood. Backbone and spinal canal forming. No eyes, nose or external ears visible. Digestive system beginning to form. Small buds which will eventually become arms and legs are present.

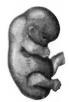

At end of eight weeks

About 1⅛ inches long.
Weighs about ¹/₃₀ ounce.
Face and features forming; eyelids fused.
Limbs beginning to show distinct divisions into arms, elbows, forearm and hand, thigh, knee, lower leg, and foot.
Distinct umbilical cord formed.
Long bones and internal organs developing.
Tail-like process disappears.

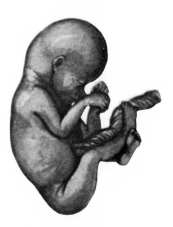

At end of twelve weeks

About 3 inches long.
Weighs about 1 ounce.
Arms, hands, fingers and legs, feet, toes fully formed. Nails on digits beginning to develop.
External ears are present.
Tooth sockets and buds forming in the jawbones.
Eyes almost fully developed, but lids still fused.

Fig. 5-2. Growth of the fetus the first three months. (Courtesy Carnation Co., Los Angeles, Calif.)

after all! This amniotic sac is commonly known as the bag of waters or "the membranes." Normally, it persists intact until the time of labor and delivery.

THE FETUS (Figs. 5-2 to 5-5)

At the end of 8 weeks of growth, the embryo is recognizable as a small, unfinished human, and its name is changed to fetus, meaning "young one." It is less than 2 inches long and weighs a fraction of an ounce. Although rudimentary, body systems are formed and working. The calcified skeleton has even begun to be established.

At 12 weeks. By the close of the third month the sex of the fetus may be clearly discerned if it is directly inspected. Needless to say, there is always considerable curiosity regarding the sex of the developing fetus. However, there is still no *completely* safe way to discover its sex before birth. Nevertheless, a technique has been introduced that now makes possible sex identification before delivery if it is genetically important. Amniotic fluid is aspirated from the bag of waters and examined for cellular content and chromosome determination. (See Fig. 5-7.)

The fetus is most susceptible to malformation from the effects of maternal drug ingestion, radiation, or infection in the first trimester when basic organs and systems are being formed. It is even possible for certain drugs to distort fetal development within 11 days of conception, before the woman realizes that she may be pregnant. Drugs or conditions that produce fetal structural defects are termed *teratogenic.* They are currently the object of much concern and study.

At 16 weeks. At 16 weeks' *gestation,* or pregnancy, the fetus has increased considerably in size. It is approximately 6 inches long and weighs about 4 ounces. The uterus

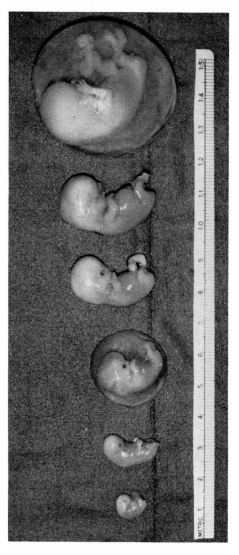

Fig. 5-3. Progressive growth of the human fetus (measured in centimeters). Two amniotic sacs are pictured still intact. (Courtesy Jeanne I. Miller, M.D., Modesto, Calif.)

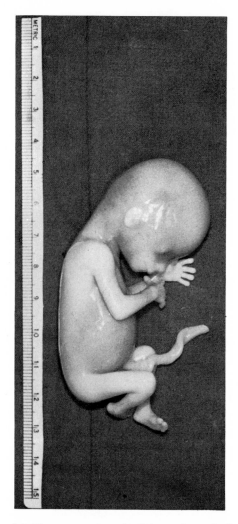

Fig. 5-4. Fetus approximately 7.5 cm. (3 inches) long at almost 3 months' gestation. (Courtesy Jeanne I. Miller, M.D., Modesto, Calif.)

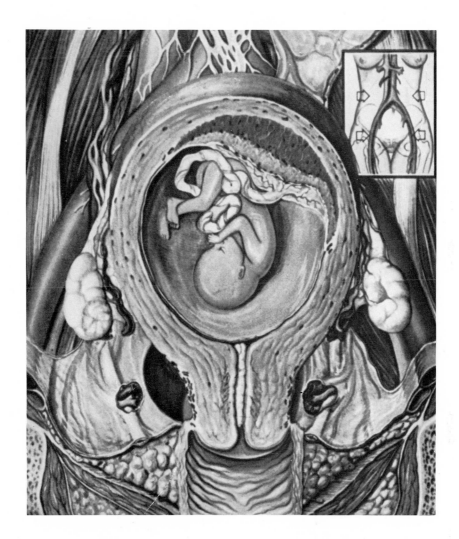

THE UTERUS:

>The fetus may develop within the uterus head down as shown or
>head up, and it may rotate completely before birth. It lives
>throughout its uterine life within the "bag of waters." The
>fluid filling this sac serves many purposes. It prevents the
>walls of the uterus from cramping the fetus and acts as an
>excellent shock-absorber. At term, there is usually about a
>quart of amniotic fluid.

Fig. 5-5. Pelvic relationships in early pregnancy, frontal view. (Courtesy Carnation Co., Los Angeles, Calif.)

will be correspondingly larger, and mother's maternity clothes may make their debut. At about 16 to 18 weeks, expectant mothers usually report feelings of life known as *quickening*. Elbows, feet, and hands punch and twitch as the fetus attempts more vigorous exercise in its confining temporary home.

At 20 weeks. The fetus is about 10 inches long and weighs approximately 8 ounces at this time time. The examining physician may begin to listen for the fetal heart tone, which, although present before, was too faint to be heard.

Some state laws declare that the legal threshold of viability is 24 weeks' gestation; others use 20 weeks as the lower limit. However, the true length of a pregnancy may be difficult to determine and can lead to moral-ethical dilemmas involving the rights and responsibilities of the parents and the community, as well as consideration for the life and well-being of the developing infant. Infants diagnosed as less than 24 weeks' gestation have made postnatal respiratory efforts. Special neonatal care units employing exceptional techniques supporting and/or monitoring body warmth, ventilation, cardiac function, and nutrition have been able to save fetuses of increasingly shorter gestations. Nevertheless, when all births are evaluated, such survivals still must be considered a rare occurrence. (See a brief discussion of premature care on pp. 221-226.)

The characteristics of the premature and his so-called grip on life depend on his genetic endowment, the length and quality of

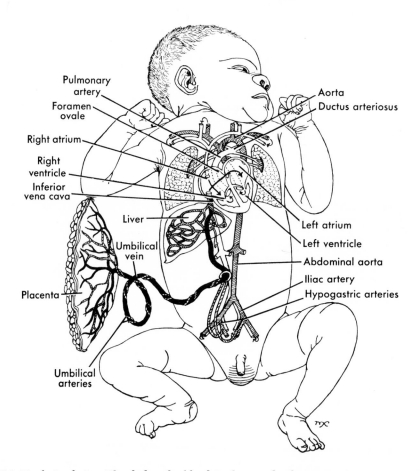

Fig. 5-6. Fetal circulation. The darker the blood in the vessels, the greater its oxygen content. (See text for blood-flow pattern.)

his prenatal environment, and his immediate postnatal care. Each additional day the fetus is able to remain in the uterus until maturity is reached, at a little less than 40 weeks of gestation, is of benefit. Each day increases its ability to withstand the demands of extrauterine life and to adjust to the tremendous circulatory, respiratory, and digestive alterations that must take place at birth.

Fetal circulation

A diagram of fetal circulation is shown in Fig. 5-6 to give a better understanding of the circulorespiratory changes. The umbilical vein extends from the placenta to the fetus, entering the body at the umbilicus. It travels upward, branching through the liver to eventually join the inferior vena cava. There its richly oxygenated blood mixes with the oxygen-poor blood flowing from the lower extremities and abdominal cavity toward the heart. The blood enters the heart via the right artium, as in postnatal circulation, but because the pulmonary circulation is unnecessary to oxygenation, much of the blood entering the heart from the inferior vena cava crosses directly to the left atrium through the fetal shunt, or interatrial opening, called the *foramen ovale*. This blood then is guided into the usual circulation pattern, left atrium → left ventricle → aorta.

Blood entering the right atrium from the superior vena cava, draining the head and upper extremities, flows for the most part into the right ventricle and is eventually pushed into the pulmonary artery. However, the trip to the lungs is superfluous at this time, and another shunt, the *ductus arteriosus*, is employed. This short duct leads from the pulmonary artery to the aorta. Relatively little blood flows to the lung fields and back to the left heart via the pulmonary veins.

The blood flow down the aorta is eventually channeled into the iliac arteries to the hypogastric arteries that join with the umbilical arteries leading to the umbilical cord and placenta.

The pulmonary circulation becomes established within a relatively short time after birth. The umbilical cord is cut and clamped, and the blood vessels it contains

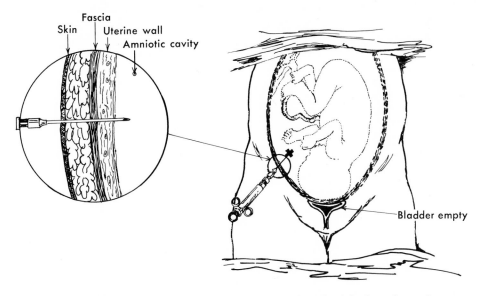

Fig. 5-7. Amniocentesis—a diagnostic tool. To help lessen the risk of fetal or placental trauma, ultrasound or amniography may be used to localize intrauterine structures before the insertion of the needle. Amniocentesis is usually performed for genetic analysis between the fourteenth and eighteenth weeks of gestation.

become occluded. As a result of the changes in thoracic pressures initiated by postnatal expansion of the lungs, the foramen ovale begins to close, and the ductus arteriosus collapses and becomes a ligament within a period of days or weeks.

Methods of evaluating the fetus

Because the maturity of an infant is so important to his survival outside the uterus, increased techniques to determine the state of his intrauterine growth, as well as his general health in utero, have been very welcome. Tests that help assess maturity by examination of amniotic fluid aspirated with sterile precautions transabdominally from the amniotic sac (amniocentesis, Fig. 5-7) are: the lecithin-sphingomyelin ratio and foam tests to evaluate respiratory maturation, the creatinine level to judge renal development, and bilirubin assay. (Bilirubin usually disappears from amniotic fluid by the thirty-sixth week of gestation.) Also available is ultrasonography, which can detect biparietal skull diameters as an esti-

mate of growth. An x-ray film could also reveal this information, but unlike ultrasound, it is potentially dangerous to the fetus in early gestation. Serial estriol determinations taken from blood or urine collections may also help to determine the function of the fetal-placental unit. Analysis of amniotic fluid for increased bilirubin pigments in cases of Rh incompatibility may be lifesaving. Some genetically determined diseases can also be identified in utero by amniotic fluid analysis. During labor the immediate status of the baby may be evaluated through simultaneous monitoring of the fetal heart rate and contraction patterns and, in certain cases, by fetal blood sampling.

• • •

Interest in the developing fetus has accelerated in recent years. A new branch of medicine, "fetology" or "perinatology" has developed. Even now, the time is envisioned when these small patients may undergo numerous corrective procedures.

6

Signs and symptoms of pregnancy

All the activity initiated within the uterus with the onset of pregnancy cannot be kept a secret for long. Widespread changes take place in the body, creating various signs and symptoms that possess varying degrees of importance in the diagnosis of pregnancy. These signs and symptoms are usually arranged, according to their accuracy, into three groups: the presumptive, probable, and positive signs of pregnancy.

PRESUMPTIVE SIGNS

The presumptive signs or symptoms of pregnancy are those that, taken by themselves, could easily be an indication of other conditions.

Amenorrhea. Although absence of menses may be an early sign of developing pregnancy, it certainly is not always. Amenorrhea may occur as a result of sudden changes in environment or occupation, emotional upset, malnutrition, fatigue, hormonal disorders, and the menopause.

Nausea and vomiting (particularly in the morning). Nausea and vomiting, presumably the results of changes in hormone levels in the body in the first weeks of pregnancy, are obviously not confined to this cause, since they are a common accompaniment of gastrointestinal tract irritation and emotional stress.

Frequent urination. Frequent voidings, usually of small amounts, are common during the first and last weeks of pregnancy because of the particular pressure of the uterus on the bladder. But frequency may also be present because of excitement, large fluid intakes, or irritation of the urinary tract.

Breast changes. Tingling, swelling, and tenderness involving the breasts are also found rather early in pregnancy. But a minimal amount of such symptoms may be experienced during each menstrual cycle just before menses. Color changes causing a deepening of pigmentation in the breast or production of breast secretion (colostrum) are considered good signs of pregnancy in a woman who has not been pregnant previously but have little value in a woman who has had children recently or has been nursing. Tiny nodules on the nipple and areola, which are enlarged lubricating glands called tubercles of Montgomery, are often seen.

Quickening. Quickening, meaning the first time life or fetal movement is felt by the mother, can sometimes be imitated by peristalsis or gas and wrongly interpreted. By the time quickening is felt (at approximately 16 to 18 weeks) other more definite signs should be manifest.

Fatigue. Fatigue, often included on the list, is a very widespread complaint even in nonpregnant women.

PROBABLE SIGNS

The probable signs of pregnancy are more certain, but not infallible. They usually include the following: changes in the shape of the abdomen, changes in the reproductive organs, and positive pregnancy tests.

Changes in shape of abdomen. Increases in abdominal size may be accompanied by pink to purplish "stretch marks" known technically as *striae gravidarum*. It is now thought that their presence is probably more related to increases in the production in or sensitivity to adrenocortical hormones during pregnancy than to gain in weight alone. Such skin changes are also noted in patients with Cushing's disease and, to a lesser degree, with sudden marked weight

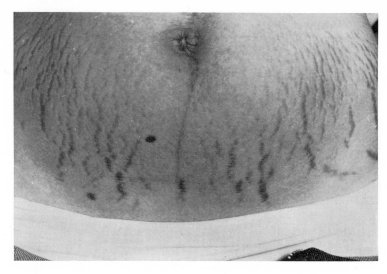

Fig. 6-1. Striae (stretch marks). (Courtesy Mercy Hospital and Medical Center, San Diego, Calif.)

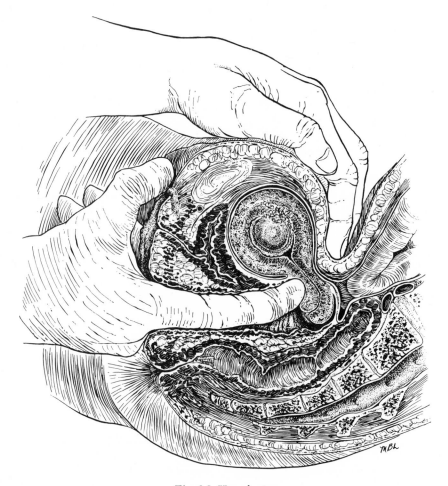

Fig. 6-2. Hegar's sign.

gains unassociated with pregnancy. Unfortunately, the contour of one's abdomen may depend on dietary willpower rather than gestation. It may also be influenced by the growth of tumors. The development of a dark line extending from the sternum to the pubis in the midline, called the *linea nigra,* is considered by some a probable sign if the patient has not been pregnant before. This line is most often seen in brunettes.

Changes in reproductive organs. The enlargement of the uterus, rather than an increase in abdominal circumference, is a more definitive sign of pregnancy. Nevertheless, uterine tumors or inflammation may cause an increase in size. Because of the increase in blood supply to the area at about 8 to 10 weeks after conception, a violet tinge to the cervical and vaginal mucous membranes can be detected *(Chadwick's sign).* Since such a color change may occur in any condition causing pelvic congestion, some authors list it as only a presumptive sign. At about 6 to 8 weeks' gestation, a special softening of the region of the uterus between the body and the cervix, called the *isthmus,* occurs. It is determined by a simultaneous abdominal and vaginal examination, a bimanual examination illustrated in Fig. 6-2. This softening is termed "Hegar's sign."

Basal body temperature elevation. This is one of the earliest diagnostic observations possible and is considered to have 97% accuracy. However, in order for this basal or waking temperature to have meaning, the patient must have taken her temperature consistently, using proper technique both before and after ovulation to detect the persistent relative increase in basal readings. (For interpretation of the temperature readings, see p. 177.)

Positive biological and immunochemical pregnancy tests. Pregnancy tests are based on the fact that the chorionic villi of an implanted ovum or of the developing placenta secrete a gonadotropic hormone, which is excreted in detectable amounts in the urine. The first tests were biological. A concentrated amount of urine obtained from a morning specimen, voided after a period of fluid limitation, was injected into a laboratory animal. The animal was then observed for changes in its reproductive cycle. Rabbits, mice, and frogs were used.

More recently, immunochemical tests that no longer require laboratory animals have been perfected. The presence of human chorionic gonadotrophic hormone causes certain changes in the test materials that may be read in minutes or hours, depending on the individual test selected. These tests are reactive much earlier than those employing animals, sometimes as early as 4 days after the expected date of menstruation. However, because they are only about 95% to 98% accurate, with possibilities of both false negatives and false positives, all these positive pregnancy tests are considered "probable" and not "positive" signs of pregnancy.

Other less-used methods of testing for possible pregnancy involve the administration of progesterone or prostigmine for 2 or 3 days. If lack of menses is *not* due to pregnancy, menstrual flow will appear when the medications are stopped. If pregnancy is present, no flow is initiated. In order for the test to be valid, prior menstrual periods must have been normal and regular. Still other tests are possible; however, they must be done at certain intervals by skilled examiners. They involve the evaluation of different types of cells obtained from a vaginal smear or the microscopic study of dried cervical mucus for the presence or absence of fernlike patterns normally inhibited by the hormonal changes of gestation. Pregnancy tests are generally not used just to satisfy curiosity —time will do that. A firm diagnosis of pregnancy can usually be made after the eighth week. But in those fairly rare cases when a pregnancy outside the uterine cavity (ectopic pregnancy) or an abnormal growth of the fertilized ovum, or *zygote,* called *hydatidiform mole,* is suspected or pelvic surgery is contemplated, pregnancy tests are of real diagnostic value.

Text continued on p. 44.

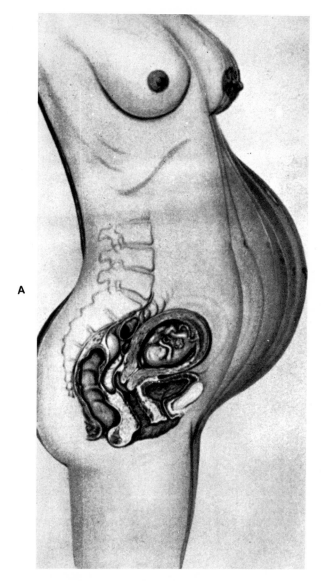

A

Your baby is now about 3 inches long and weighs about 1 ounce. It may continue to develop in the position shown or may turn or rotate frequently. The uterus begins to enlarge with the growing fetus and can now be felt extending about halfway up to the umbilicus.

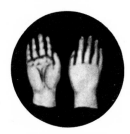

Baby's hands are fully formed even at 12 weeks with fingers and nails all distinctly present.

Fig. 6-3. Growth of the fetus within the mother, with progressive silhouette changes. **A,** Pregnancy of 3 calendar months. **B,** Pregnancy at 5 calendar months. **C,** Pregnancy at 7 calendar months. **D,** Pregnancy at 9 calendar months. (Courtesy Carnation Co., Los Angeles, Calif.)

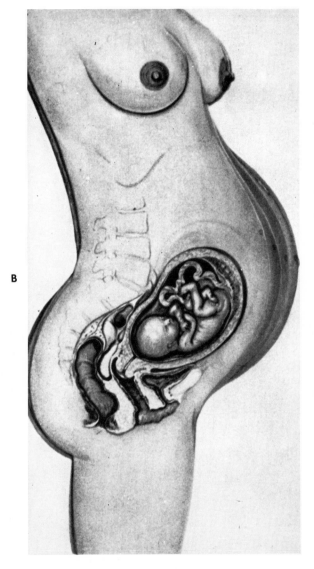

B

5th
month

Your baby measures about 10-12 inches long and weighs from ½ to 1 pound. It is still bright red. Its increased size now brings the dome of the uterus to the level of the umbilicus. The internal organs are maturing at astonishing speed but the lungs are insufficiently developed to cope with conditions outside the uterus.

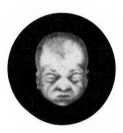

The eyelids are still completely fused at the end of five months. Some hair may be present on the head.

Continued.

Fig. 6-3, cont'd. For legend see opposite page.

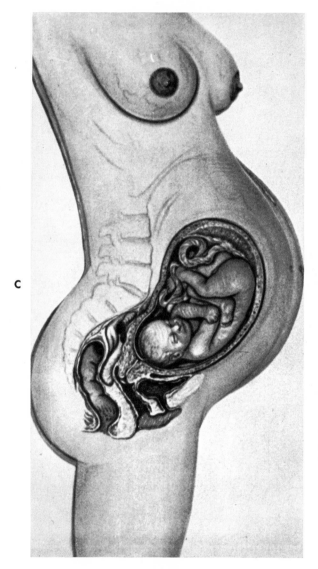

7th
month

The baby's weight has about doubled since last month and it is about 3 inches longer. However, it still looks quite red, is covered with wrinkles which will eventually be erased by fat. At seven months the premature baby at this stage has a fair chance for survival in nurseries cared for by skilled physicians and nurses.

C

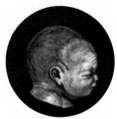

The seven month baby is wrinkled and red.

Fig. 6-3, cont'd. For legend see p. 40.

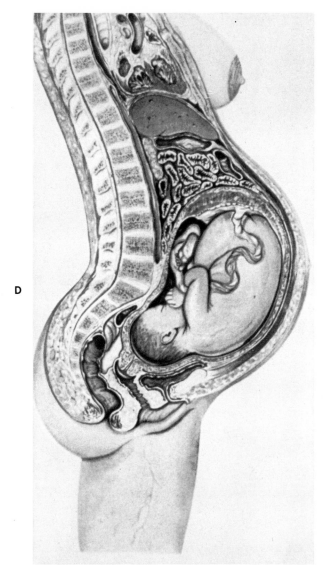

D

9th
month

At birth or full term the baby weighs on an average about 7 pounds if a girl and 7 ½ pounds if a boy. Its length is about 20 inches. Its skin is white or pink but still coated with the creamy coating. The fine downy hair has largely disappeared. Fingernails may protrude beyond the ends of the fingers.

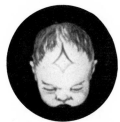

The size of the soft spot between bones of the skull varies considerably from one child to another but generally will close within 12 to 18 months.

Fig. 6-3, cont'd. For legend see p. 40.

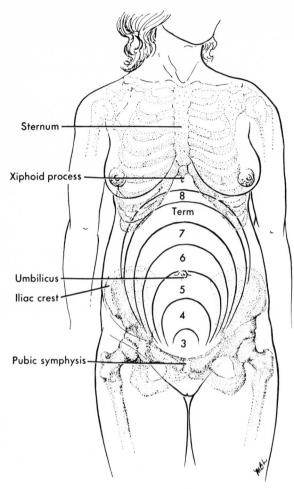

Sternum

Xiphoid process

8

Term

7

6

Umbilicus

5

Iliac crest

4

3

Pubic symphysis

Fig. 6-4. Progressive growth of the fundus during pregnancy, measured in calendar months. Note that the fundus is lower at term than at 8 months' gestation.

POSITIVE SIGNS

There are three positive signs of pregnancy.

1. Presence of a fetal heart tone, usually heard after 4½ calendar months by conventional auscultation with a standard fetoscope. (Up to the fifth calendar month the fetal heart is best heard at the center of the pubic hair line. Fetal heart tones have been detected as early as 10 weeks after conception using ultrasonic or Doppler effect techniques. The presence of the so-called uterine souffle is not diagnostic. This swishlike tone, which is at the same rate as the maternal pulse, originates from the pulsating uterine arteries and not from the placenta itself and may also be heard in the presence of large vascular pelvic tumors.)
2. Fetal movement detected by a trained examiner
3. Visualization of the fetal skeleton on x-ray film (avoided during early pregnancy because of the possibility of radiation damage to the fetus) or use of ultrasonography, which is more expensive and less available but without radiation risk

PROGRESSIVE FETAL GROWTH
(Figs. 6-3 and 6-4)

With the growth of the embryo and fetus, there are progressive changes in the contours and silhouette of the expectant mother. The fundus, or top of the uterus, is felt about halfway between the top of the pubic bone and the umbilicus at approximately 3 calendar months. It is found at the umbilicus at about 5 calendar months. Near term, it is almost at the level of the tip of the sternum. A woman expecting her first baby usually experiences a sudden relief from shortness of breath about 2 weeks before her delivery when the fetus "drops," and *lightening* occurs, taking pressure off the diaphragm.

The increasing size of her temporary boarder puts greater demands on her respiratory, circulatory, and urinary systems. Her intestines and stomach suffer from crowding and compression. Increasing size necessitates changes in wardrobe, creates a typical posture of pregnancy, and finally makes the heretofore simple process of tying shoes almost impossible.

In some women a bronze-type pigmentation, or heightening of color, probably caused by different hormonal levels, appears on the face, especially over the nose and forehead. This has been called *chloasma*, or the *mask of pregnancy*. But, as we have seen, progressive fetal growth is really impossible to mask. There is no such thing as a light case of pregnancy!

7

Prenatal care

When she suspects she is pregnant, a women should consult a physician to gain optimum care even during the early months of pregnancy. Since women are not certain that they will become pregnant and often are not aware of the fact of pregnancy until several weeks of gestation have elapsed, the earliest prenatal care is always the responsibility of the woman herself. Her general health habits and physical condition before a physician is ever consulted are of considerable importance. When the diagnosis of pregnancy is established, provision for regular medical supervision and suitable plans for the baby's arrival must be made.

In the physician's office and in the hospital, an expectant mother is given certain professional labels by the staff to help in anticipating her needs and to briefly describe her obstetrical past. This terminology, with certain modifications, is used throughout her care. It consists of a series of prefixes and suffixes to help describe the number of times the patient has been pregnant and the number of times she has carried a child to a viable age. The word elements are as follows:

gravida (a suffix) the number of pregnancies a woman has had. The term comes from the same root as gravity, which causes us to have weight. Pregnancy brings weight, too.

para (a suffix) the number of deliveries of infants a woman has had weighing 500 grams or more or, if weight is unknown, the number having an estimated gestational age of 20 completed weeks or more, whether born living or dead. In most areas the birth of twins or triplets would only be considered as one delivery. Both abdominal and vaginal deliveries are recorded in "para" counts.

nul (a prefix) means none. A *nulligravida* has never been pregnant. A *nullipara* has never delivered a viable child.

prim (a prefix) from primary or first. Combined with gravida, it reads *primigravida* and means a woman who is having or has had one pregnancy. Combined with para, it reads *primipara* and technically means a woman who has had one delivery of a viable child. However, once she is admitted into the labor-delivery suite, attending nurses usually refer to a woman who is carrying her first child but is not yet delivered as a primipara or "primip" to differentiate her from a woman who has been through the birth process.

mult (a prefix) meaning many or at least more than one. Combined with gravida it reads *multigravida* and means a woman who has had more than one pregnancy. Combined with para it reads *multipara* or "multip" and technically means a woman who has borne two or more viable infants. Actually, in the labor-delivery suite the term is applied to a woman who has delivered one viable child or more, to differentiate her from a "first timer." Sometimes women who have had six or more viable deliveries are called "grandmultips."

GOALS AND IMPORTANCE OF PRENATAL CARE

The term "antepartal or prenatal care" as used by doctors and nurses refers to the planned examination, observation, and guidance of an expectant mother. It is well to remember that the extension of prenatal care is probably the primary factor in the improvement of maternal morbidity and mortality statistics. Society needs to appreciate its importance. The goals are as follows:

1. A pregnancy with a minimum of mental and physical discomfort and a maximum of gratification
2. A delivery under the best circumstances possible
3. A normal, well baby
4. The establishment of good health habits benefiting all the family

45

5. A smooth, guided postpartum adjustment

For many years the overall goals of prenatal care have probably remained much the same, but interpretation of these goals and the methods for accomplishing them are undergoing continual change and accelerated expansion. In the beginnings of so-called modern medicine in the late 1800's and early 1900's, the focus of the doctor and nurse in attendance was on the physical needs of the parturient. Later, the psychological aspects of her needs drew deserved attention. More recently, the physical and psychosocial needs of the entire family unit, as well as the needs of the patient, have been emphasized as we concern ourselves with the concept of "family-centered maternity care."*

For example, goals 1 and 2 above underline the need for better health delivery systems that would encourage socioeconomically disadvantaged urban and rural clients to receive needed care and vital health instruction. Because of financial strain, transportation difficulties, child care problems, or fear and distrust of the established depersonalized and fragmented institutional management, they may not have sufficiently obtained or used these facilities. These goals also imply for many parents more knowledge of the processes of pregnancy and childbirth and more participation in and control over these processes than were requested by recent previous generations. Goal 3 now allows more legally permitted decision making than ever before as genetic counselling and abortion services become increasingly accessible. Goal 4 may encompass not only physical health but emotional well-being, knowledge and appreciation of life processes, and a sense of responsible personhood, which considers individual differ-

ences as well as the common good. Future parents, consumers of maternity care, today do not wish to be treated all alike. They wish to have comprehensive care that will allow them certain choices and variations of expression within the context of safety. "A smooth, guided postpartum adjustment" entails more knowledge of childcraft and parenting skills and more premeditated control of family composition.*

THE FIRST VISIT

Usually prenatal care is formally begun shortly after the second menstrual period is missed. But in a broader sense, a woman is being prepared for her experience of childbearing and nurturing long before she steps into the physician's office. Her basic physique was determined by her parents before her birth. Her environment has left its physical and emotional imprint. Her own family circle and close friends have greatly influenced her attitude toward pregnancy and the challenges and responsibilities of motherhood. In a very real sense, prenatal care, negative or positive, has gone on in the life of a young woman long before she becomes pregnant. Today there is much controversy regarding the need for sex education, what should be taught by whom, and at what age level. Sex education and preparation for marriage and parenthood are taught—sometimes negatively by default. Children and young people do not live in a vacuum.

But enough philosophizing. What, in more detail, does formal prenatal care entail? Perhaps it would be easiest to describe the visits of the future mother to the physician's office. In most cases the most lengthy visit she makes is her first.

The first visit to the physician is usually a particular time of stress. Some women

---

*Walker, L.: Providing more relevant maternity services, J. Obstet. Gynecol. Neonatal Nurs. 3:34-36, March-April, 1974.

*Jordan, A. D.: Evaluation of a family-centered maternity care hospital program, J. Obstet. Gynecol. Neonatal Nurs. 2:13-35, Jan.-Feb., 1973; 2:15-27, March-April, 1973; 2:15-22, May-June, 1973.

are very concerned because they want very much to be pregnant. Some are anxious about the nature of the examination and the tests to be made. Others may be concerned because they had not planned to have a child. Family financial problems may be mounting. A number of small children may already be part of the family, stairstep style, and the mother may feel for a while like the proverbial "old woman in the shoe." Health problems at home may cause worry. Previous unfortunate obstetrical experiences and half-believed gossip concerning pregnancy and childbirth may nag. The marriage may be undergoing a period of instability or even dissolution. All these possible situations tend to heighten the emotional content of the visit.

Setting and "climate"

The "climate" of the first as well as subsequent visits to the doctor is all important. A nurse who has the responsibility of greeting and caring for these patients has a key position. A cordial, respectful environment in which the patient feels personally important to the office staff and physician is a goal to be sought.

Preparation for the visit is usually made by a telephone call to the office. At this time it is customary for a new patient to be asked to bring a sample of the first voided urine on the day of the appointment if her visit will be made early in the morning. When the time of the appointment arrives, it is hoped that the prospective patient will not have to wait too long, but because of the very nature of a physician's practice, which deals with the unscheduled flights of "Mr. Stork," some waiting is almost unavoidable. However, some of this time can often be put to excellent use. The nurse or receptionist can start to make contact with the patient and make her feel welcome. Brief information cards for office use may be completed. Frequently changed, attractive bulletin boards may emphasize nutrition and meal planning, mental health practices, good grooming, maternity wardrobe styles, and approved courses in preparation for childbirth and child care. Up-to-date pamphlets on maternal and child care may also be available. Not all reading material should be pregnancy oriented, however. Just because a woman is pregnant does not mean that is all she wants to think about! When waits are protracted, an offer of coffee or fruit juice may be appreciated. The way to the public rest room should be clearly indicated, since frequent urination is an often encountered annoyance, and general nervousness will usually exaggerate this symptom. Just before the pelvic examination, the patient should have an opportunity to empty her bladder to ease the examination and to allow a more accurate measurement of the height of the fundus.

Vital signs and history

Before actually seeing the physician the patient is usually weighed and her temperature, pulse, and respiration are checked by the nurse. In some clinics, nurses may also take the blood pressures and medical and obstetrical histories of new patients, but many practitioners prefer to complete the blood pressures and the histories themselves. A carefully secured history is very important in helping to determine any special emphasis needed in the care of the patient. What previous medical or surgical difficulties has she had? Any problems involving mental or emotional instability? Any family problems that may affect her toleration of the stress of pregnancy? A record of previous pregnancies and their outcome is extremely important in indicating need for special emphasis in prenatal care. One method of coding the results of previous pregnancies involves the use of four consecutive digits. The first refers to the number of full-term deliveries, the second to the number of premature births, the third to abortions, and the fourth to children now living. Using this code, what would 3215 mean? Many physicians believe that the time spent in recording the historical data is well worth the greater opportunity to evaluate the patient and her child.

The period of gestation

Pelvic examination

The visit usually continues with the determination of the presence of pregnancy. Each physician has his own routine, but it is our opinion that the pelvic examination should be done first in the schedule of the physical to alleviate the additional anxiety of waiting and avoid a filling bladder! The nurse, by her manner and efficiency, can help the patient immensely.

Preparation. An adequate gown, which gives reassuring coverage but opens in such a way to make a physical examination easily possible, is desirable. A drape that makes the patient feel covered even if she is not is a real aid. The hips should extend about 1 inch over the edge of the table with the feet supported in stirrups. Various drapes may be used. A nurse should always be present during the examination to give reassurance to the patient and protect the physician from criticism. Necessary instruments should be ready (Fig. 7-1): warmed speculum, spatula or applicator, and/or vaginal pipette with rubber bulb, slides and preservative for cervical cancer detection; long swabs or cotton balls, sponge sticks, both sterile and clean rubber gloves,

lubricant, and paper tissue wipes. A good light and a convenient stool must be provided. If the patient is able to let her knees fall outward and relax, the examination will be less difficult. Having her breathe through her open mouth usually helps promote relaxation, although there is some danger of hyperventilation in very tense patients.

Progression. The pelvic examination yields considerable information. The physician first inspects the external genitalia. Next, if a Papanicolaou smear for cancer detection is desired (and it is almost always part of the routine), a warmed, but unlubricated, bivalve speculum, is inserted to reveal the cervix. Specimens of secretion may be aspirated from the posterior fornix with the pipette or secured with the applicator or spatula from the cervix and placed thinly and evenly on a slide or two. These slides must not be allowed to dry out but should immediately be placed in a fixative (usually equal parts of 95% alcohol and ether). The physician will then observe the cervix and vaginal mucosa for any abnormalities or unusual discharge. He may obtain specimens of any discharge for future study. Fungous infection caused by *Can-*

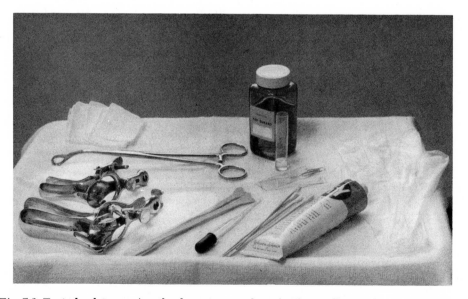

Fig. 7-1. Typical pelvic tray (sterile gloves are not shown). The small test tube contains physiological saline solution for wet mount of vaginal discharge.

dida albicans or infection initiated by microscopic animals, or protozoa, called *Trichomonas vaginalis* is fairly common. Routine culture of cervical mucus for *Neisseria gonorrhoeae*, the cause of gonorrhea, has been helpful in detecting significant numbers of so-called silent infections within certain high-risk populations. The mucosa will be checked for Chadwick's sign, a violet tinge caused by increased circulatory congestion in the area.

After general inspection of the vulva, cervix, and vagina, the speculum will be gently removed and a digital examination will be made with the lubricated gloved hand. At this time the physican will feel the size and position of the uterus and perhaps try to elicit Hegar's sign, the softening of the uterine isthmus, through vaginoabdominal pressure. He will palpate the pelvic contents to try to identify any abnormal masses or tumors. Usually before completing his examination he will attempt to measure the *diagonal conjugate* to estimate the size of the pelvic canal and will evaluate the position of the ischial spines and tuberosities. In most cases, at the end of the vaginal examination a rectal examination is carried out. Most of the time the doctor can report at the end of the pelvic examination whether or not the patient is actually pregnant.

Determination of delivery date

The most common method of determining the date of delivery involves a record of the menstrual cycle. The patient is asked to name the *first* day of her last *normal* menstrual period. The doctor then counts back 3 months and adds 7 days to calculate the estimated date of confinement (EDC). (Confinement is a rather old term used to indicate the period of labor and delivery.) For example, if a patient said that her last normal menstrual period occurred between May 7 and May 12, 1975, her EDC would be February 14, 1976. This method of calculation is called Nägele's rule. Of course, if the patient cannot remember the vital statistics involved, calculation may be more

difficult. In that case, the size of the uterus may be interpreted, or the time of the intercourse that preceded conception may be known. Occasionally, *quickening* may be used as a measurable landmark, but it is not too reliable. However, even Nägele's rule offers only an estimation. It is said that only 4% of all babies arrive "on time" using this schedule, whereas 60% appear 1 to 7 days early or late.

Complete examination

The first prenatal visit to the physician may continue with a complete physical examination, or the physician may only talk with the patient, giving appropriate guidance and information, and making arrangements for a more detailed physical examination during the following visit.

The physician is interested in much more than his patient's pelvis. He checks her blood pressure; listens to her heart and lungs; examines her mouth, eyes, ears, nose, and throat; observes and palpates her breasts, alert to any abnormalities; and perhaps inquires about her preference for feeding the infant. The abdomen is palpated with the knees flexed for greater relaxation of the abdominal wall, and the extremities are checked for bruises, swelling, and enlarged veins.

Usually at the conclusion of the physical examination, arrangements are made for the necessary laboratory tests. A sample of venous blood is drawn. A complete blood count may be ordered or perhaps a hemoglobin alone or a hematocrit to determine the amount of hemoglobin present in the blood in relation to its volume. Any pregnant woman may be or may become anemic. Dietary deficiencies of iron are common. While hemoglobin and hematocrit levels in nonpregnant women would be considered suspiciously low if less than 12 grams/100 ml. and 36% respectively, the standards of possible anemia used during pregnancy are usually less than 11 grams/100 ml. and less than 33%. The differences are due to the increased fluid content in the blood during gestation. The prenatal testing for sickle cell anemia in previously unscreened black patients is becoming more common.

A serology test for the detection of syphilis is required by law in most states. A determination of main blood group and Rh status is made to aid in maternal care in the event of hemorrhage and to detect the possibility of blood protein incompatibility, which could threaten the life of the developing fetus or infant. If the patient is found to be Rh negative, the Rh status of the baby's father should be ascertained.

Another potential threat that can now be identified by the laboratory is rubella or German measles. A history of the disease in childhood is not always reliable, since other conditions may have been incorrectly called rubella and since the disease does not always manifest a rash. The measurement of rubella antibody level in a woman's blood has recently become a premarital or prenatal legal requirement in some states. The presence of antibodies in a 1:10 or greater dilution of serum is said to indicate immunity. Some physicians in practice consider the 1:10 dilution reaction evidence of only "borderline" protection and consider the mother still at risk unless a weaker dilution (more than 1:10) demonstrates antibody levels. Pregnant women are *not* given the available immunization against rubella. There is a real possibility that the fetus could contract the deforming contagion whether or not the mother shows clinical signs of the disease. However, if immunity is considered absent, the antibody titer obtained can be used as a base line to help determine subsequent contact with the disease and the need for possible immune serum globulin or consideration of an abortion. New mothers at risk are immunized during the postpartum period only after reliable contraception techniques have been instituted. See discussion of rubella on pp. 136-137.

The urine specimen brought in the same morning or secured later at the office is tested for albumin and sugar. Many physicians order a complete urinalysis initially. .

In many patients, chest x-ray films for detection of tuberculosis are being avoided through the use of Mantoux or Tine skin testing. If the skin test is positive, then a full-sized, conventional chest x-ray film is recommended to rule out possible pathology more easily and avoid the higher amount of x-ray exposure involved in the use of photofluorographs or miniature films.

Guidance

After all these procedures have been completed, if they take place during one visit, the patient is usually tired. Long-winded instructions and explanations are not properly assimilated. Perhaps the best method of imparting needed information is through the use of some kind of prenatal instruction booklet that has been approved by or perhaps even written by the patient's doctor. Some doctors program a series of teaching films that individuals or groups can view while they are waiting to see him. Such guidance is absolutely necessary, but all of it need not come the first visit. However, some time should be spent answering questions that have been bothering the patient and giving some general instructions regarding dietary requirements and the situations that should be reported to the doctor.

Reportable signs and symptoms

The physician should indicate the signs and symptoms that must be reported in a manner that will not be too alarming to the patient. They may or may not be significant, but only qualified personnel are capable of deciding their importance and must be notified of their presence. They include the following:
1. Bleeding from the vagina at any time
2. Uncontrollable leaking of fluid from the vagina
3. Unusual abdominal pain or cramps
4. Persistent nausea or vomiting, especially in the second or third trimester

5. Persistent headache or any blurring of vision
6. Marked swelling of the ankles and especially of the hands and face
7. Painful or burning urination
8. Chills or fever

Then, armed with information, the patient may make an appointment for her next visit. Before her return she can jot down questions that come up about which she needs to be reassured.

SUBSEQUENT VISITS

During the first half of the pregnancy, expectant mothers most often visit their doctors every 3 or 4 weeks unless special needs become apparent. After 5 months, visits are usually scheduled every 2 or 3 weeks, and in the last month, checkups may be made every 1 or 2 weeks or more often.

Examination

The subsequent visits are not as long or involved. The patient is weighed by the nurse, and the blood pressure recorded. A urine specimen is checked for albumin and glucose. The urine examination for glucose, of course, is made to detect diabetes mellitus. All of the other above determinations are done to reveal the beginnings of toxemia of pregnancy. (Remember that the major signs of toxemia are elevated blood pressure, edema, excessive weight gain, and albuminuria.) The physician measures the height of the uterus to see if the pregnancy is progressing at the expected rate. He may repeat the pelvic examination during the first return visit. After about 4½ calendar months' gestation he may listen for the fetal heart tone. After 8 months' gestation he may palpate the abdomen to determine the presentation of the fetus. Hemoglobin or hematocrit levels should be repeated for all patients at least once late in pregnancy (at about 32 to 36 weeks). Those women who earlier had been found to have iron or folic acid deficiency anemias or other causes of hemoglobin reduction should, of course, be checked more frequently to determine their response to therapy.

If Rh incompatibility is a possibility, antibody titers should be done not only at the initial prenatal visit but also at 24, 28, 32, and 36 weeks' gestation, even if the patient received Rh immune globulin, such as RhoGAM, after previous pregnancies. Rising titers may indicate whether the baby is Rh positive and will alert the physician to developing erythroblastosis fetalis. A more reliable technique for evaluating fetal jeopardy related to blood factor incompatibility involves the aspiration of amniotic fluid by transabdominal needle insertion (amniocentesis) and its analysis for elevated bilirubin levels (see p. 35). Because maternal syphilitic infection may be acquired *after* a negative prenatal serology result is obtained and the disease may be transferred congenitally to the baby following the eighteenth week of gestation (when there is no longer placental shielding of the fetus from the organism causing syphilis), the prudence of securing a repeat serology test close to term is now being considered. Other laboratory evaluations of fetal and maternal health and gestational maturity are possible but would depend on the specific problems discovered.

Guidance

During the initial and return visits a feeling of trust should be built up between the patient and the physician and his staff. The physician and nurse should be able to identify areas in which the expectant mother needs special help, whether it involves need for information, reassurance in her own capacity to be a good mother, possible help in organizing her household to achieve more rest and peace of mind, or simply an interested human listener.

Nutrition

The subject of nutrition has long been considered important in prenatal care. However, it is now becoming apparent to increasing numbers of health professionals that nutrition is not only important, it is crucial in determining the health of the childbearing woman, her offspring, and perhaps even that of ongoing generations. It is imperative that girls and women consider themselves as possible prospective mothers by preparing themselves for the potential responsibility of such nurture long before a mate is selected. Their health, knowledge, and skills will profoundly influence the structure of any future family. A woman who furnishes her body with what it needs nutritionally to enjoy optimum personal health and who augments her diet as needed as a pregnancy progresses gives her child a better opportunity to be both well formed from his earliest days of development and well born as he ends his intrauterine growth period. A well-nourished mother and baby are less often the victims of obstetrical and perinatal complications, such as late toxemia of pregnancy, prematurity, low birth weight (small for dates), mental retardation, and neurological damage.

Various aids have been devised to try to help Americans eat more nourishing food according to their body build, age, activity, or special physiological needs. The National Research Council publishes peri-odically a quantitative list of calories and nutrients needed. In 1974 this list, the Recommended Daily Allowance, or RDA, was newly revised. (Table 7-1 is an abbreviated version.) The Council has indicated that a normal, healthy, pregnant woman of almost any age needs *greater amounts of calories* and every *nutrient* listed during the last half of her 40-week pregnancy than she does when not pregnant.

The daily allowance for calories has been raised from +200 in the former 1968 revision to +300. The allowance for protein has been increased from +10 grams to +30 grams. Folacin or folic acid levels were increased in the 1974 revision for the period of lactation. A specific megaloblastic anemia does occasionally occur due to folacin depletion in pregnancy. It is interesting to note that steroid contraceptives that the expectant mother may have used in the recent past may also inhibit folic acid absorption. Nondietary folic acid is often prescribed by clinicians. Thiamine and iron intakes were also elevated, while vitamin B_{12} and vitamin E allowances were lowered. Excessive vitamin intake can be dan-

Table 7-1. Food and Nutrition Board, National Academy of Sciences–National Research Council

	Age (years)	Weight (kg)	(lbs)	Height (cm)	(in)	Energy (kcal)[b]	Protein (g)	Fat-soluble vitamins				Ascorbic acid (mg)	Folacin[e] (µg)
								Vitamin A activity		Vitamin D (IU)	Vitamin E activity[d] (IU)		
								(RE)[c]	(IU)				
Recommended	11-14	44	97	155	62	2400	44	800	4000	400	12	45	400
for females	15-18	54	119	162	65	2100	48	800	4000	400	12	45	400
	19-22	58	128	162	65	2100	46	800	4000	400	12	45	400
	23-50	58	128	162	65	2000	46	800	4000		12	45	400
	51+	58	128	162	65	1800	46	800	4000		12	45	400
Pregnant						+300	+30	1000	5000	400	15	60	800
Lactating						+500	+20	1200	6000	400	15	80	600

Adapted from *Recommended Dietary Allowances*, eighth edition, publication ISBN 0-309-02216-9, Food and Nutrition

[a]The allowances are intended to provide for individual variations among most normal persons as they live in the provide other nutrients for which human requirements have been less well defined.
[c]Retinol equivalents.
[b]Kilojoules (kJ) = 4.2 × kcal.
[d]Total vitamin E activity, estimated to be 80 percent as α-tocopherol and 20 percent other tocopherols.
[e]The folacin allowances refer to dietary sources as determined by *Lactobacillus casei* assay. Pure forms of folacin may
[f]Although allowances are expressed as niacin, it is recognized that on the average 1 mg of niacin is derived from each
[g]This increased requirement cannot be met by ordinary diets; therefore, the use of supplemental iron is recommended.

gerous as well as wasteful. Routine multi-vitamin supplementation should not be necessary if a varied nutritious diet is consumed. Prescription of prenatal fluoride has not been proven to be an asset. Calcification of the permanent teeth and much of that of the deciduous teeth occurs after birth. The RDA's determined by the Council are designed to indicate safe dietary levels of selected nutrients for a wide range of normal healthy persons. Individual differences in the dietary background or obstetrical histories of expectant women may suggest the need for variations in these allowances. For example, high-risk pregnancies may need even more protein intake.

There is an increasing trend (at least among some physicians) to emphasize the quality of the pregnant woman's diet and to be less concerned about a certain total number of pounds gained. The need for quality intake is present throughout pregnancy. One can see in Fig. 7-3, which indicates the average relative-weight increase curve advocated as a pattern for evaluation by the National Academy of Sciences, Com-

mittee on Maternal Nutrition, that approximately two thirds of the weight gain occurs in the last half of pregnancy, paralleling fairly closely the baby's own weight gain curve. Quantitative increases in maternal intake are recommended for healthy, well-nourished women only in the last half of pregnancy.

Because an expectant mother cannot (as yet) go to the grocery store to purchase a package labeled "76 grams of protein" and buying many of the nutrients as pills in a bottle would be very expensive, inefficient, and unsatisfying, there needs to be a way to interpret her caloric and nutrient needs in terms of market basket commodities. For a number of years the concept of the Basic Four Food Groups and the suggested number of servings have been helpful in planning balanced family meals. These four groups—milk, meat, vegetables and fruit, and breads and cereals—only contain those foods high in leader nutrients. In the second half of pregnancy a woman needs to add more milk to her diet, to increase her intake to 3 or 4 cups of either skimmed or whole milk. Using nonfat dairy prod-

ecommended daily dietary allowances,[a] revised 1974

Water-soluble vitamins					Minerals					
Niacin[f] (mg)	Riboflavin (B₂) (mg)	Thiamin (B₁) (mg)	Vitamin B₆ (mg)	Vitamin B₁₂ (μg)	Calcium (mg)	Phosphorus (mg)	Iodine (μg)	Iron (mg)	Magnesium (mg)	Zinc (mg)
16	1.3	1.2	1.6	3.0	1200	1200	115	18	300	15
14	1.4	1.1	2.0	3.0	1200	1200	115	18	300	15
14	1.4	1.1	2.0	3.0	800	800	100	18	300	15
13	1.2	1.0	2.0	3.0	800	800	100	18	300	15
12	1.1	1.0	2.0	3.0	800	800	80	10	300	15
+2	+0.3	+0.3	2.5	4.0	1200	1200	125	18+[g]	450	20
+4	+0.5	+0.3	2.5	4.0	1200	1200	150	18	450	25

Board, National Academy of Sciences–National Research Council, Washington, D. C., 1974.
United States under usual environmental stresses. Diets should be based on a variety of common foods in order to

be effective in doses less than one fourth of the recommended dietary allowance.
0 mg of dietary tryptophan.

ucts reduces the total fat and cholesterol intake. Some fat is necessary in the diet, but it is not a scarce nutrient. Milk (and the calcium and protein it provides) is considered an important constituent of the expectant mother's diet. However, not all this requirement has to be taken without modification. The woman who does not care for milk per se is free to use flavoring, make what she does drink more concentrated in value by adding skim milk powders, use it in cooking, or select

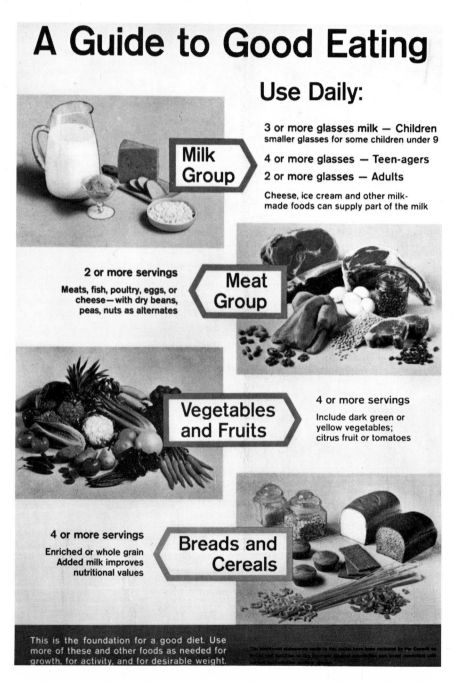

A Guide to Good Eating

Use Daily:

Milk Group

3 or more glasses milk — Children
smaller glasses for some children under 9

4 or more glasses — Teen-agers

2 or more glasses — Adults

Cheese, ice cream and other milk-made foods can supply part of the milk

Meat Group

2 or more servings

Meats, fish, poultry, eggs, or cheese—with dry beans, peas, nuts as alternates

Vegetables and Fruits

4 or more servings

Include dark green or yellow vegetables; citrus fruit or tomatoes

Breads and Cereals

4 or more servings

Enriched or whole grain Added milk improves nutritional values

This is the foundation for a good diet. Use more of these and other foods as needed for growth, for activity, and for desirable weight.

Fig. 7-2. A guide to good eating. (Courtesy National Dairy Council, Chicago, Ill.)

a milk exchange of approximate equal value for calcium. For example, 1 slice of American cheese or 1 cup of creamed cottage cheese equals ⅔ glass of milk. If she cannot tolerate milk or is having muscle cramps due to phosphorus/calcium imbalance in the blood, calcium pills may be given, but in this case a fine, relatively inexpensive source of protein is lost. Milk is also usually reinforced with vitamin D, an important consideration in climates lacking sunshine or in planning meals for those who always like the shade.

Three servings of the meat group are usually recommended during the latter part of pregnancy. This usually includes one or two eggs per day in addition to two servings of the other meat group foods listed. Eggs are recommended particularly for the rich iron source found in the yolk. Meat, eggs, even fish and poultry are expensive, but they are complete proteins, containing all the amino acids necessary for growth, repair, and development; the body cannot manufacture these protein building blocks by rearranging molecules within its own cells. The essential amino acids (eight to ten in number depending on age requirements) must be available to form new tissue within the mother's body, and they must be supplied in the diet. Such proteins are critical to the growth of the embryo and fetus as basic body systems are formed early in pregnancy and as different organs, especially the brain, undergo growth spurts in the last weeks of gestation. They are also critical for the mother if she is to maintain her health and avoid obstetrical problems such as toxemia. If legumes such as beans or peas, corn, nuts, and gelatin are used as major protein sources, they must be mixed in such a way that all essential amino acids are represented in a single meal since none of these protein sources are complete in themselves. Mixing certain incomplete proteins conscientiously or serving them with milk provides an adequate diet but is more difficult. Examples of adequate protein mixes using incomplete proteins are combinations of cornmeal and kidney beans or

whole wheat, soy beans and sesame seeds. Pure vegetarian or "vegan" diets without any animal sources, dairy products, or eggs can supply adequate protein with careful planning. But other deficiencies (for example, vitamin B_{12}) may become a problem.

High-grade biological sources of protein, such as meat, fish, poultry, milk, and eggs, contribute other nutrients as well. For example, liver, although it may not be everybody's choice, is strongly favored in the diet because of its high iron content. However, it is difficult to obtain enough iron (18 mg. or more daily) in the diet during pregnancy to prevent maternal gestational anemia and allow the fetus to lay down a reserve for hemoglobin formation during the first 3 to 4 months of life when his main source of nutrition will be milk, which is normally iron poor. The National Research Council advises the use of iron preparations to supplement expectant women's diets.

Whole grain or enriched breads and cereals provide sources of the B vitamins thiamine and niacin, as well as some iodine and iron and needed cellulose. Four or more servings are indicated. One slice of bread equals one serving. A helpful chart designed to help meet the dietary needs of pregnancy is from Sue Rodwell Williams's excellent text, *Nutrition and Diet Therapy* (Table 7-2).

Fruits and vegetables are important sources of vitamins, minerals, and roughage (if they are eaten unmodified). Constipation is a real problem for many pregnant women. The increasing pressure exerted on the bowel by the enlarging uterus, diminished intestinal tone, and decreased physical exercise have all been blamed for this trouble. The use of bulk-producing foods, including whole grain breads and cereals, and increased fluids usually helps solve the problem. A high vitamin C (ascorbic acid) intake is advised for tissue building; the fruits especially helpful are grapefruits, oranges, lemons, limes, tomatoes, strawberries, cantaloupes, green peppers, and cabbage. Two servings a day of fruits in raw, cooked, or juice forms are recommended.

Table 7-2. Daily food plan for pregnancy and lactation

Food	Nonpregnant woman or during first half of pregnancy	Second half of pregnancy	Lactation
Milk, cheese, ice cream, skimmed or buttermilk (food made with milk can supply part of requirement)	2 cups	3 to 4 cups	4 to 5 cups
Meat (lean meat, fish, poultry, cheese, occasional dried beans or peas)	1 serving (3 to 4 ounces)	2 servings (6 to 8 oz.); include liver frequently	2½ servings (8 oz.)
Eggs	1	1 to 2	1 to 2
Vegetable* (dark green or deep yellow)	1 serving	1 serving	1 to 2 servings
Vitamin C-rich food* Good source—citrus fruit, berries, cantaloupe Fair source—tomatoes, cabbage, greens, potatoes in skin	1 good source or 2 fair sources	1 good source and 1 fair source or 2 good sources	1 good source and 1 fair source or 2 good sources
Other vegetables and fruits	1 serving	2 servings	2 servings
Bread† and cereals (enriched or whole grain)	3 servings	4 to 5 servings	5 servings
Butter or fortified margarine	As desired or needed for calories	As desired or needed for calories	As desired or needed for calories

From Williams, S. R.: Nutrition and diet therapy, ed. 2, St. Louis, 1973, The C. V. Mosby Co.
*Use some raw daily.
†One slice of bread equals one serving.

Two portions of vegetables, especially dark green and yellow types, are considered optimum.

Items that contribute little or no nutrient value other than calories for energy are called "empty calorie" foods. Examples of these items are candy, cake, pie, soft drinks, spaghetti, doughnuts, and potato chips. They add pounds but contribute nothing that would assist the mother or developing child except potential heat and energy. Remember, carrying this excessive weight requires more energy, but it is infinitely better to obtain energy plus nutrients with your food.

Sometimes women during pregnancy experience special cravings for unusual foods or food combinations. Usually these desires are trivial and may be humored if they do not threaten good nutrition. However, there is a type of unusual ingestion called "pica" that is characteristic of, but not confined to, lower socioeconomic ethnic groups. Women exhibiting symptoms of pica may eat relatively large amounts of such substances as laundry starch or river clay. Such ingestions interfere with good nutrition and cause anemia.

Anything that depresses good nutritional intake, whether it be nausea and vomiting, food fads, lack of finances, alcoholism, or other personal or social problems, should be evaluated and treated to achieve good dietary prenatal care.

The restriction of salt or sodium intake has long been considered by many physicians almost part of the prenatal diet. It has been advocated in an attempt to help prevent and treat the symptoms of toxemia of pregnancy, a serious complication characterized by edema, hypertension, and albuminuria, possibly leading to convulsions and death. Toxemia of pregnancy has been a major cause of fetal, neonatal, and mater-

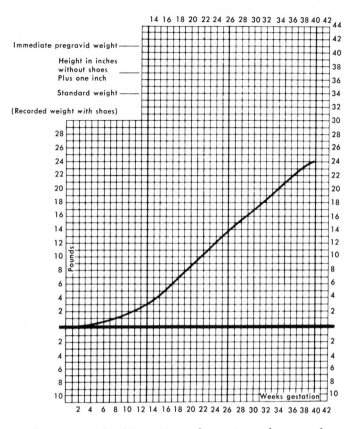

14 16 18 20 22 24 26 28 30 32 34 36 38 40 42

Immediate pregravid weight —

Height in inches
without shoes
Plus one inch —

Standard weight —

(Recorded weight *with* shoes)

Pounds

Weeks gestation

2 4 6 8 10 12 14 16 18 20 22 24 26 28 30 32 34 36 38 40 42

Fig. 7-3. Prenatal gain in weight. (From Maternal nutrition and course of pregnancy, ISBN, 0-309-01761-0, Food and Nutrition Board, National Academy of Sciences–National Research Council, Washington, D. C., 1971.)

nal mortality for many years. There has been and still is considerable controversy regarding its cause, prevention, and treatment. In the last two decades there has been increasing evidence that the type of toxemia that appears in the last trimester of pregnancy is associated with a poor nutritional (particularly low protein) intake. Some clinicians believe that malnutrition is the long-sought cause of toxemia of late pregnancy. Severe weight gain restriction, enforced weight loss through prescription of extreme, low caloric diets, limitation of sodium intake to below the "season to taste" standards, and the use of diuretics are increasingly considered to be unprofitable therapeutically and to represent even dangerous attempts at symptomatic prevention and control of this disorder. Such efforts deprive both the mother and fetus with essen-

tial nutrition and jeopardize their health and development. (See discussion of toxemia of pregnancy, pp. 143-146.)

Studies have corroborated the assertion that protein or caloric restriction below that needed physiologically for the growth of the fetus and for preparation of the maternal system in meeting the demands of pregnancy and lactation results in a smaller infant and reduction of maternal nutritional stores. Although not all big babies are healthy babies, low birth weight babies make up a disproportionate share of infant mortality. Unless the mother's prenatal and postnatal health is threatened by the known strain exerted on body systems by obesity, weight gain in itself is not detrimental and may represent only real nutritional gain or the usual increase in body fluids associated with normal pregnancy. The problem again seems to center on the quality of food intake. One woman can gain excessive weight eating "empty" calories, contributing very poor nutritional resources to herself and her child. Such a mother is a good candidate for complications such as toxemia, low birth weight, and premature deliveries. Another woman may also gain more than the norm but have a diet rich in nutrients and not suffer the same complications. Currently an average total weight gain of 10 to 12 kg. (22 to 27 pounds) is being suggested in the literature.* Some physicians have found no problems with higher gains if nutritional intake was maintained. Approximate physiological weight gain in pregnancy has been explained in the following way:

	lb.	kg.
Fetus	7.5	3.4
Placenta	1.0	.5
Amniotic fluid	2.0	.9
Uterine weight increase	2.5	1.1
Breast tissue	3.0	1.4
Blood volume	4.0	1.8
Maternal stores	4 to 8	1.8 to 3.6
Totals	24 to 28 or	10.9 to 12.7

On the average, 3 to 4 pounds are gained in the first trimester. During the remaining weeks, a weight gain of approximately a pound or less per week is considered normal (Fig. 7-3). Any sudden weight gain should be suspected as a sign of developing toxemia.

Smoking, alcohol, and other drugs

Mothers who smoke frequently bear smaller infants than do nonsmokers. In some studies late fetal and newborn mortality for infants born to cigarette smokers were significantly higher than those born to nonsmokers. Smoking may be more harmful to the unborn of women who have unfavorable obstetrical histories or socioeconomic situations.

It is interesting to note that the smaller babies of women who smoke grow faster during the 6 months following delivery than do infants of nonsmokers. This is interpreted as a response to the removal of the infant from an "inhibiting and toxic" influence in utero.* However, there is also evidence that there is a relationship between mothers who smoke excessively at home and the incidence of pneumonia and bronchitis in their babies from 6 to 9 months of age. Other possible effects, fetal or neonatal have not been sufficiently studied, but excessive smoking (more than 10 cigarettes per day) is to be discouraged. Of course, from the perspective of general maternal health, smoking is an important factor in respiratory and circulatory disease processes. Patients should be encouraged to decrease or stop the habit. The moderate use of alcohol, in itself, has not been associated with any known detrimental effects on the course of pregnancy or the health of the fetus. However, some new studies at the University of Washington indicate that severe maternal alcoholism may cause fetal malformations.†

No drug should be taken during pregnancy without the approval of the physician. Certain drugs such as corticosteriods and thalidomide are known *teratogens,* substances capable of producing fetal deformities. Others may cause hemorrhage, jaundice, neurological symptoms, and abnormal dental pigmentation. Drugs such as heroin and methadone taken during pregnancy may produce addiction in the newborn. The effects that all substances prescribed to treat illness will have on the fetus have not been determined. Then, too, effects of drugs taken during pregnancy may not become obvious in the child until years later (as the incidence of vaginal malignancy in young girls whose mothers had received diethylstilbesterol in early pregnancy to help prevent their miscarriage).

---

*American College of Obstetricians and Gynecologists: Position on nutrition and pregnancy, Chicago, Dec., 1972.

*Health consequences of smoking, Washington, D. C., Jan., 1973, Department of Health, Education, and Welfare Publication HSM 73-8704.
†Maternal alcoholism and birth defects seen related, Nurs. Care 7:34, Feb., 1974.

General hygiene

There is more to good prenatal guidance than the question of diet and smoking. The mother-to-be will undoubtedly have questions regarding many other subjects. Sometimes she wants information regarding general hygiene—the need for rest, relaxation, and exercise. Pregnant women need to conserve their resources by getting adequate rest. They may not want to actually nap in the morning and afternoon, but at least they can sit down and put their feet up! Because the bulk of the baby in later pregnancy may compress the inferior vena cava and crowd the diaphragm, resting in a flat supine position may interfere with venous blood return to the heart as well as embarrass respirations. At such a stage in pregnancy, a side-lying or Fowler's position is suggested. Walking outdoors is wonderful exercise, available to all, but often neglected. Golfing, bowling, dancing, and even swimming, when not done to the point of fatigue, are usually endorsed.

More research regarding the effects of exercise during pregnancy is needed. What sports are an asset will probably depend on the health, exercise habits, and obstetrical history of the individual. Some exercise is to be encouraged for the normal expectant mother. Curtailing the exercise of a previously active woman may be a negative factor in her physical, emotional, and mental health. Horseback riding and competitive tennis, especially singles, have been generally considered to be two sports not recommended for the usual pregnant woman until after her postpartum checkup.

Bathing. A woman is likely to perspire profusely during pregnancy, and frequent baths and showers are needed. Bathing may become a problem in late pregnancy because of the woman's awkwardness, and great care must be taken that she not fall. Some physicians recommend that tub baths not be taken during the last months for this reason and that only sponge baths be used. Some have also forbidden tub baths late in pregnancy because of the possibility of infecting the vaginal tract and uterus.

Most now consider this possibility highly unlikely.

Hair may need special attention because of the increased activity of the oil glands of the scalp. A permanent, if desired, will "take" during pregnancy.

Preparation for nursing. If the woman is planning to nurse her baby, the physician may advise certain routines to prepare her breasts for lactation. If she has inverted or flat nipples, the physician may prescribe the use of a manual breast pump or teach finger compression of the breast to draw out the nipple to make it easier for the newborn infant to grasp. He may advocate the expression of colostrum, the early breast secretion, in the last trimester of pregnancy to encourage milk production, help prevent engorgement, and toughen the nipples.

Some pregnant women, especially primigravidae, develop rather prominent pink marks called striae on the abdomen and breasts probably related to hormonal increases as well as rapid weight gain. Some people think that they are not so prominent if cocoa butter is applied to the skin. Certainly it does not hurt to use it if one does not object to the odor. These lines usually retract appreciably after pregnancy and become scarcely noticeable.

Wardrobe. Never before has a mother-to-be had an opportunity for such an attractive, versatile wardrobe as today, and since maternity patterns are also available in the fabric stores, attractive clothing need not be expensive. Maternity clothes should be lightweight, nonconstrictive, adjustable, and absorbent and should also provide a boost to the morale.

Probably more important physiologically than a cute dress or suit, however, are adequate supportive underclothes. It is especially important that the pregnant woman have good breast support to prevent fatigue and maintain a good figure. She will not be able to go through her entire pregnancy with the same size brassiere! If she plans to breast-feed her baby, nursing bras are a fine investment. A maternity corset is usually not advised. The tendency in the last few years is to counsel its use only for older multiparae if needed. Primigravidae and younger multiparae are usually told to practice certain exercises during pregnancy (especially the "pelvic rock, or tilt") that will improve posture and strengthen muscles. However, a light maternity girdle may be used with satisfaction. Specially designed garter belts are available. No constrictive round garters should be used because of interference in the blood's circulation from the legs.

If a woman has been accustomed to wearing high-heeled shoes, it will probably be difficult for her to suddenly descend to fairly flat heels. However, as pregnancy progresses and her center of gravity moves forward, she will find lower heels much less awkward and more flattering to her total silhouette. She will want to avoid shoe styles with ties or buckles, since toward the end of her 260 plus days of waiting, tying shoes will not be easy.

Dental care. The old saying "for every child a tooth" is not true. But it is a good plan for the pregnant woman to have a dental checkup during the second trimester so that plenty of time is available for any needed repairs. The gums may become swollen and exhibit a tendency to bleed in pregnancy. These symptoms are probably caused by the increase in estrogen in the body and are not necessarily related to a vitamin C deficiency. Symptoms typically recede after the eighth month. The presence of gingivitis previous to pregnancy fostered by plaque formation and malocclusion may cause the condition to become a continuing problem without care. Some women experience an annoying increase in salivation (ptyalism) in pregnancy.

Douching. Most women wonder whether they should douche or not. Normal vaginal secretions are usually intensified during pregnancy. Many physicians believe that douching should not be done routinely but only for a specific condition with a low-pressure fountain syringe, gently introduced. The individual preference of the physician concerning the specific patient should be ascertained.

Employment. Many pregnant women are employed. Whether they continue their employment and for how long depends on several factors, one of which is the type of work in which they are engaged (heavy lifting, exposure to potential hazards of radiation or chemicals, or long hours of standing without relief). The employment of pregnant women in certain occupations is often restricted by state law, policies of the individual employed (dependent on his insurance coverage, previous experience, etc.), and the health of the employee (whether she is experiencing any complications).

Recently women have been challenging disability benefit regulations and pregnancy leave rulings that require a working, expectant mother to resign her position because she has reached a certain month in her pregnancy. In 1974 the Supreme Court declared that it was unconstitutional for school boards to set an arbitrary time when women teachers must give up their jobs during pregnancy. Numerous changes in policy affecting the working pregnant woman are probably to be seen in the future.

Travel. Sometimes the question of travel presents itself. If a trip can be so arranged, it is best to travel during the middle trimester, since the expectant mother is more comfortable, the danger of abortion is not so great, and the threat of premature or unprepared-for deliveries is at a minimum. If trips must be made by car, schedules should allow for adequate rest stops and should be carefully paced. Commercial airline travel in pressurized planes is now considered as safe as other methods of transportation for this traveler. However, last minute protracted journeys close to term are to be discouraged no matter how they are made.

Marital relations

Instructions regarding sexual intercourse during pregnancy are now much more liberal than formerly. Many physicians are now allowing most couples to have sexual intercourse until full term is reached, unless the bag of waters has ruptured or discomfort is encountered. Others, believing that orgasm may initiate painful uterine contractions or premature labor, still take a more conventional approach and would limit sexual response in the last few weeks before term. If there has been a previous problem with abortion, premature birth, or bleeding during pregnancy, additional modifications in sexual life would probably be advised. Most couples find such privations stressful and may need counseling regarding alternate modes of mutual sexual gratification and other adjustments that would be helpful.

Community education resources

In many communities, classes are offered to help expectant parents prepare for the changes pregnancy and parenthood will bring. They may be sponsored by the American National Red Cross, YWCA, public health departments, adult education programs, hospitals, or groups of physicians. Participation in such approved groups is recommended, especially for primigravidae. Some classes concentrate on imparting an understanding of the basic anatomy and physiology of reproduction, what to expect during the "waiting months," what occurs during labor and delivery, how to prepare for the baby's nursery and layette, how to bathe the newborn infant, and how to prepare an artificial formula. Others emphasize exercises in training the body and mind for peak performance during pregnancy, labor, and childbirth and are usually led by a physical therapist especially interested in techniques promoting good posture, relaxation, and economy of effort (for example, the Lamaze technique, p. 123). In our opinion they are helpful to the expectant mother no matter what her preference may be regarding the use of analgesics or anesthetics.

Such informal group sessions with other couples facing similar experiences, expectations, hopes, and fears guided by competent leaders are especially helpful in assisting new prospective fathers and mothers to gain needed instruction and ego support for their changing roles.

Pregnancy and new parenthood are developmental crises for the man as well as the woman, and new self identities must be clarified and hopefully accepted. The crises may be changed or lessened when parenthood is repeated, but the sense of wonder, the expectations, and the strains recur. Adjustments are still to be made whether the child is the first or fourth. The processes of role identification are more obvious perhaps in our culture for the prospective mother. Indeed, the increasingly manifest changes in her body dramatically declare a changed status in society. Psychologists describing the focal changes during a normal woman's pregnancy usually speak of her emotional preoccupation with self, an introversion that occurs and predominates her thinking in early pregnancy. At this time, the growing baby is part of her and is yet to assume a real identity of its own. She consciously, or most often subconsciously, sorts through her feelings concerning motherhood and her early experiences with her own mother. As the pregnancy continues and her body image changes, her feelings of dependency typically grow and her focus of attention generally changes to that of the father of the child as he represents protection and continuity. Later, in the third trimester, her interest is centered on preparations for the baby, who by this time has become an unknown but acknowledged individual, and on her feelings and expectations concerning labor, delivery, and her ability to cope at that time with the demands of her body, her family, and society.

Pregnancy is normally characterized by feelings of ambivalence. One day the mother-to-be may be pleased and proud concerning her condition. The next she will be fretful and even resentful regarding the disturbance in her life that the coming baby represents. Prospective mothers and fathers need to know that these contradic-

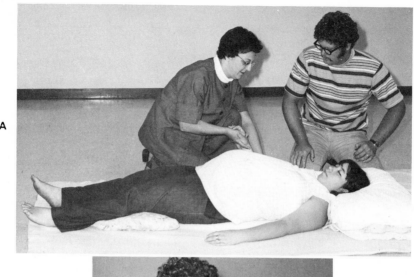

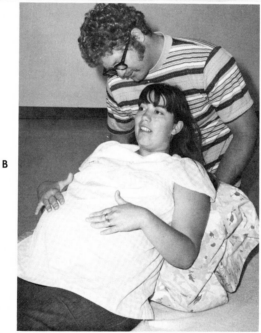

Fig. 7-4. **A,** The childbirth education instructor teaches Tom to check for muscular relaxation. **B,** Relaxation and breathing techniques such as "pant-blow" and effleurage must be practiced regularly.

tory feelings are normal. Husbands need especially to be alerted regarding the sudden mood swings and fantasies that may trouble their mates' emotional and mental equilibrium. Such knowledge will help smooth the many difficult adaptations that need to be made. Pregnancy is a developmental crisis, but it is also an opportunity for real emotional and psychological growth. Having peers and knowledgeable professional people with whom to share some of the experiences of this process is a tremendous asset.

Suggested exercises

As has been mentioned, many of the prenatal instruction groups are taught exercises to ready themselves for the demands

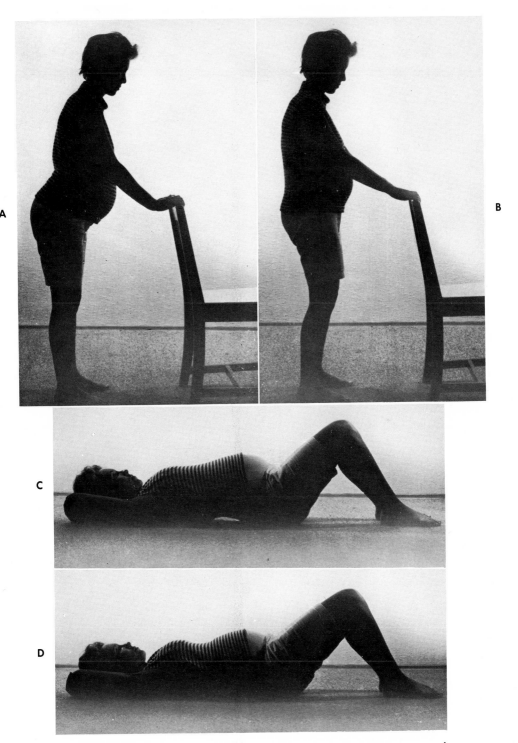

Fig. 7-5. Practice the pelvic rock standing and lying down. See posture improve!

of labor, delivery, and postpartum adjustments. The exercises will vary from group to group. Examples of four exercises that may be practiced at such sessions are included here. Modifications in breathing techniques will be found in various communities. Some classes do not teach abdominal breathing. The high chest breathing described below is now often taught, combined with slow chest breathing at the onset and end of an intense contraction in order to prevent the problems of hyperventilation. Various combinations of high chest breathing and blowing techniques are often taught for the period of transition when the cervix is nearing complete dilatation. These particular exercises are some of those described and outlined by Dr. John Seldon Miller in his very delightful and helpful *Childbirth, a Manual for Pregnancy and Delivery*. The following information is directly quoted from his instructions to the mothers-to-be:

Pelvic rock. This is the most important exercise for comfort during pregnancy. It increases the flexibility of the lower back, strengthens the abdominal muscles, and shifts your center of gravity back toward your spine. It relieves backache, improves posture, and improves your appearance in late pregnancy tremendously. It should be practiced daily as an exercise, and in addition, once learned, you should always walk and stand with the pelvis tilted forward, thus providing your baby with a cradle of bone in which to lie. Then he won't be supported by your abdominal wall nearly so much with resulting and ever increasing stretching. . . . If you will learn this, you will not need a corset to support a sagging abdominal wall and a tired back [Fig. 7-5].

First practice lying on your back, knees bent, feet flat on floor. You may put a small pillow under your head.

A. Tighten lower abdominal muscles and muscles of the buttocks. This will cause tailbone to be elevated, small of back pressed into floor. Do not lift buttocks off floor.

B. Relax abdominal and buttock muscles. As you do this, arch your back as high as you can.

C. Again tighten abdominal and buttock muscles, being sure that the small of your back presses tightly into the floor, your back becoming a straight line.

D. Do this five or six times daily. Do it before getting out of bed in the morning if your back feels stiff when you awaken.

Then practice it on your hands and knees, hands directly under the shoulders, knees under the hips.

A. Contract abdominal and buttock muscles and at the same time hump your back up as far as possible. Bend head down.

B. Slowly relax abdominal and buttock muscles and let yourself sag through the middle as you lift your head.

C. Repeat five or six times slowly.

Then practice it standing up.

A. Stand about 2 feet away from the back of a chair or other prop that is level with your hips.

B. Bend slightly forward from the hips, placing hands on chair back, elbows straight.

C. Rotate hips backward and sag with your abdominal muscles creating a real "sway back."

D. "Unlock" your knees, flexing them ever so slightly.

E. Slowly rotate hips forward, tucking buttocks under as if someone were pushing your buttocks from behind. In this position your pelvic cradle will be parallel to the floor.

F. After doing this three times, stand erect with buttocks tucked in, knees slightly flexed, arms at side, chest high. This is the ideal position for standing and walking, especially during the latter part of pregnancy. . . .

Abdominal breathing. This type of breathing utilizes the diaphragm primarily to the exclusion of the chest muscles. It is the type of breathing singers use for perfect control and will be very helpful during the first half of labor. When you breathe with your diaphragm the abdominal muscles automatically relax, thus allowing the uterus to rise during contractions without tension against the tight abdominal wall. You may practice lying down, standing or sitting.

A. Place hands on abdomen.

B. As you inhale, elevate the abdominal wall. Expand your abdomen as far as you can.

C. As you exhale, allow the abdominal muscles to go down slowly.

D. Inhalation and exhalation should be of the same length. The chest should be completely still during the abdominal breathing.

E. Work toward breathing as slowly as possible—a slow, rhythmic inhalation and exhalation.

F. As you become more adept at this type of breathing, it will require less effort for you to expand your abdomen during inhalation.

This type of breathing, together with total relaxation, will often carry you through most of the first stage of labor. When it is no longer possible or effective in keeping you comfortable, you will switch to high chest breathing. This minimizes motion of the diaphragm and abdominal muscles.

High chest breathing.

A. Place hands on lower part of rib cage.

B. Inhale and exhale completely.

C. Start rhythmic, shallow breathing at a very rapid rate, approximately 100 breaths per minute. It may be helpful to punctuate this breathing pattern, at intervals, with a deep breath and continue shallow breathing. End by inhaling and exhaling completely.

D. Practice breathing for a minute at a time. Remember, it is very important to concentrate your attention on the chest and breathing rapidly, while simultaneously maintaining a high degree of total body relaxation.

Panting. You will pant during the actual delivery of your baby, letting the uterus do the work. This will prevent you from injuring yourself and it is probably better for your baby, too. Furthermore, if the baby's head is very low during the late first stage of labor, sometimes your urge to push prematurely becomes very great. Only by panting in this circumstance can you keep from pushing. Your doctor will of course instruct you as to when it is all right to push and when it is best to pant. As simple as panting seems to be, you should practice.

A. Place hands on breastbone.

B. Open mouth, allowing jaw to hang loosely.

C. Pant, making the breastbone move up and down, Pant slowly, deeply, and rhythmically.

D. Practice for 45 seconds at a time, at least once a day.°

The layette

Provided finances are not too strained, preparing the layette for the new baby can be one of the most pleasurable duties of the expectant mother. For first timers, baby showers may also help in this regard but are not dependable. Contributors at such affairs should be told that the baby will grow, and perhaps half the group could purchase basic clothes for the 1- to 2-year old child. If the baby is not a "firstborn," then there probably will be considerable infant clothes left over from the last time. Babies usually do not wear out their clothes, but they do grow out of them.

A basic layette, at least enough to start with, consists of the following items:

°From Miller, J. S.: Childbirth, a manual for pregnancy and delivery, New York, 1963, Atheneum Publishers.

1. Six cotton shirts, short or long sleeves, depending on the weather (Stretch shirts cost more but can be worn by baby longer. Long sleeved shirts can have a fold-over cuff enclosing the hands rather than the string tie. To purchase a 3-month size is a waste of money.)

2. Four dozen cotton gauze, bird's eye or flannelette diapers if diaper service is not used; 1 dozen, if it is; or disposable diapers may be purchased.

3. Two or three plastic diaper covers, to be used only if baby does not have any skin irritation

4. Four or five long gowns, opening down the front with grip fasteners

5. Two or three sweaters with no more than 10% wool content to prevent allergic skin rash

6. Three or four soft, light receiving blankets

7. One square heavy blanket for use outdoors

8. One cap

9. Booties if it is cold

10. One bunting if in a climate requiring such protection (The tendency is to overdress rather than underdress infants.)

11. Two or three waterproof squares for protecting surfaces from baby

12. Two washclothes used just for baby

13. Six cotton sheets, two crib blankets

Basic furniture needed includes a bed (a bassinet, although pretty, is unnecessary), a firm mattress, and cover. No pillow should be used because of the danger of suffocation. Some type of chest of drawers for storage, a covered diaper pail, and a large plastic tub or, if preferred, a canvas bathinette (this, too, is a frill) will be needed. A bath tray is a great convenience, but it does not have to be expensive. Any clean tray will do. On it should be a jar of cotton balls, a jar of safety pins, a mild soap and dish, a supply of baby oil or lotion, a box of paper tissues, and perhaps baby powder. But remember, baby lotion and powder are not to be used together, and powder should be used sparingly!

Even if baby is to be nursed, there should be equipment in the home for preparing artificial feedings, if necessary. In most cases, this means six 8-ounce formula bottles, nipples, a bottle brush, a bottle sterilizer or a large pan with a lid in which the bottles will stand upright, a quart measuring cup, measuring spoons, kitchen tongs, can opener, and funnel. Do not forget that mothers can often borrow such equipment.

There are many things on the market for baby, but many of those cute eye-catching gadgets and extras require money better spent elsewhere.

What to take to the hospital

There are other things the mother should have ready before that "special date" comes due. She should consider what she will take to the hospital with her. Usually, the following list suffices:

Two nightgowns (the short type is preferred)
Robe
Slippers
Two brassieres (nursing type if breast feeding)
One sanitary belt
Toothbrush, dentifrice, brush, comb, cosmetics, and hairpins
Deodorant
Shower cap
A good book
Writing materials, stamps, birth announcements, checkbook or cash for deposit at hospital, and insurance identification if applicable

"Going home" things for baby may be brought to the hospital later.

PERSPECTIVE

The period of pregnancy is a creative, productive period in a woman's life from many points of view. It should be a happy, truly expectant interval. But how a woman reacts to the challenge of pregnancy will be, in the main, determined by her basic emotional maturity or want of it. The doc-

tor, the nurses, the clergy, and members of the community health agencies have an opportunity to help a patient mature in the understanding of herself and her role in life at this crucial time. If they help her, they are also helping the generation to come.

unit three
Suggested selected readings and references

Ademowore, A. S., Courey, N. G., and Kime, J. S.: Relationships of maternal nutrition and weight gain to newborn birthweight, Obstet. Gynecol. 39:460-464, March, 1972.

Anthony, J. E., and Benedek, T., editors: Parenthood: its psychology and psychopathology, Boston, 1970, Little, Brown and Co.

Bigelow, J., editor: Which drugs for the pregnant patient? J. Pract. Fam. Med. 8:54-66, March, 1974.

Bing, E. D.: Six practical lessons for an easier childbirth, New York, 1967, Grosset & Dunlap, Inc.

Brewer, T. H.: Human maternal-fetal nutrition, Obstet. Gynecol. 40:868-870, Dec., 1972.

Cahill, I. D.: The mother from the slum neighborhood, Columbus, Ohio, 1964, Ross Laboratories.

Chabon, I.: Awake and aware: participation in childbirth through prophylaxis, New York, 1966, The Delacorte Press.

Chez, R. A.: Prenatal care: "first, do no harm," Contemp. OB/GYN 1:9-11, Feb., 1973.

Chez, R. A., and others: The effects of drugs on the fetus, Contemp. OB/GYN 2:103-120, March, 1974.

Claypool, J., and Ferris, P.: Students' experience and the prenatal care of high-risk pregnant women, J. Nurs. Ed. 12:7-14, Nov., 1973.

Colman, A. D., and Colman, L. L.: Pregnancy: the phychological experience, New York, 1971, Herder and Herder, Inc.

Colman, A. D., and Colman, L. L.: Pregnancy as an altered state of consciousness, Birth and Fam. J. 1:7-11, Winter, 1973-74.

Dickinson-Belskie: Birth atlas, ed. 5, New York, 1968, Maternity Center Association.

Downs, F. S.: Maternal stress in primigravidas as a factor in the production of neonatal pathology, Nurs. Science 2:348, Oct., 1964.

Druckemiller, S. D.: Order out of chaos, Am. J. Nurs. 71:109-113, Jan., 1971.

Eastman, N. J., and Russell, K. P.: Expectant motherhood, ed. 5, revised, 1970, Boston, Little, Brown and Co.

Edwards, J.: Patient-oriented maternity nursing, Hosp. Top. 48:83, March, 1970.

Edwards, M.: Teaching the young and the poor, Birth and Fam. J. 1:6-10, Spring, 1974.

The effects of drugs on the fetus, Contemp. OB/GYN 2:103-120, Sept., 1973.

Ferguson-Smith: Prenatal diagnosis: new developments, Med. World News 14:70-71, Dec., 1973.

Fitzpatrick, E. E., Reeder, S. R., and Mastrianni, L.: Maternity nursing, ed. 12, Philadelphia, 1971, J. B. Lippincott Co.

Fleischman, A. R., and Chez, R. A.: Communicating with the patient for optimal perinatal care, Contemp. OB/GYN 2:91-93, April, 1974.

Gardiner, S. H.: Current needs in the delivery of OB/GYN care, J. Obstet. Gynecol. Neonatal Nurs. 1:12-13, Nov.-Dec., 1972.

Garnet, J. D.: Pregnancy in women with diabetes, Am. J. Nurs. 69:1900-1902, Sept., 1969.

Gibbs, C. E.: Rubella immunization in women: test before shooting, Am. Fam. Physician 8:145-147, Sept., 1973.

Golbus, M.: The prenatal diagnosis of genetic defects, Birth and Fam. J. 1:3-6, Winter, 1973-74.

Goodheart, B.: Sex in the schools: education or titillation? Today's Health 48:28+, Feb., 1970.

Goodlin, R. C., Keller, D. W., and Raffin, M.: Orgasm during late pregnancy, Obstet. Gynecol. 38:916-920, Dec., 1971.

Goodwin, B.: Psychoprophylaxis in childbirth. In Duffey, M., and others, editors: Current concepts in clinical nursing, vol. 3, St. Louis, 1971, The C. V. Mosby Co.

Greenhalf, J. O.: Constipation during pregnancy, Contemp. OB/GYN 2:29-31, Aug., 1973.

Gudpaille, W. J.: Is there a "too soon," Today's Health 48:34+, Feb., 1970.

Haynes, D. M.: Dental care and the pregnant patient, Contemp. OB/GYN 2:63-65, Aug., 1973.

The health consequences of smoking, Department of Health, Education and Welfare, Publication No. HSN 73-8704, Jan., 1973.

Henderson, P. A., and Henderson, V. M.: Teamwork in maternity and infant care projects, Obstet Gynecol. 39:401-406, March, 1972.

Hendrick, W.: An elderly primigravida takes a "refresher course" in obstetrics, Am. J. Nurs. 70:787, April, 1970.

Hennel, M.: Family-centered maternity nursing in practice, Nurs. Clin. North Am. 3:289, June, 1968.

Hobbins, J. C.: Sports during pregnancy, Contemp. OB/GYN 3:36-38, April, 1974.

Hungerford, M. S.: Childbirth education, Springfield, Ill., 1972, Charles C Thomas, Publisher.

Jordon, A. D.: Evaluation of a family-centered maternity care hospital program, J. Obstet. Gynecol. Neontal Nurs. 2:13-35, Jan.-Feb., 1973; 2:15-27, March-April, 1973; 2:15-22, May-June, 1973.

Kaminetzky, H. A., Newton, M., and Pritchard, J. A.: Maternal nutrition, Obstet. Gynecol. 40:773-785, Dec., 1972.

Karmel, M.: Thank you, Dr. Lamaze, Philadelphia, 1959, J. B. Lippincott Co.

Kitay, D. Z.: Assessing anemia in the pregnant patient, Contemp. OB/GYN 2:17-24, Oct., 1973.

Krugman, S., and Ward, R.: Infectious diseases of children and adults, ed. 5, St. Louis, 1973, The C. V. Mosby Co., pp. 236-253.

Lang, D. M.: Providing maternity care through a nurse-midwifery service program, Nurs. Clin. North Am. 4:509, Sept., 1969.

Larsen, G. L.: What every nurse should know about congenital syphilis, Nurs. Outlook 13:52, March, 1965.

Larson, V. L.: Stresses of the childbearing year, Am. J. Public Health 56:32, Jan., 1966.

Leppert, P., and Williams, B.: Birth films may miscarry, Am. J. Nurs. 68:2181, Oct., 1968.

Lerch, C.: Maternity nursing, ed. 2, St. Louis, 1974, The C. V. Mosby Co.

Lesser, A. J.: Progress in maternal and child health, Children Today 1:7-12, March-April, 1972.

Lubic, R. W.: What the lay person expects of maternity care: are we meeting these expectations, J. Obstet. Gynecol. Neonatal Nurs. 1:25-31, June, 1972.

Malnutrition, learning and behavior, Dairy Council Digest 44:31-36, Nov.-Dec., 1973.

Maternal alcoholism and birth defects seen related, Nurs. Care 7:34, Feb., 1974.

Maternity Center Association: A baby is born, ed. 2, New York, 1960, The Association.

Michaelson, M.: In search of sanity: man in the middle, Today's Health 48:31+, Feb., 1970.

Miller, J. S.: Childbirth, a manual for pregnancy and delivery, New York, 1963, Atheneum Publishers.

Montagu, A.: Life before birth, New York, 1964, The New American Library, Inc.

Moore, B. M.: Education for family living—what is it? Nurs. Clin. North Am. 4:359, June, 1969.

Moore, M. L.: The mother's changing needs, Briefs 32:79, May, 1968.

Moore, M. L.: The clay eaters, RN 33:44, Aug., 1970.

Nitowsky, H. M.: Prenatal diagnosis of genetic abnormality, Am. J. Nurs. 71:1551-1557, Aug., 1971.

O'Connell, E.: Hospital maternity nursing—then and now. In Bergersen, B. S., and others, editors: Current concepts in clinical nursing, vol. 2, St. Louis, 1969, The C. V. Mosby Co.

Pregnancy, aspirin, and the baby, Med. World News 15:16-17, April 5, 1974.

Preparation for childbearing, ed. 4, New York, 1972, Maternity Center Association, pp. 5-28.

Rosso, P.: Nutrition and abnormal fetal growth, Contemp. OB/GYN 2:53-54, Sept., 1973.

Rubin, R.: Cognitive style in pregnancy, Am. J. Nurs. 70:502-508, March, 1970.

Seacat, M., and Schlachter, L.: Expanded nursing role in prenatal and infant care, Am. J. Nurs. **68**:222, April, 1968.

Shank, R. E.: A chink in our armour, Nutr. Today **5**:2, Summer, 1970.

Slatin, M.: Why mothers bypass prenatal care, Am. J. Nurs. **71**:1388-1389, July, 1971.

Stone, A. R.: Cues to interpersonal distress due to pregnancy, Am. J. Nurs. **65**:88-91, Nov., 1965.

Walker, L.: Providing more relevant maternity services, J. Obstet. Gynecol. Neonatal Nurs. **3**:34-36, March-April, 1974.

When a mother smokes during pregnancy, will it affect her baby? Clin. Prediatr. **13**:485-486, June, 1974.

Williams, S. R.: Nutrition and diet therapy, St. Louis, 1973, The C. V. Mosby Co.

8

Presentations, positions, and progress

The relationship of the fetus to the obstetrical passageway is of great interest to both doctor and nurse. It will usually influence the length of labor, the preparation of the delivery room, and the type of complications possibly encountered.

Some common words are used in special ways to describe this relationship. For instance, in obstetrics one refers to the following terms: presentation, attitude, position, station, engagement, effacement, and show.

Presentation

The *presentation,* or *lie,* means the relationship of the length of the fetus to the length of the uterus. If the fetus is lying so that either the head, buttocks, or feet may be found just above or within the true pelvis, its presentation may be called longitudinal. If, instead, the body lies crosswise in the uterus, the term "transverse lie" may be used. A baby in transverse lie cannot be delivered vaginally without manipulation to a longitudinal presentation. At present, he may be delivered abdominally, since fetal manipulation or version is not always preferred or practiced with the increasing safety of the so-called cesarean section. Many times the term "presentation" is used synonymously with the phrase *presenting part,* that part of the baby which is coming through or attempting to come through the pelvic canal first. Headfirst placement is referred to as a cephalic presentation. Feet or buttocks first is termed "breech." Ap-

proximately 96% of all deliveries are headfirst, or cephalic. About 3.5% are breech. Transverse presentations account for the remaining percentage. Presentation may be determined by abdominal palpation and rectal, vaginal, ultrasonic, or x-ray examinations.

Attitude

The *attitude* refers to the degree of flexion of the body, head (Fig. 8-1), and extremities. The normal attitude is complete flexion. A well-flexed head presents the smallest cephalic diameter and fewer mechanical problems in descent and delivery. This "chin-on-chest" posture makes possible the *vertex* delivery so desired.

Position (Figs. 8-3 to 8-5)

The *position* technically is the relationship between a predetermined "point of reference or direction" on the presenting part of the fetus to the pelvic quadrants *of the mother.* It gives more detailed information about the fetus's progress as the presenting part seeks to adapt to the shape and size of the various parts of the pelvic birth canal. The maternal pelvic quadrants are identified as right and left posterior and right and left anterior (Fig. 8-2). They never change location, although the different perspectives from which they are viewed in illustrations and diagrams sometimes confuse the student. Sometimes the quadrants are seen from "below," that is, as they appear to the physician in front of

69

the delivery table ready to receive the baby. Sometimes they are viewed from "above," from the vantage point of the unborn child entering the true pelvis. In some other diagrams, students miraculously look directly through the abdominal wall to view the fetus within the canal. The point of reference, of course, will vary according to the presenting part discussed and the amount of flexion present. In the event of a well-flexed cephalic or vertex presentation the point of reference employed is the occipital bone, or occiput. It is the most accessible bone to identify in rectal or vaginal examination. The vault of the fetal skull is made up of three paired bones and one single bone separated by tough but softer membranous seams, or sutures. It is fairly easy to follow these sutures with a gloved finger after sufficient cervical dila-

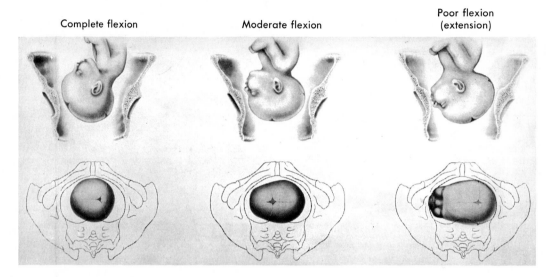

Fig. 8-1. Head diameters in various degrees of flexion. (From Phenomena of normal labor, Columbus, Ohio, 1964, Ross Laboratories, Publisher.)

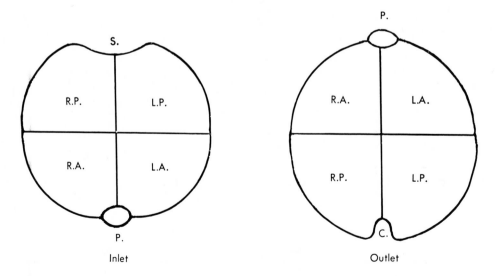

Fig. 8-2. Maternal pelvic quadrants stay the same; however, the student's perspective may change! *C,* Coccyx; *P,* pubic bone; *S,* sacrum.

tation has occurred and to determine the placement of the occiput. The sutures trace a Y, and the occiput is found between the top shafts of the Y just in back of the triangular posterior fontanel (Fig. 8-3).

To simplify reference to the various positions possible, the descriptive phrase usually begins with either right or left followed by the point of reference used and the adjectives anterior, posterior, or transverse. Thus we refer to the most common vertex position as "left occiput anterior" or, shortcutting further, L.O.A. Each presenting part has the possibility of eight positions following the same pattern. Only the middle initial or code letters representing the point of reference need be changed. For example:

1. Right occiput* anterior   R.O.A.
2. Left occiput anterior   L.O.A.
3. Right occiput posterior   R.O.P.
4. Left occiput posterior   L.O.P.
5. Right occiput transverse   R.O.T.

*Sometimes the combining form "occipito" is used instead of the noun occiput.

6. Left occiput transverse   L.O.T.
7. Occiput at sacrum   O.S.
   Occiput posterior   O.P.
8. Occiput at the pubis ⎱
   Occiput anterior   ⎰   O.A.

Note that a transverse position is *not* the same thing as a transverse presentation, or lie. The letter "O" is usually employed only in the case of well-flexed or median vertex presentations (military). In the rare cases of cephalic presentations demonstrating more deflexion, other points of reference must be sought, since the occiput is no longer available or meaningful to the examiner. In a brow presentation, the letter "F" for fronto is used, referring to the area of the anterior fontanel. Brow presentations are usually slow and difficult because of the increased diameter of the skull trying to force its way through the passageway. A cesarean section may be the procedure of choice. In cases of full extension of the head, resulting in a face presentation, the letter "M" for mentum, or chin, is seen. Face presentations, although slow, usually

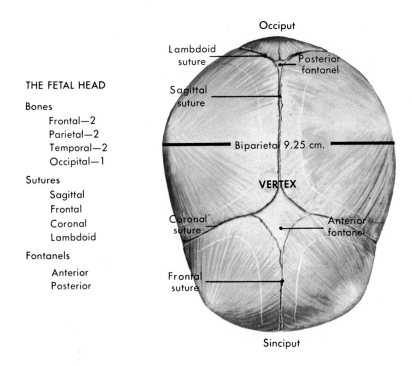

THE FETAL HEAD

Bones
    Frontal—2
    Parietal—2
    Temporal—2
    Occipital—1

Sutures
    Sagittal
    Frontal
    Coronal
    Lambdoid

Fontanels
    Anterior
    Posterior

Fig. 8-3. Fetal head—physician's map. (From Phenomena of normal labor, Columbus, Ohio, 1964, Ross Laboratories, Publisher.)

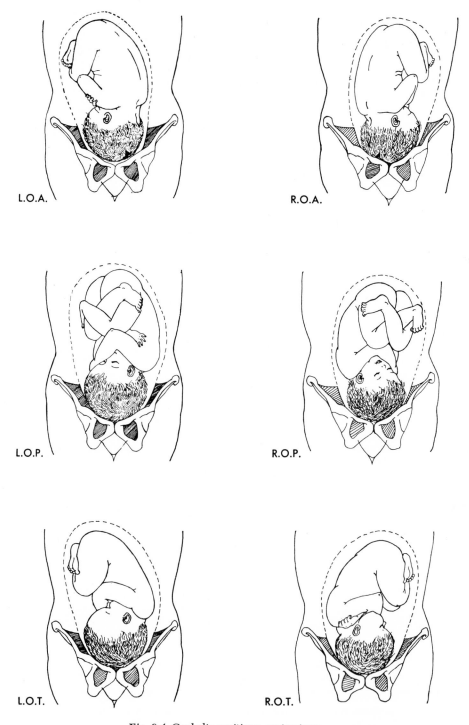

Fig. 8-4. Cephalic positions—vertex type.

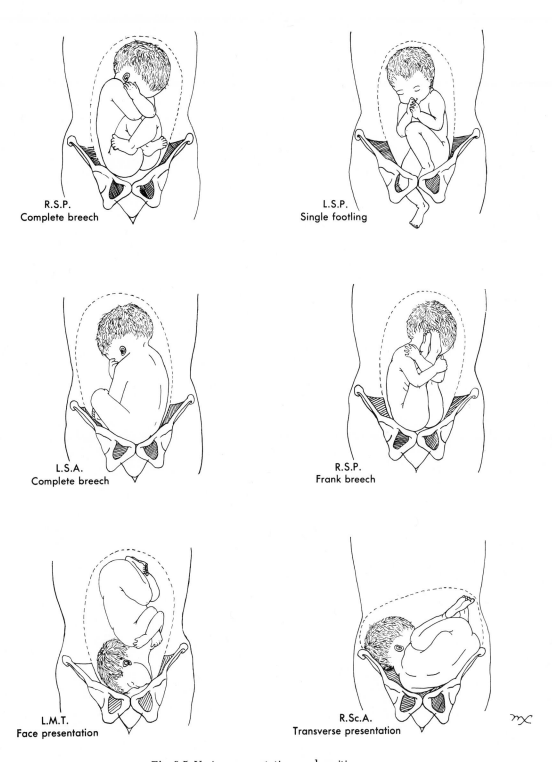

Fig. 8-5. Various presentations and positions.

terminate satisfactorily without intervention. The nursery nurse, however, will probably admit to her area a small person whose remarkable but temporary facial edema and distortion proclaim to all the staff his unorthodox entry into our world.

Breech presentations employ the sacrum or coccyx as a point of reference and the code letter "S." Characteristically, three types are described. A *complete* or *full* breech involves the flexion of the infant's legs usually tailor fashion so that the buttocks and feet appear at the vaginal opening almost simultaneously. A *frank* or *single* breech is said to occur when the thighs are flexed on the abdomen with the extended legs against the trunk and the feet against the face (sort of a foot-in-mouth posture). The term *incomplete* breech may indicate the initial appearance of either the feet or knees. The presentation of one or both feet is labeled a *single* and *double* footling respectively. Frank breech is the most commonly encountered. Breech birth is associated with a higher perinatal mortality (approximately 12%). See discussion on p. 116.

A transverse lie, sometimes called a shoulder presentation, usually employs the scapula or its upper tip, the acromion, for reference, and "Sc" or "A" is the code. The baby lying crosswise in the uterus may be positioned with his back toward the front or back of his mother. The baby's scapula, posteriorly located, indicates the position of his back. Sometimes the terms dorsoanterior or dorsoposterior may be used to clarify this. A fetus whose shoulder and head occupy the right side of the mother's pelvis and whose back is toward her front may be said to be in the right acromiodorsoanterior position, or R.A.D.A. This is an impossible presentation for normal delivery.

Station and engagement

Of course, another measurement related to the location of the fetus in the passageway is *station*. One may recall that station may be defined as the relationship of the presenting part to the ischial spines of the pelvis. When the presenting part is at the level of the spines, it is usually considered engaged, and the station is said to be 0. If the presentation is above the spines, it is usually considered high, and the station is said to be -1, -2, etc., an estimate of its location in terms of centimeters above the ischial spines. If the presenting part is below the ischial spines, we code the station as $+1$, $+2$, etc., again making the estimate in centimeters. A centimeter is a little less than ½ inch. A plus station is considered low (Fig. 8-6).

Effacement and dilatation

One should not forget that the power accomplishing the shortening and thinning (effacement) and dilatation of the cervix to an opening approximately 10 cm. (or about 4 inches) in diameter is provided by the intermittent but increasingly frequent and progressively stronger uterine contractions. It should be noted that effacement may occur rather "silently" as the result of unobtrusive contractions before the onset of more definitive, vigorous labor. This early effacement of the cervical canal is typical of the woman having her first baby. Limited cervical dilatation (approximately 1 to 3 cm.) may also take place before the onset of the "formal" labor period.

Show

Dilatation of the cervix is usually accompanied by what is called *show*. During pregnancy, the mucus-producing glands of the cervix have formed a mucoid deposit in the cervical canal that helps protect the interior of the uterus from the introduction of infection. When the cervix begins to dilate, this mucoid material is discharged. As the cervix continues to dilate, small capillaries in the cervix break and stain the mucus with blood. The faster the cervix dilates and the closer it is to complete dilatation, the more abundant and red will be the "show." However, it should not assume the proportions or characteristics of frank bleeding.

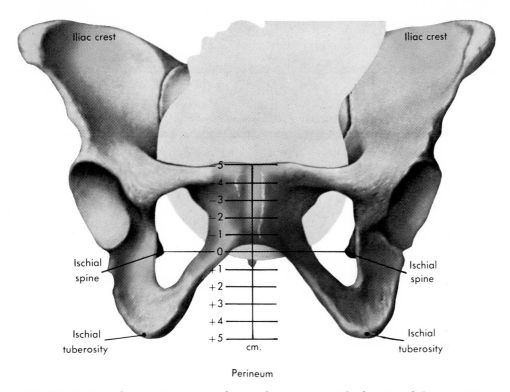

Fig. 8-6. Stations of presenting part, or degree of engagement. The location of the presenting part in relation to the level of the ischial spines is designated *station* and indicates the degree of advancement of the presenting part through the pelvis. Stations are expressed in centimeters above *(minus)* and below *(plus)* the level of the ischial spines *(zero)*. The head is usually engaged when it reaches the level of the ischial spines. (From Phenomena of normal labor, Columbus, Ohio, 1964, Ross Laboratories, Publisher.)

After complete dilatation is accomplished, then both abdominal and uterine muscles contract to push the fetus to the exterior. The mother has no control over the contractions of her uterus; they are under involuntary control. However, once dilatation is complete, she may aid immensely by pushing with her abdominal muscles when her uterus contracts to help make the fetus descend in the pelvic canal.

Thus to help determine the progress of the passenger, the physician is interested in the *presentation,* the body part that is trying to come first; the *position,* the relationship of the presenting part to the pelvic quadrants; and the *station,* the depth of the presenting part in the pelvic canal. If he knows these things plus the relative size of the pelvis and fetus, the condition of the soft tissue uterine exit called the cervix, and

the quality and frequency of the uterine contractions providing the power, he has a good basis for his evaluation of the progress of the labor and the mechanisms involved.

MECHANISM OF LABOR

Textbooks usually speak of the cardinal movements in the mechanism of labor. In the vertex delivery they usually include the following: descent, flexion, engagement, internal rotation, extension, external rotation, and expulsion. The first *four* movements are not necessarily in order, since flexion may be present before descent and increase thereafter. Descent and internal rotation will also continue after engagement. These mechanisms may occur concurrently and defy a 1-2-3 order (Fig. 8-7).

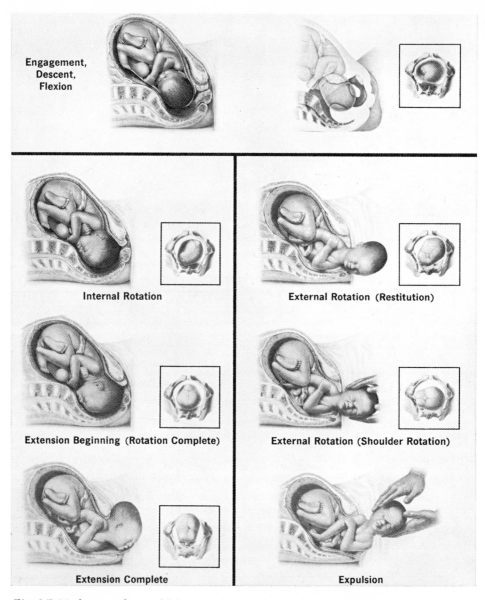

Fig. 8-7. Mechanism of normal labor, L.O.A. position. (From Nursing education aid, No. 13, Columbus, Ohio, 1964, Ross Laboratories, Publisher.)

Descent, flexion, and engagement

In the case of a primipara,* a woman bearing her first baby, *descent* of the fetus into the true pelvis usually occurs about 2 weeks before the actual birth of the child. This descent is referred to as *lightening* and results in *engagement*, or passage of the largest diameter of the presenting part into the pelvic canal. Lay people remark about this change in fetal location by the phrase "the baby has dropped." The expectant mother, with less pressure on her dia-

---

*The words "primipara" and "multipara" in this section are used from the delivery-labor room perspective. More correct would be the terms "primigravida" and "primipara," but these are seldom employed in areas where we have worked.

phragm, happily finds that she can breathe more freely. The increased tilt and lowered location of the fetus produce a characteristic change in the maternal silhouette. In the case of a multipara, a woman who has borne one or more children, descent and engagement may not occur until actual dilatation of the neck of the uterus, or cervix, begins.

Internal rotation

The amount of *internal rotation* necessary will depend on the position of the fetus and the way the head rotates to accommodate itself to the changing diameters of the pelvis. The most common rotation is that which involves the turning of the head to occiput anterior position. If the fetus begins its descent in L.O.T. or L.O.A. position, this rotation represents only a short distance of 45 to 90 degrees. If however, the internal rotation involves moving from a posterior position, it may mean a turn of 135 degrees. For this reason posterior positions usually entail a longer labor and more lower back discomfort for the mother, who will usually appreciate a nurse's firm, cool, intermittent sacral support. Occasionally, instead of rotating to an anterior position the occiput turns to the sacrum, and the child is born in O.S. position. This mode of delivery is usually slower and more dangerous to the maternal tissues. More often, the occiput will complete the longer rotation from the posterior position to the pubis. Sometimes the occiput lingers unduly in the posterior position or stops its rotation in transverse. The former situation is called "persistent posterior" and the latter a "transverse arrest." This can occur at almost any station or depth in the pelvic canal and may necessitate manual rotation or the use of rotation forceps by the obstetrician.

Extension

In a vertex delivery the head is delivered by *extension*. During descent it is normally forced into a flexed attitude by the pressure of the cervix, pelvic walls and floor. Once the occiput has rotated to anterior position and occupies the pubic arch, the head cannot make any further progress unless extension is accomplished. Because of this extension plus the natural curve of the lower pelvis, the head is born pushing upward out of the vaginal canal. The rate of extension is gently controlled by the doctor. If the bag of waters (membranes) has not previously broken during labor, it must be artificially broken now by the doctor to avoid aspiration of amniotic fluid. To prevent uncontrolled tearing of the perineum, an episiotomy, or surgical incision extending the soft tissue vaginal opening, may be executed by the doctor just before the birth of the head.

External rotation (restitution, shoulder rotation) and expulsion

When the perineum slides over the chin of the baby and temporarily only the neck occupies the outlet, more room is available to the infant for head movement. Usually without coaxing by the physician, the back of the baby's head will then turn to line up with his back, revealing the baby's position just before internal rotation of the head took place. This movement is called *restitution.* The turning movement of the head usually continues and influences the location of the back, helping to line up the unborn shoulders just beneath the pubis in anteroposterior position. This process of alignment is called *shoulder rotation.* Usually the top of the anterior shoulder is next seen just under the pubis—generally aided by the physician, who may exert gentle but firm downward traction on the head. Then the head is gently raised to clear the posterior shoulder, and the entire body follows without any particular difficulty. *Expulsion* of the infant is accomplished.

THE THREE STAGES OF LABOR

Labor is classically divided into three stages:

1. Stage one begins with the onset of regular, definitive labor contractions, which begin the effacement and dila-

Table 8-1. Stages of labor

	First stage	Second stage	Third stage
Primipara	8 to 20 hours	30 minutes to 2 hours	5 to 20 minutes (usually aided by oxytocics or manual pressure)
Multipara	3 to 8 hours	20 minutes to 1½ hours	5 to 20 minutes (usually aided by oxytocics or manual pressure)

stage *longest*

tation of the cervix and ends when dilatation is complete—10 cm.

2. Stage two begins with complete dilatation of the cervix and ends with the birth of the baby. *Expulsion*

3. Stage three begins with the birth of the baby and ends with the expulsion of the afterbirth, or placenta and membranes.

Approximate relationships

A wise nurse or doctor makes no specific predictions regarding the length of the stages of labor. However, Table 8-1 may be of some aid in estimating possible time intervals. Labor lengths for both primiparae and multiparae have decreased in the last generation. A graph called the Friedman Labor Curve, which relates the progress of cervical dilatation to duration of labor, indicates 12 hours as the average "primip" first stage of labor and about 7 hours as the average "multip" first stage of labor. A labor *without letup* lasting more than 24 hours is usually considered extended. The mother and baby must be evaluated carefully for exhaustion or distress.

Third stage: special considerations

The third stage of labor is characterized by the separation of the placenta and its expulsion.

Placental separation. Separation of the placenta from the uterine wall is accomplished by the contraction of the uterus. The site of the placental attachment suddenly becomes reduced, but the placenta itself remains the same size, causing a separation of the two structures. The placenta slides down into the lower portion of the uterus and vagina. The physician watches for signs of placental separation, which include the following:

1. The rise of the uterus to the umbilicus or above—pushed up by the bulky placenta in the vagina

2. The increased firmness and rounded shape of the fundus

3. The lengthening of the exposed umbilical cord at the exterior as the placenta descends

4. The sudden appearance of moderate temporary vaginal bleeding originating from the site of the placental attachment at the time of separation

Placental expulsion. After the placenta is separated it may be pushed out by the mother as uterine contractions resume, and she is again instructed to "bear down," or, more commonly, she is assisted by the physician who carefully exerts abdominal pressure on the fundus from above, causing the placenta's expulsion. At times the physician may elect to help deliver the placenta through cautious intravaginal, intrauterine, or abdominal maneuvers. Manual extraction may be a necessity in cases of abnormally retained placenta or excessive uterine bleeding. Some physicians routinely carry out manual palpation of the uterine cavity after the delivery of the placenta in an effort to make sure that it is normal and empty. Visual inspection of the cervix is part of the usual follow-up. The expelled placenta is checked for abnormality and completeness.

The third stage of labor and those hours immediately following are probably the most dangerous for the mother because it is during this time that hemorrhages most often occur. In an effort to speed the separation of the placenta and lessen blood loss, oxytocics, medications that help contract the uterus, are often employed in the delivery room. The medications used will depend on the time during the delivery sequence that their action is desired, the condition of the patient, the anesthesia used, and the personal preferences of the attending physician.

The satisfactory completion of the mechanism of labor and delivery as seen in all three stages is cause for congratulation. However, the whole drama of birth and adjustment is not completed—only Act I.

9

Labor and delivery

Normally, the onset of labor is the anticipated climax of 9 months of very constructive waiting. Under normal conditions each day has better prepared the fetus to make the transition from intrauterine to extrauterine existence smoothly, without undue strain. As the time of labor and delivery approaches, the mother should be alerted to certain "get set" signs, and she should be instructed when to call the physician and come to the hospital.

SIGNS OF IMPENDING LABOR

Several signs and symptoms usually precede the onset of true labor—the opening of the cervix and expulsion of the baby and placenta. These hints of things to come are usually welcome. At the end of a full-term pregnancy the mother is quite willing to relinquish her lively and bulky boarder; however, she also has feelings of anxiety as she considers the actual period of labor and delivery.

Lightening. In a woman bearing her first infant, usually about 2 weeks before delivery a relative change in fetal location may be suddenly apparent. As the fetus "drops" into the true pelvis (a process called *lightening*) and the presenting part "becomes engaged" (the largest diameter of the presenting part passes the pelvic brim), she finds herself able to breathe more freely with less pressure on the diaphragm. Doctors expect primigravidae (women pregnant for the first time) to experience lightening and engagement before true labor begins. If it does not occur, the possibility of too small a pelvic inlet or too large a presenting part (fetal-pelvic disproportion) may be considered. Women who have borne children previously may not undergo

lightening until just before or during true labor.

Frequent urination. The woman may also find, alas, greater pressure on her bladder and may be troubled with *frequent urination.*

Energy. Many women experience a phenomenal "burst of energy" just before going into labor and want to clean the whole house. They should be advised to resist the impulse.

Uterine contractions. The uterus contracts and relaxes intermittently all during pregnancy, but its contractions are usually mild and not detected by the mother-to-be. However, in the last few weeks of waiting, these uterine contractions may become quite annoying, and contrary to what some texts declare, may be painful. The most discouraging aspect about these contractions of late pregnancy is that they are often only a rehearsal for the real thing. They do not serve to dilate the cervix and, therefore, are called false labor, or Braxton Hicks' contractions, after the British obstetrician who described them. Characteristics of false labor contrasted with true labor contractions include the following:

1. The duration of the contraction remains about the same, not becoming appreciably longer or more intensive as do true contractions.
2. The period between contractions remains quite long and irregular. True contractions are regular, with a gradually decreasing interval.
3. Pressure or pain is felt primarily in the abdomen rather than in the small of the back.
4. Walking can be tolerated during the contraction. In fact, walking may help

relieve discomfort, whereas true labor contractions may be intensified by ambulation.

5. Show, or the appearance of a mucoid vaginal discharge tinged with blood, is absent in false labor but is usually present in true labor.
6. On rectal or vaginal examination the cervix is usually found to be long and closed in false labor but is effacing or dilating in true labor.

An expectant mother should be counseled to contact her physician about the onset of labor if (1) contractions are regular, becoming increasingly frequent and intensive; (2) show is present; or (3) the bag of waters, or membranes, ruptures.

THE TRIP TO THE HOSPITAL

When the woman is instructed to go to the hospital depends on her reported progress, the distance she must travel, how many babies she has had, and the history of her previous labors. Usually, physicians want all their patients to be admitted as soon as the bag of waters ruptures or show appears. If these signs are absent, admission is advised when the contractions of primigravidae are regular at about 7-minute intervals. In the case of mothers who previously have had one baby or more, physicians usually want them hospitalized when contractions have achieved some regularity, but they do not wait until a certain frequency is reached. Women who have previously experienced a full-term normal delivery usually deliver more rapidly than those who have not. They are not encouraged to wait at home too long. If the onset of labor is suspected, the prospective mother should eat nothing and limit her intake of fluids until evaluated by the doctor to prevent possible aspiration at the time of delivery.

It is hoped that the ride to the hospital will not turn into a race or be complicated with too many obstacles. Certainly, it is best to be able to be admitted without rush and confusion. Detailed planning for the journey should be made. The patient should

be told by her physician or his office nurse before her entry what the admission procedures involve so that she may be more prepared for what will transpire.

HOSPITAL ADMISSION

Admission directly to the labor room unit with a minimum of front office procedure is desirable. Usually only one signature is needed, that of the patient herself, for permission to perform the routine procedures necessary during labor and delivery. "Routine procedures" do not include a cesarean section. The husband or other accompanying family member may help complete any other office admittance procedure needed while the patient is being cared for in the labor room area. Answers to study questionnaires indicate that a number of prospective fathers resent being sent to the admission desk to complete lengthy forms at a time when they feel that they can be supportive to their wives. Preadmission arrangements to obtain as much information as possible regarding the physical, mental, and social status of the patient and the expectations and desires of the parents, as they may affect their labor delivery experiences, are to be encouraged. If brief information sheets could be filled out before admission by the patient and the clinic or office personnel and forwarded with the current prenatal record close to term, it would seem that the individual needs and preferences of the patient and her family might be better understood and considered. The so-called assembly line maternity care of many hospitals has caused some patients to feel more like objects than human beings. A few have so resented or feared hospitalization experiences that they seek alternatives to a hospital delivery.

All women harbor anxiety regarding their hospital experience. Some patients are very nervous and fearful. The nursing staff should do everything in its power to alleviate this anxiety and make the patient feel welcome and secure. A gracious welcome to the patient and her accompanying family makes a lasting impression. Unfortunately, so does a rude, thoughtless, or disorganized admission experience. The patient does not want to hear about the current problems of the maternity service, past obstetrical experiences of former patients, or the personal histories of her attending nurse. Such recitals are indiscreet, impolite, and worrisome to the patient and her family. The members of the immediate family should be shown a place where they can comfortably wait during the completion of the admission procedures. Ideally, this would include provision for a public telephone, magazines, perhaps a small, automatic coin-operated canteen for refreshments, and a television set. Once the admission is completed, most hospitals encourage visitation of the patient by her immediate family during labor. However, most limit this contact to one person at the bedside at one time.

Role of vocational or practical nurse

The trained vocational nurse, as a part of the maternity staff, can make a real contribution to the well-being of the patient and her family. Under the supervision of an experienced registered nurse, she can render valuable assistance to the department and the patient. We believe that the use of the prepared licensed vocational nurse (LVN or LPN) in nonsupervisory capacities in this department is legitimate and desirable but that it is a misuse of personnel to expect her to assume the role of a charge nurse or, on the other hand, to delegate to her only those duties that can be accomplished by workers with less training.

The vocational nurse can provide valuable assistance in the admittance of the patient to the labor-delivery suite. After the patient arrives at the hosiptal, she is usually taken by wheelchair to the labor room area. The nurse helps the patient remove her clothes and put on a hospital gown and encourages the return of her clothes to her home. She makes special note of valuables, such as watches and eyeglasses. If the bag of waters has ruptured, the patient should

not be allowed up. As soon as possible the patient is properly identified, preferably by use of a banding technique. If such a technique is used, the band should be carefully checked with the patient, who is initially asked, "What is your name?" The nurse asks the name of the attending physician and secures the patient's prenatal record if one is present at the hospital. With the supervising registered nurse, she may read the record to determine as much as possible about this patient before continuing with the admission. Important factors to check are (1) the obstetrical history—number of viable births she has had, previous difficulties, the rapidity of former labors, and Rh status; (2) the record of the current pregnancy—serology result, the expected date of confinement, and any known allergies; (3) plans for the labor and delivery—type of anesthesia, if desired, whether she has attended childbirth education classes, accommodations preferred, method selected for feeding the infant, and name of the doctor to care for the baby; and (4) marital status and, if it is questionable, plans for the baby, which should be determined with the utmost tact and discretion by one staff member only so that the patient need not be troubled by needless repetition of questions. Some of the necessary admission information will, by its very nature, be absent from the prenatal record. The admitting nurse must inquire when the contractions (if any) began, if any show has been noted, and if the bag of waters is known to have broken. The staff should know if the patient has recently eaten. In some maternity services a voided urine specimen is routinely obtained for urinalysis at the time of admission. In others, a specimen is secured on admission only if prenatal history prompts the physician to order it. A specimen may be obtained by catheterization just prior to delivery. Some maternity services include weighing the patient in their admission procedure. Although most of the time a call will have previously been received from the attending physician regarding the admission, in some situations the nurse may want to know if the patient has contacted the doctor and if she has been examined by him. She will take the patient's temperature, pulse, and respiration. She will determine the blood pressure, in the absence of a contraction, and time the duration, interval, and intensity of her contractions. She will listen for and count the fetal heart rate and note the presence of amniotic fluid drainage and/or any show.

Role of the registered nurse

The registered nurse having overall responsibility for the case greets the patient, noting any special needs. She palpates the patient's abdomen, evaluates contractions, and examines the patient rectally or vaginally, depending on local policy, to determine fetal station and presentation, the dilatation and effacement of the cervix, and the condition of the membranes and position of the fetus. These last two are sometimes difficult or impossible to discern through the rectal-vaginal wall. If the rectum is not empty of feces, the results of the examination may be questionable. The position of the cervix may make the estimation of dilatation difficult. The patient's condition, progress, and reaction to labor are evaluated. The individual orders of the attending physician are consulted regarding types of analgesia and anesthesia and the expected delivery room setup. If no previous arrangement is known, the physician is called regarding the arrival of the patient at the maternity service, and any unusual vital signs and pertinent information gained from the rectal examination and other evaluations of the patient are relayed.

Unless the presence of true labor is doubted, a perineal shave of some type is usually carried out. Whether or not an enema is given will depend on the progress and condition of the patient and her doctor's desires. Vitamin K is no longer given at the time of admission since it is uncertain that the infant will receive a protective dosage. If analgesia is ordered, side rails should be in place. Which staff member carries out the necessary admission procedures depends on the patient's condition and needs.

Procedures

Principles of the admission procedures should be discussed. It is impossible to describe in detail an admission that fits the needs of every hospital. There are many ways to accomplish similar aims. However, certain principles are followed in every good maternity service no matter where it may be. We will now discuss the admission shave, or "prep," the labor room enema, the timing of contractions, and the determination of fetal heart tone.

PERINEAL SHAVE

Purpose: To cleanse the external genitalia in preparation for delivery by shaving the pubic and/or perineal hair with an antiseptic and/or sudsing solution and safety razor in order to:
1. Prevent infection
2. Make possible episiotomy repair easier
3. Aid in postpartum observation and care of the area

Setup: Provides individual equipment for each patient or equipment that is used in such a way that no cross infection can take place. Provision should be made for:
1. Privacy
2. Adequate lighting
3. A waterproof pad under the patient's hips to protect the bed
4. A supply of clean, warm water
5. A sudsing antiseptic solution
6. A sharp safety razor
7. Two or three clean dry cotton balls or gauze compresses to help pull back on the skin as it is being shaved and to clean the labial folds
8. An irrigation pitcher and/or folded soft paper or cloth towels to help rinse off the soapy solution and dry the area
9. Several paper towels or a plastic sack to receive the waste in a convenient manner and intermittently help to clean off the razor
10. Clean plastic gloves for the nurse's use during the procedure

Procedure (Complete or partial shaves may be ordered. Partial shaves exclude the pubic hair.):
1. If possible, place light (wall or gooseneck lamp) on opposite side of bed from where you will stand so that no shadows are cast.
2. Screen the patient. The sheet may be over

the lower legs and feet; the gown is turned up to just above the perineal hairline giving adequate space to work.

3. Have the patient bend her knees and drop her legs sideways—heels toward one another. Lather the pubic hair (if it is to be removed) and, creating tension on the skin with a dry compress with one hand, shave with the other, placing your razor approximately at a 30-degree angle to the skin. Begin at the pubis and shave toward the perineum. Be sure to remove *all* hairs from the labia and cleanse away any collection of smegma (cellular debris found especially in the labial folds). Avoid getting any solution into the vagina. Wipe off prepped area with soft towel, having folds dampened with water to remove the solution, which may be irritating. Use a different surface for each stroke (or irrigate the area) and dry with second soft towel, using same technique, never returning to the vulva after passing over the rectal area.

4. When the preparation of the perineal area is complete, turn the patient on her side to finish the perianal region. Probably the most important area to clear is between the vagina and anus, the *true* perineum, because this is the area cut during an episiotomy. Wipe off any residual solution.

5. Have your first "prep" checked so that you are certain what is expected of you. Even if it is your first "prep," you should not impress the fact on your anxious patient!

6. During the prep, if possible, try to gauge the frequency and quality of any contractions the patient may have, as well as how she is tolerating them. Report any vaginal discharge as to character and amount.
   Note: No perineal pads are worn during labor to cut down on the possibility of vulvar contamination resulting from the pad passing from the rectal to the vaginal area. However, the patient may have absorbent, protective bed pads under her hips.

DELIVERY ROOM ENEMA TECHNIQUE

Purpose: To empty the colon of feces in order to:
1. Help assure a clean delivery and prevent infection
2. Encourage contractions
3. Possibly provide more passageway for the child
4. Facilitate rectal examinations during labor

Setup:
1. Enema can or bag with appropriate tubing and clamp
2. Lubricant (K-Y jelly)
3. Protector for bed

4. Bedpan and tissue for patients not getting up
5. Paper towels to receive used tube
6. Ordered solution—a tap water or a soap solution enema made of water and castile soap may be used. The solution should feel moderately warm. Fill the can and give as much as can be tolerated—usually about half (1,000 ml.).
   Note: Some physicians order the prepackaged phosphate enemas, which may be given in less time with less discomfort to the patient. Some believe that the results are not as satisfactory, however.

Procedure:
1. Explain procedure to patient.
2. Screen patient and place her in Sims's position on left side if possible. Drape with a sheet.
3. Place protector under hips.
4. Expel air from tubing.
5. Gently insert the lubricated tube approximately 2 inches, telling patient to take a deep breath and bear down slightly; insert 2 inches more. (Occasionally, because of the position of the fetal head, more tubing must be inserted.) Hemorrhoids are common during pregnancy. Extra care and lubrication are necessary during the insertion if they are present. Hold the enema bag or can no higher than 18 inches from the rectum.
6. Stop the procedure when air is in danger of entering the tube via the enema can when it is almost empty.
7. If cramping results, you may clamp off the tube momentarily and lower the can. Instruct patient to breathe rapidly through an open mouth, "Pant like a puppy." Stop flow temporarily during a contraction.
8. Clamp tube and withdraw.
9. Leave pan and tissue with patient if she cannot get up to expel the enema. She may be placed on the bedpan. Instructions should be given regarding proper use of tissue, that is, to wipe from front to back and discard! In some maternity services, cotton balls or antiseptic-impregnated towelettes are used, or perineal irrigations are administered following the enema. Patients are not allowed up if:
   a. Disoriented, sedated, weak, or in advanced labor.
   b. Membranes are ruptured (there is danger of prolapse of cord).
10. Be sure necessary supplies are always replaced. Enema cans are sterilized between each patient or disposable units are used.
11. Additional information.
    a. Enemas are not usually ordered for pri-

miparous patients after a dilatation of 6 to 8 cm. or for multiparae above 4 to 5 cm. dilatation to avoid expulsion of the enema during delivery.

   b. Enemas should not be given to a frankly bleeding patient, since this will further encourage bleeding.

TIMING OBSTETRICAL CONTRACTIONS

Purpose:

1. To help evaluate the efforts of the uterus to dilate the cervix and expel the baby and to aid in determining the progress of the labor
2. To detect any abnormalities such as lack of uterine relaxation, which may reveal the onset of complications
3. To reassure the patient and her family by your presence and interest and, at the same time, to help her better support her labor by:
   a. Encouraging and listening
   b. Rubbing her back or providing sacral support as desired
   c. Helping with relaxation, breathing, or pushing techniques as needed
   d. Moistening her lips and offering oral hygiene
   e. Changing pillowcases and replacing bed pads
   f. Watching for signs of the patient's changing needs (for example, the beginning of the second stage of labor)

Procedure:

1. Before going to the bedside, if possible, learn about each patient individually.
   a. Number of pregnancies and viable deliveries
   b. Her marital status and any special arrangements for the baby
   c. Whether she has attended childbirth education classes
   d. Any special complications or problems anticipated
2. The fact that you are feeling her uterus, as it contracts and relaxes under the abdominal wall, to measure her progress in labor should be explained unless she has previously had contractions timed.
3. Your hands should be clean and not too cold.
4. The term "contractions" should be used, not *pains*. Not all contractions are painful. Use of the word "pain" may interfere with maternal conditioning for childbirth.
5. If the pregnancy is full term, the fundus, where the strongest muscular contraction can be felt, will be located just above the umbilicus. The nurse's hand should rest

lightly there to best detect the uterine contractions.

6. When the uterus contracts, it gradually becomes hard. The degree of hardness is called the *intensity* of a contraction. As the uterus contracts and the uterine muscle fibers shorten, the uterus may be seen or felt to rise in the abdominal cavity. It then gradually relaxes. The time that the uterus is discernibly firm or tight is called the contraction's *duration*. Usually contractions are easier to feel on multiparae than primiparae because of differences in abdominal muscle tone.
7. The term *"interval"* in the timing of contractions is used a bit differently than sometimes supposed. When one is asked to time the interval of a contraction, one times from the beginning of one contraction to the beginning of the following contraction.
8. The time between contractions is called the relaxation time a period equally important. If the relaxation time is very short or nonexistent, the baby may suffer from lack of oxygen. A continuously contracted, hard uterus may be a symptom of abruptio placentae. Between contractions the fingers should be able to depress the abdominal wall, a sensation similar to depressing a foam rubber pillow.
9. The contraction and relaxation periods and the interval have often been diagramed as shown in Fig. 9-1. The straight line represents complete relaxation, and the curved line the actual state of the uterine musculature.
10. There is usually a relationship between the duration and frequency of uterine contractions and the dilatation of the cervix. It follows *somewhat* the pattern shown in Table 9-1 (1 inch = 2.5 cm.).

Table 9-1. Usual uterine contraction and dilatation relationships

Cervical dilatation	Contraction	
	Duration	Interval
1. Fingertip to 2 cm.	20-30 seconds	6-8 minutes
2. 2 cm. → 4 cm.	30-35 seconds	5-6 minutes
3. 4 cm. → 6 cm.	40-50 seconds	4-5 minutes
4. 6 cm. → 8 cm.	45-60 seconds	3-4 minutes
5. 8 cm. → 10 cm.	50-80 seconds	2-3 minutes
(Most difficult period, fatigue, nausea, vomiting, irregular, intensive contractions)		(Tends to be irregular)

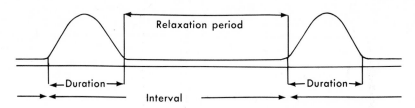

Fig. 9-1. Diagram of the contraction and relaxation of the pregnant uterus.

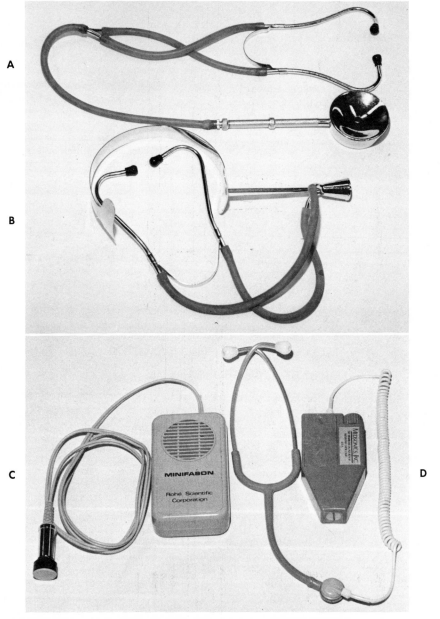

Fig. 9-2. A, Leffscope; **B,** DeLee-Hollis head scope; **C,** ultrasonic fetoscope, amplifies FHR so that it may be heard by all in area; **D,** ultrasonic fetoscope, transmits FHR via ear pieces.

11. Recording of observations of contractions would include duration, interval, and intensity, as well as possible patient tolerance. For example, "Contractions q 5 minutes for 35 seconds, mild in character. Using abdominal breathing effectively."

FETAL HEART RATE EVALUATION

Purpose:

1. To help detect the presence of fetal life at the time of admission
2. To detect possible fetal distress

Equipment needed: Continuous recorded monitoring of the FHR would be ideal for all laboring patients, since fairly recent research has indicated that intermittent "spot checks" of the FHR using standard fetoscopes, especially as has been classically taught, is in most instances inadequate for detecting *early* fetal distress.* However, appropriate electronic equipment, though increasingly available, is still not generally accessible or feasible for all laboring hospital patients. Therefore we will discuss the use of widely employed manual fetoscopes and only briefly describe more sophisticated electronic monitors, which may record contraction patterns as well as fetal heart activity simultaneously.

*Manually held monitors—*used intermittently:

1. The Leffscope—a stethoscope with a large, heavily weighted bell (Fig. 9-2, A)
2. The DeLee-Hollis head scope (Fig. 9-2, B)
3. An ordinary stethoscope equipped with rubber bands to prevent the sound distortion that results when handling the bell directly
4. Various "lubricated" ultrasonic fetoscopes, which may amplify the FHR (Fig. 9-2, C and D), held in the examiner's hand against the abdominal wall

Procedure:

1. Explain that you are checking the fetus by listening to its heartbeat.
2. Listen to the FHR immediately following a contraction; or better yet, if your patient will allow you, listen during, as well as immediately following, the contraction to hear the heartbeat adequately. (This procedure is a departure from the older method, which advised waiting 30 seconds after the end of a contraction before listening for the FHR.) This may enable you to possibly detect late deceleration of the heartbeat, a condition thought to be related to

*Hon, E. H.: An introduction to fetal heart rate monitoring, Los Angeles, 1973, Postgraduate Division, University of Southern California, School of Medicine.

fetal distress due to uteroplacental insufficiency. (See Fig. 9-5.) However, the pressure exerted on the abdominal wall during a contraction by the manual fetoscope is uncomfortable and annoying to mothers and not easily tolerated by many. For this reason, a monitor attached to the mother is superior to manually held types, and listening immediately following a contraction will probably be the more frequent observation pattern used. Listen 30 to 60 seconds if possible. Multiply as necessary to obtain the rate for 1 minute. Every separate beat heard should be counted. It will usually sound like a little watch. At first much concentration will be needed to hear it.

3. Be sure that friction noises from the fingers or the abdominal surface do not distort the sounds. Keep your fingers off the bell. Press firmly on the abdominal wall.
4. The area where the FHR may be heard the best is related to the following:

   a. *Presentation.* In headfirst or cephalic presentations the FHR is found in the lower abdominal quadrants, below the umbilicus. In breech presentations, the FHR is usually found at the level of the umbilicus or above.

   b. *Position.* If the back of the infant is toward the mother's left (L.O.A. or L.O.P. position), the FHR will probably be heard best on the mother's left. If it points to her right, the FHR will, in most cases, be heard best on her right. Just because a FHR can be heard in more than one place does not necessarily mean that more than one baby is involved. However, you may want to check by having another nurse listen simultaneously, using a finger-wagging technique to be sure that the rate heard in both areas is the same.

   c. *Station.* As internal rotation and descent occur, the location of the FHR changes, swinging gradually from the right or left quadrants to the midline and dropping until, immediately before delivery, it is found just above the pubic bone.

5. It is recommended that the FHR be taken frequently during labor at half-hour intervals or less in the first stage of labor. In the event of problems, it would be checked more frequently. The mother should be told at the time of admittance that a frequent check of the FHR is routine. Early in labor she or her husband may enjoy listening once, too.
6. A rate that is too rapid or especially too slow is considered a sign of fetal distress.

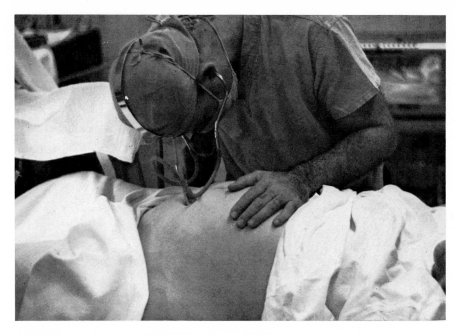

Fig. 9-3. Physician listens to the fetal heart rate (FHR) shortly before delivery. Note the location of the scope on the abdominal wall. (Courtesy Grossmont Hospital and Martin M. Greenberg, M.D., La Mesa, Calif.)

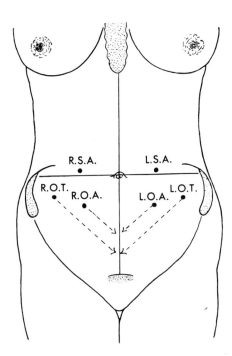

Fig. 9-4. Fetal heart tone locations on the abdominal wall indicating possible corresponding fetal positions and the effects of the internal rotation of the fetus.

Normal FHR is usually considered to be 120 to 160 beats per minute. A fetal heart rate under 100 beats per minute usually signals definite distress. However, even though the heart rate with or without the pressure of a contraction *may* at no time leave the normal range, significant periods of deceleration or slowing may occur undetected unless the labor is continuously monitored. Hon, a prominent investigator of fetal heart action, states that contrary to previously accepted belief, slowing of the FHR does not accompany all uterine contractions and that it is *not normal* for the FHR to slow with contractions. He has described three types of fetal cardiac deceleration according to their sequential relationships to uterine contractions. (See Fig. 9-5 for descriptions, explanations, and possible therapeutic interventions.)

a. Early fetal cardiac deceleration starts at the onset of a contraction and occurs only at the same time as the contraction. This pattern is probably due to head compression and increase in the intracranial pressure of the infant. As far as is known, this pattern is harmless. It does not call for any intervention on the part of the obstetrical team.

b. The late deceleration pattern, which is characterized by a slowing of the fetal

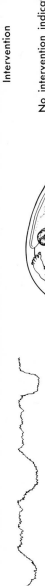

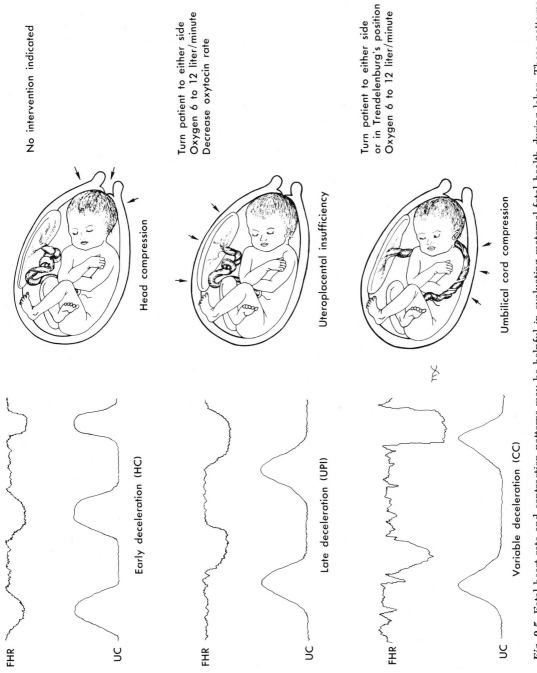

Fig. 9-5. Fetal heart rate and contraction patterns may be helpful in evaluating maternal-fetal health during labor. These patterns accurately recorded have been found worthy of study.

heart after the peak, or acme, of the uterine contraction and regularly reflects the waveform of the uterine contractions, may be found first within the normal FHR range of 120 to 160 beats per minute. As fetal distress increases, the range and frequency of the FHR deceleration increases. This pattern is frequently associated with uterine hyperactivity caused by oxytocin administration, maternal hypotension, or various high-risk pregnancies. Obstetrical interventions to decrease or eliminate fetal distress include: decreasing the rate of oxytocin administration, providing oxygen by mask or cannula to the mother at 6 to 12 liter/minute and turning the mother to either side.

c. The variable deceleration pattern is characterized by a periodic, unpredictable slowing of the FHR that shows neither a consistent sequential relationship to the uterine contractions nor a regular repetitive range or duration. This type of pattern is considered the result of umbilical cord compression. Changes in maternal posture, to either side or to Trendelenburg's position, are recommended interventions.

If either late or variable deceleration persists for 30 minutes after the above interventions have been carried out,

Hon recommends operative termination of the labor.

Note: Marked irregularity of FHR *may* be significant, but a certain amount of irregularity in the so-called baseline FHR (the rate determined either before labor begins or during labor in a 10-minute interval exclusive of any periodic slowdown) is now considered to be an indication of a well-developed, healthy, cardiac nervous control system. Continuously monitored, a FHR displaying *no* baseline irregularity is a signal of fetal distress. Patterns of irregularity are often difficult to assess when the classical intermittent methods of evaluation are used. (See Figs. 9-6 to 9-8 for other types of monitors that may be useful.)

7. Other sounds may be heard in the mother's abdomen as well. *Don't be confused.*

a. The maternal pulse may be heard. You should guard against reporting the maternal pulse as the FHR by feeling the mother's radial pulse at the same time as you are listening with a fetoscope. They should be different rhythms and rates.

b. The increased sound of the pulsation of the uterine arteries can sometimes be identified. This "sh" sound with the same rhythm as the maternal pulse has

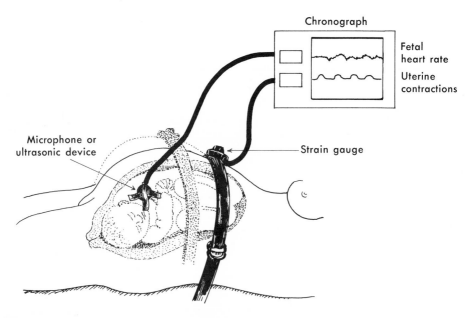

Fig. 9-6. External fetal heart and contraction monitoring is nonintrusive. Usually the supine position is the most satisfactory for recording. This posture may be difficult for the patient to maintain.

been called the placental souffle, or whistle. Sometimes the FHR can be heard at the same time in the background. Move the fetoscope about an inch, and you will probably hear the FHR better. The identification of a placental souffle does not guarantee that the fetus is alive.

c. Rarely you can hear a sort of soft, whistling sound occurring at the same rate as the fetal heart rate. This has been called the funic souffle, or cord whistle. Some think it is caused by a compression of the cord. Its presence indicates fetal life.

d. Many mothers-to-be are hungry, so you may hear peristalsis!

e. Occasionally, fetal hiccups may be de-

tected. More properly, these may be felt rather than heard.

Monitors attached to mother and/or fetus for extended or continuous use:

1. Sensors attached to the maternal abdomen to detect the mechanical energy of the fetal heartbeat. These may produce instantaneous visual or audible signals, and when appropriately equipped, they may produce permanent written records. They may be used early in labor before significant cervical dilatation or rupture of the bag of waters. They are simple to use, and there has been no known fetal injury related to their use. However, the position of the sensors may need frequent attention as labor

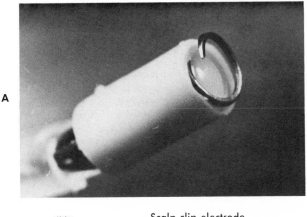

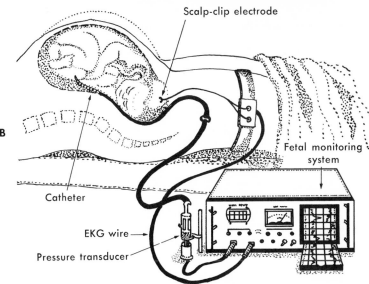

Fig. 9-7. **A,** Spiral electrode sometimes used to attach FHR monitor to fetal presentation. **B,** Internal fetal heart and contraction monitoring indicates the fetal EKG and the intensity as well as the frequency of uterine contractions. It provides more information but is an intrusive procedure. (**A,** Courtesy Corometrics Medical Systems, Inc., Wallingford, Conn.)

becomes more advanced and accuracy of the recording becomes more difficult to obtain. These FHR sensors may be combined with an externally placed diaphragm that is capable of recording the frequency of uterine contractions when held in place with abdominal strapping. Examples are:

    a. Small amplifying microphones (phonocardiography)

    b. Ultrasonic or Doppler-type instruments that produce characteristic reflected sound waves more clearly and accurately than phonocardiography

2. Fetal electrocardiography to detect the electrical energy associated with fetal heartbeat.

    a. Indirect fetal electrocardiography is possible with electrodes attached to the abdominal wall. It can be used well in early labor, but considerable "electrical

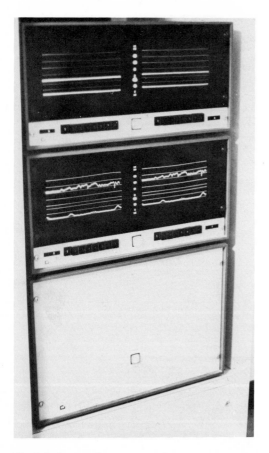

Fig. 9-8. A central monitor, such as might be seen at a nurse's station, displays FHR and contraction patterns of different patients in labor. (Courtesy Corometrics Medical Systems, Inc., Wallingford, Conn.)

noise" may be generated with patient movement during advanced labor, and the recording obtained is inferior to that of direct monitoring.

    b. Direct fetal electrocardiography requires ruptured membranes, 1 to 2 cm. of cervical dilatation, and a presenting part no higher than −2 station. A physician usually attaches the electrode vaginally to the presenting part (scalp or buttock) penetrating the epidermis by a tiny metal spiral or clip. Infection and soft tissue injury are possibilities but have not been significant problems.

3. Uterine contraction patterns interpreted by pressure exerted on a catheter inserted cervically into the uterus just beyond the parietal diameter of the fetal head may be viewed and recorded concurrently with the FHR. This arrangement, of course, greatly improves the ability to diagnose correctly early fetal distress.

Signs of fetal distress: Fetal distress may also manifest itself by the passage of meconium-stained amniotic fluid when the baby is in cephalic presentation; however, this sign is not consistently reliable. The onset of exaggerated fetal movement has at times also been considered a clue of difficulty. Recently in the presence of FHR and contraction patterns that denote possible distress, fetal scalp vein sampling has been used to try to confirm fetal jeopardy. The presence of an acid-base imbalance in the form of pH values below 7.20 indicates *fetal acidosis.*

CONTINUING CARE AND PREPARATION

Once admission is completed, unless delivery is imminent, there is a prolonged period of waiting and observation in which the physical and emotional support of the patient and preparation for her delivery are paramount. Usually, the presence of her mother, husband, or another family member at the bedside is a source of support. Quite often the husband or another family member may have trained to be the patient's labor coach and, as such, is extremely important in sustaining the morale and comfort of the parturient. If such visitation is not supportive or if it appears to antagonize or upset the patient, such observations should be reported to the charge nurse or doctor. Sometimes arrangements can be made for the visitor to have a "rest"!

Early labor

The patient in early labor (usually defined as up to 4 cm. dilatation) is characteristically alert, talkative, and nervous. She is usually most eager to cooperate with the doctor and nursing staff in attendance and responds readily to a calm, cheerful nurse who seems genuinely interested in her welfare. Her contractions, although perhaps uncomfortable, are tolerable. If her membranes are not ruptured, her contractions are not too frequent or intensive, and show is not too remarkable, she will probably appreciate being able to be up and around for a while and not automatically confined to her bed just because she has been admitted to the hospital. It has been found that when she does rest in bed, there is less interference with maternal and fetal circulation, increased urinary function, and greater uterine efficiency if she reclines on her left side. However, it is true that a number of nursing observations and procedures (determining fetal heart rate, checking the dilatation or perineum) are more easily carried out if the patient turns to the supine position intermittently. Later in labor, during transition and while the mother is pushing, the supine position is preferred. If the patient will be supine for an appreciable length of time, the head of the bed should be elevated approximately 30° to prevent circulatory and respiratory disturbances. She should conserve her physical and nervous energy for the more demanding period of labor to come. Her temperature, pulse, respiration, and blood pressure should be taken at least every 4 hours, oftener if individual history or indications warrant it. Fetal heart tone should be checked at approximately half-hour intervals or less. The amount and character of any show or amniotic drainage, if present, should be noted.

Rupture of the membranes (spontaneous)

If the bag of waters breaks at any time while the patient is in the labor area (if not ruptured before admission), she should be instructed not to get out of bed or sit up steeply. Most visitors should be asked to step out while the nurse inspects the perineum for signs of a prolapsed cord or, in the case of advanced labor, evaluates signs of the advance of the presenting part (bulging perineum, appearance of the fetal scalp) and the amount and color of the amniotic fluid. If there is any meconium (infant stool) in the fluid, staining it a brownish yellow to gray-black, it should be reported immediately. Meconium-stained amniotic fluid in the case of cephalic presentation is considered a sign of fetal distress—the response of the fetus to oxygen lack. Such staining in the case of a breech presentation is usually not considered significant, since the pressure exerted on a breech during its passage through the pelvic canal may cause the discharge of meconium, and no real fetal distress may be involved. The appearance of old, dark blood or bright red, frank bleeding at any time during labor should also be reported. The fetal heart tone should be taken right after the rupture of the membranes to try to detect possible cord prolapse. The fact that the bag of waters appears to have ruptured should be reported to the head nurse immediately. Contractions should be frequently evaluated, depending on the progress the patient seems to be making.

Evaluation of progress

Rectal examination. Proof of the progress is usually gained through rectal (Fig. 9-9) or vaginal examinations. A nurse may perform either rectal or vaginal examinations or both if properly instructed, depending on the policies of the hospital for which she works and the wishes of the physicians involved. These examinations should be kept to a minimum because of the discomfort caused by the patient, and, in the case of vaginal examinations, the possibility of introduction of infection. Student nurses are not routinely taught the techniques of rectal examination. Student nurses in programs leading to registration are sometimes taught when it is known that they are es-

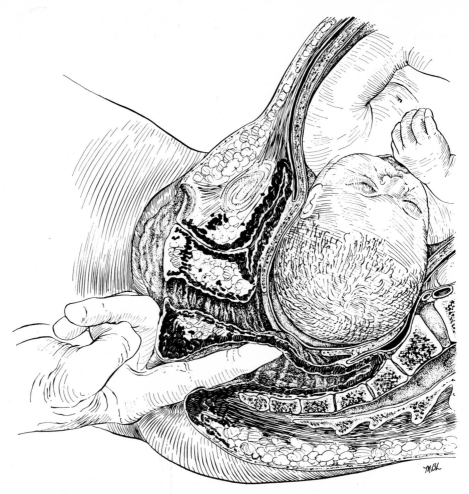

Fig. 9-9. Midsagittal section of the pelvis showing a rectal examination during labor. Note how the fingers are held away from the vagina to prevent contamination.

pecially interested in the delivery room area and want to continue working in obstetrics after graduation. To instruct all students in the techniques would be useless because unless they are practiced frequently, the ability to interpret what is felt is never obtained in the first place or is easily lost. In addition, the patient would have the discomfort of duplicate examinations. The LVN or LPN is rarely given the responsibility of performing rectal exams. This is usually considered the duty of the registered nurse. However, she may be asked to assist a doctor when he examines a patient rectally. She does so by making sure that a supply of clean rectal gloves

and lubricant is available and by chaperoning the patient and helping her to relax during an examination. Usually, if the patient drops her knees toward the outside and breathes deeply through her open mouth during the digital examination, it helps. Squeezing the nurse's hand seems to give some great satisfaction, too! After the examinations, the patient's rectal area should be cleansed of any leftover lubricant, and she should be encouraged as much as the circumstances permit.

Vaginal examination. The physician, and at times the RN, may perform a vaginal examination. The LVN or LPN may assist.

PROCEDURE. The way this procedure is

carried out differs from institution to institution and physician to physician. In some instances, the patient is cleansed and draped as for delivery, and the doctor may scrub his hands with a brush before putting on sterile gloves. In other hospitals, the preparation may not be so elaborate. However, it seems to us that certain principles should always be observed. The vulva should be cleansed of any soil. The examiner's hands should be carefully washed. A sterile examining glove should be used. A sterile lubricant and disinfectant should be poured over the gloved fingers and vulva. Care should be taken in inserting the fingers not to touch anything but the actual vaginal canal, so that organisms from anal or other areas are not introduced into the canal. A vaginal examination can reveal information not detected by a rectal examination because the cervix and presenting part are felt directly by the fingers and not through the rectovaginal wall. It may help greatly in the determination of the type of presentation, position, and the condition of the bag of waters.

RUPTURE OF THE MEMBRANES (ARTIFICIAL). At times, in an effort to induce or hasten labor, the doctor will artificially rupture the membranes during a vaginal examination. This is done, however only under certain conditions. The cervix should be effaced, and some dilatation must be present. The head should be engaged. The doctor ordinarily uses a sterile instrument with a small clawlike end, such as an Allis or Iowa or special plastic hook. He ruptures the membranes between contractions and lets the fluid flow slowly out past his fingers to avoid having the cord swept out of place by a sudden gush of "water." Prolapse of the cord and its subsequent pinching between the presenting part and the bony pelvis is a complication to be feared and watched for. Immediately after the membranes have ruptured, the fetal heart tone should be taken to determine any distress of the fetus. The actual rupture of the bag causes no pain because there are no nerves in the membranes, but the pressure exerted

in order to do the vaginal examination and to position the instrument may cause the patient some discomfort. She should be especially encouraged during this period. If rupture of the membranes is anticipated at the time of a vaginal examination, the patient should be placed on several bed-protecting pads to catch the drainage. Some advocate placing the patient on a bedpan; however, the patient's discomfort is usually increased in such a position. The approximate amount (small, moderate, or large) of fluid expelled and its color should be noted and recorded. Remember, the appearance of meconium in the amniotic fluid during a head presentation is interpreted as a sign of fetal distress. After the examination, the patient should be made as comfortable as possible. The excess lubricant should be wiped from the vulva, using good technique (wiping from front to back with no return of a used sponge to the vaginal region). Dry protective bed pads should be in place. The patient should be instructed to stay in bed.

Intensified labor: characteristics and care

As labor progresses, the patient experiences more frequent and intensive contractions. More and more her attention is focused on meeting their demands on her physical and psychological resources. If she has had training in relaxation and breathing techniques, these usually are of great aid. Abdominal and high chest breathing are described in Chapter 7, p. 64. If a laboring patient has had no previous training in these techniques, she may still benefit by some simple instruction in abdominal breathing. This usually eases the discomfort markedly. Rapid breathing techniques can also be taught; but if the mother-to-be is unfamiliar with the method, she is likely to hyperventilate, and the normal proportion of oxygen to carbon dioxide in the blood will be upset. She may feel lightheaded, and her fingers may begin to tingle. Such side effects should be avoided. If they appear, it may help if she breathes into a paper bag. The patient should be especially encouraged, and signs of her progress and condition should be frequently shared with responsible family members.

Probably the most difficult time during the labor and delivery is that period just preceding complete dilatation, the period of approximately 8 to 10 cm. dilatation. The laboring patient is now fatigued and usually discouraged. She wonders if she is ever going to have her baby and worries about her performance when she does. Although analgesics such as meperidine hydrochloride (Demerol) and tranquilizers such as hydroxyzine (Atarax) may have been given, she still may be fretful concerning the outcome of her labor. Her contractions may be irregular, at times seeming to come "one right after another." Nausea and vomiting are common. She is usually most grateful for the presence of the nurse or labor coach, who can help tremendously by offering firm back rubs, sacral support, cool, fresh pillowcases, damp clean gauze sponges to ease the dry mouth, oral hygiene, or a cool cloth on the forehead. Husbands and mothers can often help with these simple methods of relieving distress. The nurse should offer the bedpan at intervals to the patient and be sure her bladder does not become distended. Distention may delay labor or, rarely, cause laceration of the bladder.

Signs of the second stage of labor

During this period, the patient needs to be frequently evaluated concerning the possibility of the onset of the second stage of labor, the period of expulsion. The doctor and other delivery room personnel should be kept informed of the patient's progress. The second stage will ordinarily be heralded by (1) an increase in show, (2) an involuntary urge on the part of the patient to push or bear down with each contraction as the presenting part escapes the cervix and descends, (3) the fetal heart tone usually being heard just above the pubic bone in head presentations, and (4)

late signs, including the bulging of the perineum, the dilatation of the anus, and the appearance of caput, or the fetal scalp (Fig. 9-10). It is fervently hoped that a multipara will be in the delivery room and adequately prepared for the actual delivery before these last signs manifest themselves. Usually, multiparae are transferred to the delivery room at about 8 cm. dilatation to avoid a last minute race. However, women bearing their first babies, many times are not transferred to the delivery room proper before these last signs appear, since the period between complete dilatation and the delivery of the infant may be relatively protracted in the case of a primipara. Many hospitals in the United States now welcome husbands in the delivery room.

These hospitals have changed previous policies to allow fathers in the delivery room, especially those men who have attended childbirth education classes. The excitement and wonder of the occasion is appropriately shared with this most significant family member. The father sits at the head of the delivery table, encouraging the mother in her efforts and watching with her

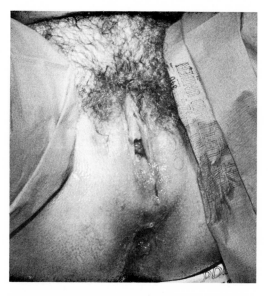

Fig. 9-10. Note bulging of perineum and appearance of fetal head (caput). (Courtesy Grossmont Hospital and Martin M. Greenberg, M.D., La Mesa, Calif.)

the progress of the delivery in a mirror attached overhead. For most couples, sharing the moment of birth together appears to create a "natural high" that they never forget. However, the father will previously agree to leave in the event of special problems where his presence is thought to compromise the best interests of the patient. Not all men want to see their children born, but for those who do, it seems to be a memorable, positive experience.

Pushing

Although she may wish to do so, a laboring patient should not be encouraged by the nurse to bear down or push before complete dilatation of the cervix is determined. To do so could cause greater fatigue for the mother, greater strain on the fetus, and possible injury to the cervix. Once complete dilatation has taken place, however, and all preparations for the delivery are made, pushing will be recommended. Unless experienced, the patient will probably have to be taught how to push to use her energy most efficiently. Most patients are quite relieved by pushing and cooperate well in following instructions, if they are not confused by too many instructors. The following aids and advice have been found to work well:

1. The patient is positioned on her back with her knees flexed. She may want to grasp her legs or the side rails or hand supports while pushing. The patient should be instructed to take a deep breath and blow it all out as she begins to feel a contraction. She then takes a second deep breath, which she holds.

2. She should close her mouth, put her chin on her chest, and bear down in the same manner as she would to move her bowels. If there are no contraindications, she is usually helped in this endeavor by being raised about 45° by the nurse's or coach's hand and arm under her pillow.

3. If she "runs out of air" before the contraction finishes, she should be encouraged to take another deep breath and continue pushing. Short pushes are ineffectual.

4. Between contractions, she should be allowed to rest. The nurse may observe that once the second stage of labor has been entered, the contractions, although forceful, may be less frequent. There may be intervals of 3 to 4 minutes. This gives the working mother a welcome bit of respite. She may even snooze a bit between contractions.

Preparation of the delivery room
(Figs. 9-11 to 9-14)

Before the second stage of labor is reached, the delivery room should be prepared for the actual birth of the baby. The responsibility of its preparation may be that of a trained vocational nurse. Hers is an important responsibility. To execute it correctly, she must have a clear concept of the principles of sterile technique, know where supplies are kept, know the patient's

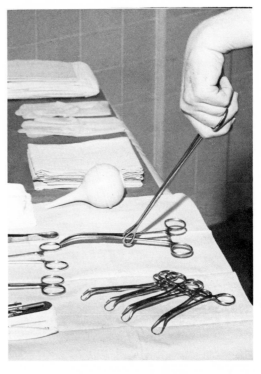

Fig. 9-11. Lifting sterile instruments. For beginners this is a good grip. The instrument is balanced and the hand is far from the surface of the table. (Courtesy Grossmont Hospital, La Mesa, Calif.)

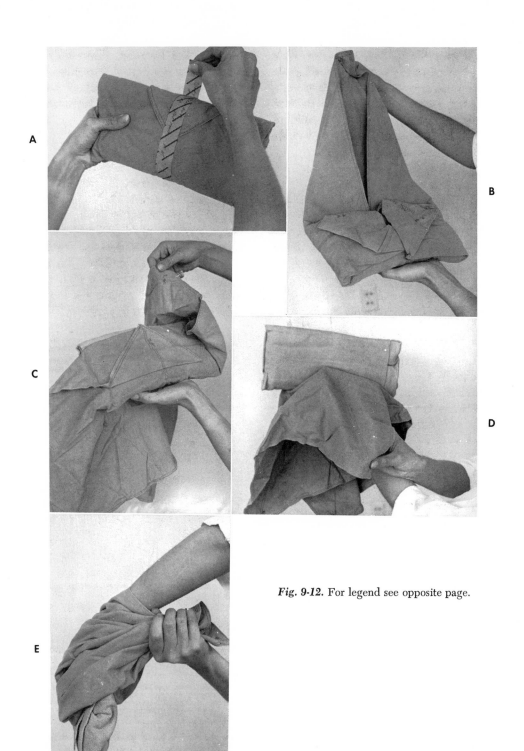

Fig. 9-12. For legend see opposite page.

special needs and the attending physician's desires. She should have some idea when the room will be needed so that she can plan her work. The actual preparation of the delivery room will vary in different maternity services, but the basic needs to be met and the principles employed will be the same.

Capsule review of principles and practice of aseptic technique

The practice of asepsis is not really difficult if the appropriate equipment and supplies are available and conscientious, knowledgeable persons are involved in their use and care. It is, however, a very serious responsibility. It involves evaluation of the area environment, including the nurses' dress and personal health problems that may possibly threaten the safety of the patient. Four simple rules sum up aseptic technique:

1. Know what is sterile.
2. Know what is not sterile.
3. Keep the two apart.
4. Remedy contamination immediately.*

Using transfer forceps. The use of transfer forceps in the handling of sterile supplies is as safe as the technique employed for their care. The forceps and their holding canister are steam sterilized periodi-

---
*Hoeller, M. L.: Surgical technology: basis for clinical practice, ed. 3, St. Louis, 1974, The C. V. Mosby Co.

cally. The holding canister is filled with an antiseptic solution to maintain the sterility of the lifts. When these forceps are used, care should be taken not to touch the ends of the instrument on any exposed inner side of the holding canister, since the area above the level of solution cannot be considered sterile because of prolonged exposure to the air. Some specially designed forceps and canister combinations include a lid, which reduces the danger of this complication. Sterile transfer forceps should not be held below the level of the waist, and the points should always be pointed down.

General considerations. Review the methods of unwrapping and placing supplies (Fig. 9-12). When approaching a sterile field to add sterile supplies, take care to avoid accidentally brushing or touching the area. When passing a sterile field, keep a safe distance away and, if possible, face the field. Never turn your back on a sterile area. Avoid turning your back toward an associate who is gowned and masked in a sterile manner.

If contamination of a sterile area does occur, the event must be immediately reported. It is no terrible sin to contaminate, although it is unfortunate. It is a sin to contaminate a sterile field, know it, and do nothing about it when something could be done. No one at the time may see those organisms introduced into the sterile area, but later on the patient may feel the effects of their insidious activity. Everyone on the

Fig. 9-12. Opening sterile packages. **A,** Remove the heat-sensitive tape closing the package and check the tape for color change. Start unwrapping the package with the point of the wrapper facing you. In this way the part of the package next to you will remain covered and protected for the longest period possible. **B,** Pull back the point and let it drop down after assuring yourself that the outside of the dangling wrapper will not contaminate any possible nearby sterile surface. **C,** Pull back the two side folds by the little turnbacks designed for your use. Uncover the end on the side of the supporting under hand first, then the side next to the active hand. If you are preparing the inner package for a drop onto a sterile surface, stabilizing the pack by bringing your thumb over the top of the wrapper before completely exposing the inner pack is sometimes very helpful. **D,** Pull back the last fold covering the inner wrap to expose the sterile surface. The inner pack can now be picked up by a gloved associate or it can be "scooted" onto a sterile table while the ends of the outer wrapper are held back to prevent contamination. **E,** If the hand-thumb grip is used, the pack can be dropped in the manner pictured. Care must be taken not to get too close to a sterile table or field while adding supplies. (Courtesy Grossmont Hospital, La Mesa, Calif.)

medical-nursing team should be glad to have breaks in technique or inadvertent contamination called to their attention in order to correct the situation.

DELIVERY ROOM SETUP REMINDER

Purpose: The purpose of this procedure is three-fold:

1. To provide an aseptic field for the anticipated delivery and subsequent newborn infant and maternal care.
2. To assure the convenient placement and operation of all necessary articles to promote safety, speed, and confidence on the part of the staff in behalf of the physical and emotional care of the mother and child.
3. To aid in the necessary legal and statistical recording of the event.

Setup:

1. Personal preparation
   a. Secure information.
      (1) Which doctor (for glove size, etc.)
      (2) Which delivery room
      (3) Type of anesthesia to be used, if any anticipated
      (4) Special problems involving the patient (Rh-negative, preeclampsia, varicosities of the extremities, etc.)
      (5) Approximate time the room is needed
   b. Wash hands.
   c. Put on mask. Be sure all your hair is covered by a cap. Remember, you should not wear clothes worn in areas outside the labor-delivery suite in the delivery room proper.
   d. Review in your mind the principles of sterile technique.
      Remember:
      (1) Touch sterile supplies only with sterile equipment!
      (2) As you handle the sterile transfer forceps, keep the points down and your knuckles away from the sterile surface being prepared.
      (3) As you work, keep back from the sterile tables. Never turn your back on a nearby sterile area.
2. Put out necessary sterile packs. Check outside tapes on packs for proof of sterilization if this type of tape is used. Check dates on packs to avoid outdated materials. Usually included are:
   a. The basic delivery pack with drapes and materials used on the patient or to accomplish the delivery. One such setup includes these sterile supplies:
      (1) Two drapes for the delivery supply table
      (2) One gown for the nurse caring for the baby
      (3) One drape for the interior of the incubator
      (4) One baby blanket
      (5) One gown and towel for the doctor
      (6) One set of drapes for the patient
         (a) One under-buttocks drape and pad
         (b) Two leggings
         (c) One abdominal drape
      (7) Two perineal pads
      (8) Four extra sterile towels
      (9) Eight gauze compresses
      (10) One gauze vaginal plug
      (11) One urine specimen bottle
      (12) One medicine glass for local anesthesia (if used)
      (13) One cord clamp
      (14) One sterilization indicator, which should be checked early in the arrangement of the supplies for the proper color change

   Note: Added to these materials will be the following sterile articles:
   One pair gloves
   One aspirator bulb
   One catheter (if catheterization is desired)
   Appropriate needles and suture
   One tube in which to collect and store cord blood for possible tests of the neonate in case of special need later
   One tube for cord blood for Coombs, hemoglobin, reticulocyte count, and bilirubin determinations if the patient is Rh negative

   b. The instrument pack (unless instruments are taken directly from a sterilizer). A typical pack may include:
      (1) One pair suture scissors
      (2) One pair episiotomy scissors
      } Because these are sharp and may become dull with autoclaving, they may be wrapped separately.
      (3) Two curved Kelly's, for clamping the cord
      (4) Four towel clips to help secure the drapes
      (5) One needle holder
      (6) One tissue forceps
      (7) Two straight Kelly's
      } To help in any repair necessary
      (8) Two transfer forceps (pick-ups, ring forceps, sponge sticks)

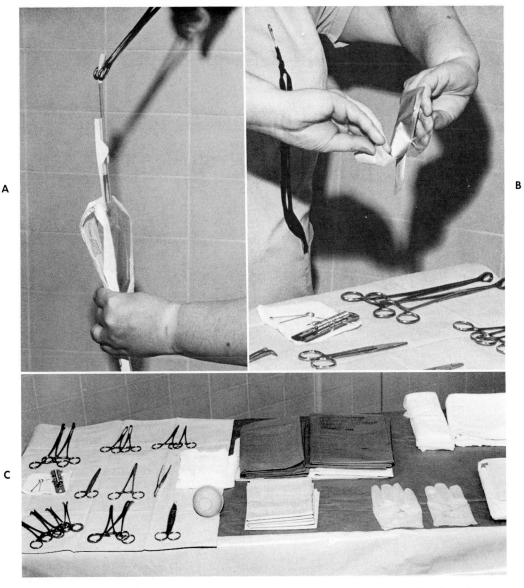

Fig. 9-13. **A,** Extracting a sterile catheter from a commercially prepared peel-back package, **B,** Dropping sterile suture from a commercially prepared peel-back package. **C,** One way to set up a basic delivery room table. (Courtesy Grossmont Hospital, La Mesa, Calif.)

(9) Two Allis clamps to help break the amniotic sac or aid in the repair of the perineum

Note: Other instruments may be requested (Gelpi retractor, Pelvi-fix retractor, etc.).

c. The basin-set pack, used to provide a sterile basin for the placenta and a sterile basin for lubricating obstetrical forceps, rinsing gloved hands, or cleansing the patient.

d. The perineal preparation tray will usually provide:
(1) A cleansing solution
(2) Sterile gauze sponges
(3) Sterile gloves or sponge sticks
(4) An antiseptic to be used on the skin after the cleansing of the area

e. The spinal anesthesia tray (if appropriate) will usually contain:
(1) Two sterile towels
(2) Four gauze compresses

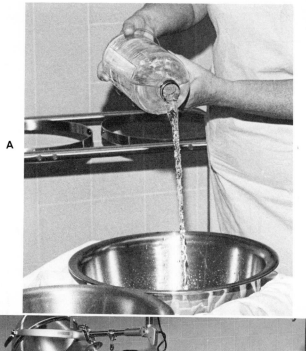

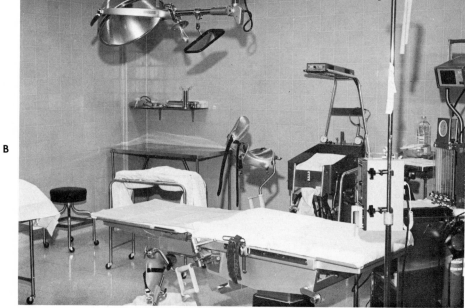

Fig. 9-14. **A,** When pouring sterile water into the "splash basin," hold the bottle high. **B,** The delivery room in readiness. Note covered sterile table and basins. Anesthesia machine with EKG apparatus for mother. Overhead warmer for baby. (Courtesy Grossmont Hospital, La Mesa, Calif.)

(3) One cup for antiseptic
(4) Three small sponges and sponge forceps for applying the antiseptic
(5) One syringe
(6) Several sizes of spinal needles plus stylets

Note: Added to this tray at the time it is opened for actual use are the doctor's gloves and the ordered anesthetic and antiseptic

f. Any indicated obstetrical forceps are usually placed conveniently (still wrapped) in the room until called for, except Piper forceps used in breech deliveries for the aftercoming head. Piper forceps are usually unwrapped previously and placed on the supply table.

g. At the time of the delivery the necessary records are brought into the room for completion, and the identification procedures for mother and child are carried out.

Transfer and immediate predelivery care

The transfer of the patient to the delivery room should be as smooth as possible. If the patient has a strong desire to push and it is not appropriate activity at the time, she should be advised to pant through her open mouth. Care should be taken in the transfer of the patient from bed to cart to delivery table. In some maternity services, the bed itself is momentarily wheeled into the delivery room to avoid one change and speed the process. The patient can usually help considerably in the move to the delivery table if the staff is able to wait until a contraction is not present.

While the patient is being prepared in the delivery room, the doctor may be dressing and scrubbing for the administration of the spinal anesthesia, if used (analgesia and anesthesia are discussed in Chapter 10), or for the delivery proper. The circulating nurse will uncover the sterile table and basin set and turn on the necessary operative lights. If no spinal anesthesia is used, the doctor usually advises the staff when he wants his patient placed in dorsal lithotomy position with her legs in supports.

Positioning

It is ideal to have two nurses assist in positioning, although it can be accomplished by one. To prevent strain on the patient's back, both legs should be raised or lowered at the same time. Coaching her to bend her knees as her legs are raised helps. Remember, if crutch or stirrup-type legs supports are used, you fit the supports to the patient, you do not fit the patient to the supports! The wrists of the patient may

be gently secured while she is on the table in order to prevent contamination of the sterile field and not primarily to restrict movement. Most modern delivery tables have some method of dividing in half, temporarily eliminating the foot portion of the table to allow the buttocks to hang over the end of the upper part of the table and the doctor to stand directly in front of the perineum. As soon as the patient's legs are adequately secured in the supports, the table is so adjusted. This is called "dropping," or "breaking the table."

Delivery in lithotomy position is not an anatomical necessity, but it is the position that is associated with the use of spinal or general anesthesia and is most familiar to physicians in the United States. In some cultures, the mother delivers her infant in squatting position. In parts of Europe a modified Fowlers' position is typically used with flexion and abduction of the lower extremities. These postures allow gravity to aid the mother in her efforts to push the baby to the outside world.

Sterile perineal preparation

As soon as the table is dropped, the circulating nurse cleanses the abdomen, thighs, and complete perineal area with a soap or antiseptic solution. This procedure is the so-called "sterile prep." Again, it is carried out in different ways in different institutions. It may involve sterile gloving or the use of sterile forceps or sponge sticks (Fig. 9-15). The principles are the same; the purpose is to help prevent infection and increase the visibility of the area involved. In performing the "prep" to prevent contamination of the birth canal, care should be taken that no sponge is used in the anal-rectal area and then returned to the vulvar region. Usually the first sponge is used to cleanse side to side from the pubic bone to the umbilicus. It is then discarded. The second and third are used to cleanse the thighs with an up-and-down motion from the labia majora to the midthigh. Each is discarded directly after use. The fourth and fifth are used to clean the labia on the right and left

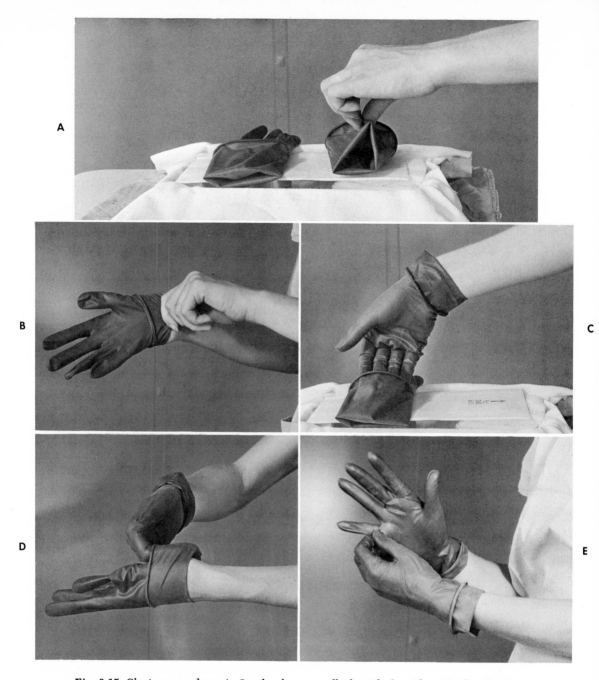

Fig. 9-15. Gloving procedure. **A,** Sterile gloves usually lie side by side with the thumbs on top at the outside edges, the left glove on the left and the right glove on the right. Pick up the glove by pinching the cuff folded down over the palm of the glove. If right-handed, slide on the right-hand glove first. Your bare fingers may touch any area of the glove that represents the inside of the glove. **B,** Slide your hand in with a rotating motion while pulling on the turned down cuff. **C,** Pick up the second glove with your gloved hand by sliding your sterile fingers *under* the turned down cuff. **D,** Place your other hand into the glove, sliding and rotating your hand as you pull out and up against the inside of the cuff with your gloved fingers. Keep your thumb back out of the way. Remember, your arm and the top of the cuff are contaminated and must not be touched with your fingers. When only gloves are worn, it is permissible to retain narrow cuffs at the tops of the gloves, but they, of course, are not sterile and should not be treated as such. **E,** After you are gloved you may adjust the fingers. Learning to glove takes time, patience, and usually more than one pair of gloves. (Courtesy Grossmont Hospital, La Mesa, Calif.)

of the vagina, avoiding the rectum, and then discarded. The last cleansing sponge passes directly over the vagina and anus. The patient is then usually rinsed and dried in a similar manner and sprayed or painted with an antiseptic. The purpose of the prep should be kept in mind. The object is not to go through so many prescribed motions but to get the patient clean. On the other hand, it must be performed rather swiftly, or the baby may be there before one is through. The gowned doctor is usually ready to drape for delivery as soon as the nurse is finished. Care should be taken to see that his hands or gown are not contaminated as she completes her "prep."

Draping

During the draping procedure, the circulating nurse provides a stool for the doctor, pushes the sterile supply table and double basin rack into position, adjusts the light, unwraps the forceps if they are desired, secures any additional supplies if needed, and begins her record of the delivery.

After the patient is draped, no part of the exposed side of the sterile linen (or paper) covering the patient should be touched by anyone not properly gloved or gowned. If pressure must be exerted on the abdomen by a "nonsterile attendant" for any reason, she must reach under the sterile drape, avoiding the exposed perineum to accomplish her task. After the baby is born, if he is placed on his mother's abdomen, she may reach under the covering drape and, using the drape as a hand guard, hold on to an infant arm or leg to help give support while he is aspirated or the cord is tied. Babies can be very slippery.

Delivery

Forceps and episiotomies

If the mother is bearing her first infant, many doctors will assist her efforts by employing outlet forceps to lift out the baby's head. This assist may also be given to multiparae. The forceps are applied after an episiotomy or planned incision of the perineum is performed and the bladder emp-

tied by catheterization. Many times the episiotomy and judicious use of forceps considerably shorten the second stage of labor, especially when the use of general anesthesia makes it difficult or impossible for the patient herself to help push the baby. It also may avoid injury to the maternal perineum and the baby's skull. An episiotomy may be cut from the vaginal opening straight down toward, but not extending into, the rectum (midline). It may be cut at 5 or 7 o'clock position from the vaginal opening to extend sideways away from the anus (lateral). It may originate in the midline just above the anus, but then angle to the left or right (mediolateral). The use of outlet (elective low) forceps is quite common. A midforceps is occasionally applied. The use of a high forceps is never recommended in modern obstetrics. It is too dangerous to mother and baby. Many babies are born without any previous episiotomy or forceps application. Catheterization prior to delivery has become less common.

Delivery mechanisms (Figs. 9-18 and 9-19)

If forceps are not used for the complete delivery of the head, it may be delivered manually between contractions by slow gentle extension. If the mother is awake and able, she may be asked to bear down between contractions to facilitate the actual passage of the head from the vaginal canal. After the head is delivered, the doctor checks to see if the umbilical cord is wound around the baby's neck. If it is, it must be slipped over the baby's head or clamped and cut to avoid strangulation or excessive pulling. Even before the entire body of the baby is delivered, the mouth may be aspirated to clear the airway. In order to deliver the shoulders, the doctor usually turns the baby's head to the side so that the occiput lines up with his back. He may then gently but firmly pull down to deliver the top (anterior) shoulder and then gently pull up to deliver the bottom (posterior) shoulder. Before one scarcely

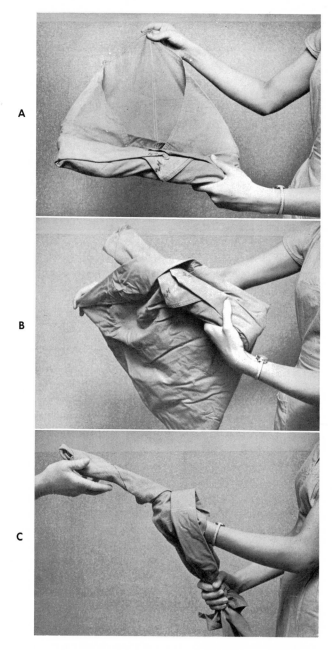

Fig. 9-16. Steps in unwrapping sterile forceps to hand to the physician. **A,** Grasp one end of the package, remove outer tape, and unwind outer wrapper. **B,** Pull back the inner turnback at the top of the package and continue to uncover the inner wrap (rather like peeling a banana!). **C,** Grasp carefully all dangling ends of the outer wrap and pull them out of the way toward your wrist. Do not touch the inner wrap! (Courtesy Grossmont Hospital, La Mesa, Calif.)

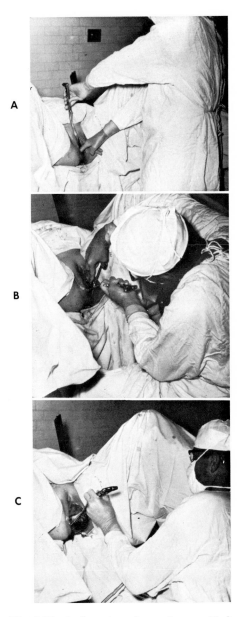

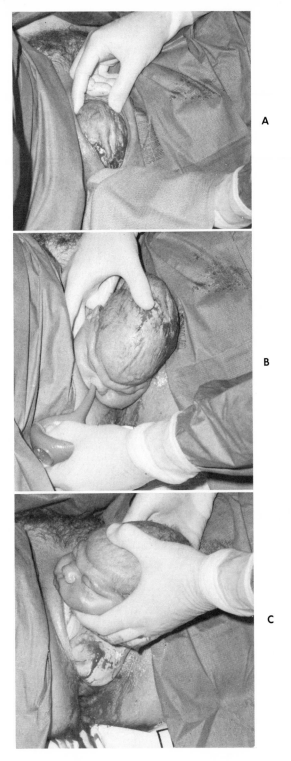

Fig. 9-17. A, Insertion of one forceps blade. B, A midline episiotomy (one blade of the forceps has been inserted). C, Use of outlet forceps. (Courtesy Wayne B. Henderson, M.D., San Diego, Calif.)

Fig. 9-18. Delivery sequence L.O.A.: A, Crowning; B, delivery of head and clearing of airway; C, delivery of posterior shoulder. (Courtesy Grossmont Hospital and Mark A. Treger, M.D., La Mesa, Calif.)

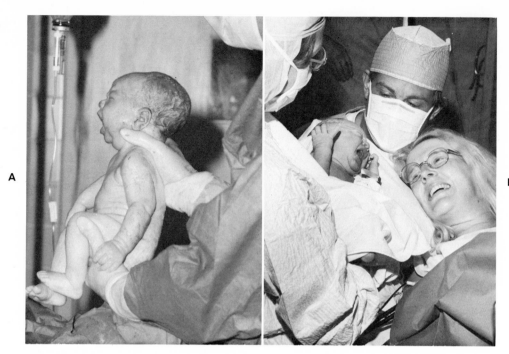

A   **B**

Fig. 9-19. A long-awaited personal introduction! It's good to have Father there for this special moment. (Courtesy Grossmont Hospital, Mark A. Treger, M.D., and Martin M. Greenberg, M.D., La Mesa, Calif.)

realizes it, all of the baby has been born. Further aspiration of the airway may be necessary, but normally the infant cries very soon. His umbilical cord is tied or clamped and cut, and he is handed to the nurse for further care in such a way as to protect the doctor's gloves and make a safe transfer.

The baby

Immediate care. The period immediately after birth is hazardous for the baby. Many adjustments must be made in his body to fit him for his new environment. He should be placed on his side and carefully and frequently observed. The nurse caring for the newborn infant should have freshly washed hands and wear a clean overgown. The nurse must provide warmth (usually in the form of an incubator, heated blanket, or a radiant infant warmer), observe his color and breathing pattern, and attach the identification approved by the hospital. During the same period of time, she

usually performs the prophylaxis prescribed to prevent gonorrheal infection of the eyes. Silver nitrate, 1%, is used followed by a rinse of sterile physiological saline or distilled water.* Due to sensitivity problems, penicillin is now used less often.

Apgar evaluation. If the Apgar method of evaluating the newborn infant is used, the infant should also be scored for heart rate, respiratory effort, muscle tone, reflex irritability, and color, 1 and 5 minutes after birth. This scoring may be done by the physician, anesthesiologist, or the nurse; but the nurse is thought by some to be the more "impartial and available" observer, especially for the 5-minutes evaluation. The Apgar score is used in follow-up stud-

---

*There seems to be lack of agreement regarding the eye rinse to use after AgNO$_3$ instillation. Some nurseries employ saline because it forms a precipitate (silver chloride), which more quickly inactivates the irritating AgNO$_3$. Others consider the precipitate itself to be irritating and prefer to use water.

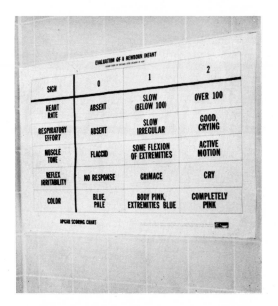

Fig. 9-20. Prominently displayed on the walls of a delivery room is the Apgar Scoring Chart. (From Apgar, V.: J.A.M.A. **168**:1988, 1958.)

ies of the child and is important in many research inquiries. Infants receiving a score of 7 to 10 are considered vigorous. Scores 4 to 6 are considered to denote mild to moderate depression, while 0 to 4 indicates severe depression. The highest score that can be given is 10. Dr. Apgar believed that few newborn infants conscientiously scored deserve a first rating totaling 10. She believed that few babies are completely pink 1 minute after birth (Fig. 9-20).

Third stage of labor
Use of oxytocics

In most cases, some form of oxytocic is ordered after the birth of the baby and/or after the delivery of the placenta. Oxytocin (Pitocin) hastens the delivery of the placenta. After delivery of the placenta, a form of ergot helps the uterus clamp down for a relatively long period to help prevent postpartum hemorrhage.

Delivery of the placenta (Fig. 9-21)

After it has separated from the uterine wall, the placenta may be delivered through the bearing down efforts of the mother if she is awake, or it may be expressed by the manual pressure exerted by the doctor on the fundus, or top of the uterus, through the abdominal wall. This must be done very carefully, and only when the placenta has separated and the fundus is firm. Otherwise, hemorrhage or inversion, a turning inside-out of the uterus, may occur, a grave obstetrical complication.

Signs of placental separation are (1) the rising of the uterus to or above the umbilicus, (2) the rounding out and firming up of the fundus, (3) the lengthening of the umbilical cord outside the vulva, and (4) a small gush of blood to the exterior. The placenta should be inspected to see if it was delivered in its entirety. Some doctors also perform an internal palpation of the uterus to assure themselves of its condition. In some hospitals, placentas that have not become contaminated with stool or were not born of women whose pregnancies were complicated by infectious disease, fever, or premature rupture of the membranes are saved and later processed by a pharmaceutical concern to extract the immune globulin they contain.

Immediate postpartum care
Lacerations

After the delivery of the placenta, any necessary perineal repair can be made (Fig. 9-22). Generally the same anesthetic used for a delivery can be employed. Some times a local anesthetic is administered. If this is used, the doctor will need a syringe (usually Pitkin), some infiltration needles, and the local anesthetic of choice as well as the usual materials involved in a perineal repair. He will want to sit down and be provided with a good light.

In spite of precautions, lacerations or episiotomy extensions will occasionally occur. Some maternal tissues tear more easily than others. Very large babies or unusual positions are a special threat to the perineum. Lacerations of the perineum are described as first, second, or third degree. First-degree lacerations, involving a tear in the mucous membrane and skin only, are fairly common and usually of no permanent consequence. Second-degree lacerations include a tear into the muscles of the perineal block, but exclude the rectal sphincter. Adequately repaired, they usually heal well with little problem. Third-degree lacerations, which by definition involve the circular anal sphincter muscle, however, are more difficult to repair and may result in permanent damage to the perineum and sphincter (review the anatomy of the pelvic floor). Lacerations may involve areas other than the true perineum. Tears of the labia, interior vaginal wall, and cervix are not uncommon. All these areas should be inspected for such possibilities after a delivery.

If repair is nonexistent, inadequate, or improper, the patient is soon a possible candidate for hemorrhage, hematoma, and/ or infection.

Later, as the weeks and years pass, certain pelvic displacements and malfunctions may show themselves. The patient may be troubled with urinary or fecal incontinence, or she may suffer from a sagging of the pelvic musculature. When the tissue wall between the bladder and the vagina becomes abnormally relaxed, usually because of previous injury, the bladder drops out of place and pushes the anterior vaginal wall backward. The resulting abnormal condition is called a *cystocele*. A similar hernia-type abnormality involving the rectovaginal wall and a falling forward of the rectum is what is known as a *rectocele*. Small rectoceles or cystoceles are usually asymptomatic and are not surgically repaired. Large abnormalities of this type, however, may cause such complaints as a "dragging sensation" in the pelvis and such conditions as stress incontinence, urinary retention, and cystitis in the case of cystocele or constipation and hemorrhoids in the case of rectocele. A vaginal repair of these difficulties, or colporrhaphy, may be performed. If both a bladder and a rectal prolapse are surgically treated, the procedure is often called an A and P (anterior-

posterior) repair. *Prolapse*, or a falling out of place of the uterus, often accompanies these other displacements. Occasionally, abnormal canals or tracts between two body cavities or a body cavity and the exterior develop as a result of obstetrical injury. These tracts, most often found between the vagina and the urethra or the vagina and the rectum are termed *fistulas* and are very difficult to eliminate. An adequate

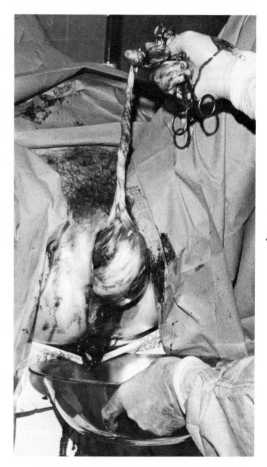

A

Fig. 9-21. **A,** Delivery of the placenta, or afterbirth. **B,** Maternal side showing cotyledons and membranes pulled to one side. The cord attaches on the opposite side. If this side appears first at the outlet, the placenta is said to have separated by Duncan's mechanism. **C,** Fetal side showing insertion of the cord. If this side appears first at the outlet, the placental separation is by Schultz's mechanism. (Courtesy Grossmont Hospital and Martin M. Greenberg, M.D., La Mesa, Calif.)

early repair of any obstetrical injuries to the passageway or its supports is very important to continuing good health.

After delivery, during perineal inspection and repair, the mother is customarily shown her baby; then he may be taken to the nursery with the appropriate records of the delivery. If she is not alert, definite arrangement should be made for her to see the infant later as soon as she is able.

With the termination of the repair and the cleansing of the perineum, if needed, the head and foot of the delivery table are again realigned, and the patient's legs removed from the stirrups or supports. The perineal pads are attached, and a warm, clean hospital gown replaces the one worn by the patient during delivery. She is covered by a warm blanket. In some maternity services any initial preparation of the

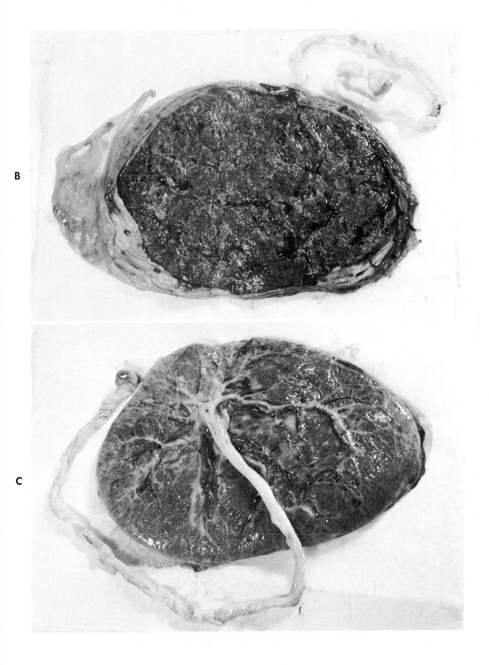

B

C

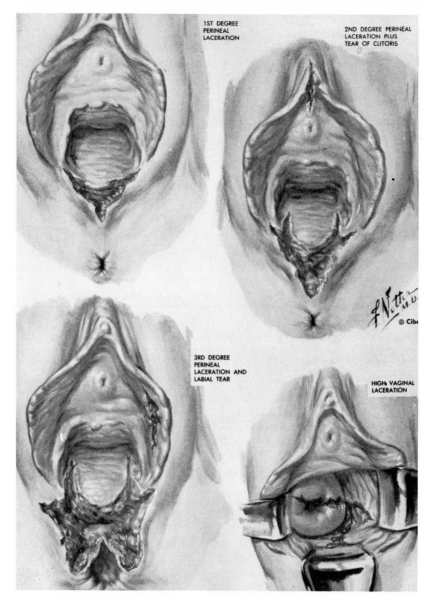

Fig. 9-22. Obstetrical lacerations—vagina, perineum, and vulva. (From The CIBA collection of medical illustrations, by Frank H. Netter, M.D. Copyright CIBA.)

breasts of nursing mothers is done at this time also. Some doctors allow their patients to nurse their babies while still on the delivery table or in the delivery room if the baby is in good condition and free of excessive mucus and the new mother is alert and so wishes. The nursing of a baby directly following delivery of the placenta has a physiological basis, since stimulation

of the breasts causes the uterus to contract and helps prevent blood loss when other means of control are not available (something to remember in a disaster situation). The early establishment of an intimate mother-child relationship involving touch and nourishment is also considered one way to promote positive maternal emotions or maternal attachment. For some mothers who are not troubled by the relative lack of privacy and are not too tired, this opportunity may be cherished.

Observation

All during this early postpartum period, the patient is being observed for excessive bleeding and signs of shock. The blood pressure and pulse are frequently determined and the respirations observed. The uterus is palpated frequently to discover any relaxation of the fundus. If an intravenous infusion is in place (often used in conjunction with spinal anesthesia), it is carefully watched for rate of administration and possible infiltration. Many of these infusions contain an oxytocic and should not be given rapidly. Great care should be exercised that the needle is not dislodged during the transfer of the patient from the delivery table. Several hands may be needed for this project if the patient has an intravenous infusion and is temporarily unable to use her legs properly because of the lingering effects of spinal anesthesia, or the staff may be fortunate in having a mechanical aid for the patient transfer. The newly delivered mother may remain in the delivery room suite for a specified time for close observation near equipment that may be needed, or she may be transferred to a special postpartum recovery room. At the time of her various changes in location, special attention should be given to the transfer of her personal belongings. Family members should see her as soon after delivery as is appropriate, although they are not encouraged to have a long visit. Mother needs her rest!

Special situations

Because questions always develop concerning them, we will now take time to consider some special situations that occasionally arise in the labor-delivery sequence.

Precipitate delivery

First to be considered is what is termed "precipitate delivery." This means a delivery that occurs with such speed and in such a situation that proper preparation and medical supervision of the event are lacking. A multipara with a relaxed perineal floor may have an extremely short period of expulsion. Two or three powerful contractions may cause the baby to appear with considerable rapidity. In this case, the nurse may be the only one at the bedside or delivery table to assist the patient. In no instance should she leave the patient alone. If it is obvious that the baby would be born before the delivery room is reached (for example, the patient is a para iii and the head is almost delivered), the nurse should do the best she can with what she has at hand. If present, any family member usually should be asked to step outside the room. The call light should be turned on. If there is time and it is available, an antiseptic lubricant may be poured over the perineum. The nurse should wash her hands or put on sterile gloves and have a few towels handy.

Birth of the head. The baby's head should not be forcibly held back, since this may cause fetal distress and aspiration, but it should be restrained to prevent a rapid exit from the vaginal canal. This restraint can usually be achieved by allowing the baby to deliver slowly against a guiding hand placed on the top of the advancing head. The fingers of the nurse should not enter the vagina. If the bag of waters is not broken, it must be pinched or torn to release the fluid and protect the baby from aspiration. The actual delivery of the head should be accomplished between contractions, with the mother panting or lightly bearing down as needed to assist. As soon as the head is born, the nurse should wipe off the face and check to determine whether the cord is around the neck. If it is, she should slip it over the head or shoulders to prevent choking. Rarely it may be too tight to slip over with the fingers. If this happens, it is hoped that sterile clamps and scissors are available in the labor room or that a staff member has answered the light and brought the emergency pack containing the clamps and scissors necessary to cut the cord! The mother should firmly be instructed to pant through her open mouth and not push during this interval.

External rotation and expulsion. After the head is delivered and wiped and the location of the cord is determined, many times the rest of the child's body delivers without further assistance. However, if there seems to be no further progress or if the back of the head has not already turned toward the mother's thigh, it can be turned in the direction of least resistance to line up with the child's back. There is no need to hurry. Next, the head should gently but firmly be directed downward to deliver the top shoulder. After the top shoulder is expelled, the baby is lifted up toward the pubic bone to release the bottom shoulder. The rest of the child is delivered without any particular problem. Before the expulsion of the shoulders, it is sometimes very helpful if the mother's hips can be elevated (or the foot portion of the table lowered a few inches) by another person in order to give more room for the gentle up-and-down maneuvers described and to help keep the baby's face free of vaginal and anal drainage.

Immediate care of the baby. After the complete birth of the baby, care should be exercised that the airway be cleared. The baby should not lie in a puddle of amniotic fluid where aspiration can take place. He should be held upside down to "drain" without any tension being placed on the umbilical cord. After the airway is clear, he may be gently stimulated to cry, if necessary, and placed on his mothers' abdomen —head slightly lower than his body. (Most of these babies cry immediately.) He should be wrapped in a towel or blanket for warmth. There is no haste to cut the cord, or for that matter to deliver the placenta. The cord can wait until proper sterile equipment is available. Usually the physician, who in the meantime has been contacted by the staff, completes the delivery of the placenta and repairs any possible lacerations. A calm, reassuring manner on

the part of the nurse (even if she doesn't really feel so calm) is very helpful to the patient and all concerned.

Usually no great permanent harm results from such an event, but every effort should be made to prevent its occurring. All patients should be frequently evaluated for progress during labor. Signs of the approach of the second stage of labor should not be ignored. In such deliveries, the advantages of antisepsis and asepsis are largely lost, there is greater danger of injury to the maternal tissues, danger of aspiration and injury to the baby, and acute embarrassment for the patient, not to mention the nurse.

Summary. Principles of emergency unprepared delivery, no matter where it takes place, include the following:

1. Keep contaminating articles, including fingers, from the birth canal and provide as clean a delivery area as possible.
2. Help the head deliver slowly against a clean towel or hand and allow its delivery between contractions to prevent perineal lacerations.
3. Allow the normal mechanism of labor to take place with a minimum of interference.
4. Hold the newborn infant upside down to clear the airway—no tension on the cord.
5. Gently stimulate the infant to breathe, if necessary, after placing the child on the mother's abdomen.
6. Provide warmth for the newborn infant.
7. Wait for sterile supplies to be available to cut the cord.
8. Wait for delivery of the placenta unless professional aid is very long in arriving or excessive bleeding occurs. However if no professional help is forthcoming, if the signs of separation of the placenta have occurred, if the uterus is firm, and if the mother experiences a return of contractions, she may be asked to bear down to deliver the placenta. It should be supported

114

as it is born so that the membranes are not torn. It should be saved for later evaluation by a doctor.

Induction of labor

At times in the labor suite there may be admitted a mother-to-be who is not in labor at all. She has come on appointment to have her labor induced.

Reasons for induction. There may be several reasons for an induction of labor: (1) a problem with erythroblastosis fetalis may have developed, (2) the mother may be diabetic, (3) the mother may have increasing symptoms of toxemia, or (4) the baby may be *definitely* late in arriving (postmaturity). Occasionally, induction is planned for the convenience of the patient or the doctor, although this is not usually considered a valid reason.

Methods and care. Candidates for induction of labor must be selected carefully, since it is not a procedure totally without risk to the mother and baby. In the past, prescriptions of castor oil and/or warm enemas were often made to start labor. But there are two main ways of inducing labor in the hospital today: the administration of pituitary hormones or their synthetic substitutes (most commonly Pitocin) and/or the artificial rupture of the membranes. The latter procedure alone is now less frequently performed. Unless the uterus is ready for labor, it will not occur. The cervix must at least be partially effaced and soft and pliable. If the membranes are artificially ruptured and labor does not begin within 24 hours, the possibility of introducing infection must be faced. Posterior pituitary extract is very powerful and can cause violent uterine contractions. For this reason, mothers receiving this medication must be closely watched with very frequent checks of contraction patterns, fetal heart tone, and blood pressure. Today oxytocin (Pitocin) is probably most often administered by intravenous drip (usually 10 units of Pitocin per 1,000 ml. of 5% glucose in water). The rate of flow is usually ordered by the physician, who should be in the area while his patient is receiving such treatment.

Cesarean section

With the decreasing risk involved in the performance of cesarean section, the removal of the child through an incision in the abdominal and uterine walls, the operation is used more frequently in modern obstetrics.

Reasons for cesarean section. Sometimes patients admitted to the labor area will unexpectedly demonstrate symptoms that will advise the emergency use of the procedure: conditions such as placentae abruptio, placenta previa, fetal-pelvic disproportion, abnormal presentations, prolapsed cord, or uterine inertia (failure of the uterus to contract sufficiently to continue progress in labor). The most common cause for cesarean section in the United States, however, is not usually an emergency, but a previous cesarean section. It can be scheduled days in advance. But conditions that indicate acute fetal distress or maternal jeopardy demand the prompt and rapid preparation of the patient once the condition has been discovered and the course of action determined. A patient scheduled for an emergency cesarean section is subjected to much in a very few minutes. Everything should be done with as much calmness and dispatch as possible. The patient's morale should be supported as much as possible, because, if she is alert, she will probably be very frightened.

Preparation. The following procedures are routinely carried out:

1. Signing of the operative permit by the patient or responsible party
2. An abdominal-perineal prep, which starts at the nipple line and includes the entire abdomen from side to side as well as the perineal and rectal areas
3. Insertion of an indwelling catheter—sometimes done in surgery after anesthesia
4. Blood type and crossmatch and hemoglobin determination

115

5. Removal of any hairpins or hard objects from the hair; application of a surgical cap; removal of any extra jewelry, glasses, contact lenses, etc., to be given to the family; taping of wedding and engagement rings to the fingers, but not so as to impede circulation
6. Removal and safekeeping of any removable dentures
7. Removal of any nail polish from at least two or three fingers of each hand, in order that the anesthetist can check for cyanosis of the nail beds
8. Preoperative medications as ordered

The patient is given nothing by mouth as soon as cesarean section is contemplated, if this measure has not been instituted previously. An infusion may be started, although usually intravenous therapy is begun in the area where the actual section will take place.

Patients may be transferred to the operating room suite for surgery, or a delivery room may be prepared for the procedure. During all the busy preparations, any family members present should not be forgotten, and provision should be made for them to wait in as much mental and physical comfort as possible.

Discussion of the care of a cesarean patient after delivery is included in the section of the book treating the postpartum period.

Breech presentation

Another situation that is fairly often part of the labor-delivery experience is a breech presentation.

Incidence. You will recall that breech births make up approximately 3% of all deliveries. In former years, considerable effort was exerted in trying to turn these babies to a cephalic presentation before the onset of labor. Many were turned without too much difficulty only to revert back to a breech before the time of labor. Many practitioners now believe that if a baby is found to be a breech it is because of a valid anatomical or physiological reason,

and there are fewer attempts to turn the child (a process called version).

Complications. Although a breech presentation would probably not be considered an abnormality, it involves more risk to the infant than a cephalic birth, and the mother is likely to have a longer and more tiring labor. As a rule there is greater possibility of prolapse of the umbilical cord during breech labor, and during the delivery of the body of the baby, it may be compressed against the pelvic outlet. The baby may try to take a breath before his head has been born and aspirate tenacious vaginal secretions. Occasionally, trouble is encountered in the extraction of the arms. Sometimes an unexpectedly large head may cause concern, and cerebral damage may occur. Although few maternity services today routinely provide a sterile scrub nurse in the delivery room, many physicians appreciate and request the help of such a nurse at the time of breech delivery. Such an attendant usually helps support the baby's body or may, when instructed, apply fundal pressure when it comes time for the delivery of the head. A special type of forceps called "Pipers" applied to the aftercoming head may be used at the time of a breech birth. They should always be on the sterile supply table when a breech delivery is anticipated. The delivery of the head is many times accomplished in such a way that the baby almost seems to do a guided half somersault over the mother's abdomen. A rather deep episiotomy is customary in breech deliveries. The baby may have edematous or bruised genitalia. In a minority of cases the doctor may elect to perform a cesarean section because of the general condition, history, or age of a patient.

Twins

Twins are another interesting feature of the obstetrical department. They occur about once every ninety pregnancies. There are two types of twins—fraternal and identical. Fraternal twins are the result of two simultaneous pregnancies developing from

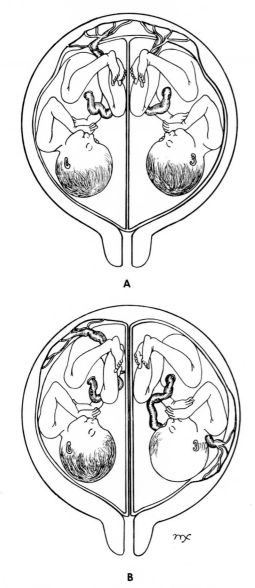

A

B

Fig. 9-23. **A,** Identical twins; **B,** fraternal twins. Note differences in construction of amniotic sacs.

the fertilization of two separate ova by two distinct spermatozoa. They do not resemble one another any more than siblings resemble one another. They may be of the same sex or of opposite sexes. The placental circulation of each fetus is separate, although the adjoining placentas may be fused. Each fetus develops within its own amniotic and chorionic sac.

Identical twins result from the division of one fertilized ovum into two identical halves, which develop into two similar individuals of the same sex. The placental circulation is shared by the attachment of two umbilical cords. Each infant is encased in a separate amniotic sac but shares the chorionic sac with his twin. Fraternal twins are more common than those classified as identical. Approximately 54% of twins are premature, and the risk of intracranial hemorrhage, developmental respiratory distress syndrome, and other neonatal difficulties is high. Mortality for a second twin is about three times higher than it is for his sibling, probably because of a greater incidence of malpresentations. Thus the nursery should be alerted when a twin birth is anticipated. Occasionally, such an event is not anticipated, and the family, doctor, and nurse are surprised to receive a "bonus baby."

Preparations and complications. When twinning is expected, two sets of identifications should be ready with double newborn record sheets. Two sterile baby receiving blankets, two cord clamps, and two aspirator bulbs should be available. In almost half of all twin births, both infants are cephalic presentations, but any combination of presentations and positions may exist. Occasionally, the babies' relative positions may cause problems in their delivery. Mothers of twins are more likely to suffer from toxemia of pregnancy and placenta previa and, because of the greater distention of the uterus, are more often victims of postpartum hemorrhage.

• • •

The nurse's experience in the labor-delivery room area can be a very satisfying, rewarding type of nursing. If skilled in the art of human relations and the observations and procedural techniques necessary to care for her patients, she can play an indispensable and gratifying role in a very crucial period in the life of a family. The alert student in this area can learn much and gain an appreciation and reverence of life that she will never forget.

10
Analgesia and anesthesia

METHODS OF PAIN RELIEF

One should not leave the subject of modern childbirth without at least discussing briefly the most common methods being used to make the experience of labor and delivery easier and more comfortable for the mother. The methods practiced may differ considerably from one locale to another. As we have seen, these methods involve more than the administration of drugs; they also include ways available to help the patient to better understand the process of childbirth and to consciously cooperate with what her body is trying to accomplish. In most cases a clean, calm, quiet, dimmed environment, attention to the techniques of relaxation, the application of sacral support, the close supervision and encouragement of a concerned nursing staff and attending physician, and the companionship of those she loves will greatly decrease the need for the administration of analgesic and anesthetic drugs.

Key vocabulary

Five words perhaps should be defined for use before a discussion of pain-relieving drugs is attempted.

amnesic a technique or medication that causes memory loss of varying degrees.
analgesic a technique or medication that reduces or eliminates pain.
anesthetic a technique or medication that partially or completely eliminates sensation or feeling. It may be local in extent or general, producing unconsciousness.
hypnotic a technique or medication that causes sleep.
sedative or *tranquilizer* a technique or medication that relieves anxiety and quiets the patient.

Obstetrical analgesia (first stage of labor)

The prescription and administration of analgesic drugs during the first stage of labor is not without difficulty but is highly rewarding.

Special considerations

The physician must consider that he is caring for two patients. He must realize that many analgesics have a hypnotic effect not only on the mother but also on her unborn baby. He must so calculate the dosage and time of administration so that the baby will not be "sleepy" at the time of his birth and too drowsy to want to breathe on his own. Before delivery, the sleepiness of the fetus is not so crucial, because he does not have to breathe; he gets all of his oxygen from the mother. But after birth this oxygen supply is no longer available. Failure to breathe or respiratory depression results in a condition known as asphyxia neonatorum. If a premature delivery is expected, the mother will be encouraged to carry through her labor with a minimum amount of analgesia. Some antagonistic medications, for example, nalorphine (Nalline) and levallorphan (Lorfan), are now available to counteract the depressant action of drugs containing morphine and its derivatives on the newborn infant's respiratory system. However, doctors do not like to be forced to use them, because they may be ineffective, and occasionally they cause effects opposite from those desired and further depress the infant.

Another consideration that must be made in the adminstration of drugs during the first stage of labor is the possible effect of the medication on the progress of the labor.

Given too soon, many analgesics may unnecessarily slow down or even stop contractions. Most physicians do not wish to give any drug before approximately 4 cm. dilatation has been achieved. Many patients will not need medication prior to or even after this dilatation has been reached.

Hypnotics and amnesics: effects and side effects

Many times, more than one drug will be used to gain the desired result. For example, the analgesic meperidine hydrochloride (Demerol) and the tranquilizer hydroxyzine (Atarax) are often given together with usually excellent results. The combination makes both medications more effective than they would be if given alone.

If an amnesic or hypnotic drug is given without an analgesic in the presence of pain, great restlessness can be produced in the patient. Amnesics such as scopolamine are usually accompanied by pain-relieving drugs such as meperidine hydrochloride. Scopolamine reduces anxiety and promotes amnesia for the period of labor. It is also used because it helps to dry the oral and bronchial secretions in preparation for future inhalation anesthesia and combats vagus nerve stimulation, which can cause irregularities in the heartbeat. However, the liberal use of the drug with barbiturate hypnotics such as pentobarbital sodium (Nembutal) or, at times, analgesics may cause disorientation. Many patients so medicated do not remember their labors, but their nurses usually do. Often the patients are so restless that it is difficult to minister to their needs. They require constant supervision to avoid injury in the labor room, and many hands may be rallied to place them in position for delivery. True, the patients are spared discomfort, but they also lose much of the creative feeling of having consciously participated in the drama of labor and usually are not sufficiently alert for many hours to welcome their babies after they arrive. Still, this method of pain relief during labor is followed by a few physicians.

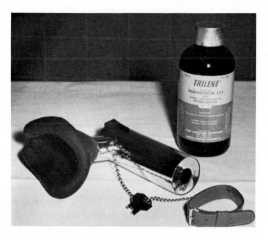

Fig. 10-1. The Duke inhaler used for self-administration of trichloroethylene (Trilene). (Courtesy Grossmont Hospital, La Mesa, Calif.)

Trichloroethylene (Trilene) inhalations (Fig. 10-1)

Occasionally, a type of inhalation analgesia that is controlled by the patient herself, is offered during the latter part of the first stage of labor. This is trichloroethylene (Trilene), a clear, blue liquid that readily assumes the form of a gas. It is placed in a cylinder that is equipped with a mask and a wrist attachment (the Duke inhaler). As the approach of a contraction is detected, the patient puts the mask to her face and breathes deeply. As the patient momentarily loses consciousness, her grip on the mask weakens, and the administration of the tricholorethylene comes to an end until needed again. The nurse should never "assist" the patient in holding the apparatus over her face because this may result in overdosage. Trichloroethylene may cause heartbeat irregularities, and it has the disadvantage of lingering in the body. A patient who has recently received it should not receive other anesthetics through a gas machine that employs soda lime to absorb carbon dioxide. Such use can cause the formation of very toxic gases. Trichloroethylene is often used in conjunction with local anesthetics, especially when trained anesthetists or anesthesiologists are not available. For the most part, inhalation therapy is restricted to use in the second stage of labor.

Obstetrical analgesia and anesthesia (second and third stages of labor)
General anesthesia

In obstetrics, a general anesthetic, if used, is typically inhaled (Fig. 10-2), although occasionally it may be administred intravenously.

Special considerations. When inhalation anesthesia is planned, it is very important to know how recently the patient has eaten because there is real danger of aspiration, obstruction of the airway (asphyxiation), and/or pneumonia. For the same reasons, it is also important to remove any gum or movable dentures from the mouth. Many gases used during anesthesia either support burning or are explosive. For this reason,

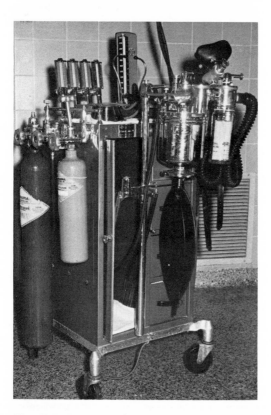

Fig. 10-2. One type of anesthetic machine. Gases commonly administered are nitrous oxide, cyclopropane, and oxygen. (Courtesy Grossmont Hospital, La Mesa, Calif.)

delivery room nurses should routinely wear conductive footwear and clothing that will not build up static electricity and cause a spark. Nylon uniforms and underwear are not allowed. All equipment in the delivery room and the floor itself must be grounded. Periodic checks for conductivity must be made. Unnecessary, purposeless movement in the delivery room is discouraged; it is confusing and a possible explosion hazard. With the exception of the anesthetist, personnel should stay away from the gas machine or locale of gas administration during a delivery, since gases are concentrated in this area. Danger of explosion is probably greatest just at emergence (the completion of gas administration). During the period when a patient is being put to sleep (the period of induction), the delivery room should be as quiet as possible to make the induction smooth without patient distraction. Undue confusion and noise should also be avoided at the time of emergence.

All inhaled anesthetics, if given in sufficient concentration, will eventually pass the placental barrier to produce symptoms in the child. Therefore, they should not be started too far in advance of the expected birth of the infant. It is said that there is usually a margin of about 8 minutes before gas passes the placental barrier. General anesthetics may be accompanied or followed by nausea and vomiting. For this reason, it is routine to give a progressing patient in labor nothing by mouth. The nurse should be prepared for such problems and not offer unrestricted amounts of fluid or any solid food too soon after delivery. In case of vomiting, the patient's head should be turned to the side. Even better, if possible, is the maintenance of a side position.

Ether and chloroform, although still used in various areas of the United States, are not often administered in a hospital obstetrical area. Other medications are more advantageous and safe, although these newer agents may necessitate more complicated equipment and more trained personnel for their administration. Anesthesia is the province of the trained physician, anesthesiologist, or nurse-anesthetist. Nurses should not attempt to function in this area without skilled advanced training. The administration of anesthesia is not a nursing function.

The gases most often used in modern obstetrics in a hospital setting are oxygen, nitrous oxide, and cyclopropane. Oxygen must always be mixed with anesthetics to supply the body needs of the mother and her unborn child.

Nitrous oxide. Nitrous oxide (laughing gas) with oxygen is often given for analgesic effect in the period of expulsion during contractions. Administered in low percentages, it relieves the mother but still allows her to bear down with her contractions. Nitrous oxide may support combustion but is nonexplosive.

Cyclopropane. Cyclopropane is a useful fast-acting gas that produces fairly good muscular relaxation and allows a high oxygen concentration with a wide margin of safety for the mother and child. However, it is extremely explosive and may produce laryngospasm and heart irregularities. The danger of explosion persists after delivery in the immediate postpartum period because the gas is expelled from the body through the respiratory tract. Therefore, smoking should not be permitted in the postpartum room of this patient after her delivery.

Regional and local anesthesia

Regional anesthetics have enjoyed considerable popularity in recent years.

Saddle block. The use of low spinal, or "saddle," anesthesia has been particularly successful. The patient is supported on the edge of the delivery table in a sitting position or lies on her side with her back arched forward. The physician, using sterile technique, inserts a long spinal needle between the vertebrae at about the level of the iliac crests. The needle tip is placed in the subarachnoid space below the spinal cord proper. Its position is identified by the appearance of cerebrospinal fluid dripping from the needle's hub. Between contractions, an anesthetic that is heavier than the

cerebrospinal fluid is injected into the subarachnoid space. Examples of anesthetics used include hexylcaine hydrochloride (Cyclaine), tetracaine hydrochloride (Pontocaine), and lidocaine (Xylocaine). The patient must be kept supported in a sitting position for 30 seconds after its instillation. She is then positioned flat on her back with only her head and shoulders elevated on two pillows. Her legs are then placed in stirrups. Such timing and positioning help localize the anesthetic at the correct level in the spinal canal (Fig. 10-3).

Low spinal, or saddle-type, anesthesia deadens the abdominal and pelvic area below the umbilicus, and it usually affects the legs and feet as well. Classically, a "saddle" is only supposed to affect those areas of the body that would be touched by a saddle if a person were riding horseback. In practice, the anesthesia is usually more extensive. It begins to take effect immediately and gains maximum potency in about 8 to 10 minutes. How long it lasts depends on the medication used (1 to 3 hours). Because of vertebral abnormalities not all women can have spinal anesthet-

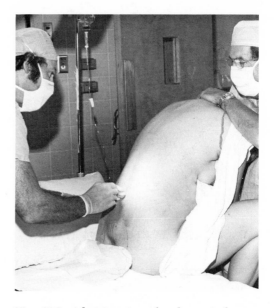

Fig. 10-3. Administration of a low spinal anesthetic. (Courtesy Grossmont Hospital, and Martin M. Greenberg, M.D., La Mesa, Calif.)

ics. A few are allergic to the type of medications usually injected. Sometimes lack of time or medical personnel able to do the lumbar puncture required precludes the use of a spinal anesthetic.

Much has been said about the aftereffects of spinal anesthesia. The so-called "spinal headache" is a complication often feared by patients. In fact, we have heard physicians counsel that the word "saddle" be used exclusively with patients because of anxiety that may have been previously built up concerning spinals. Actually, low spinal, or saddle, anesthesia does not deserve the poor reputation that it has in the minds of some members of the public. The incidence of postdelivery spinal headache has been estimated at less than 5% and is decreasing with the adoption of different techniques (for example the use of an intravenous infusion to promote better hydration of the patient and the insertion of only small-bore spinal needles to cut down on the possibility of cerebrospinal fluid leakage). Whether keeping the patient flat during the postdelivery period helps is debatable. Spinal anesthesia does entail certain other inconveniences, however. The mother must sit quietly while the procedure is carried out. This is difficult to do during the second stage of labor, even with the support of an understanding nurse. Saddle anesthesia does not stop contractions, but the patient does not feel them. She finds it difficult to push properly, and many times outlet forceps are used. Occasionally, a patient may experience a drop in blood pressure that may affect the baby's oxygen supply, or she may suffer from respiratory problems because of a high level of anesthesia. In the postpartum period the patient may find it more difficult to void spontaneously.

In the minds of many practitioners the negative aspects of this type of anesthesia are outweighed by its positive aspects. The baby is not in danger of being put to sleep by the anesthetic and of having a difficult time breathing at birth because of its action. The mother is awake. If she desires, she may see her baby born. She can hear his first cry—a real thrill. The regional anesthetics are safer than "gas" for a patient who has recently eaten, since nausea and vomiting during and after their use are minimal.

Other types of regional anesthesia. Other types of regional anesthetics are available. In considerable vogue for a time was *continuous caudal anesthesia,* or one-shot caudal, which introduces anesthetic agents into the sacral canal, where significant nerves travel outside the meninges or spinal cord coverings. In another kind called the lumbar epidural block, the drug is injected into the peridural space between the lumbar vertebrae. These types of anesthetics can be used for pain relief during the latter part of the first stage of labor as well as during the second and third stages. However, their use involves the constant attention of an anesthetist and special apparatus. Maternal hypotension, if uncorrected, may adversely affect the fetus. In the hands of the unskilled it can be dangerous, but this observation can be made of almost any nursing or medical procedure!

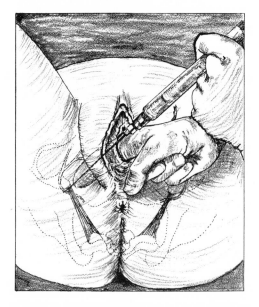

Fig. 10-4. Pudendal block using a transvaginal approach. Relaxation of the perineal muscles and anesthesia of the skin of the perineum occur in a few minutes.

Pudendal block. Local anesthesia using direct infiltration of the perineal tissues or infiltration of those local nerve centers that serve to relay sensation initiated in the perineal area to the brain is probably the safest anesthesia for both mother and baby available today. A popular technique blocks four separate nerves by infiltration of a medication into specific areas using a long needle. It may be used in conjunction with nitrous oxide very satisfactorily. It is called a *pudendal block.* With its use, an episiotomy may be performed or outlet forceps applied. However, some women do not experience the relief they desire. This technique often causes some temporary bruising of the perineum.

Paracervical block. Another type of regional anesthetic that has been used less frequently but is favored in certain cases by individual physicians is the paracervical block. Approximately 10 ml. of local anesthetic is injected into the lateral fornices of the vagina at the junctions of the vaginal wall and cervix that correspond to the 3 and 9 o'clock positions on the face of a watch. This injection, usually performed with a special needle guard to prevent inadvertent deep infiltration, interrupts the sensory impulses traveling from the uterus to the spinal cord in the paracervical area. Anesthesia relieving the discomfort of uterine contractions develops in 3 to 5 minutes and may last approximately 1 to 2 hours. However, the procedure does not anesthetize perineal tissue and in most instances is not considered sufficient in itself to meet the total needs of the patient during the second and third stages of labor.

The paracervical block may be performed in the delivery or labor room when the patient has completed a cervical dilatation of more than 4 and less than 8 cm. Most patients report considerable benefit. When properly done, the technique, barring personal idiosyncrasies to the anesthetic employed, should have no adverse effect on the mother or child. However, when injections are repeated, temporary slowing of the fetal heart rate has been reported. Fetal heart tone should be checked frequently. Maternal blood pressure should also be taken regularly to detect possible medication reactions.

EDUCATION FOR CHILDBIRTH

Modern trends in obstetrics favor a more alert patient during labor who is able to participate with dignity in her experience of childbirth. To this end there have been greater efforts made to educate the woman for her role, both psychologically and physically. Courses have been instituted to teach helpful techniques in posture, breathing, and relaxation, as well as to impart basic information to the expectant mother. Many times her husband also attends the sessions in order to better understand and aid his wife.

The late English obstetrician Dr. Grantly Dick Read probably popularized the term "natural childbirth" in his book *Childbirth Without Fear.* In his writings and lectures he stressed that much of the fear felt by mothers-to-be was caused by a lack of knowledge of what was really happening and an ensuing feeling of helplessness. He declared that fear builds tension and that tension eventually produces pain. Because of this, much of his effort was spent in educating the future mother and prescribing exercises to better fit her body for labor and delivery. He stated that "Elation, relaxation, amnesia and exultation are the four pillars of parturition upon which the conduct of labor depends."[*] All his instruction was designed to strengthen these "pillars."

In 1952 the French obstetrician Fernand Lamaze became intrigued with the labor and delivery techniques based on Pavlov's theories of conditioned response that he had observed during a visit to the Soviet Union. When he returned to Paris, he introduced "psychoprophylactic" concepts into his practice to better prepare his patients for their maternity experiences and to assist them in a conscious, rewarding partici-

---

[*]From Read, G. D.: Childbirth without fear, ed. 2, New York, 1953, Harper & Row, Publishers.

pation in the birth of their children. Much of what he emphasized was also stressed by Dr. Read. However, the relaxation taught by Dr. Lamaze is based on the principle that a high level of concentrated cerebral activity can inhibit the reception of other stimuli. That is, the mind (psycho) could be induced to prevent (prophylaxis) the reception of unpleasant and painful sensations. Using the Lamaze techniques, the patient is educated (conditioned) to respond neuromuscularly to specific verbal cues. Intense preoccupation with certain muscular tension and release patterns, respiratory movements, and massage helps to attain these goals. A specially prepared labor coach, or "monitrice," may be assigned to assist and support the patient in her efforts to utilize her training, or more often her husband fills the role.

The monitrice, if present, the patient's husband, and the entire labor-delivery room staff should work as a team for the realization of a constructive, dignified, aware, satisfying parturition. The attending nurses should be calm, cheerful, and knowledgeable concerning the aims of the techniques employed. The details of the exercises used may differ but it is helpful if the delivery room nurses acquaint themselves with the psychoprophylactic programs that may be available in their communities and how the women have been taught. The mothers so trained for labor need nursing support and encouragement. The patient needs a nurse who will enhance, not disturb, her concentration during contractions; help evaluate and aid relaxation; render sacral support or pressure as directed; share information regarding progress in labor; and be sincerely complimentary of the idealism and efforts manifested by the patient and her husband. In addition, the nurse should render the other nursing care services and watchful observation that all laboring patients require. Occasionally, symptoms of hyperventilation may be associated with some of the rapid-breathing techniques used. The patient may complain of tingling of the hands and feet, which causes her an-

noyance and loss of concentration. Slowing respirations or breathing into a paper bag helps relieve these problems. Symptoms related to hyperventilation have not been as frequent since rapid-breathing patterns have been modified to include slower acceleration and deceleration periods and shallower respirations. The absence of all forms of drug-induced analgesia or anesthesia is not a prerequisite of either the Read or Lamaze method, although this interpretation has been made. However, many patients do not use any drugs.

Those who have evaluated psychoprophylactic techniques (cared for patients who were prepared as recommended or used them themselves) usually believe they are of real value. The breathing and relaxation exercises, patterned light massage (effleurage), visual focal point, and the mental and physical conditioning that such team efforts involve represent helpful tools that many mothers can profitably employ as they face the task of childbirth. If a laboring mother decides to use other "tools" (such as analgesia, tranquilizers, or anesthetics) in addition, she should not feel herself to be a failure or guilty of "betraying a concept." She is not a competitor in a contest. She is a participant in an experience.

The main problem in using these techniques seems to be in securing enough time and personnel to adequately prepare the patient. The patient herself may find it difficult to attend instruction classes. Many people do not agree that these methods of caring for the childbearing woman are truly "natural childbirth." They look on them as "intensive education and preparation for childbirth." Some patients respond very well to the conditioning offered; others have personal histories or personality structures that make constructive participation in labor and delivery such as Read and Lamaze recommended very difficult or impossible. Both methods are advised only for those undergoing a normal labor and delivery. For those qualified candidates able to seek out a sympathetic practitioner and to undertake the intensive preparation involved, such a management of labor and delivery can bring many enduring rewards, not the least of which is a characteristically noisy, pink, new member of the family.

More information regarding childbirth education can be obtained from the American Society of Psychoprophylaxis in Obstetrics (ASPO), P.O. Box 17186, Charlotte, North Carolina, 28211, or the International Childbirth Education Association, ICEA Secretary, P.O. Box 5852, Milwaukee, Wisconsin, 53220.

Hypnosis and acupuncture

No discussion of obstetrical analgesia and anesthesia can be undertaken without mentioning the possibilities of hypnosis and acupuncture. Admittedly the possibilities exist for the use of hypnotic suggestion in obstetrics, but little scientific research has been done in the field. It appears that candidates for hypnosis need to be selected carefully in order to avoid occasional untoward psychological reactions. More experience and training are needed before hypnosis can be evaluated as a method of pain relief in obstetrics. Limited experimentation with acupuncture for obstetrical patients in the United States has been carried out at the University of California, San Francisco, with mixed results.* Certainly these two approaches to pain relief are fascinating topics and may one day be more than subjects of conversation.

From the foregoing it must be evident to the reader that no perfect means of pain relief applicable to all patients and situations has been found. But it is also clear that the physician has at his disposal many agents of worth, which, when used judiciously and backed up by good nursing care, will assist the patient tremendously.

---

*Shearer, M. H.: Obstetrical acupuncture, Birth and Fam. J. 1:14-18, Spring, 1974.

unit four
Suggested selected readings and references

Babies have fathers, too, Am. J. Nurs. 71:1980-1981, Oct., 1971.

Bond, S.: Reevaluating positions for labor—lateral vs. supine, J. Obstet. Gynecol. Neonatal Nurs. 2:29-31, Nov.-Dec., 1973.

Case, L. L.: Ultrasound monitoring of mother and fetus, Am. J. Nurs. 72:725-727, April, 1972.

Cassidy, J. E.: A nurse looks at childbirth anxiety, J. Obstet. Gynecol. Neonatal Nurs. 3:52-54, Jan.-Feb., 1974.

Clark, L.: Introducing mother and baby, Am. J. Nurs. 74:1483-1484, Aug., 1974.

Edwards, M. E.: Unattended home births, Am. J. Nurs. 73:1332-1335, Aug., 1973.

Estey, G. P.: Natural childbirth—word from a mother, Am. J. Nurs. 69:1453-1454, July, 1969.

Fleming, G.: Delivering a happy father, Am. J. Nurs. 72:949, May, 1972.

Friedman, D. D.: Childbirth education for the adolescent, Birth and Fam. J. 1:11-13, Spring, 1974.

Gause, R. W.: Multiple pregnancies: diagnosis, delivery and problems of development, J. Obstet. Gynecol. Neonatal Nurs. 1:22-26, Sept.-Oct., 1972.

Greiss, F. C., Jr.: Obstetric anesthesia, Am. J. Nurs. 71:67-69, Jan., 1971.

Howard, R. E., and Marie, Sr. J.: Initial experience with a prepared childbirth program, J. Obstet. Gynecol. Neonatal Nurs. 1:30-34, Sept.-Oct., 1972.

Hutchinson, S., and Shemdin, M. A.: Anxiety, ecstasy, and the nurse's role, RN 34:36-39+, Nov., 1971.

Kopp, L. M.: Ordeal or ideal—the second stage of labor, Am. J. Nurs. 71:1140-1143, June, 1971.

Lasater, C.: Electronic monitoring of mother and fetus, Am. J. Nurs. 72:728-730, April, 1972.

Lerch, C.: Maternity nursing, ed. 2, St. Louis, 1974, The C. V. Mosby Co., pp. 177-210.

O'Neill, S. K.: Childbirth by the book, RN 36:42-44, July, 1973.

Petty, C.: No more home deliveries! RN 35:42-43+, Oct., 1972.

Preparation for childbearing, ed. 4, New York, 1972, Maternity Center Association.

Rice, G. T.: Recognition and treatment of intrapartal fetal distress, J. Obstet. Gynecol. Neonatal Nurs. 1:15-22, July-Aug., 1972.

Rich, O. J.: How does the patient use the nurse during labor? In Duffy, M., Anderson, E. H., Bergersen, B. S., Lohr, M., and Rose, J. H., editors: Current concepts in clinical nursing, vol. 3, St. Louis, 1971, The C. V. Mosby Co.

Rising, S. S.: The fourth stage of labor, Am. J. Nurs. 74:870-874, May, 1974.

Russin, A. W., and others: Electronic monitoring of the fetus, Am. J. Nurs. 74:1294-1299, July, 1974.

Sasmor, J. L.: Stress adaptation: a theory for childbirth education, J. Obstet. Gynecol. Neonatal Nurs. 2:48-50, Nov.-Dec., 1973.

Sasmor, J. L., Castor, C. R., and Hassid, P.: The childbirth team during labor, Am. J. Nurs. 73: 444-447, March, 1973.

Shearer, M. H.: Fetal monitoring: do the benefits outweigh the drawbacks? Birth and Fam. J. 1:12-18, Winter, 1973-74.

Shearer, M. H.: Obstetrical acupuncture, Birth and Fam. J. 1:14-18, Spring, 1974.

Smith, B. A., Robert, M. P., and Mona, K. S.: The transition phase of labor, Am. J. Nurs. 73:448-450, March, 1973.

Wright, W. C.: Continuous lumbar epidural block for labor and delivery, Contemp. OB/GYN 3: 111-114, Feb., 1974.

Complications associated with pregnancy and delivery

11

Minor problems of pregnancy

Once upon a time there was a French obstetrician named Mauriceau who declared that pregnancy was a disease of 9 months' duration. Although today we do not like the term "disease" applied to normal pregnancy, a number of minor discomforts may be associated with this period of waiting. Some were mentioned in Chapter 7. Now let us take a more detailed look at those discomforts and others not previously discussed.

Digestive difficulties

Nausea and vomiting. Probably the first discomfort noted by many pregnant women is nausea and vomiting—particularly in the morning, although it may occur at any time. Remember that it is a presumptive signal of pregnancy. This temporary condition is experienced by approximately 60% of pregnant women in the first trimester. It is said to be linked with the great hormonal changes in the body at the onset of pregnancy or a decreased glycogen reserve. Emotional factors may also enter into the cause and effect relationship. The most successful preventative seems to be eating more frequent small meals instead of three rather large meals as is our custom. Liquids are tolerated better if taken between, instead of with, meals. Eating something dry and high in carbohydrate value, like a few crackers or a piece of toast, before getting up also seems to help. Some physicians

may prescribe certain gastrointestinal tranquilizers that are also commonly used to combat motion sickness on boats and planes—medications such as dimenhydrinate (Dramamine). However, any use of medication by a pregnant woman must be carefully evaluated for need and closely supervised. Some medications may affect fetal development adversely. If the nausea persists and becomes severe, threatening the nutrition of the mother, then it is considered a rather serious complication called *hyperemesis gravidarum,* and it may necessitate hospitalization, the administration of intravenous feedings, and perhaps in some cases psychiatric counseling.

Other digestive complaints may be voiced by the pregnant woman, and considering the compression of the internal organs caused by the growth of the fetus, plus the hormonal changes in her body, it should not be surprising that such complaints may occur.

Heartburn. Heartburn, or *pyrosis,* an uncomfortable burning sensation felt behind the sternum often accompanied by gas and acid regurgitation into the esophagus, has nothing to do with the heart. It only feels that way. Heartburn becomes more common as pregnancy advances and is thought to be related to decreased peristalsis and the pressure of the growing fetus. For this reason, lying flat directly after eating is not recommended. Since the ingestion of fat in-

127

hibits the secretion of stomach acid, a small amount of butter or cream taken about 20 minutes *before* eating and at the onset of nausea may be considered. It can also be prevented or lessened if gas-forming foods, such as cabbage, cauliflower, Brussels sprouts, onions, cucumbers, radishes, turnips, and dried beans, are avoided. More frequent, smaller, leisurely meals are also recommended. With the physician's approval, an antacid such as Maalox (a mixture of magnesium and aluminum hydroxides) may be used.

Constipation. Constipation may also be a problem, especially if the woman has had such difficulty before pregnancy. Four things may help: a diet that includes plenty of roughage, abundant fluids, regular exercise, and a consistent time of day set aside for evacuation when she does not have to

hurry. Mild laxatives may also be used, but an expectant mother should check with her doctor regarding the type and frequency of such medication. Taking a laxative is one way labor might be initiated.

Circulatory difficulties

Varicosities. Many pregnant women suffer from *varicosities*, also called varices, or varicose veins. They most often occur in the lower extremities and rectal area but may also occasionally involve the vulva and groin. These are surface veins, the walls of which are thin and greatly enlarged. They may appear as a swollen, purple, knotted network just under the skin. The affected lower extremities tire easily. The swollen veins may be more than a cosmetic problem, since occasionally they may be injured, rupture, and bleed or become

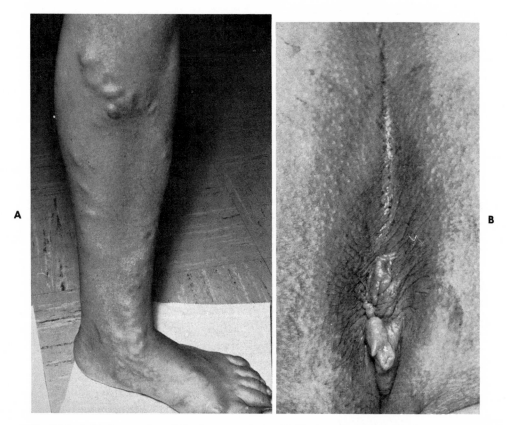

A

B

Fig. 11-1. **A,** Varicose veins of the lower extremity. **B,** Varicosities of the rectal area (hemorrhoids). (Courtesy Mercy Hospital and Medical Center, San Diego, Calif.)

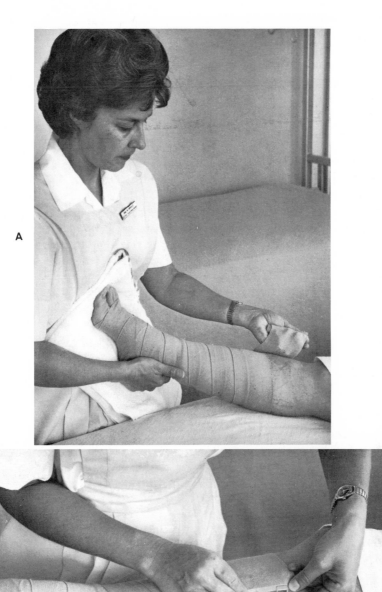

Fig. 11-2. **A,** When elastic bandage is put around the lower leg, even tension is desired. **B,** Two types of fasteners are shown.

the point of origin for a blood clot, or thrombus. Most patients find relief by the application of elastic stockings or bandages that give the legs support and stimulate return circulation to the heart. If elastic bandages are used, they should be applied from the footup, with an even tension, in order not to become in themselves obstructions to circulation. Ideally they are applied after the patient has had her legs elevated several minutes to drain the swollen veins. Because of mechanical interference in the return circulation of blood by the growing fetus, edema of the legs is fairly common in late pregnancy. Swelling and fatigue will be less if the pregnant woman can avoid standing for protracted periods and especially if she can lie down at intervals and elevate her feet above the level of her head. Round garters should never be worn. Pooling of the blood in the lower part of the body plus dilatation of the surface blood vessels may be one cause of the faintness experienced by many expectant mothers (Figs. 11-1 and 11-2).

Hemorrhoids. Rectal varicosities are termed "hemorrhoids." They may be external or internal. They are produced or aggravated by the pressure of the developing fetus and/or constipation. They can be quite painful and occasionally become thrombosed or bleed. Most of the time surgical treatment is not contemplated during pregnancy, because the condition usually disappears or vastly improves after delivery. Attention should be paid to the prevention of constipation. Witch hazel compresses or analgesic ointments such as dibucaine (Nupercainal) may help. Warm water sitz baths may also aid.

Muscle cramps

Muscle cramps are often experienced during pregnancy; they usually involve the calf muscle and can be agonizing. They are said to result from an imbalance in calcium and phosphorus in the body causing a form of *tetany.* Immediate treatment consists of straightening the leg by pushing down on the knee and pushing the ball of the foot

up toward the knee. Preventive therapy includes increased calcium intake in the form of calcium lactate or gluconate with increased vitamin D intake. Some physicians using this regimen may limit the woman's intake of milk because of its high phosphorus content. Others will continue to recommend a quart of milk per day but prescribe small quantities of aluminum hydroxide gel (Amphojel) in the diet to prevent the assimilation of excess phosphorus into the body.

Leukorrhea

Increased mucoid vaginal drainage found in pregnancy is caused by the increased activity of the cervical glands. However, profuse, white, cream-colored, or yellowish foul-smelling drainage or vulvar itching or burning is abnormal and should be checked by the physician. A number of conditions can cause such a discharge, which is called *leukorrhea.*

Trichomonas vaginalis. Trichomonas vaginalis, a microscopic animal, is a common cause of leukorrhea. This organism may inhabit the vaginal canal without causing noticeable symptoms. However, during pregnancy the changes in the pH, or acidity-alkalinity, of the vagina may cause *Trichomonas vaginalis* to multiply rapidly and create annoying signs and symptoms. Typically these are an irritating, profuse, yellow vaginal discharge and vulvar itching or burning. The motile organism may be identified under the microscope in a hanging drop slide or occasionally by culture methods. *Trichomonas* is quite difficult to combat locally because of the structure of the vaginal folds, and many types of treatment have been attempted. However, metronidazole (Flagyl) in oral or suppository form has been quite successfully prescribed, though some authorities do not recommend it during the first trimester of pregnancy and urge "discretion" in its use. Infected husbands should be treated as well.

Candida albicans. Monilia albicans, or *Candida albicans* as it is more commonly called now, is another cause of leukorrhea.

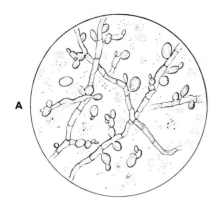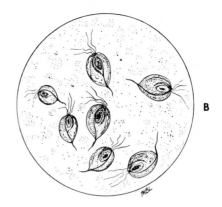

Fig. 11-3. Microscopic views. **A,** *Candida (Monilia) albicans,* a fungus. **B,** *Trichomonas vaginalis,* a protozoon, or microscopic animal.

This organism is a fungus or yeast and is quite easily diagnosed by direct microscopic examination of the discharge or by culture techniques (Fig. 11-3). A *Candida* vaginal infection produces a cheesy, whitish discharge and local irritation. Like *Trichomonas, Candida albicans* can inhabit the body without any apparent signs or symptoms being produced, but under certain conditions (especially with the use of broad-spectrum antibiotics) it may spread tremendously. The old remedy consisted of locally applying 1% gentian violet. The antibiotic nystatin has proved quite effective. It is given to prevent monilial overgrowth when broad-spectrum antibiotics are prescribed or to treat a current infection. The relationship of *Candida albicans* and thrush is discussed in Chapter 15.

Gonorrhea. It should not be forgotten that gonorrhea is still, unfortunately, an important disease in the community. Its incidence is increasing, particularly in the younger age groups. Profuse, purulent, yellow or greenish yellow vaginal drainage may signal the presence of the causative gonococcus. Particularly characteristic in such an instance is the involvement of the urethra, causing painful voiding. Gonorrhea may be cured by doses of penicillin or sulfonamide drugs. Sterility (caused by inflammation of the fallopian tubes) or even a threat to the patient's life because of a more widespread infection may be the result of poor or in-

adequate treatment. The disease confers no immunity and may be contracted repeatedly. The danger of blindness in the newborn infant of an infected mother has been discussed on p. 108.

Other causes. Leukorrhea may also be a symptom of the presence of cervical pathology such as polyps (fleshy growths), inflammation, and, occasionally, malignant changes. It can also be seen as a result of foreign body irritation in the vaginal tract.

Douching. Occasionally, as part of the treatment of leukorrhea, careful douching is advised if the pregnancy is not of more than 5 months' duration. If such advice is given (it should be given only by a physician), the nurse should be able to help the patient by giving more detailed or repeated instructions. Many times women are hesitant or embarrassed to admit they would like more information about the technique of douching. Some may not realize that they are not proceeding properly. Following are some factors that should be mentioned:

1. A fountain-type syringe with bag, tubing, and curved plastic or hard-rubber tip should be used. A bulb syringe is not efficient in treating the vaginal mucosa, and cases of air embolism introduced by the use of the bulb during pregnancy, although rare, have been reported in the literature.

2. All equipment should be personal and clean.
3. The douche is probably more effective if done in a reclining position in the bathtub or on a bedpan, but it can also be done on the toilet. It should be administered only under low pressure. The bag should be no more than 18 inches above the hips.
4. Before douching, the external genitalia should be carefully washed so that organisms are not introduced into the vagina during the procedure. Care should be taken to wash first the genitalia and then the rectal area to avoid contamination.
5. The solution ordered should be warm but not hot. If powder or crystals are to be added to water to make the solution, they should be added and mixed in a container other than the douche can or bag to assure uniform distribution. One to two quarts of solution are needed.
6. The air should be expelled from the tubing before insertion.
7. The douche tip should be lubricated with water or water-soluble jelly. Insertion of the douche tip should be *down* and *back* to follow the angle of the vaginal canal if the patient is in modified dorsal lithotomy position (legs flexed and pulled up slightly toward the chest, with the knees dropped toward the outside). The douche tip should be inserted no more than 3 inches. The labia may be closed around the douche nozzle, if the solution is retained, only until there is a slight feeling of distention. The solution should be allowed to escape intermittently, four or five times during the procedure to protect against excessive pressure.
8. The irrigation usually takes about 5 minutes. Afterward all equipment, including the tub, if used, should be carefully cleaned.

12

Major problems of pregnancy and delivery

HIGH-RISK PREGNANCIES

Certain characteristics or conditions of the prospective mother or her child cause situations of jeopardy. Some of these can be detected at the onset or shortly after the beginning of a gestation. Such pregnancies are termed "high risk." Examples of high-risk pregnancies include: unmarried young girls (less than 18 years of age); women bearing their first child, twins, or having had more than 4 children; members of poor socioeconomic groups; women who have had difficult obstetrical histories; and those who have coincidental illnesses (for example, diabetes, heart or renal disease) or problems particularly associated with their pregnant state, such as toxemia. Some of these patients are being referred to regional obstetrical intensive care centers where specialists and sophisticated equipment are available. These centers are commonly associated with high-risk or special care nurseries capable of caring for the endangered newborn in the best manner possible. The maternal, fetal, and infant mortality for many of these conditions have improved with the use of these facilities.

Diabetes mellitus

Glucose in the urine during pregnancy is not always a symptom of diabetes but should always be evaluated. Diabetic mothers need special care in meeting their metabolic requirements and in controlling their disease. Insulin requirements during pregnancy often fluctuate. In early pregnancy the need for insulin may decrease slightly, but generally, more insulin is needed. Periodic fasting and 2-hour postmeal blood glucose level examinations help monitor control. The most common cause of fetal death associated with this disease is maternal diabetic acidosis.

A large proportion of diabetic mothers develop toxemia. They are more likely to have large babies and mechanical problems in the passage of their children. Placental insufficiency, perhaps related to degenerative vascular changes associated with diabetes, may cause the increase in births of stillborn and premature babies and hydramnios encountered by these patients. Bed rest is many times recommended after the thirty-fourth week to improve intrauterine blood flow. The response of the fetal heart to the trial administration of oxytocin (oxytocin stress test) can also be of help in deciding when termination of the pregnancy should be planned. Diminished placental function may be detected during pregnancy through periodic serial evaluations of the amount of estriol in a 24-hour urine specimen. If tests of fetal lung maturity (L/S ratio or foam test) show that the danger of respiratory distress syndrome (RDS) is minimal or past, the physician may elect to try to initiate labor before term or perform a cesarean section, depending on the individual case involved. Children of diabetic mothers are more likely to suffer from RDS because, despite their relatively heavy birth weights, they are often immature. After birth, these infants frequently show symptoms of lowered glucose level (hypoglycemia) probably due to overactive pancreatic function initiated in utero because of a high glucose environment. Congenital defects are more common in these infants. For a more detailed discussion of diabetes, the reader is referred to the pediatric section of this book.

Cardiac problems

Patients with cardiac disease are also individually evaluated to determine their capacity to tolerate a vaginal or abdominal delivery. They should be watched for any sign of possible heart failure. Such signals include increasing shortness of breath, cough, and rapid pulse.

Urinary problems

The pregnant patient with urinary tract disease is a real challenge to medical management, especially when kidney function is impaired. Pregnancy in itself puts a strain on the urinary system. The developing uterus may pinch or kink the ureters (particularly the one on the right because of the usual location of the uterus). Stoppage of normal urinary flow predisposes the system to infection (pyelonephritis). Infections are often caused by colon bacilli, but other organisms may also be responsible. If the kidneys are already damaged by previous pathology, the added load imposed by the excretion of fetal waste may be significant. Infection of the kidney may manifest itself in several ways: chills and fever, lower back pain, pain on voiding, as well as a urinalysis characterized by the presence of numerous white blood cells, bacteria, and, in more severe cases, perhaps red blood cells and albumin. Infection of the kidney usually responds well to such measures as bed rest, forced fluids, the application of heat to the lower back, and some type of antibiotic therapy. When hospitalized, these patients are routinely on intake and output and have frequent blood pressure and daily weight determinations. Daily urinalysis is often ordered. Not all urinary tract or kidney disease is infectious. If it is, it is not always contagious in the usual sense. Many patients do not need isolation precautions to protect others. They themselves, however, must be protected from respiratory infections that may worsen their condition. Renal disease may be inflammatory or degenerative. It is closely connected with the condition of the blood supply to the kidneys, and any continuous process that interferes with this supply will, in time, present symptoms. Conversely, any significant damage to the kidney will reflect itself in a change in the circulatory system, particularly an elevation of the blood pressure as more and more pressure is exerted in an attempt to maintain adequate filtrations. The onset of significant hypertension is related to a worsening prognosis for both the fetus and mother. Patients whose renal disease is not caused by a current infection (for example, those suffering from glomerulonephritis) receive much the same nursing care as those with a diagnosed bacterial invasion, and antibiotics are often given prophylactically. Chronic or advanced renal disease should be frequently evaluated by renal function tests. It may pose a real threat to both the mother and her unborn child.

Syphilis

Many states, although not all, require a premarital blood test to detect syphilis. A complete prenatal examination always includes a serological test for detection of syphilis, although the results may occasionally render false negatives or positives. At one time it was believed that the problem of syphilis had been largely solved because of these precautions and the successful introduction of the antibiotics in its treatment. Many so-called L clinics, so named for *lues,* another name for syphilis, were closed. Education of the public and the related necessary casework regarding the venereal diseases (principally syphilis and gonorrhea), which were responding so well to penicillin therapy, were not continued with the same diligence. Health workers were then very much concerned to find that national morbidity for syphilis had risen sharply. The reported cases of gonorrhea had also increased alarmingly. These increases were caused in part by the ill-founded sense of security regarding venereal disease and the cutbacks in federal, state, and local budgets helping in its control. They were also symptoms of the growing lack of purpose, restlessness, family breakdown, and moral laxity and resulting promiscuity, which have unhappily become major problems of twentieth century society.

Transmission. It should also be understood, however, that not all persons with a diagnosis of syphilis have been guilty of irresponsible conduct. The infectious agent, a corkscrewlike organism, or spirochete, called *Treponema pallidum* may also infect the innocent. A blameless marriage partner may contract the disease. The organism invades microscopic breaks in the mucous membranes. A fetus is susceptible to the mother's disease after the beginning of the fifth month of pregnancy. Up to that time a placental barrier exists that protects the fetus. Syphilis may be acquired through accidental inoculation by contaminated needles or exposure to infectious skin lesions on the part of professional personnel or other contacts, but this later source of infection is rare. The infective organism cannot live for more than a few hours in an environment deprived of moisture, and it is destroyed by drying. It is also killed by many chemicals, including soap.

Stages. The disease is divided into three different stages of development or progression. The first stage or period of initial body response usually manifests itself from 10 days to 10 weeks after exposure. The average time is 3 weeks. The characteristic lesion of the first stage of the disease is a relatively hard, raised, painless area crowned by a craterlike depression found at the area of entry known as a *chancre*. This lesion is not always seen, however. Sometimes it seems to be actually absent. At other times it is present but hidden from view in the folds of the vaginal or urethral canals. Rarely, the chancre may develop on the lips or breast. The chancre is highly infectious. The spirochete may be identified in its secretions in dark-field microscopic studies. However, at this time the serology test is usually negative. The chancre disappears after 3 to 8 weeks. The uninformed victim may think that the prob-

lem has also disappeared, but such is not the way of syphilis. The organisms have been multiplying and spreading throughout the body. Usually not long after the chancre vanishes, the patient discovers other difficulties, and their advent signals the beginning of the second stage of the infection.

The second stage of syphilis is characterized by a bronze or rose-colored rash often called *rose spots.* Flattened, moist, wartlike lesions called *mucous patches,* or *condylomata lata,* may also appear on the skin and mucous membranes. These are very infectious, containing the spirochete. The patient does not feel well and may have headache, sore throat, and aching joints and muscles. There may be spotty loss of hair. These signs and symptoms may, after several weeks, fade away never to return in the same way, or they may reappear at irregular intervals for a period up to 3 to 4 years. During the second stage of syphilis the serology test is routinely positive.

The third stage of the disease may occur anywhere from 2 to 20 years after the initial contact with the spirochete. Although the disease is present, it may produce no visible symptoms. About 20% of those patients in the tertiary stage do develop widespread serious disorders that interfere greatly with life. Soft tumors called *gummas* develop in the tissues and may ulcerate or form abscesses. Vital centers such as the brain, spinal cord, large blood vessels, and heart are often damaged. There may be gastrointestinal symptoms. A patient may become mentally ill; such mental illness is called *generalized paresis.* He may be unable to walk normally because of central nervous system disease, and he has a typical body-jarring gait. The patient is usually not infectious at this stage. Routinely the serology test is positive. Adequate treatment with penicillin in the first or second stages brings an optimistic prognosis. Results of treatment in the third stage are questionable.

Congenital syphilis. The prenatal serology examination has been quite successful in warding off congenital syphilis by establishing treatment before the infant is affected. Some physicians repeat these blood tests later in pregnancy to combat developing infection and fetal damage. The disease may be prevented prenatally by treating the affected mother for syphilis before the eighteenth week of pregnancy.

The syphilitic baby may not be delivered alive. The untreated syphilitic mother characteristically has a high abortion rate. If born alive, the innocent child may suffer from various problems. Probably the most common characteristic of the syphilitic infant is the presence of a thick, almost continuous, sometimes blood-tinged nasal discharge associated with a sniffling sound on respiration. For this reason the manifestation is called "snuffles." The skin, especially over the palms of the hands and soles of the feet, may be blistered and peeling. There may be sore fissures around the lips and anus. The joints are sometimes very tender. The liver and spleen are usually enlarged. The causative organism has been found in some of the skin lesions and such a syphilitic infant should be isolated. Fortunately such full-blown cases of congenital syphilis are not common now in the United States. Other more permanent but later appearing signs of the one-time presence of congenital syphilis are notched teeth, "Hutchinson's teeth," and a so-called saddle nose. Penicillin is again the drug of choice in the treatment of congenital syphilis.

Gonorrhea

Gonorrhea is the most common venereal infection. In fact, it is the most common contagious disease. (See p. 523, Fig. 33-3.) In many communities it has now reached epidemic proportions, particularly among the teen-age and young adult population. Many city and county health departments accept minors for free venereal disease diagnosis and treatment confidentially, without parental consent, relying on their right under law to care for persons of all ages suffering from communicable diseases.

However, not all states have laws that permit private and hospital physicians to treat minors for venereal disease without parental consent. Gonorrhea is caused by a coffee bean–shaped diplococcus, *Neisseria gonorrhoeae*. In females it typically produces an irritating purulent vaginal discharge and, since it often infects the Skene glands, may initiate burning on urination. The disease may spread up the reproductive tract and bring inflammatory changes. It may cause abnormal narrowing of the fallopian tubes and may be responsible finally for ectopic pregnancy (a pregnancy that develops outside the normal uterine placement) or sterility. In males it generally produces a urethral irritation or discharge. However, asymptomatic carriers of either sex are possible. Gonorrhea may also become a more generalized infection spread through the bloodstream and lymphatic system. It is not innocuous, occasionally causing serious complications, spreading abscesses, arthritis, and other inflammations in both sexes. It responds well to treatment with sulfonamides or penicillin. Gonorrhea may be contracted by common use of infected articles such as towels, clothing, or bathroom fixtures. These are the means by which some children may acquire a gonorrheal vaginitis. Infection of the eyes through contact at birth or later is a real possibility. Prophylactic newborn eye care is a legal requirement in most states because of this possibility.

Rubella

German, or 3-day measles, technically known as *rubella*, is in itself a rather mild disease, but it has a deservedly bad reputation associated with pregnancy. If an expectant mother develops the disease in the first trimester (3 months) of her pregnancy or even soon thereafter, it is possible that her infant will be seriously damaged by the causative virus' action on the fragile developing fetal tissues. The effect of the disease on the baby is influenced by the time of its onset. The disease can cause heart defects, congenital cataracts, deafness, mental retardation, bone diseases, and blood abnormalities. Young girls have been counseled in the past to purposely expose themselves to rubella before marriage in order to reduce the risk of fetal complications during pregnancy. Now a safe and effective vaccine against the rubella virus is available. It has been used chiefly to immunize preschool and school-age children. This procedure will substantially reduce the number of susceptible persons remaining in the population who may serve as a reservoir of the virus for another outbreak. Immunization of adult women is not now recommended unless there is no possibility of pregnancy, since the vaccine's effect on an undetected embryo or fetus is unknown. The susceptibility of a woman to rubella can be tested by a blood test that measures antibody formation. In some states this test has been made a requirement for marriage licensure. Infants who have been infected with the disease are themselves infective and should be isolated.

Tuberculosis

Tuberculosis, although not as common as formerly, is still a maternal-child health problem because the disease may be worsened by pregnancy and postpartum demands, and it may be contracted fairly easily by the newborn infant. Rarely, cases of infection of the fetus have been reported. A pregnant woman with tuberculosis should be under close medical supervision. Drug therapy and newer surgical techniques have made the outlook for tuberculosis patients much more optimistic. As a rule, gas anesthetics at the time of delivery are avoided. The infected mother should not breast-feed her infant because of his great susceptibility to the disease.

DISEASES ASSOCIATED WITH PREGNANCY

The following complications are so grouped because they are of major importance and are associated only with pregnancy, labor, and delivery. They are not always preventable or predictable.

Hemorrhagic complications

The threat of hemorrhage is a very real consideration during all periods of pregnancy, delivery, and even postpartum. In the months of gestation, vaginal bleeding is always considered a potential menace to both the fetus and the mother. Hemorrhage, you will remember, is the most common complication of pregnancy.

Abortion

Spotting or bleeding during the early months is usually related to *abortion*, defined as loss of the fetus before viability. It does not in itself imply any illegal proceedings.

Types. Abortions may be *spontaneous,* without any premeditation (called miscarriages by the public), or they may be *induced.* Most communities identify two types of induced abortion: legal abortions, which are done with the consent of society after medical consultation, and criminal abortions, which have no legal sanction. The problem of criminal abortion is one of the factors that has brought about a change in the laws governing legalized abortion.

Other terminology is also used in describing an abortion. Physicians and nurses often use the adjectives "threatened" and "inevitable." A *threatened abortion* may possibly be halted. It may declare itself by uterine cramping or intermittent backache and spotting, but the loss of blood is relatively small, and the cervical opening remains closed. An *inevitable abortion* is characterized by severe or persistent contractions, moderate to abundant blood loss, and dilatation of the cervix. Loss of the fetus cannot be prevented. An *incomplete abortion* refers to the retention of some of the products of conception, most commonly a portion of the placenta. The uterus usually must be emptied by a mechanical dilatation of the cervix and gentle scraping of its walls by a curet. Such a procedure is called a dilatation and curettage, or "D and C." If it must take place at all, a *complete abortion* is desirable. In the case of a complete abortion, all the products of the pregnancy are eliminated from the uterus. Usually patients with the diagnosis of threatened or inevitable abortion are admitted to the gynecological service. However, if the viability of the fetus is debatable, the patient may be placed on the obstetrical service.

Women who have lost more than three pregnancies at about the same stage of development are said to be victims of *habitual abortion*. Sometimes a very young fetus will die in the uterus and remain there 2 months or longer before it is expelled, either through spontaneous processes or medical or surgical intervention. Such a situation is declared a *missed abortion*. In such cases the placenta usually remains attached to the uterine wall for an extended period of time, and the amniotic fluid is gradually absorbed, producing a type of fetal mummification or even petrification.

Nursing care. The nursing care of a woman diagnosed as having a nontherapeutic abortion would routinely include bed rest; observation for uterine cramping and loss of amniotic fluid; temperature, pulse, and blood pressure records; careful determination of the presence and amount of vaginal bleeding (the physician may wish all pads and soiled linen saved to evaluate the extent of blood loss); and watchfulness to secure any passed tissue for diagnosis. Periodic checks for fetal heart tone should be performed if the fetus is over 4½ months' gestation. Vigilance for an elevation of temperature should be maintained. Orders would probably include hemoglobin and hematocrit checks, sedation, and hormonal therapy, depending on the condition of the patient. The use of progesterone may help maintain the pregnancy. Iron medication or blood transfusions may be indicated. Antibiotics may be employed. Inevitable abortion may be speeded by the use of drugs (oxytocics) to stimulate the uterus to contract or by surgical intervention, especially in the presence of hemorrhage. A patient who aborts must continue to be closely observed for complications for several hours or days, depending on her general condition and the circumstances of her loss.

About 50% of all threatened abortions terminate as abortions. A large percentage of such fetal loss is associated with some defect in the developing child. Spontaneous abortion seems to be one way that nature tries to rectify a basic error.

The nursing care of a patient undergoing a voluntary legal abortion in the hospital setting will be determined by the condition of the patient, the length of her pregnancy, and the method used by the physician to terminate her pregnancy. Termination may be secured by dilatation and curettage, aspiration techniques, or intra-amniotic saline injections. (See Chapter 14.)

Nurses caring for patients receiving hypertonic intra-amniotic salt injections should observe their patients carefully for signs of saline injection into the bloodstream: localized burning or painful sensations, thirst, nausea and vomiting, and excessive blood sodium levels revealed by mental confusion, changes in the level of consciousness, and shock. Resuscitation equipment should be readily available.

Because of recent changes in the interpretation and content of abortion laws, nurses working in gynecological, delivery, and operating room areas may be requested more frequently to assist in the process of legal abortion. If the scruples of a nurse would dictate that she not participate, she may decline her services if by so doing she is not jeopardizing the immediate health or life of a mother (for example, she could secure another nurse to assist for whom abortion did not pose the same ethical problem). However, the nurse who declines to participate may be risking the loss of her employment.

Ectopic pregnancy

The term "ectopic pregnancy" refers to any pregnancy that does not occupy the uterine cavity proper. In the vast majority of pregnancies the migrating egg is fertilized by the sperm in the fallopian tube and nests or implants rather high on the walls of the uterine cavity. However, because of the anatomy and physiology involved, this progression does not always occur. Sometimes the tubes are abnormally narrow. This narrowing, or stenosis, may occur because of inflammation or tumor formation, or it may be congenital in origin. The tube may allow the sperm to ascend but be too narrow to allow the passage of the fertil-

ized egg into the uterus. The egg may develop in the tube and cause rupture or eventually drop out the end to perish. In rare cases, it may continue growing as an abdominal pregnancy, which in unusual cases produces a full-term child who may survive if delivered through an abdominal incision. Pregnancies have also been found trying to develop in the ovary. The danger

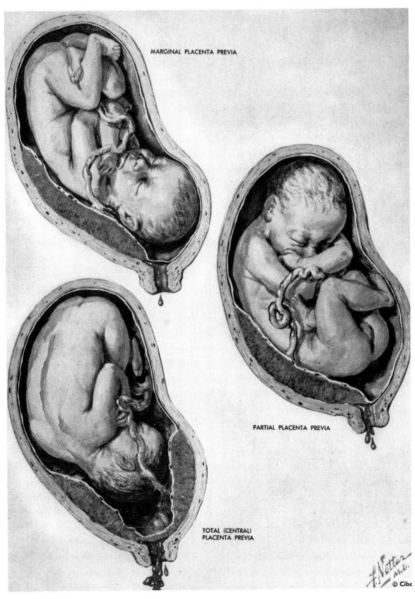

Fig. 12-1. Placenta previa. (From The CIBA collection of medical illustrations, by Frank H. Netter, M.D. Copyright CIBA.)

of hemorrhage in ectopic pregnancy is very serious. The amount of vaginal bleeding observed does not always reveal the true condition of the patient, since much blood loss can be hidden within the abdominal cavity. An ectopic pregnancy is most often tubal. There is a higher incidence of ectopic pregnancies associated with failure of intrauterine contraceptive devices.

Symptoms. If tubal rupture or abortion occurs, the patient, who may or may not consider herself to be in early pregnancy, characteristically suffers severe knifelike pain in either lower abdominal quadrant. This may or may not be followed by spotting or bleeding.

The signs of shock that develop are out of proportion to the amount of blood loss apparent. The patient may exhibit the classic signs of circulatory shock: pallor; cold, clammy skin; rapid, weak pulse, which will slow if shock deepens; falling blood pressure (a systolic reading of 90 or under is usually considered "shock" depending on previous readings obtained); apprehension; loss of consciousness; and dilated pupils. Rapid surgical treatment and blood loss replacement are usually indicated. Estimates vary, but ectopic pregnancy is more common than usually supposed, occurring approximately once in 200 to 250 pregnancies. It terminates almost invariably with fetal loss, and the maternal mortality is alarmingly high.

Placenta previa

Two main types of obstetrical hemorrhage are associated with the location of the placenta and its attachment. In the condition known as *placenta previa,* the placenta implants low on the interior of the uterine wall. It may cover or impinge on the cervical opening. In the latter part of pregnancy, the uterine contractions, which are always taking place to some degree although they are not always felt by the mother, may loosen the attachment of this abnormally positioned placenta and cause bright red, painless bleeding. The presence of placenta previa in other cases may not

be detected until the onset of true labor and the dilatation of the cervical canal. Because of the relative safety of cesarean section today, it is usually the treatment of choice. However, if the placenta is not implanted too low, bleeding is minimal, and the fetus is well but premature, some obstetricians may adopt a "wait and see" attitude and eventually deliver the patient vaginally. The use of electronic fetal monitors has been of real aid in detecting fetal problems in this instance.

Infection and embolus are other possible complications of placenta previa that should be considered. Many hospitals now practice the "double setup technique" when treating a patient with placenta previa. Because vaginal or rectal examinations may worsen any bleeding present but are considered necessary for proper evaluation, these procedures may be delayed until preparations are completed for either a cesarean or a vaginal delivery in the same location as needed. X-ray diagnosis and detection of a low placental insertion by the use of radioactive tracers or ultrasonic techniques are increasingly available. Placenta previa is more common in women who are multiparous (Fig. 12-1).

Abruptio placentae

The other type of hemorrhage related to placental attachment is one resulting from *abruptio placentae,* or placentae abruptio, also called premature separation of the placenta. In this condition the placenta is implanted in the correct place, but for some reason—high blood pressure, sometimes as part of the toxemia of pregnancy syndrome, vitamin C and folic acid deficiency, local injury, hormonal imbalance, etc.—it becomes detached. Although its name implies that the detachment occurs suddenly, this is not always the case. Separation of the placenta from the uterine wall may occur over a period of time. Detachment may occur first at the center of the placenta, resulting in hidden hemorrhage at first, or it may begin at the rim or outer portion, causing vaginal bleeding of varying amounts.

Old blood, which has been trapped behind the separating placenta, appears dark when it finally escapes from the vaginal canal. Fresh bleeding usually is bright red in color. Bleeding from a premature separation of a normally implanted placenta may be severe enough to cause rapid maternal circulatory shock and danger to the fetus (Fig. 12-2).

Symptoms. The first signs of abruptio placentae during labor may be an alteration in the contraction pattern. The contractions are very strong and almost constant. Little relaxation period, if any, is detected. The uterus becomes boardlike, may enlarge with retained hemorrhage, and seems quite tender. There may or may not be external bleeding from the vagina.

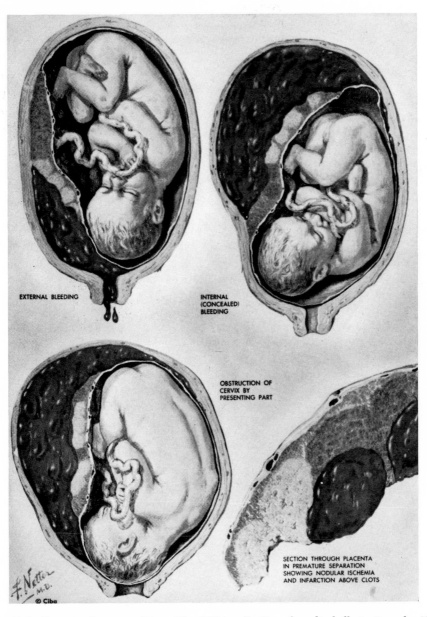

EXTERNAL BLEEDING

INTERNAL (CONCEALED) BLEEDING

OBSTRUCTION OF CERVIX BY PRESENTING PART

SECTION THROUGH PLACENTA IN PREMATURE SEPARATION SHOWING NODULAR ISCHEMIA AND INFARCTION ABOVE CLOTS

Fig. 12-2. Abruptio placentae. (From The CIBA collection of medical illustrations, by Frank H. Netter, M.D. Copyright CIBA.)

The fetal heart tone is either greatly accelerated or slowing. (Normal rate is approximately 120 to 160 per minute.) Electronic monitoring techniques are encouraged in suspect cases. The fetus, in its struggle to obtain more oxygen, may be very restless and active. If the amniotic sac, or bag of waters, is ruptured, meconium may appear in the amniotic fluid—another sign of fetal distress. As shock from blood loss develops, the blood pressure falls, and the pulse increases and weakens. Abruptio placentae in its more severe forms is an obstetrical emergency. The treatment often, although not inevitably, includes delivery by cesarean section and blood replacement. A serious complication of abruptio placentae that has been encountered often enough to warrant mention is the development of afibrinogenemia, or an abnormally low fibrinogen level in the blood that makes normal blood clotting impossible. Treatment may include fibrinogen replacement, an expensive but lifesaving technique.

Hydatidiform mole

Another complication that may produce hemorrhage, although it is characterized by a much more unusual series of signs and symptoms, is called *hydatidiform mole* (usually shortened to hydatid mole). In this condition, for some unknown reason the fertilized ovum deteriorates, and instead of producing a fetus and normal placenta, an abnormal tissue develops, which usually does not include any clearly defined fetal structures. At times this tissue may resemble a cluster of small grapes, or it may be of tapioca consistency. Its presence may be suspected when a pregnancy seems to be growing abnormally rapidly (a 3-month pregnancy may equal the size of a 5-month gestation), when no fetal heart tone or movement is detected, and nausea and vomiting are excessive or persistent. Vaginal bleeding may be intermittent. Ultrasonic diagnosis is possible. No fetal skeleton is demonstrated. If part of the abnormal tissue is expelled from the uterus, pathological examination is indicated. This

growth rarely may erode the uterus and cause rupture. If not totally expelled or carefully removed, it occasionally becomes malignant, spreading to the lungs and other body parts. After the mole's removal, pregnancy tests are continued to see if any tissue is still active in the body and producing hormones. In the event of the diagnosis of hydatid mole, physicians may consider the advisability of removal of the uterus (hysterectomy) because of the possibility of the development of a malignant tumor, choriocarcinoma. Spreading choriocarcinoma, it is wonderful to relate, is usually curable by the use of anticancer chemicals such as methotrexate and dactinomycin.

Other causes

The causes of obstetrical hemorrhage previously discussed—abortion, ectopic pregnancy, placenta previa, placentae abruptio, and hydatidiform mole—are those that most often occur during pregnancy or early labor. However, they are not the only causes of significant blood loss associated with childbirth. Obstetrical laceration—vaginal, perineal, or cervical—and uterine inertia (abnormal postpartal relaxation of the uterus) leading to excessive bleeding from the site of former placental attachment can be important intrapartal and postpartal complications.

Care of the bleeding patient

Before leaving the topic of blood loss during pregnancy and labor, let us review the care of bleeding patients. Here are some important "do's" and "don't's" that all nurses should know. Although licensed vocational or practical nurses (LVN's or LPN's) should not have the total responsibility in such cases, they should understand the following basic considerations:

1. Never give a bleeding patient an enema as part of the "routine admit." Never examine a bleeding patient rectally or vaginally. The physician performs the examination if he wishes. Unnecessary manipulation of the area may increase the bleeding (especially

in cases of placenta previa). Keep the patient on bed rest and give no food or fluids until ordered otherwise.

2. Observe the patient carefully and frequently:

   a. Take frequent pulse and blood pressure determinations. Systolic blood pressure readings of 90 or below are usually indicative of shock, but remember that a hypertensive patient may not have a pressure reading so low that it would routinely indicate shock but may still be suffering from what would be, for them, hypotension. Compare, if possible, the results obtained with the patient's blood pressure reading on her prenatal record. Check for rising pulse.

   b. Check for type and amount of vaginal bleeding and/or amniotic drainage. If it is possible, save the evidences of bleeding for evaluation by the physician.

   c. Check the fetal heart tone every 15 to 30 minutes, depending on the patient's condition. Remember, distress is related to irregularity and speed (too slow or too fast). (The normal fetal heart tone averages 120 to 160 beats per minute. Rates of 100 or below definitely indicate distress.) An unusually active fetus may signal difficulty.

   d. Estimate the character of the contraction and relaxation period by frequent timing. Check for any special uterine pain or tenderness and for poor or absent uterine relaxation.

3. Keep the charge nurse and physician informed of changes in the patient.

4. Expect possible orders for intravenous fluids, hematocrit or hemoglobin determinations, and cross match for blood transfusion. Record intake and output. Know if any religious scruples would preclude transfusion (for example, if the patient is a Jehovah's Witness).

5. Maintain a calm, supportive manner, sensitive to the appearance as well as the reality of the situation.

Toxemias of pregnancy (Fig. 12-3)

One of the most common causes of maternal mortality is not, in itself, primarily a hemorrhagic disease, but it may finally contribute to the development of hemorrhage. Hypertension associated with toxemia of pregnancy may initiate abruptio placentae or, in severe cases, be seen with localized hemorrhages in the maternal liver, brain, and other organs. Sometimes one sees references to the toxemias of pregnancy, a purposeful use of the plural because the general health histories of the patients and pathological changes encountered are not always similar. Usually classifications of toxemias of pregnancy refer to complications occurring that include two or more of these classical signs: excessive weight gain produced by hidden or observed *edema, hypertension,* and the appearance of protein (albumin or globulin) in the urine (proteinuria). In severe cases, coma and convulsions may also occur.

Such signs that have an onset after 24 weeks' gestation are referred to as "acute," "true," or "metabolic toxemia of late pregnancy." Hypertension or kidney disease that predates or is worsened by the presence of pregnancy is generally considered as a second, separate category of complications. Toxemia that includes the occurrence of coma or convulsion is called *eclampsia.* In the absence of these neurological signs the disease is termed *preeclampsia.* Preeclampsia occurs in about 7% of obstetrical patients. Its incidence is greater in young primigravidae, and among women with twin gestations, in low socioeconomic groups, and others with poor nutritional intake.

Long among the first three causes of maternal mortality, all the toxemias of pregnancy (excluding those relatively few cases associated with abortion) accounted for

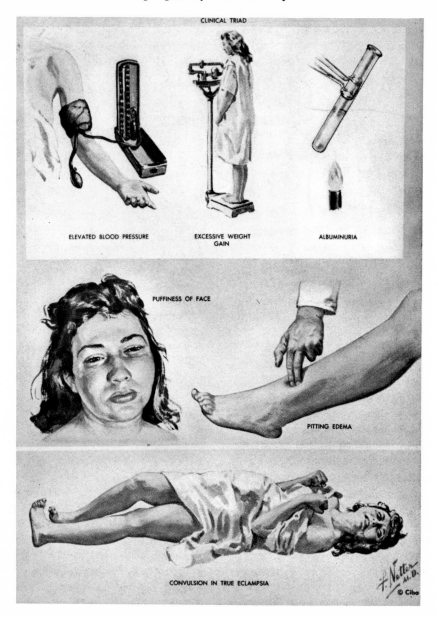

Fig. 12-3. Acute toxemia of pregnancy; symptomatology of preeclampsia and eclampsia. (From The CIBA collection of medical illustrations, by Frank H. Netter, M.D. Copyright CIBA.)

111 of the 477 recorded maternal deaths in the United States in 1973.*

*U. S. Department of Health, Education, and Welfare, Public Health Service. Monthly vital statistics report from the National Center for Health Statistics, vol. 23, No. 11, Suppl. 2, Feb. 10, 1975, p. 18. (Preliminary figures.)

Pathology. There is no lack of theories regarding the causes and mechanisms of toxemia of late pregnancy. A limited list includes explanations involving uterine overdistention, lack of normal blood supply to uterine and placental tissues, psychological factors, and malnutrition. Most references state that the cause is unknown. Probably the most popular hypothesis currently is that mechanical factors impede the development of a proper blood flow to the uterus and its contents and that this circulatory lack (uterine ischemia) favors the production of substances that raise the systemic blood pressure and cause the other characteristic symptoms of the disease. Dr. T. H. Brewer* has been most instrumental in promoting the concept that malnutrition is the underlying cause of the problem of toxemia. He believes that malnutrition, particularly protein deprivation, in pregnant women causes impaired liver function, which in turn interferes with the synthesis of albumin, the metabolism of the increased output of progesterone and estrogen characteristic of pregnancy, and normal hepatic detoxification processes. In his writings he cites the low serum protein levels found in many such patients as a cause of the typical edema, lowered blood volume, and reduced placental blood flow, which trigger a compensatory hypertension and kidney pathology. He especially condemns broad calorie restriction, protein-poor and salt-deficient diets, and diuretics in the treatment of symptoms, believing that they increase the threat to both mother and child.

As the disease progresses, edema and spasm of the blood vessels may sometimes be detected by ophthalmoscopic examination of the fundus of the eye. Visual problems may occur. Edema of the brain associated with headache, nausea, disorientation, and other disorders may eventually cause coma and convulsions. If the patient dies, her death is usually caused by cerebral hemorrhage, congestive heart failure with pulmonary edema, or the complications of operative maneuvers. Fetal death or damage is more frequent. Reduced placental circulation, secondary to lowered blood volume and low serum protein levels may play a role in the production of the low birth weight infant typically associated with this disorder. Eclampsia has an overall mortality of 7%.

Symptoms. Hypertension is usually the first sign detected. Several systolic blood pressure readings during a period of at least 6 hours, of 140 mm. Hg or above or a rise of 30 mm. Hg or more beyond the known overall normal level of the patient in question is significant. Also, diastolic readings of 90 mm. Hg or above or 15 mm. above the patient's usual diastolic pressure are noteworthy. A weight gain of over 1 pound a week during the last 12 weeks of gestation is thought to be suspicious, signaling fluid retention. Edema of the face and hands is more significant than swelling of the ankles, which afflicts most pregnant women to some degree in the last weeks of waiting. Since most women do not have the tools or the ability to take their own blood pressure, they should be told to report persistent headache, dizziness, or spots before the eyes, which may be symptoms of hypertension and edema of the retina. Other significant signs and symptoms of developing or worsening toxemia may be vomiting, epigastric pain, and decreased urine production.

Treatment. Treatment of preeclampsia or acute toxemia of pregnancy depends on the severity of the symptoms encountered and the philosophies of the physician. Regular, adequate prenatal care is the best insurance for control of the complication. In cases of mild toxemia, if a patient is conscientious in carrying out her physician's instructions, all treatment may be possible on an outpatient basis, but many physicians prefer to hospitalize their patients until symptoms are controlled. Treatment is directed toward relieving the edema and hypertension and restoring normal kidney function. Bed rest in a side-lying position to increase placental blood flow, with mild sedation, is usually helpful in decreasing blood pressure. Improvement of the diet emphasizing high-quality protein, vitamin, and mineral intake, and avoidance of empty calories is to be encouraged. Salt restriction, while still prescribed by some, is recom-

---

*Brewer, T. H.: Metabolic toxemia of late pregnancy, Springfield, Ill., 1966, Charles C Thomas, Publisher.

mended with less conviction of its therapeutic role. Other doctors consider salt a necessary ingredient in the diet and allow foods seasoned to taste. Diuretics are increasingly considered to be of no value and capable of causing harm to the toxemic patient and the fetus.

When hospitalized, these patients are usually placed on bed rest in a quiet room. Valium or sedatives, usually phenobarbital, make bed rest more tolerable. Blood pressures and FHR's are taken at least every 4 hours. A daily weight determination and urinalysis are common. Intake and output should be observed. The patients are questioned regarding the appearance of any symptoms such as headache, blurred vision, abdominal pain, or nausea. The treatment of toxemia of late pregnancy is, at this time, for many physicians as controversial as its proposed causes. However, all agree that delivery of a viable child as soon as possible is the best therapy. The rationale of treatment is to improve the condition of the mother to allow a vaginal or abdominal delivery at term. However, if her condition continues to deteriorate, induction of labor or a cesarean section may be carried out.

Preeclampsia may be defined as "severe" if one or more of the following signs and symptoms are present: blood pressure of 160/110 or more, albuminuria 3+ or more, urinary output of less than 400 ml. per 24 hours, cerebral or visual disturbances, pulmonary edema, or cyanosis. In the event of severe preeclampsia, the room should be dimmed, and the toxemia tray containing a padded tongue blade, airway, percussion hammer (to test reflexes), emergency sedative, and diuretic drugs with appropriate equipment for their administration should be close at hand. An oxygen mask or cannula, a suction apparatus, and possibly emergency tracheostomy equipment should be nearby.

Fortunately, the incidence of convulsion is rare today. However, this does not mean that the nurse can consider the possibility so remote that no precautions are taken. Abdominal pain, apprehension, twitchings,

and hyperirritability of the muscles often precede convulsions. As soon as a convulsion manifests itself, a padded tongue blade or soft, rolled washcloth may be placed in the patient's open mouth between the teeth to prevent biting the tongue and help maintain an airway. If possible, the head should be turned to the side. Suctioning is rarely necessary. During the periods of rigidity and muscle contraction, the patient should be restrained only enough to keep her from hurting herself or rolling off the bed. The sides of the bed should be padded with pillows. Be aware that babies have been suddenly born during a convulsive episode. An eclamptic patient should never be left alone. Certain patients may convulse in response to loud noises, jarring of the bed, or bright lights. Conversation should be minimal.

To measure urinary output and character more accurately, an indwelling catheter is often inserted and attached to a urinometer. The blood pressure cuff is left in place. Frequent pulse and respiration checks are made. The patient is heavily sedated. Magnesium sulfate is frequently used. A temperature elevation is often associated with the onset of eclampsia. Rectal or axillary temperatures should be taken.

As soon as the patient's convulsions are controlled, the condition of the fetus (if the seizures occur before delivery) is ascertained, and plans for the birth are considered. The patient may deliver spontaneously. If the progress of labor is sufficient and the condition of the patients (mother and fetus) is satisfactory, vaginal delivery may be the procedure of choice. After delivery of the baby, the possibility of convulsion diminishes with the passage of time. Convulsion 72 hours after delivery is very rare.

Rupture of the uterus

Rupture of the gravid uterus may occur during late pregnancy but is most often reported during labor and delivery. The nurse should know under what circumstances this emergency is most likely to occur, the signs and symptoms most often seen, and the usual treatment pursued.

Uterine rupture is most frequently associated with previous uterine surgery (e.g., cesarean sections, myomectomies), injudicious application of obstetrical forceps, a tempestuous or prolonged obstructed labor (e.g., fetal-pelvic disproportion) grand-multiparity, and the use of oxytocin.

Typically, the patient experiences a period of strong, almost unremitting contractions that, in spite of their force, produce little progress in the descent of the fetus in the birth canal. The uterus becomes extremely tender, and a weakening of its lower segment may cause a distention above the pubic bone, which may simulate the appearance of a full bladder. At the moment of rupture the patient may exclaim that she had a sharp pain and "felt something giving way." If rupture is complete, that is, the wall of the uterus is torn through, contractions will suddenly cease. The patient, after experiencing momentary relief from the pain, will usually quickly develop signs of profound circulatory shock due to intraabdominal hemorrhage. Some of this blood loss may be visible vaginally. Signs and symptoms of rupture depend on the extent and depth of the tear, the location of the fetus, and the stage of labor in which the complication occurs. Occasionally, the onset of symptoms will be delayed. Almost all the unborn babies and one third of their affected mothers die. Treatment usually consists of immediate laparotomy, possible hysterectomy, antibiotics, and massive blood transfusions.

Amniotic fluid embolism

A complication that few women survive involves the spontaneous, accidental infusion of amniotic fluid into the endocervical or uterine veins after the bag of waters has ruptured. This may occur anytime during the labor-delivery and immediate postpartum period but has been most often reported near the end of the first stage of labor. Amniotic fluid containing particles of meconium, vernix, and lanugo may enter the large blood sinuses in the placenta through defects in the placental attachment. These emboli gain access to the mother's general circulation and lodge in the lungs. Although the entire disastrous mechanism is not clear, it would seem that this foreign matter also produces profound shock and intravascular clotting, leading to lowered fibrinogen levels in the blood and subsequent hemorrhage. It is important to note that this complication is more frequently associated with tumultuous uterine contractions and has been described in an excessively disproportionate number of cases in which oxytocin has been administered to initiate or stimulate labor.

Symptoms manifest themselves suddenly. The patient may complain of chest pain or dyspnea and become extremely restless and cyanotic, occasionally expectorating frothy, blood-tinged mucus. Profound circulatory shock from hemorrhage may occur rapidly. Fetal death may result, and maternal death is almost always the outcome. It is good to know that this complication is rare—occurring only once in several thousand deliveries. Emergency care includes intravenous administration of fibrinogen, blood, and other fluids and oxygen therapy. If the baby is not yet born, he is delivered as soon as possible.

Prolapse of the cord

When the umbilical cord precedes the presenting part of the fetus during labor so that the blood circulating within the vessels of the cord may be clamped off against the pelvis by the continued advance of the fetus down the birth canal, an obstetrical emergency exists. This condition, termed prolapse of the cord, occurs in approximately 0.4% of labors. It is typically associated with certain types of fetal presentations, maternal pelvic contours, or labor situations. For example, the nurse should be aware that this complication is more frequent during labors involving multiple pregnancies, and in footling, breech, or shoulder presentations. It is more common when pelvic distortion or asymmetry is present. To prevent prolapse of the cord, patients in labor whose fetal presentations are not engaged should not ambulate or sit up steeply after cervical dilatation has advanced. A sudden gush of amniotic fluid may push the cord down into the vagina or to the exterior. This is one of the reasons the fetal heart tone is always taken after the bag of waters ruptures spontaneously or is ruptured artificially by the physician. Sometimes the cord is clearly visible outside the vaginal canal. In other instances it has prolapsed but is not visible. It may only be felt. As long as pulsations are detected, blood is flowing in the cord. Periodic checks of the fetal heart tone are necessary, since any compression of the cord would usually cause detectable, abnormal alterations in its rhythm or rate. A constantly monitored patient with cord compression may characteristically reveal variable deceleration patterns. Other signs associated with fetal distress could be the passage of meconium in the case of a cephalic presentation and sudden agitated fetal activity.

Treatment is directed toward removing any real or potential pressure on the prolapsed cord by applying vaginal or abdominal pressure to push the baby away from the cord or by a steep head-down or knee-chest position. Close observation of the fetal heart tone is maintained. A fetal heart monitor would be very helpful. The nurse should never attempt to replace the cord. The administration of oxygen is not thought to aid the baby if oxygenation of the mother is adequate, since oxygen concentrations would already be maximal even if the supply system, the cord, is in jeopardy. Usually the only feasible treatment is cesarean section, carried out as quickly as possible—preferably within 30 minutes.

Premature labor and delivery

A baby born before the end of the thirty-seventh week of gestation is considered premature. The incidence of a baby born "before his time" represents a special threat to the life or future health of the infant, special physical, psychological, and eco-

nomic stress on the family, and a challenge to community resources. Premature babies are more likely to suffer trauma during birth, to be victims of respiratory distress syndrome and other problems, and to require longer supportive hospital care.

For these reasons, in most cases, attempts would be made to halt a premature labor. Bed rest and sedation may inhibit progression, but other drugs may be used to quiet uterine contractions. Among them are intravenous infusions of isoxsuprine hydrochloride (Vasodilan) or ethyl alcohol in a 5% dextrose solution. The alcohol is thought to reduce the release of oxytocin, a hormone that stimulates the uterus to contract, into the circulation. However, if there is evidence of intrauterine infection, hemorrhage, or cervical dilation beyond 4 cm., these efforts would not be appropriate.

If labor cannot be terminated, little analgesic medication is given because the premature infant's body cannot detoxify drugs well, and his respirations when born must not be depressed. Spinal-type anesthesia may be given at delivery. A deep episiotomy may be performed to minimize head compression at expulsion. The nursery must be notified of an impending premature birth. Ideally, a pediatrician particularly skilled in the immediate care of immature newborns would be present at the delivery. Transport to a special intensive care nursery may be indicated.

Special attention to the psychological needs of the mother is essential. Her labor is all the more demanding and difficult because her body is not prepared for the event, the outlook is precarious, and analgesic aids are minimal.

ILLEGITIMATE PREGNANCIES AND TEEN-AGE MOTHERHOOD

Other problems meriting our consideration as nurses may be related to special circumstances surrounding the events of pregnancy, delivery, and the responsibilities of parenthood. They may not be physiological or anatomical problems per se, but they represent situations that may be associated

148

with certain obstetrical complications and may profoundly affect the entire experience of the patient and her future adjustment to life's challenges. Two such situations that are creating increasing concern in our society are teen-age parenthood and illegitimate pregnancies. Although the two need not be related, they often are.

Current statistics are difficult to obtain, but in 1968 the largest number of illegitimate births occurred in the 15- to 19-year-old group (158,000),* an increase of 18% since 1965. Since the Supreme Court decision, which made abortion in the first trimester of pregnancy a private decision of the patient and the doctor, and since the age of majority has been lowered in certain states and the parental consent for medical care for minors is undergoing revision,† actual illegitimacy figures may have decreased for this age group in some localities. The use of contraceptive devices may also be a factor. However, many of these teen-agers choose not to use contraceptive techniques. Many teen-age marriages take place after pregnancy has occurred. The divorce rate for these unions is very high. This is not meant to imply that there are no successful marriages begun in teen-age years. It does, however, reveal that the chances for a satisfactory, continuing family relationship are slim. Teen-age marriages in modern American society too often are an attempt to solve or escape problems too serious and complex to be corrected by a wedding ring.

Many factors may be related to the incidence of early marriage or illegitimate births. These factors most often involve family conflicts, social and economic deprivation, individual psychological problems, and/or a lack of education and appreciation regarding the role and responsibilities

of sexuality in the family and society. Communities are now becoming more aware of the needs of the young parent, married or not. Not long ago few services were available to meet these needs. Some programs have been instituted in recent years that make it possible for the pregnant girl's formal education to continue. These programs also may supervise prenatal care; prepare the girls for their experiences during pregnancy, labor, and delivery; possibly increase mothering skills; and assist them with needed personal and vocational planning. In the instance of illegitimate birth, attempts are made to avoid a defeating repetition of similar behavior. A few agencies make efforts to work with the unwed father, as well as the mother.

Physicians and nurses are learning more about the needs of the teen-age obstetrical patient, both in and out of the hospital setting. Needless to say, most teen-age maternity patients need a great deal of supportive care, careful instruction, and explanation to enable them to gain constructively from their experiences. A punitive attitude toward these patients on the part of the nursing staff does not aid the individual girls or help solve the larger problems involved.

The nurse should realize that the incidence of toxemia of pregnancy is higher in this age group, especially for girls in their early teens from lower socioeconomic backgrounds. This increased incidence may be related to the poor dietary management exhibited by many of these young girls. These patients also have an especially large number of low-weight babies. The delivery room nurse will be interested to know that teen-age multiparae are more prone to precipitate labor than any other group of obstetrical patients. For the teen-ager who has experienced a forced marriage or an illegitimate pregnancy, the trauma of the situation is mainly psychological. Her misdirected search for identity, freedom, love, or recognition places her in a role for which she is ill prepared, faced with decisions the outcome of which will

---

*Juhasz, A. M.: Unmarried adolescent parent. Adolescence 9:263, Summer, 1974.
†Maternal and Child Health Service: Report on promoting the health of mothers and children, FY 1973, U. S. Department of Health, Education, and Welfare, Health Services Administration, Maternal and Child Health Service, Rockville, Md., p. 7.

unavoidably influence her the rest of her life. (See section on the unwed mother, p. 169.)

• • •

This unit, with its rather dismal recital of the minor and major complications of pregnancy and labor, may seem frightening to the student anticipating marriage and founding a family. She may be reassured. It is the purpose of a text to point out the unusual as well as the commonplace. It is the business of a nurse to know about the possibility of these problems although some of them she may never encounter—either personally or professionally.

unit five
Suggested selected readings and references

Anderson, G. V., moderator: Symposium: ob-gyn emergencies, part 2, Contemp. OB/GYN 2:75-96, Aug., 1973.

Beckner, F. J.: How do you respond to the unwed mother, RN 33:46-53, Aug., 1970.

Bond, S.: Reevaluating positions for labor—lateral vs. supine, J. Obstet. Gynecol. Neonatal Nurs. 2:29-31, Nov.-Dec., 1973.

Brewer, T. H.: Metabolic toxemia of late pregnancy, Springfield, Ill., 1966, Charles C Thomas, Publisher.

Case, L. L.: Ultrasound monitoring of mother and fetus, Am. J. Nurs. 72:725-727, April, 1972.

Chez, R. A., editor: The Shirodkar procedure: managing the incompetent cervix, Contemp. OB/GYN 3:137-139, May, 1974.

Committee on Youth, American Academy of Pediatrics: Statement on "teenage pregnancy and the problem of abortions," J. Obstet. Gynecol. Neonatal Nurs. 1:55, Sept.-Oct., 1972.

Conklin, M. M.: DIC in the pregnant patient, J. Obstet. Gynecol. Neonatal Nurs. 3:29-32, May-June, 1974.

Curtis, F. L.: Observations of unwed pregnant adolescents, Am. J. Nurs. 74:100-102, Jan., 1974.

Curtis, F. L.: The pregnant adolescent, Nursing '74 3:77-79, March, 1974.

Fort, A. T.: The obstetrics emergency: management of the injured gravida, Contemp. OB/GYN 3:41-46, Feb., 1974.

The great eclampsia mystery, or the case of the empty plaque, Med. World News, pp. 41-52, July 20, 1973.

Gregory, M. G., and Clayton, E. M.: Amniotic fluid embolism, Obstet. Gynecol. 42:236-244, Aug., 1973.

Kelly, J. V.: Use of the vacuum extractor for delivery, Contemp. OB/GYN 2:69-73, Dec., 1973.

Lasater, C.: Electronic monitoring of mother and fetus, Am. J. Nurs. 72:728-730, April, 1972.

Lerch, C.: Maternity nursing, ed. 2, St. Louis, 1974, The C. V. Mosby Co., pp. 212-241.

Lindheimer, M. D., and Katz, A. I.: The high-risk pregnancy: managing the patient with renal disease, Contemp. OB/GYN 3:49-55, Jan., 1974.

Lindheimer, M. D., and Katz, A. I.: Major problems in dealing with minors, Contemp. OB/GYN 1:14-32, Feb., 1973.

Mestman, J. H.: Medical management of the pregnant diabetic patient, Contemp. OB/GYN 1:61-64, Jan., 1973.

Milic, A., and Adamsons, K.: Fetal blood sampling, Am. J. Nurs. 68:2149-2152, Oct., 1968.

Nelson, S. A.: School-age parents, Children Today 2:31-40, March-April, 1973.

Prenatal clinic for teen-agers provides a comprehensive program, University of Pennsylvania Hospital, Contemp. OB/GYN 3:79-87, March, 1974.

Rice, G. T.: Recognition and treatment of intrapartal fetal distress, J. Obstet. Gynecol. Neonatal Nurs. 1:15-22, July-Aug., 1972.

Russin, A. W., and others: Electronic monitoring of the fetus, Am. J. Nurs. 74:1294-1299, July, 1974.

Shearer, M. H.: Fetal monitoring: do the benefits outweigh the drawbacks? Birth and Fam. J. 1:12-18, Winter, 1973-74.

Symposium: nutrition and the pregnant patient, Contemp. OB/GYN 5:110-146, Feb., 1975.

Williams, S. R.: Nutrition and diet therapy, ed. 2, St. Louis, 1973, The C. V. Mosby Co., pp. 372-373.

Postpartal and population problems

13

The postpartal period

The postpartal period, or puerperium, is usually considered to be the interval extending from the birth of the baby until 6 weeks after. It is characterized by the return of the reproductive organs to their approximate prepregnant positions and the development of lactation. Of course, some mothers, not wishing or unable to nurse their babies, do not experience the full development of this latter characteristic. The return of the reproductive organs to the nonpregnant state is called the process of *involution*.

ADMISSION
Preparation and transfer

The basic care of the postpartum patient is an extension of the care given in the delivery room after delivery. The patient arriving in the postpartum area is put to bed in a unit previously prepared for her. The bed will be turned down, and bed protectors will be in place to catch extra vaginal drainage. Near at hand will be a sphygmomanometer, stethoscope, and individual unit equipment such as towel and washcloth set, wash and emesis basins, soap, bedpan, back care lotion, breast and perineal pads, and newspapers or paper bags for pad discard. If the patient has an intravenous infusion, some sort of support for the bottle will also be needed.

The transfer of the patient from the stretcher to the bed may require two or three people, depending on her condition and the equipment available. Side rails are applied. Before the delivery room nurse leaves the area she checks the patient's fundus and vaginal flow to determine if the uterus is firm and makes sure that any pertinent information concerning the patient is told the postpartum charge nurse as she transfers the patient's records. Care is taken to properly oversee the patient's personal effects and not to lose anything in transit.

Observation

The postpartum nurse continues to check the condition of the patient every 15 to 20 minutes for at least 2 hours to determine the following (Fig. 13-1):
1. Blood pressure, pulse, and respiration
2. Type and amount of vaginal discharge (lochia) and the appearance of the perineum
3. Consistency and location of the fundus
4. Signs of urinary distention
5. General condition of the patient: color, feel of her skin (warm or cold, dry or clammy), level of consciousness (drowsy, apprehensive, unresponsive), and the presence of nausea or vomiting
6. Any special complaints or requests (pain, need to call husband, etc.)
7. Rate of flow and condition of any infusion present

Observation for signs of hemorrhage

Blood pressure, pulse, and general condition. Occasionally the blood pressure will

151

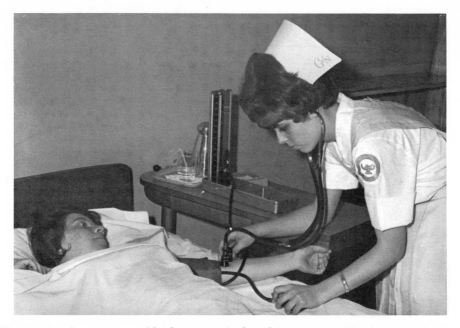

Fig. 13-1. Another postpartum blood pressure check. Pulse, respiration, blood pressure, fundus, and lochial checks should be made every 15 to 20 minutes. (Courtesy Grossmont Hospital, La Mesa, Calif.)

be elevated at the time of transfer. This condition may be the result of the excitement of the delivery and seeing the baby. It may be related to the type of oxytocic the patient received or is still receiving by intravenous feeding. It may be a sign of toxemia. All elevations over 130 mm. Hg systolic or 90 mm. Hg diastolic should be reported orally to the charge nurse.

The blood pressure may be low. Any pressure 100 mm. Hg systolic or below should definitely be reported. Other pressures that may not be that low but are not hypertensive and continue to fall should be reported for evaluation. Many patients with a systolic reading of 90 mm. Hg or below are going into circulatory collapse or shock. Such a falling blood pressure would be accompanied by an initially rising pulse. However, if the patient continues in shock, the pulse will gradually slow, weaken, and have a thready quality. Abnormally dilated pupils, pale, cyanotic, or clammy skin, apprehension, and an unconscious state are also signs of shock.

Some postpartum patients have a rela-

tively slow pulse, but it has a good quality and is not associated with other signs of shock. This pulse rate (usually in the 60's) is not significant.

Lochia. The attending nurse is also interested in the amount of vaginal drainage, or *lochia.* As she checks the patient's drainage, she is sure to check under the patient's hips, since much of the drainage may not be observed on the perineal pad but seeks lower dependent areas. Immediately after delivery the lochia should be moderate in quantity and dark or bright red in color— a quality called *rubra.* (About 2 days later the lochia changes to a pinkish brown, called *serosa.*) The patient will usually wear two perineal pads that have to be changed once or at the most twice during her routine 2-hour postpartum check. These should always be removed and applied from front to back to avoid contamination of the perineum. The saturation of a greater number of pads would be considered abnormally excessive. When estimating blood loss and its significance, the general condition and size of the patient must be evalu-

152

ated. Usually a 450 to 500 ml. blood loss is considered hemorrhage.

Fundus. The first consideration related to blood loss is the condition of the uterus. Is the fundus firm and contracted? Is it at or below the umbilicus? If a fundus is large, soft, or boggy (seems to contain excess blood), it should be gently massaged with a circular motion until firm, while one hand is held against the top of the pubic bone to prevent the uterus from being inverted or prolapsed. If clots are suspected, once the fundus is *firm* it may be gently grasped and positioned in the middle of the abdomen. Pressure is then exerted in the direction of the pelvic canal to push out to the exterior the clots that were emptied from the uterus into the lower uterine segment and vagina during the period of massage. Students should not attempt to express clots alone until instructed individually. In the event of excessive vaginal bleeding, massage is the first measure employed to control vaginal hemorrhage.

It is surprising how quickly the uterus responds to simple massage in most cases. The nurse can easily feel the uterine muscle tighten. This tightening of the uterine muscle to make a firm fundus is essential. It pinches off the large vessels that brought blood to and from the placental sinuses before the placenta separated and was delivered.

Postpartum hemorrhage. In cases in which the uterus does not contract or remain contracted, the presence of placental fragments in the uterus may be suspected. If bleeding continues to be excessive and the uterus remains firm, a cause other than uterine relaxation must be sought to explain the blood loss. Excessive bleeding may develop because of a previously undetected cervical or vaginal laceration, or it could be the result of a defective suture or repair. In many cases of abnormal bleeding the patient will be returned to the delivery room to facilitate inspection of the uterus and vaginal canal. In some cases a dilatation and curettage of the uterus or the insertion of vaginal or, more rarely, uterine packing

may be undertaken. If no lacerations or abnormal tissue retention are evident, treatment is usually confined to the administration of additional oxytocics such as ergot or its modification, methylergonovine (Methergine). Such treatment will combat the lethargy of the uterine muscles known as uterine inertia. Blood transfusions may be required. Patients who have had many children, multiple or frequent pregnancies, large babies, or long or induced labors should be especially observed for the development of uterine inertia.

The location and consistency of the fundus are important. A high, soft fundus makes nurses think of possible uterine bleeding; a high, firm fundus more often indicates urinary retention. A distended bladder, located just below the uterus, will cause the fundus to rise (usually to one side and most often to the right). After the completion of the third stage of a normal full-term labor, the fundus should be found below or possibly just at the umbilicus. Any higher position is suspect.

The position of the fundus is usually coded by counting finger widths above or below the umbilicus in the following manner. If the fundus (which usually feels somewhat like a large cantaloupe through the abdominal wall) is two finger widths above the level of the umbilicus, it is recorded as +2. If it is located one finger width below the level of the umbilicus, it is recorded as −1. A recording of 0 may indicate that the fundus is found at the level of the umbilicus, but usually nurses write "@ umbilicus." A typical record of the condition of the fundus would be "Fundus: firm −2 central." The first day after delivery the fundus is usually felt at the umbilicus or below at −1 or even −2 position. The location of the fundus may be influenced by the size of the patient's baby, the condition of her uterine muscle, the content of the urinary bladder, and such abnormal conditions as retained placental fragments and the development of uterine infection. Normally the uterus undergoes involution at the rate of about one finger width a day.

153

At the end of 10 days it is usually down behind the pubic bone again and not palpable (Fig. 13-2).

Multiparae often complain of "after-cramps" caused by the contraction of the uterus in the process of involution. They are more often bothered by cramping than are primiparae, who usually possess better muscle tone. Nursing mothers may experience more aftercramps because of the stimulation of the uterus during the process of nursing. Mild analgesics usually relieve the discomfort.

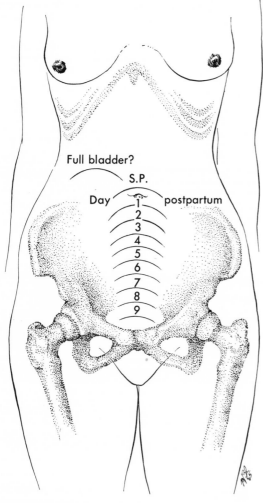

Fig. 13-2. Involution of the uterus, showing the various positions of the fundus. *S.P.*, Level just after separation of the placenta from the uterine wall before its delivery.

Observation for signs of urinary distention

The most common cause of a high fundus is a full bladder. Even when a woman is catheterized just before delivery, she may have a full bladder fairly soon after admittance to the postpartum area, especially if she is receiving or has had intravenous infusions. Routine catheterization just before delivery is being done much less frequently.

Other signs of urinary distention are a puffy area just above the pubic bone, complaints by the patient that she feels she should void but cannot, or the voiding of small amounts—less than 200 ml. This is called "dribbling" and usually indicates a full bladder that is capable of contracting only partially to release limited amounts of urine. A distended bladder is to be avoided because it jeopardizes normal bladder tone and may lead to the development of residual urine, an amount that routinely remains in the bladder and is not voided. Residual urine may become an excellent medium for bacterial multiplication. A distended bladder may also interfere with the normal contraction of the uterus and predispose the patient to hemorrhage. A distended bladder may be painful and add to the aftercramping experienced by some patients.

Encouraging voiding. Voidings of postpartum patients are usually measured until two voidings of over 300 ml. are recorded and a fundus check after the voidings indicates that the patient is emptying her bladder well. To check the efficiency of a bladder the physician will sometimes order a catheterization for residual urine. It is important that all the equipment necessary be at the patient's bedside before she voids so that the catheterization may proceed without delay.

If a patient is suspected of having a full bladder, every effort should be made to help her void without resorting to catheterization, which may cause inflammation even in the best of circumstances, especially if repeated. Several techniques to encourage voiding may be useful.

If the patient cannot get up to the bathroom because of her general condition, because she has delivered too recently, or because she has had a saddle type of anesthesia and does not as yet have an ambulation order, the problem of initiating natural voiding is more difficult. Many patients find it difficult to use the bedpan. The time that physicians allow their patients to ambulate postpartum differs widely. Patients who have received spinal anesthesia may be kept in bed, flat or with a pillow, for a period of 6 to 24 hours after delivery. The restriction in ambulation and posture is chiefly an effort to reduce the possibility of "spinal headache." Whether the restriction actually prevents the headache, however, has been debated. Patients who have had a general anesthetic are usually ambulated at the end of 8 hours. Those who have had local or no anesthetic usually are allowed up with aid as soon as they wish. Sometimes if a physician knows that a choice must be made between catheterization and probable success in voiding, he will choose to order earlier ambulation. "Saddle" patients also have more problems voiding because they have lost normal feeling in the bladder area.

If a bedpan must be used, it should be warmed. Patients who have had a saddle type of anesthesia may be raised just enough so that their hips are not higher than their heads while positioned on the pan. Privacy should be maintained, and, if possible, water should be left running into a washbowl to provide psychological stimulation. If an order is available, giving a "pain pill" such as oxycodone (Percodan) about 20 minutes before the bedpan is offered often helps solve the problem. Having the patient blow bubbles through a straw into a glass of water or pretend to blow up a balloon while she is on the bedpan sometimes helps relax the sphincter muscle. Pouring a measured amount of warm water over the perineum may help the patient void. If not, it will help clean off the area prior to catheterization. Encouraging the patient to drink *large* amounts of fluid before she has voided normally will, at times,

add to rather than relieve the problem and is not recommended.

Catheterization technique. If none of the preceding methods bring about the desired result, catheterization must be carried out. The nurse should know whether a specimen should be saved for laboratory analysis. The technique of catheterization and the materials used will differ from hospital to hospital. The following instructions are only general in character to make allowances for the different setups used, but they include principles that should be understood as well as review information for the student.

CATHETERIZATION: POSTPARTUM AREA

Purposes:
1. To relieve urinary distention
2. To obtain a "sterile" specimen for laboratory examination
3. To check for residual urine not expelled at the time of voiding (In this case the catheterization must be done immediately after the patient voids.)
4. To instill medications into the bladder
5. To maintain an emptied bladder during surgical procedures—generally with the use of a retention catheter (Foley)

Materials needed:
1. A sterile tray containing:
   a. A drape (to provide a field)
   b. Antiseptic and cotton balls for cleansing
   c. One or two No. 14 straight catheters
   d. Lubricant
2. Gloves
3. Adhesive tape and rubber band
4. Provision for the collection of the urine obtained; specimen bottle, if needed. If an indwelling catheter is ordered, add the following sterile equipment:
   a. No. 14 Foley catheter
   b. Five-milliliter syringe filled with sterile saline
   c. Drainage tubing and bottle or bag
   d. Safety pin
5. A protective bedpad under the patient's hips
6. A good light, well placed
7. A bath blanket for adequate draping (The diamond drape is recommended.)
8. Paper for perineal pad disposal
9. Perineal pads
10. Waste basin or plastic bag

Procedure:
1. Check the physician's orders regarding catheterization.
2. Assemble and position equipment.
3. Explain in simple terms what is going to be

done for the patient and that she will feel better as a result of the procedure.

4. Provide privacy and *lighting*.
5. Wash your hands, remove the perineal pads; wash your hand again and drape the patient.
6. Carry out routine perineal care if indicated.
7. Actual catheterization:
    a. Open the sterile tray, conveniently located.
    b. Lift the perineal drape to expose area.
    c. Make provision for the disposal of waste and collection of urine.
    d. Put on sterile gloves.
    e. Lubricate catheter, if not already done. (Do not occlude eyes.)
    f. Prepare cotton balls with antiseptic if not done previously. (How and when this is done will depend on the packaging available.)
    g. Place sterile field up to patient and position sterile tray.
    h. Expose the upper vestibule.
        (1) With the hand closest to the patient's head as you stand facing the bedside, gently part the labia majora *and minora* to expose the upper vestibule.
        (2) You *must* get sufficient exposure to identify the urethral meatus, but you must be gentle. Remember, many patient's have stitches in the true perineum just below the vagina.
        (3) Some of the newly delivered "saddle" patients will have little feeling in the area; others will be very sensitive.
        (4) *Remember*, once your hand has touched the patient, it is contaminated.
        (5) Sometimes, holding the labia back with a cotton ball under one supporting finger helps maintain the position.
        (6) Technically, if you let the labia close after having washed the crucial area with antiseptic, the area must be rewashed, since it has been contaminated by the enfolding tissue; therefore, it is important to maintain the labia in a drawnback position.
    i. Gently cleanse the upper vestibule:
        (1) Gently wipe down one side of the urethra; discard ball in waste disposal. Some techniques provide a forceps on which to mount the ball. Others use a forceps for picking up and inserting the catheter.
        (2) Gently wipe down the other side of the urethra; discard ball.

(3) Gently but firmly cleanse the urethra (wiping down with the cotton ball at the same time as you lift up against the tissue with your other hand; this helps smooth the area immediately surrounding the meatus and visualize the urethra). The urethra is usually located midline, just above the vaginal opening, and may look like a little slit, dimple, or inverted V. Use more cotton balls as necessary.

(4) Guard your fingers against touching the tissue or drainage while cleansing the area with your "sterile hand."

j. Insertion of the catheter:
    (1) Pick up the catheter about 3 inches from the tip.
    (2) Ask your patient to take a deep breath at the moment of insertion. This distracts her and helps loosen the urethral sphincter.
    (3) The female urethra is about 1½ inches long. No more than 4 inches of the catheter should ever be inserted, to avoid bladder puncture. If obstruction is encountered, the catheter should never be forced. There may be an abnormality of the canal (presence of a tumor, stricture, etc.), or you may not have properly identified the meatus.
    (4) A slight downward incline of the catheter may aid insertion as the urethral canal slopes downward when the patient is in dorsal recumbent position.
    (5) Urinary flow should come within a few seconds. If it does not, ask the patient to cough and *gently* press on the area above the pubis; this may start the flow. If it still does not appear, reposition the catheter, pulling it out slightly. If it still does not come, you may be in the vaginal canal instead of the urethra, or your patient may have an empty bladder!
    (6) Any time you touch a nonsterile object, perineal tissue that has not been antiseptically prepared, or the vaginal canal with a urinary catheter, it is contaminated, and another sterile catheter must be used.
    (7) If 600 to 700 ml. of urine are collected and the bladder is still not empty, most physicians do not object if you clamp off the catheter in a sterile manner, tape it to the inside of the thigh, and return to drain

and remove it in half an hour. (Removing a large amount of urine suddenly by artificial means may cause shock.) It is better not to have a bladder become distended with such an amount of urine in the first place. However, if the bladder does contain more urine, the preceding is perhaps the best procedure.

(8) If a Foley insertion is ordered, inflate the bulb with the sterile saline solution as soon as the catheter is in place. Gently tug on the Foley catheter to make sure it is positioned correctly and the bulb is inflated. Connect the drainage tubing attached to a collection bottle or bag. Stabilize the catheter by a strip of adhesive tape attached to the inner thigh of the leg that is farther away from the doorway of the patient's room. Lead the tubing underneath the patient's knee or over her thigh (according to her physician's preference) and over the side of the bed to the collecting bag or bottle. Stabilize the drainage tubing, using a safety pin and rubber band attached to the sheet to assure direct gravity drainage to the urine collector. There should be no dependent loops in the tubing. All patients with an indwelling catheter are on intake and output determinations.

k. Always measure the amount of urine obtained and record it. Note also the color of the urine. Note whether a catheter was left in place and if a specimen was obtained and sent to the laboratory.

l. When withdrawing a catheter, pinch the tube and ask the patient to take a deep breath.

m. Make the patient comfortable; dry and straighten her legs before caring for equipment or measuring output.

n. If the procedure was carried out for distention, the patient's ability to void should continue to be evaluated. She should still be on "output" and any complaints of frequent or painful urination reported.

o. A few physicians desire the instillation of a prophylactic urinary antiseptic just before the withdrawal of the catheter at the conclusion of a catheterization.

CONTINUING CARE

The need for good aseptic technique during all procedures in the postpartum area is readily understood when one realizes that within the uterine cavity, easily accessible to microorganisms from the exterior, is an open "wound," the former place of placental attachment. This diminishing, but still easily infected, area is well supplied with veins and arteries. It provides an ideal entry into the general body circulation and the possibility of septicemia.

Infection is still a threat if we are not enlightened and conscientious in our techniques. In fact, although our maternal death rate is falling, the early 1973 statistical reports for the United States list sepsis (infection) of childbirth and the puerperium as the second cause of maternal mortality.

Perineal care

Postpartum perineal cleansing is given in countless ways in maternity services across the nation. Techniques range from the use of separate sterile irrigation setups by a masked nurse each time needed by the patient, to teaching the mother which way to wipe with a clean washcloth. The acceptance of a technique should be based on whether it is safe, adequate, simple, inexpensive, and aesthetically satisfying to all concerned. The principles involved in perineal care should be the same whether it is done by the nurse or the patient herself.

Perineal cleansing

Perineal cleansing is performed to prevent infection, eliminate odor, observe the area and lochial flow, and ease the patient. Any equipment used by the patient should be absolutely clean and should not be used by another. Equipment used by more than one patient should be sterilized between patients. Hands should be washed before and after care. Care should be taught in cleansing the perineum and in removing and applying perineal pads so that soil cannot be introduced to the vulva. This means, for both nurse and patient, stroking from front to back once only with each cotton ball or cleansing surface. It means that the nurse will routinely remove and apply perineal pads from front to back, but this is a bit hard for mother to do! It is better to teach her to attach both ends to her sanitary belt, and then draw the belt up snugly into place so that the pad will not slip. The pad should be changed each time she uses the toilet. Some maternity services issue plastic squeeze bottles for antiseptic solution or warm tap water plus cellulose wipes to each mother for self-care. Others issue pitchers and furnish appropriate solutions. Still others provide individually wrapped, moist towelettes impregnated with rapidly drying antiseptic. Whatever is offered, the principles must be understood. No "pour-off" technique should be used if the patient has a vaginal packing. The patient will be cleansed with moist cotton balls or towelettes instead.

Episiotomy and first- and second-degree lacerations

For patients who have had episiotomies or laceration repairs, perineal care usually involves more than just cleansing. In these cases many hospitals also provide an antiseptic, analgesic perineal spray such as Dermoplast or ethyl aminobenzoate (Americaine). Most maternity services also routinely offer a perineal heat lamp several times a day for 20-minute intervals. The heat lamp is used to improve circulation, promote healing, and ease discomfort. It is usually not applied until several hours after delivery because it may stimulate additional bleeding if given too early. When heat lamps are applied, care must be taken that they are no less than 18 inches from the perineum. A 60-watt lamp is used. The thighs of blondes, redheads, or other fair-skinned patients should always be draped before the lamp is used.

Patients with standard episiotomies and first- and second-degree lacerations usually respond very well to the combination of irrigation, heat lamp, and analgesic spray offered. However, many such women still would prefer to stand rather than sit during periods of waiting. Advising the mother to tense her buttocks and tuck in her pelvis before sitting down often helps.

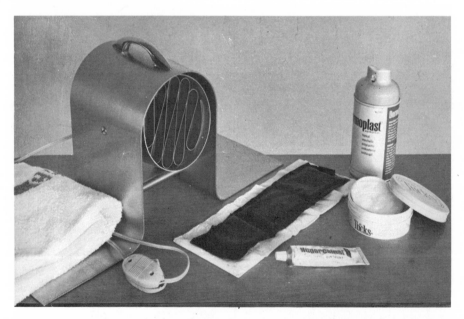

Fig. 13-3. Aids in relieving perineal discomfort through local application: the perineal lamp (the hood is draped with a towel when used), a perineal ice pack (unwrapped for better viewing), Nupercainal anesthetic ointment, Dermoplast antiseptic-anesthetic spray, and Tucks (lightweight witch-hazel–impregnated compresses). (Courtesy Grossmont Hospital, La Mesa, Calif.)

Other local analgesics may also be ordered, such as dibucaine (Nupercainal) ointment and witch-hazel compresses such as Tucks (Fig. 13-3).

Third-degree lacerations

Mothers who have had third-degree perineal lacerations (extending into the rectal sphincter) may need more help. Great caution must be exercised in giving patients who have had such problems any type of enema, suppository, or cathartic, since the suture line may not only involve the sphincter but also may extend into the rectum itself. Oral analgesics may be needed.

Application of cold to the perineum

Occasionally a patient has a swollen perineum after delivery, or a physician may consider swelling of the perineal tissues likely in a certain case. An order for the application of cold compresses or ice packs may be written. An ice pack should be wrapped with sterile, waterproof material and a fairly thin, sterile, absorbent outer layer and applied directly to the perineum. This must be done to protect the patient against cross infection and still render the cold desired by the physician. It may be held in place by an encircling sanitary pad. Various perineal ice packs are now available. They need to be fairly comfortable, durable, and able to provide cold for reasonable periods. If no such pads are available to the nurse, she may fill a rubber glove with cracked ice and water, close it tightly and wrap it in a light, disinfected plastic covering and a sterile towel. Ice packs must be changed frequently. The perineal area should be frequently observed for developing hematoma or increased swelling.

Ambulation

As previously stated, the ambulation of the postpartum patient is determined by the orders of the attending physician. His orders depend on the type of anesthetic given during delivery and the general condition of the patient. Early judicious ambulation of postpartum patients lessens the incidence of respiratory, circulatory, and urinary problems, helps prevent constipation, and promotes the rapid return of strength. But whenever the patient is first allowed out of bed, *the nurse should not leave her alone!* These patients often become dizzy and faint. If the patient does become faint, ease her onto a chair, her bed, or even gently to the floor, but do not leave her to seek help. If she is on a chair, support her with her head lowered to her knees. No matter how many days post partum, the nurse should always evaluate her ambulating patient.

The first time the postpartum patient gets up she may experience a sudden temporary gush of vaginal discharge. If it is dark red, it is not significant. It reflects the patient's change in posture after being several hours recumbent when the uterine drainage was not as efficient.

Bath and breast care procedures

The postpartum bed bath given the afternoon or morning after delivery is a procedure designed to permit observation and instruction as well as provide comfort and protection against infection. The postpartum patient is likely to perspire profusely. It is one way the body has to rid itself of excess fluids. In most cases mothers have only one such bed bath during their hospital stay. On succeeding mornings they take showers.

The postpartum bed bath differs from the routine bed-bath procedure followed in other hospital areas. It recognizes that the new mother's body includes two areas that are easily infected; the breasts and the perineum, which leads to the internal reproductive tract. If initial breast care is not given to nursing mothers in the delivery room area, it will be incorporated into this bath. Following is a suggested postpartum bath procedure.

POSTPARTUM BATH PROCEDURE

Materials:
1. Clean wash basin
2. Two clean washcloths and a towel

159

3. Soap
4. Bath blanket
5. Clean supportive bra or breast binder
6. Breast pads

Procedure: After the preliminaries necessary before all bed baths, including washing one's hands:

1. Start washing the breast area first, whether the mother is nursing or not. Often only clear water is used to help prevent the formation of cracked nipples.
   a. Wash in a circular manner from the nipple outward.
   b. Instruct the mother to follow this same order of bathing during her shower the next day.

c. If the mother is planning to nurse, especially observe the nipples for inversion, fissures, and cleanliness.
d. Dry the area and cover with a clean towel. If mother is nursing, exposure of the nipples to the air for short periods (15 minutes) will help maintain healthy tissue. The application of lanolin following air exposure and nursing is advocated by many.

2. Continue the bath by washing the face, neck, hands, arms, axillae, abdomen, and back.
3. Give a back rub. This is much appreciated!
4. Apply bra or breast binder and breast pads.

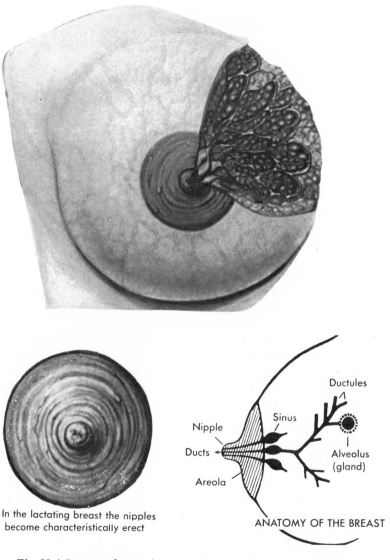

In the lactating breast the nipples become characteristically erect

ANATOMY OF THE BREAST

Fig. 13-4. Lactating breast. (Courtesy Carnation Co., Los Angeles, Calif.)

a. If patients may wear their own bras, be sure they are large enough and clean. Otherwise, apply a supporting breast binder until the patient can have another bra brought in.

b. All patients should have some type of adequate breast support and breast pads whether they are nursing or not.

c. In applying the bra or binder, be sure the breasts are not pushed down against the chest wall. They should be elevated and lifted toward the opposite shoulder.

5. Wash the feet and legs; do not rub vigorously or massage because of the danger of embolus.

6. Perineal care is usually done at the completion of the bath as a separate procedure. At this time the prinicples of perineal self-care are taught.

Anatomy of the breasts

A greater understanding of the basics of breast care, the technique of nursing an infant, and the principles involved in pumping the breasts may be gained at this time by a brief description of the anatomy involved.

The breasts, or mammary glands, are

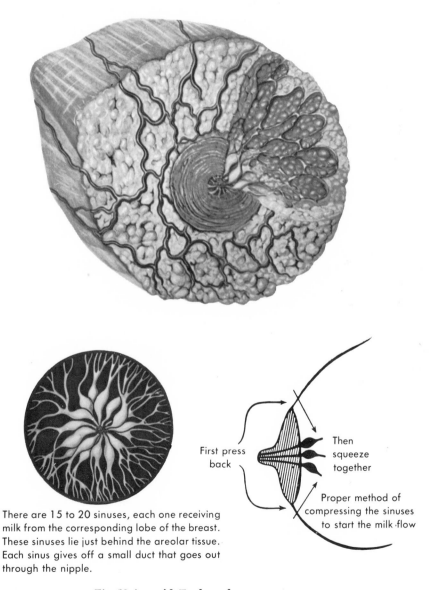

There are 15 to 20 sinuses, each one receiving milk from the corresponding lobe of the breast. These sinuses lie just behind the areolar tissue. Each sinus gives off a small duct that goes out through the nipple.

First press back

Then squeeze together

Proper method of compressing the sinuses to start the milk flow

Fig. 13-4, cont'd. For legend see opposite page.

normally two in number. Each breast is divided into segments, or lobes, which in turn are divided into lobules (smaller lobes). These contain the actual milk-producing glands known as *acini,* or alveoli—as indicated in Fig. 13-4. The breasts are richly supplied with blood vessels, lymphatics, and nerves.

Each segment of the breast radiates from the central colored portion known as the *areola,* which in turn rings the sensitive erectile tissue known as the *nipple.* Milk ducts from the acini travel toward the areola and open out onto the surface of the nipples. There are usually 15 to 20 such openings on one nipple.

As each major milk duct approaches the areola, it widens temporarily, forming a small reservoir, or sinus. When a mother pumps her breasts manually, she obtains the best flow if she first presses the breast tissue back with her thumb and fingers and then squeezes the breast. Properly holding the breast with one hand during nursing not only allows the baby to breathe more comfortably but also encourages the secretion of milk.

When the order is given that a mother's breasts be pumped, it is usually done to maintain or encourage her milk supply. It is not advised routinely to relieve engorgement in nonnursing mothers, since emptying the breasts stimulates more milk production.

Breast engorgement

Breast engorgement may occur about the third day post partum and is often regarded by mothers as the result of the "milk coming in." However, not all the tenderness and swelling results from the presence of more milk. It is, for the most part, the result of the increased venous and lymphatic congestion in the breast tissue.

Engorgement may be avoided or lessened by breast massage techniques and manual expression of colostrum during the prenatal period. It also will be greatly reduced or eliminated by frequent early (on demand) feedings of the newborn. With engorgement, the breasts may feel hard and nodular. Lay people often call this "caked breasts." This uncomfortable and painful condition can sometimes be eased for nursing mothers by the manual expression of a small amount of milk or, if necessary, the short-term use of nipple shields to make it less difficult for the baby to "latch on" and nurse. Good breast support worn continuously, the ordered intermittent application of ice "caps" or warm, moist compresses, or the use of an oxytocin nasal spray prescribed to enhance the letdown reflex and the flow of milk may be helpful. Analgesic drugs may also be prescribed to relieve the pain. Nonnursing mothers may be made more comfortable by supportive bras, the application of ice "caps," analgesics, and the prescription of oral estrogenic or androgenic compounds, such as stilbestrol and cholorotrianisene (Tace). A single intramuscular injection of testosterone enanthate (Deladumone OB) (best given from late first stage to the third stage of labor) may have been prescribed.

Pumping the breasts

A mother may pump her breasts manually as described or use a hand or electric pump as shown in Fig. 13-5. Whatever method is used, she should be supported comfortably in a sitting or side position with her hands and breasts freshly washed. Any equipment that would touch her breasts should have been sterilized before use. If the milk is to be saved for the baby, it should be collected in a sterile container, using aseptic technique. The mother should be instructed how to empty her breasts using the method that is ordered or preferred. If the electric breast pump is used, the nurse must make sure that the suction is not too great. It should be increased gradually. Four to 6 inches of pressure is plenty! A record of the amount of milk obtained should be kept in the patient's chart. Mothers sometimes are distressed at the color of their milk. They should be assured that human breast milk looks weaker or

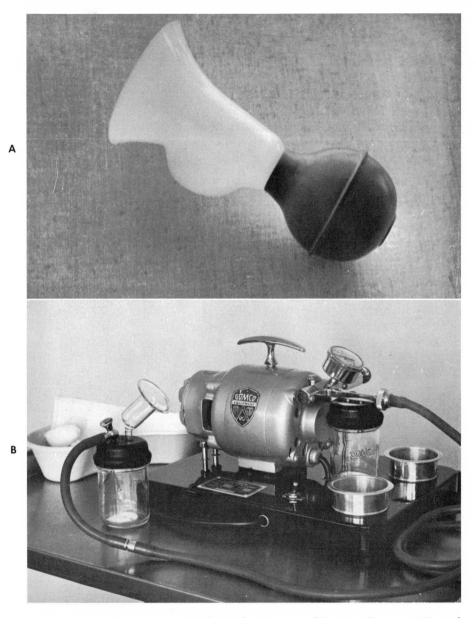

Fig. 13-5. A, Hand breast pump. **B,** Electric breast pump. (Courtesy Grossmont Hospital, La Mesa, Calif.)

more bluish than cow's milk but that it is perfectly suited for baby.

Breast infections

Infections of the breast are not as common today as formerly, but occasionally they still occur. Most infections are introduced at the nipple area, which may be fissured or cracked because of poor nursing techniques or exceptionally fragile breast tissue. If such a complication develops, it is usually not found while the patient is in the postpartum area because of early discharge practices. It becomes the subject of an office call and, rarely, an admission to another part of the hospital for excision and drainage of an abscess. Fortunately, most cases of infectious mastitis do not pro-

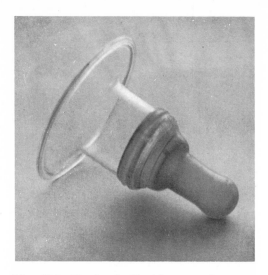

Fig. 13-6. Nipple shield. (Courtesy Grossmont Hospital, La Mesa, Calif.)

gress as far as abscess formation. The nurse should always observe the patient's breasts or inquire about their condition. Signs of inflammation or cracked and bleeding nipples should always be reported. For the latter, a nipple shield (Fig. 13-6) is sometimes ordered, and periodic exposure to warm air (perhaps the local use of a hair dryer) and application of an antiseptic analgesic breast cream may be advised. Breast infections are most often caused by the organism *Staphylococcus aureus.* Any patient with such an infection should be isolated and moved from the maternity service. The application of cold or heat to the breasts may be ordered. The treatment prescribed will depend on the stage of the infection. Systemic antibiotics are commonly given.

Elimination

Constipation may be a problem to the postpartum patient; it may be caused by diminished intestinal and abdominal muscle tone. Physicians often order a mild laxative the evening of the first or second postpartum day. If this medication does not produce results, a suppository or a gentle enema is often scheduled. Since many of these patients suffer from hemorrhoids or have adjacent episiotomy or laceration repairs, one must be very careful in the insertion of the suppository or well-lubricated enema tip. Early ambulation, increased fluids, and a diet containing roughage may prevent constipation. If stools are difficult to pass, a stool softener may be prescribed.

Supportive care and educational opportunities
Aims of postpartal hospitalization

The postpartal hospital stay should ideally provide safety, rest, and constructive encouragement to the recent parturient. However, in some areas the actual hospitalization period is so brief that it is quite difficult to realize the ideal. Brief postpartal hospital experiences are largely motivated by economics and availability of accommodations. It is not unusual in some maternity services to see a mother going home with her baby 2 days or less after her delivery date. Discharge in the third postpartum day is almost routine in many parts of the United States. The pendulum has swung a long way since the time of mother or grandmother, when 5 and 10 days passed by before the new mother stirred from her bed!

The fact that the pendulum of postpartum management needed to swing is not debated. Certainly early ambulation and self-care techniques have reduced the incidence of many complications associated with prolonged bed rest, such as thrombophlebitis, pneumonia, and subinvolution of the uterus. However, the shortened postpartal stay necessitates a prenatal reevaluation of the needs of the new mother and her provisions for help in the home setting. The average primipara has had less opportunity than her counterpart of past generations to learn the arts and crafts of child care in her own family circle while growing up. In many cases her first responsible contact with a newborn infant arrives the day she takes her own baby home from the hospital. Many times she has adequate and loving help at home. Too many times she does not.

Educational resources

There do not seem to be enough hours in the hospital day to teach a new mother what she needs to know about herself and her baby and still give her sufficient time to regain her strength and composure. Of course, in the case of a multipara perhaps educational needs are not as great, but the primipara cannot gain the assurance desired in a 3-day period even if hospital classes and practice sessions could be held all day long and she could attend them all.

At present the answer seems to lie in the introduction of parent-craft courses into the school curriculum, greater utilization of the prenatal courses offered by community agencies such as the YWCA, Red Cross, or public health departments, wider involvement of the visiting nurse, greater availability of rooming-in facilities in hospitals, and a greater awareness on the part of all postpartum staff members of their teaching roles.

The vocational nurse may not find herself involved in any formalized classroom teaching, but the quality of nursing care given, the importance she places on personal hygiene (her own and her patient's), and the skill she develops in observing, listening to, and responding to her patient's needs will make her an important teacher nonetheless.

Of course, in places where postpartum stays are longer and facilities and staff are available, actual classes in baby care, bathing, formula preparation, and nursing techniques may be offered to mothers. Some maternity departments are considering starting closed-circuit TV classes. If the prerequisites are present, the maternity department should not neglect its opportunity.

Rooming-in

The so-called rooming-in plan is especially well adapted to provide learning opportunities for the new mother who desires to have this closer contact with her infant. The baby is kept at the mother's bedside or in an adjoining cubicle close at

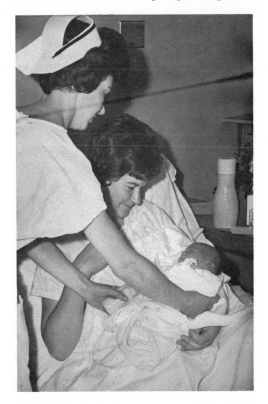

Fig. 13-7. Nurses can do a great deal to reassure new mothers. (Courtesy Grossmont Hospital, La Mesa, Calif.)

hand most of the day. If the mother so desires, her baby may be returned to a special part of the newborn nursery for the night or specified periods. A nursery nurse may be assigned to go to the patient's unit, bathe the baby, and help with any questions that the mother may have. She may return at feeding times and when called to assist in any way necessary. As the mother feels stronger and more confident, she is invited to participate in her child's care. The postpartum nurse washes her hands and wears an overgown when caring for the mother, her unit, or the baby. Visitors are usually restricted to the father. He must wear an overgown during the visit and wash his hands when entering. In this way he, too, is able to know his child better before discharge. Rooming-in is not desired by all parents. Some mothers, especially multiparae, welcome the brief period when they will have little direct responsibility for child care. Others may feel too tired to have the baby at the bedside for extended visits. This method of care however, when available, offers excellent teaching and learning possibilities.

. . .

The new mother is usually an exceptionally good source of questions. Some the nurse will be able to answer immediately. Others she must refer to the physician.

One of the first things the mother wishes to investigate after she has seen her baby and recovered some of her strength is her own weight loss. She is usually dissatisfied with her initial loss the first time she steps on the scale and needs to be reassured that under normal conditions she will approximate her prepregnant weight in about 1 month. However, to help regain a good figure, she must regulate her caloric intake to her metabolic needs. The weight gained during pregnancy in normal conditions is caused by the size of the infant, the weight of the placenta (about 1 pound), the amniotic fluid (about 2 pounds), the increased size of the uterus (about 2 pounds), breast enlargement (about 3 pounds), and increased circulating and tissue fluids and reserves.

Sometimes students are a bit taken aback when they see postpartum patients ambulating for the first time. They confide to one another that Mrs. Smith does not look as though she has delivered yet! Multiparae, because of the repeated stretching of the abdominal muscles, particularly need time and effort to regain a nonpregnant-appearing shape. Occasionally a hernia develops because of the separation of the rectus abdominus muscles, which are supposed to support the adbominal contents. This condition adds to the "pregnant look." A number of years ago the use of straight or many-tailed scultetus abdominal binders for support was common. Now they are not often ordered unless the abdomen is particularly pendulous. If a scultetus binder is ordered in the postpartum period, it should

be applied upside down with the wrapping starting at the top to avoid forcing the uterus up and out of place.

Nowadays it is thought better to rely on the abdominal muscles for support and to build up their strength instead of advocating indiscriminate use of abdominal binders. Various postpartum exercises are recommended to restore muscle tone as well as improve circulation, promote involution, and regain general strength. These exercises are graded according to difficulty, ranging from deep breathing and gentle range of motion to pelvic tilts, leg lifts, and the knee-chest position. The progression of exercises should be directed by the attending physician because some may be too strenuous or even dangerous if done too early. (The knee-chest position done in early puerperium has been associated with a few cases of air embolism.)

Mothers often ask what they may do when they return home. They should be advised to increase their activities gradually, avoid fatigue, lifting heavy objects and older children, and climbing stairs. They should be encouraged to have midmorning and midafternoon rest periods. There is a tendency for a newly delivered mother to try to do too much and then regret it. Even while in the hospital the provision for rest is sometimes limited. Nurses should make every effort to provide their patients with a restful environment. Showers and shampoos at home are allowed as soon as desired. Many physicians allow tub bathing equally as early. Douches and intercourse should be deferred until the routine postpartum checkup by the physician is completed, usually at the end of 6 weeks.

In the interim, patients should be made to feel welcome to contact their physicians if any problems arise. Accessible and knowledgeable nursing staff members, a good physician-patient chat, and the distribution of printed instructions and hints for a smooth adjustment to life with baby before discharge helps solve some of the predictable difficulties. Problems that should be reported when noted include pain or localized tenderness in the legs, increased vaginal flow, painful breasts or cracked nipples, painful urination, backache, and fever.

In the case of nonnursing mothers, menses usually return in 5 to 8 weeks. The nursing mother may not experience menstruation until several weeks after the weaning of her infant. This does not mean, however, that she cannot become pregnant during this period.

Discharge

The discharge of the mother and child from the maternity service is an exciting time for the family. A calm and, literally, collected patient the morning of discharge is rather the exception despite all efforts to smooth the departure. Before the patient leaves, any instructions concerning the mother or baby to be carried out after discharge must be clarified.

The baby is brought to the room after

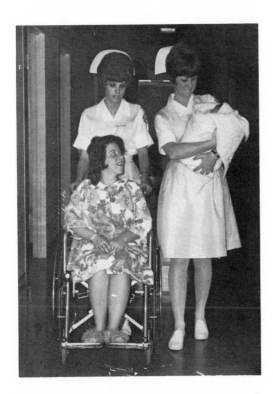

Fig. 13-8. Soon you'll be in your own little bed!

all other arrangements have been completed and the mother is ready to go. Her bags are packed, and she is dressed as she wishes to travel home. Great care should be taken that all her belongings leave with her.

The baby is identified again and dressed for the short trip outdoors to the car. The mother is usually discharged in a wheelchair. The nursing staff sincerely wish to both a "bon voyage."

SPECIAL CONSIDERATIONS

Postpartum hemorrhage, the most common, serious problem in postpartum, has been previously discussed on pp. 1, 2 and 153.

Toxemia of pregnancy has been discussed on pp. 143 to 146.

The cesarean section patient

Let us now discuss some of the exceptional conditions that students encounter in their postpartum experience. First, let us consider the patient who has had a cesarean section. In many hospitals such a patient is kept in a recovery room for several hours before returning to general nursing care. If her cesarean section was anticipated, she may have been admitted initially to the postpartum unit and prepared for surgery by its staff. For information regarding the preparation of a patient for cesarean section, see p. 115, where the topic was discussed in relation to complications of labor and delivery.

The physical care of the postcesarean section patient is similar to that of any patient who has had abdominal surgery. However, in addition, this patient has become a mother. She needs special attention to her postpartal needs.

Nursing care

Immediate observation. The care she receives on transfer is an extension of the postoperative care she received in surgery or the recovery room. Blood pressure, pulse, and respiration rate should be taken at least every 20 minutes for a minimum of 2 hours and until stable. Students are again reminded that a systolic blood pressure reading of 90 mm. Hg or below is usually considered a sign of circulatory shock. A falling blood pressure and a rising pulse are among the first signs of difficulty. Other signs of shock include pallor, cold, clammy skin, apprehension, disorientation or unresponsive behavior, and dilated pupils. But do not wait to observe all the classic signs of shock before seeking help. As is the case with all surgery patients, the dressing should be observed for drainage and any staining reported. The abdominal dressing is not the only site to be watched for signs of hemorrhage, however, The lochia must be observed and evaluated. As a rule cesarean section patients have less lochial flow. After the placenta is extracted during surgery the uterus is inspected and gently sponged, emptying the cavity of some of the drainage that would otherwise be expelled vaginally. The fundus is not routinely palpated because of the presence of the dressing and the recent incision, but its height may be gently measured.

The patient usually receives intravenous fluids during the first 24 to 48 hours. The first ordered fluids may contain an oxytocic to cause the uterus to contract. The intravenous infusion should be frequently observed for rate of flow and signs of infiltration. An indwelling Foley catheter is usually maintained for 24 hours or until the intravenous fluids are discontinued. The catheter should be checked for rate of flow and the type of urine being expelled. The tubing should be stabilized and without dependent loops.

Psychological and postpartal support. Though the initial physical care of the new cesarean section patient is perhaps one's primary priority, the emotional and maternal needs of the patient must not be forgotten. According to her strength and desires, she should be given opportunity to see and handle her infant. Communication with the nursery should be frequent. If the infant can be brought to the bedside for care by the nursery nurse, perhaps this

should be considered. Often the "section patient" feels very isolated and fearful regarding her offspring.

Dietary considerations. At first, the patient is usually given nothing by mouth, and then she is gradually given a progressive surgical diet based on her toleration of oral feedings. This would mean progressing from sips of water to a clear liquid, a soft diet, and then to a regular diet, over a period of approximately 3 to 4 days. Because of their reputations as gas formers, milk, ice water, and citrus juices are many times omitted from the diet along with other notorious foodstuffs such as green peppers, cauliflower, and Brussel sprouts. Some observers believe that drinking through straws may also increase flatus. A new surgical patient or a patient with an intravenous infusion or an indwelling catheter should be on intake and output determinations.

Ambulation. Although orders to get the patient out of bed may not be written until the day after surgery, planned movement in bed should be carried out. The patient is periodically encouraged to breathe deeply and cough as soon as she is put to bed from surgery. She is turned at least every 2 hours. How long she remains flat depends on the anesthetic used (usually spinal), her general condition, and her physician's orders. When she is first allowed out of bed, she should briefly dangle her feet and then stand and march in place; during the second attempt, she walks with the nurse's support. Walking the patient to a chair two steps away for a 15-minute period of sitting is not considered the best interpretation of "ambulate the patient"! The sitting position does not aid the circulation in the lower extremities. It is very important to follow orders for progressive ambulation. Just because a patient is hesitant does not mean that ambulation should not be carried out. The nurse does not need to reiterate all the complications that the physician is seeking to avoid by early ambulation. Usually if she simply states that it will help the patient feel stronger faster and help prevent or relieve flatus, the needed motivation will be provided.

Abdominal distention. Abdominal distention caused by trapped flatus can be quite distressing to any patient who has undergone abdominal surgery. Many times it is the chief complaint of the cesarean section patient. Although medications such as morphine or meperidine hydrochloride (Demerol) may be used for postoperative pain, it is still much better to try to eliminate the distention. As part of her care the nurse should evaluate the condition of the abdomen. Is the area just above the dressing hard, bloated, and tender, or is it soft and relatively flat? Ambulating the patient may help relieve distention—so may intermittent, small enemas, the Harris flush technique, or insertion of a rectal tube. Also helpful are suppositories, laxatives, or the use of neostigmine. Occasionally, strange to say, the use of carbonated drinks helps the patient to "bring up air" more easily and gain relief. In severe cases a nasal gastric tube connected to suction may be inserted.

Sutures. The cesarean patient will receive perineal irrigations for cleanliness and comfort, but no sprays or heat lamps are used, since there are no sutures in the perineal area. But there are abdominal sutures, clips, or adhesive "butterflies" that are usually removed about the fifth or sixth postoperative day.

Complications

Cesarean sections result in a relatively low maternal mortality—less than 0.2%. Neonatal mortality, however, is quite high. The results depend on the condition of the mother and the fetus, the equipment available, and the skill of the operator and nursing staff. The most common serious maternal complications reported are thrombosis and embolism. Occasionally afibrinogenemia complicates the recovery. Most physicians advise no more than three cesarean sections for one patient, although more have been performed. Many physicians believe that once a cesarean section has been performed, subsequent pregnancies should be delivered abdominally because of the danger of rupture of the previous uterine scar. Others believe that a trial labor is justified if obstetrical indications for cesarean section do not persist.

The sorrowing mother

Not all mothers admitted to the postpartum area leave with healthy babies. Some leave without a child because the infant did not survive birth or died in the early hours of life. Some leave alone because their infant is premature or has some abnormality. Still others leave alone because they are not going to keep their babies; They will be placed for adoption. It is especially sad when a new mother who has waited for her child with anticipation finds that for all her waiting and care there is either no child or a child with gross deformities. Mothers of stillborns are usually placed in an area where they will be far from the nursery and away from baby traffic. Supportive nurses who are available, who listen, who recognize the stages of mourning, and respond to the patient's cues, by touch or voice, will be much needed by these women.

Nurses on the postpartum floor should be alerted by the nursery when a baby is not "doing well." Good communications between the nursing and medical staffs concerning what has been told patients regarding their infants is essential. Discretion should be practiced by all nursing personnel.

The unwed mother

At times, conditions surrounding pregnancy and delivery call for "confidential" or "no information" treatment of a patient. For numerous reasons, knowledge of the presence of the patient in the hospital may not be wished to be shared. The patient may be unmarried. Her child may have been conceived before marriage took place. Her husband may not have fathered the child. A patient may simply want a quiet hospital period without undue publicity attached to legitimate pregnancy. Some of these patients will choose to have their babies adopted; others will keep them. "Confidential" or "no information" patients are often cared for in a separate unit or wing.

Several community agencies are engaged in helping the unwed mother and her child. The Salvation Army operates residential and casework facilities as do the Florence Crittenton Homes and various church-related and public organizations, although with changing attitudes and mores, special homes for these maternity patients are less frequently used. Public welfare departments assist with adoption arrangements when desired. It is not the function of the nurse to judge patients who have illegitimate pregnancies. Her function is to meet these patients' postpartum needs as much as possible. The circumstances in which most of these patients find themselves are symptoms and not the cause of basic difficulties in their lives. The nurse may privately disapprove of the conduct of such a patient, but she should not reject the patient herself. This patient needs kindness probably as never before. Constructive help from professional social work personnel to aid the patient in facing the situation and evaluating its causes is indicated (see p. 148).

Postpartum "blues"

As body hormonal levels change and the responsibilities of an enlarging family and infant care rather suddenly make themselves felt, most newly delivered women experience at least some degree of depression, commonly called postpartum "blues." The nurse may enter a patient's room for a routine check and find her previously exuberant mother trying to wipe away some tears. While providing some tissues and gently asking what she may do to help, the nurse is often told that the patient does not really know why she is crying. "The tears just come." The knowledge that mothers sometimes are a bit depressed after delivery is usually reassuring to the patient. "Blues" commonly are not prolonged.

Postpartum psychosis

Labor and delivery is often a physically and emotionally exhausting period even for the normal, healthy woman. For a small minority the entire period of pregnancy is a great strain because of other basic unresolved psychological problems. During the postpartum period these patients may show the development of definite signs of mental illness. They may become withdrawn and disinterested or belligerent and suspicious. They are often victims of unreasonable fears. In severe cases they may become dangerous to themselves and others. Any signs of such behavior or inability to cope with reality should be reported and evaluated by the patient's physician. Psychiatric help may be indicated. Many times these patients have had histories of previous emotional instability or mental illness.

Puerperal infection

The term "puerperal infection" may be used to describe any infection of the reproductive tract during the puerperium. However, more technically speaking, a patient has been considered to have a puerperal infection if she has a fever of 100.4° F. or more on 2 successive days during the first 10 days post partum, excluding the first 24 hours—unless another source of the temperature rise is determined. However, this definition has been found to be inadequate by critics, since many infections may be masked by the use of antibiotics.

The appearance of a puerperal infection is always a serious development. It may involve the perineum proper, the uterine lining (endometritis), or the pelvic area outside the uterus (parametritis). It may extend via blood vessels and lymphatics to areas relatively far removed, as in the case of septic thrombophlebitis of the leg. It is most often localized, but it can become a generalized peritonitis or septicemia. It can be caused by several different organisms, but the usual microorganism implicated is the streptococcus or staphylococcus. If such an unfortunate complication should occur, all effort should be made to determine the original source of the infection. Such detective work involves a knowledge of the history of the patient, the personal health of attending personnel and visitors, and the nursing and medical techniques used.

Accompanying signs and symptoms

Along with the appearance of fever, pelvic infection is often accompanied by abdominal tenderness or pain, foul-smelling lochial drainage, an abnormally large uterus, and the presence of chills. The patient may complain of general malaise and lack of appetite and display a rise in pulse rate. Such signs and symptoms should be reported immediately. Detection of a puerperal infection should initiate isolation procedure and again, if possible, the removal of the patient from the maternity service proper. Such a diagnosis may also affect the nursing procedures in the care of the infant, and the infant would not be allowed to visit his mother.

Treatment of a case of puerperal infection will depend on the extent of involvement. Antibiotics to which the causative organisms are sensitive will be ordered. In cases of pelvic infection the patient will most often be placed in Fowler's position to encourage drainage of the affected area.

Extension of infection

Observation for signs of the extension of the infection or generalized peritonitis should be constant. Such indications would be increased abdominal tenderness and distention and nausea and vomiting, as well as the previously listed symptoms.

Thrombophlebitis. Not all cases of thrombophlebitis involve the presence of infection, but many do. Clots may form anywhere in the body where a slowdown in circulation, a repair of damaged tissue, or a plugging of bleeding vessels occurs. During the postpartum period, clots or thrombi may form in the pelvis or the lower extremities. They may stay localized and interfere with local circulation, set up areas of inflammation, or actually become foci of in-

fection. Rarely, they may break away from the original site of formation and travel about in the circulation. Then they are called emboli (singular, embolus). These clots are particularly dangerous because they may enter some small but vital vessel and cause grave damage or even sudden death. This most often occurs in the case of an embolus or emboli to the lung field or brain.

A common site of thrombophlebitis is the thigh or calf. Sometimes circulation is so impeded that the leg swells considerably, is extremely painful, and may demonstrate red streaks or locally inflamed areas. The skin may be so tense that it appears particularly white. The appearance of the enlarged white extremity gave femoral thrombophlebitis its oldtime lay name of "milkleg." It often occurred at the time of engorgement and to the uninformed appeared to be white because it was "full of milk."

Treatment of femoral thrombophlebitis varies considerably depending on the philosophy and experiences of the physician in charge. Some will order elevation and the application of heat with a heat cradle or pad. Others will order ice packs. Antibiotics may be indicated. Some may prescribe anticoagulants to cut down on the formation of further thrombi. The nurse must recognize that use of anticoagulants on a postpartum patient increases the possibility of postpartum hemorrhage significantly. Her observations of any abnormal bleeding would need to be quickly reported. Blood pressure would need to be taken periodically. Prothrombin determinations by the laboratory would be expected.

An order for Ace bandages or other elastic-type leg supports is common. Applied correctly, they help speed the venous circulation back to the heart and discourage the formation of clots. No massage of the legs is permitted for fear of dislodging previously formed clots. Ambulation is only ordered dependent on the day-by-day progress of the patient revealed by the presence or absence of fever and her general condition. Thrombophlebitis may occur in

171

all degrees of severity. Some physicians automatically order Ace bandages applied to the legs of their patients who have had difficulties with varicosities, as a preventive measure.

· · ·

The postpartum stay is brief in many parts of the United States. However, the nurse can do much, even in this short interval, to aid the patient to face her increased responsibilities with added knowledge, skill, energy, and assurance.

14

Population, ecology, and reproduction

Any text focused on maternal and child health published in the decade of the 70's would be neglecting a crucial area of concern and controversy if it did not include at least a brief consideration of the topics of population, natural resources, and environmental protection. These subjects are vitally linked with such obstetrical and pediatric interests as genetic counseling, birth planning, abortion, sterilization, fertility, and adoption. Because discussion of birth planning has often been part of postpartal counseling, these topics are included in this unit. However, it is readily understood that they represent a much broader area of concern, involving more than this particular interval in an individual's life.

For many centuries, some of these subjects were deemed either irrelevant, irreverent, or simply outside the possibility of human control. The idea that the entire earth could become seriously impoverished or poisoned by mankind was foreign to most human thought. A rather simple optimism existed that as one resource became scarce, another would be prepared to take its place. Problems of ecology, such as the balance of nature, were considered to be largely theoretical or curiosities of only local importance.

Now, of course, one can hardly pick up a popular magazine or scientific journal without encountering a discussion of some aspect of this very complex problem. In fact, some people have already grown weary of the theme and request a respite. Some believe that the ecological crisis has been overstated and is being used to divert attention from other international and domestic issues that cannot afford to be slighted. However, the wish to avoid appropriate analysis and any subsequent necessary action must not be granted if we are to be reckoned responsible ancestors by those who live after us.

Let us consider some of the factors that have made those engaged in predicting the shape of tomorrow's world extremely uneasy. They revolve about the realization that although the earth's resources are finite, or limited, the demands for her bounty are steadily increasing (Fig. 14-1). Note that the world population projected by the United Nations for the year 2000 is more than twice that of 1960. The reason for this vast increase is the decrease in infant and maternal mortality and the lengthening of the average life-span. Also sobering is the prediction that the major areas experiencing this population growth will be the underdeveloped countries, where often a large percentage of the people already live on the border of starvation. Although some have expressed the opinion that methods will be found to substantially increase food production and provide the nourishment necessary, a look at the current doubling time of our planet's population should cause us to reject this theory. It is presently estimated that our current world population, barring intervention, will double in approximately 35 years. The doubling time for the population of the United States was estimated in 1974 to be 100 years. Even if interplanetary colonization were soon feasible, we would, at this rate, still eventually face an unmanageable population growth.*

Other threats to earth's inhabitants besides starvation should be identified. An in-

---

*Ehrlich, P. R.: The population bomb, New York, 1968, Ballantine Books, Inc., pp. 17-26.

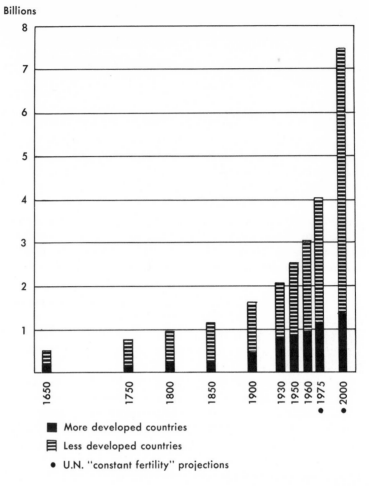

Billions

Fig. 14-1. Growth of world population. (Courtesy Planned Parenthood-World Population, New York, N. Y.) Note: according to the Population Reference Bureau, Washington, D. C., world population by the year 2000 is estimated (as of August, 1974) to reach about 6.5 billion persons. Reduction in population growth rates occurred chiefly in the more developed countries.

creasing population uses more and more raw materials of all kinds. When the supply of an article is limited, intense competitive activity may develop in an effort to obtain its control. A nation whose population is rapidly increasing and whose vital resources are curtailed has frequently become a militant nation. As peoples double and triple in number, both goods and services are stretched to the point where they can no longer meet basic human needs, and more mental and physical illness is to be anticipated. Is mankind expecting famine, war, and disease to automatically solve our

population problem? There must be other more acceptable alternatives! To preserve a worthwhile world for our children these should be intensively and extensively explored.

The options would all seem to involve a conscious, orderly limitation of the number of persons who are to inherit our earth. Such a limitation may be achieved in various ways, and there is much debate regarding the efficiency and morality of the techniques employed. The basic methods, all of which have been used at some time, are (1) abstinence, (2) contraception, (3) premeditated abortion, (4) sterilization, (5) infanticide, and (6) adult murder.

Attitudes, both public and private, concerning the desirability and methods of birth planning have undergone considerable modification in the last 40 years. Changes have been particularly marked in the last decade. Of the methods just listed, infanticide and adult murder are, of course, unacceptable to all. Abstinence, although very efficient when practiced, appears difficult to maintain. Its use within the context of marriage, except for special circumstances for agreed periods, may be questioned. Three methods seem to have gained some acceptance by segments of modern society today. They are contraception, abortion, and sterilization.

All human beings do not accept the same explanation of the origin and meaning of life, nor do they agree concerning the order of life's priorities. A number of diverse codes of behavior or morality of varying usefulness to present society and the individual are observed. When the morality of an individual or group clashes significantly with the concepts of right or wrong held by another person or group, the parties involved may label the activities of the other "immoral." In reality, probably any evaluation of human conduct considered controversial would include more than the two points of view. Indeed, one might say that in addition to the perspectives of those persons engaged in a dispute, there is also the perspective of truth that some would declare is reserved to God alone.

Philosophical differences in viewpoint cause various groups or individuals to endorse, tolerate, or condemn certain techniques of population control or family planning. These philosophical considerations include convictions regarding (1) the ultimate purpose and potential of the individual and mankind as a whole, (2) how the developmental state of the unborn child affects his status as a person or soul, (3) the rights of the unborn vis-à-vis those who have already begun extrauterine existence, (4) the purposes of the marriage relation-

ship and sexual intercourse, (5) the responsibility and ability of the individual to make and implement decisions involving personal conduct, and (6) the role of Diety in the affairs of man.

Various religious groups have spoken regarding these matters at different times. Though most agree concerning the importance of the population problem, they are not agreed regarding the morality of the methods proposed to ease it. Because of the size and structure of the Roman Catholic Church and the historical authority of the papacy, the encyclical letter of Pope Paul VI, Humanae Vitae, or "Of Human Life," has been much discussed. Within this document, Pope Paul states that ". . . the Church, calling men back to the observance of the norms of the natural law, as interpreted by their constant doctrine, teaches that each and every marriage act . . . must remain open to the transmission of life." He does, however, recognize that "if . . . there are serious motives to space out births, which derive from the physical or psychological conditions of husband and wife, or from external conditions, it is then licit to take into account the natural rhythms . . . for the use of marriage in the infecund periods only. . . ."* Periodic abstinence or continence of married couples is approved. Premeditated abortion, even for therapeutic reasons, and sterilization of either sex is prohibited. There continues to be much dialogue concerning these considerations in the Catholic church today. Evangelical Christian and Jewish representatives, though usually assuming positions of greater acceptance and in numerous instances endorsing birth planning, are not of "one mind"— lacking unity regarding the propriety of different contraceptive techniques and the practices of abortion and sterilization.

CONTRACEPTION

Contraceptive techniques or methods used to temporarily prevent birth are usu-

---

*From Encyclical Letter of Pope Paul VI: Of human life, 1968.

ally considered to fall into three main categories: (1) those that prevent fertilization, (2) those that prevent ovulation, and (3) those that prevent implantation. Strictly speaking, the last is not a method of contraception, since the egg may be fertilized but unable to embed itself into the uterine lining to maintain life.

The first efforts to limit birth were designed to prevent fertilization. These methods included premature withdrawal of the penis before ejaculation during intercourse (coitus interruptus), the selection of infertile periods for sexual relations, and the use of various kinds of barriers by the man or woman to prevent the entry of the sperm through the cervical opening. Barrier techniques included the use of the penile sheath, "prophylactic," or condom, the insertion of various cervical caps or diaphragms, and/or the application of spermicidal chemicals. The method that involves the prevention of ovulation is the use of "the pill" for which there are numerous chemical formulas. Although the mechanism is not clear, the intrauterine contraceptive devices seem to help prevent the implantation of a fertilized egg. A brief description of these methods follows.

Methods used to prevent conception

1. Coitus interruptus (withdrawal, "being careful"). This is probably the oldest type of birth control practiced. It has been accused of being related to the incidence of pelvic congestion and frigidity in females and enlargement of the prostate and impotence in males. However, these charges have not been proved, and the method is used by many couples.

2. The "rhythm technique." This method depends on the identification of the infecund period of each individual woman's menstrual cycle, which is best determined by an extended, careful calendar history of her menses and her basal body temperature patterns. Such combined procedures are prudent, since menstrual cycles differ so much from woman to woman and, indeed, at various times in the experience of one woman. Ovulation may not always be correctly detected even with the help of these procedures. The use of a calendar alone to estimate the time of ovulation or the period of greatest fertility reduces protection considerably. Any calculation of an infecund period must consider that spermatozoa live approximately 72 hours after deposit and that an ovum is available for fertilization for an estimated 24 hours. This method involves temporary abstinence during the period of risk. The Catholic Marriage Advisory Council recommends the inclusion of days 10 through 19 of the menstrual cycle. The detection of ovulation by changes in basal body temperature is illustrated in Fig. 14-2.

3. Condom. The most widely used birth control device in the world, the condom was probably first employed to prevent the spread of venereal disease. It must be carefully applied to the penis after erection. It can be used in conjunction with chemical contraceptives, which may also serve as lubricants.

4. Cervical caps and diaphragms. Use of these devices was first reported in the 1800's. Cervical caps may be made of rubber, metal, or plastic. They fit closely over the cervix. Diaphragms are latex domes with spring rims (Fig. 14-3). They are positioned over the cervix between the pubic bone and posterior vaginal wall. Both devices must be used in conjunction with spermicidal cream or jelly. They hold these chemicals in place over the mouth of the uterus. Caps and diaphragms must be fitted by a doctor or technician. The patient's ability to insert them properly must be checked, and detailed education regarding their use is necessary. Because of anatomical differences not all women can be fitted satisfactorily. Some women find it distasteful to insert the device. These barriers are most effective when inserted no longer than 1 hour before intercourse, since the spermicidal application becomes less powerful with the passing of time, and should remain in place at least 6 hours after intercourse.

176

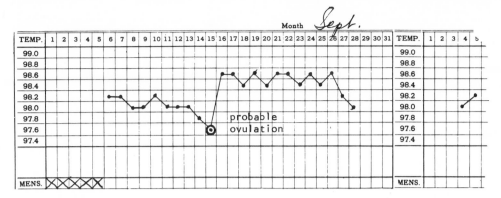

Month *Sept.*

TEMP.	1	2	3	4	5	6	7	8	9	10	11	12	13	14	15	16	17	18	19	20	21	22	23	24	25	26	27	28	29	30	31	TEMP.	1	2	3	4	5
99.0																																99.0					
98.8																																98.8					
98.6																																98.6					
98.4																																98.4					
98.2																																98.2					
98.0																																98.0					
97.8												probable																				97.8					
97.6												ovulation																				97.6					
97.4																																97.4					
MENS.																																MENS.					

Fig. 14-2. Basal body temperature graph. Normally, ovulation is signaled by a drop in basal body temperature of about half a degree Fahrenheit followed by a rise of 1 degree or more. This relative elevation continues until about 2 days before the menstrual flow reappears. If pregnancy occurs, the temperature remains within a relatively high range. Basal body temperatures must be taken consistently, either rectally or vaginally before *any* activity directly on awakening each morning.

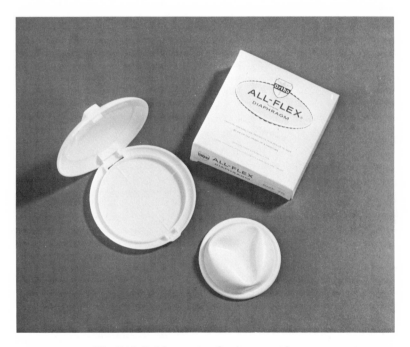

Fig. 14-3. Rubber spring diaphragm with case.

5. Chemical contraceptives used alone. These substances are available in the form of creams, jellies, suppositories, foams, and aerosols. They must be applied immediately before sexual relations and be allowed to remain in the vagina for 6 hours after intercourse. Couples sometimes complain that they are irritating to tissues and "messy" to use.

6. Vaginal sponges. These may be made of natural or synthetic materials and have been used in conjunction with spermicidal chemicals. They may be bulky and possibly irritating.

7. Douches. Vaginal irrigations are not recommended as a means of contraception. Sperm may enter the cervix 10 to 90 seconds after ejaculation. Douching may help to force sperm into the uterus.

Methods used to prevent ovulation

In recent years various combinations of estrogens and progesterone-like compounds have been introduced in tablet form that, when taken orally as directed, are designed to prevent the escape of the ovum from the ovary. They simulate pregnancy in this regard. Another associated action of these substances that help prevent pregnancy in the rare instances when ovulation is not inhibited involves the decrease in and the thickening of cervical mucus, making the uterus less hospitable to spermatozoa. "The pill" was first accepted for general use by prescription in the United States in 1960. It is now the most popular method of contraception in this country. If the standard technique of administration is followed, a woman is given a special dispenser to help her keep a record of her medication. She takes one tablet every day, beginning the fifth day of her monthly flow, for 20 or 21 days (depending on the type of pill); then she discontinues the tablets. Usually menstrual-like vaginal bleeding results from 1 to 3 days later. She begins her medication again on the fifth day of this period. There are three main types of pills and programs that may be prescribed. One prescription uses one type of tablet (the combination) that includes both estrogens and progesterones throughout. The second includes two types of tablets to be taken in special sequence—first an estrogen only, then the last five days, a combined pill like those previously described. The third type is the all-progestin Mini Pill (norethindrone), which is taken *every* day. Perhaps it should not technically be placed in this category, since it does not necessarily inhibit ovulation but seems to prevent sperm transport by causing cervical mucus to thicken. Irregular menstrual-type bleeding will occur. If it seems excessive or prolonged or if pregnancy is suspected, a physician should be consulted. It is claimed to be 96% effective. The so-called morning-after pill designed to be taken after unprotected intercourse often contains diethylstilbestral in large doses. It has not been sufficiently studied at this time to comment regarding its safety or efficacy. It may cause considerable nausea.

Frequently reported problems associated with oral contraception include nausea, occasional vomiting, breast tenderness, acne, headache, increased weight gain, and irregular vaginal bleeding. Paradoxically, however, some women are placed on the pill, not primarily for contraceptive protection, but because its use may eliminate or reduce dysmenorrhea and symptoms of premenstrual tension. It may also improve acne. Although an increased incidence of blood clot formation and embolism has not been demonstrated conclusively, it is possible that certain women may be more susceptible. Research investigating its hypertensive effects is now in progress.

Disadvantages involved in its use also include (1) the need for ability and motivation to proceed with its administration faithfully, (2) its expense, and (3) possible interference in lactation, causing insufficient milk supply and unknown absorption of the drug by the baby. However, some physicians are prescribing low-dose contraceptives to lactating mothers. Advantages include its high reliability, the fact that its use is removed from the actual sex act, and the patient's ability to stop therapy and conceive.

Methods that may prevent implantation

Authorities are not agreed as to how the intrauterine devices (IUD) may prevent birth. It would seem, however, that the mechanism involved interferes in some way with the fertilization process, the readiness of a fertilized ovum to implant, and/or the ability of the uterine wall to receive the egg. IUD's are not new, but only within the last decade have they been used with much success. Those inserted in the early 1900's

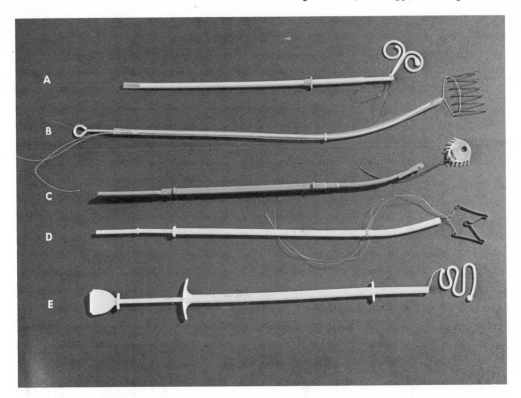

Fig. 14-4. Various types of intrauterine devices with their inserters. *A*, Saf-T-Coil; *B*, Majzlin spring; *C*, Dalkon shield; *D*, "M" device; *E*, Lippes loop. The Majzlin Spring is not currently being marketed.

often caused tissue damage and infection because of their placement or design. Their use was largely abandoned by physicians. However, since the advent of polyethylene and improved designs, including the tiny 7-shaped copper-containing "7 cu" IUD, they have been a particularly popular method for controlling birth in populations who lack the finances, skill, or opportunity to use other techniques. IUD's must be positioned by a proficient physician or technician. They may still be associated with uterine cramping and bleeding and, in rare instances, infection and perforation. (Because there have been four fatalities caused by spontaneous septic abortion among women using the Dalkon shield, this IUD is now undergoing special investigation. The Majzlin spring has been withdrawn from the market because of instances in which it had embedded itself in the uterine wall. However, considering the many IUD's that

have been inserted, the incidence of complications appears to be quite low—less than that reported for "the pill.") IUD's may be spontaneously expelled. However, once inserted they require little care and unless expelled, they may remain in place for months or years without untoward symptoms. Ectopic pregnancies occur more frequently among wearers of IUD's than among pregnant women in general not because the device causes these abnormally placed pregnancies but because it prevents uterine pregnancy much more efficiently than extrauterine gestation. Occasionally, failure of the device may be noted in the delivery room when it is identified by the attending obstetrician after the birth of a baby (Fig. 14-4).

Reliability of contraceptive methods

An evaluation of the efficiency or reliability of the various methods of contraception is difficult to present in statistical terms because in some instances data collection and analysis have posed particular problems. However, all discussions consulted considered oral contraception the most effective. (Some writers claimed 100% success when the pill was "taken as prescribed.")* All discussions also rated the IUD as second-most reliable. Contraceptive techniques perhaps can be ranked for effectiveness as follows, with the recognition that more research is needed:

Most reliable	"The pill"
Highly reliable	Intrauterine devices
	Condom
	Diaphragm with jelly or cream
	Cervical cap
Moderately reliable	Aerosol vaginal foam
	Rhythm, using basal body temperature
	Jelly or cream alone (non-foaming)
	Suppositories
	Intravaginal tablets (foaming and nonfoaming)
Less reliable	Withdrawal
	Rhythm (calendar computation)
	Vaginal sponge
Least reliable	Douche

It is plain that there is no perfect method applicable to all persons and circumstances, and research continues. Equally clear is the trite observation that a method must be used consistently to be effective. It is important to note that the maternal death rate associated with pregnancy and delivery is greater than that associated with the use of any of the types of contraceptives previously discussed and more than that of legal first-trimester abortion.

ABORTION

If a pregnancy occurs that for medical, psychiatric, economic, or social reasons is unwanted by those who would have the responsibility of bearing and caring for the child, the possibility of terminating the in-

---

*Guttmacher, A. F.: Birth control and love, New York, 1969, The Macmillan Co., p. 35.

trauterine life before it is supposedly capable of extrauterine survival is sometimes considered. Until 1967 the only way that a woman could procure a legal abortion in most states was through a statement of medical agreement that continuation of the pregnancy would be a threat to her life. (A few states also considered the *health* of the mother in the wording of relevant legislation.) Laws condemning abortion were written approximately a hundred years ago when the operation was dangerous, even under the best auspices, and in unskilled hands was often catastrophic. Community concepts concerning population growth, the roles of women and children, and meanings and rules surrounding sex, pregnancy, and childbirth also influenced this legislation. In the 1967 to 1973 interval several states modified their statutes to include other reasons for abortion: the mother's physical and mental health, probable serious deformity of the baby, and cases of incest or rape. A few made abortion, with certain reservations, a private decision between a woman and her physician.

In January, 1973, the United States Supreme Court in a vote of 7 to 2 ruled that the state may not intervene with the decision of a woman and her physician to undergo an abortion during the first trimester of pregnancy. However, during the last 6 calendar months the state may regulate and monitor medical practice associated with abortion to protect the health (mental or physical) of the mother. The court further stipulated that only in the last 12 weeks of pregnancy do the states have the authority to prohibit abortion in cases not threatening the health or life of the mother.

The judicial decision has not been unchallenged, and practical compliance to the law appears uneven although 25 attorneys general simply declared their former state legislation "null and void." Organizations such as the Right to Life Committee and the National Youth Pro-Life Coalition, which favor abortion only when the mother's life is in danger, are supporting efforts to overturn the Supreme Court decision by a constitutional amendment as well as other anti-abortion legislation. Meanwhile the National Abortion Rights Action League (N.A.R.A.L.) is working to maintain and expand the impact of the 1973 court action. In April, 1973, a Louis Harris survey indicated that 52% of U. S. citizens supported the court in its decision of legalizing abortions in the first trimester; 41% opposed it, and 7% were undecided.

First-trimester abortions may be performed in doctors' offices, separate clinics, or hospitals. Abortions occurring later are carried out in hospitals. Medical personnel should be familiar with the regulating laws of the area where they practice. The question of professional participation in abortion when not done for obvious health needs of the mother is emotionally charged, morally disturbing, and legally complex for many. As the legal abortion rate has risen, maternal and infant mortality rates have dipped, but reported embryonic and fetal deaths have, of course, climbed.

Nurses should be familiar with the laws of the area in which they practice and how they have been interpreted. Legal sanctions regarding this problem are currently undergoing rapid change.

The following methods of abortion are employed in hospital settings if the pregnancy is of less than 3 months' duration:

1. Dilatation and curettage. The cervical canal is progressively dilated, and the products of conception are gently scraped from their uterine attachments.

2. Aspiration. The uterine contents are dislodged by the use of a specially designed suction catheter. The procedure is rapid (approximately 5 minutes), and blood loss is minimal. It is now the most common method used with the least complications.

Methods used if the pregnancy is of greater duration are as follows:

1. Intra-amniotic instillations. Techniques vary. Amniotic fluid is withdrawn from the bag of waters by a vaginal or abdominal approach. This fluid is usually replaced by an equal amount of approximately 200 ml. concentrated (20%) saline solution. An antibiotic may also be instilled. The hypertonic salt solution kills the fetus and usually initiates uterine contractions within a day or two. Complications have included inflammation of the uterine lining, retained products of conception, hemorrhage, and cardiovascular collapse. The risks of mortality are not negligible.

2. Hysterotomy. This is a type of cesarean section, but it is performed when a nonviable fetus is judged present. It usually involves a hospitalization and recovery period similar to that of a patient who has had a cesarean section.

Obviously, interruption of a pregnancy after 3 months is a more difficult and hazardous procedure. The poor and uneducated are more likely to be second-trimester abortion patients. The psychological impact of abortion, though perhaps not immediately apparent, is a critical consideration. Clearly, contraception is a better solution than abortion. The nursing care of the patient who has had an abortion is briefly discussed in Chapter 12.

STERILIZATION

In some instances an individual or couple, for health, genetic or social considerations, may wish to permanently discontinue the capacity to have children. Any process that produces this result may be termed "sterilization." The written consent of a spouse, although not usually a legal requirement, may be requested by the hospital or physician. Such procedures may be performed without interfering with the ability to participate in sexual relations or diminishing any masculine or feminine characteristics previously present.

Either the male or female may be sterilized. Women may now be sterilized by the occlusion of the fallopian tubes by electrocoagulation while the physician observes the operative site through a laparoscope introduced into the abdominal cavity. It may be performed in the hospital on an in- or out-patient basis. It is considered effective, inexpensive, with a low complication rate. Sterilization of the male by vas ligation or vasectomy is accomplished without entry into the abdominal cavity. It may be an office procedure. Twin surgical incisions are often made in the area where the scrotum joins the body, just over the vas. The ducts are tied and separated. Portions may be excised. After the operation the male does not become sterile immediately, and follow-up sperm counts should be made to determine when contraceptive techniques are unnecessary.

Although sterilization procedures are performed to be permanent, occasionally a man or woman may regret his or her decision. In some cases the tubes may be rejoined and reproductive ability regained, but sterilization should be viewed initially as a lasting intervention. Occasional spontaneous failures of sterilization techniques have been reported, but attempts to provide temporary sterility using various devices have been disappointing.

• • •

This section has been a discussion of methods used to limit population. That they can be successful is probably demonstrated by the decline in birth rate shown in Fig. 14-5. In some instances birth control has been used to control the types, as well as the number, of persons living in our world. The power to control population is staggering in magnitude and implies the application of value judgments that would seem beyond the ethical capacity of small influential groups. It is hoped that voluntary action based on intensive research and education will be forthcoming and that the democratic process of action through representation will continue to function.

GENETIC COUNSELING

One fairly recent attempt to advise individuals of the probable inherited potential of their offspring and thus make possible more enlightened decisions regarding family size is the establishment of genetic counseling services. There is no coercive action associated with the information given. What persons do with the knowledge they

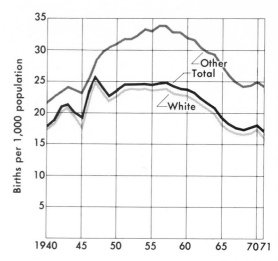

Fig. 14-5. U. S. birth rates: 1940-1971 (1971 figures are provisional). Source: Maternal and Child Health Project, George Washington University, using data from National Center for Health Statistics. (From Maternal and Child Health Service reports on: Promoting the health of mothers and children, FY 1973, Washington, D. C., U. S. Department of Health, Education, and Welfare.)

gain is a personal choice. Through the use of the services of a genetic counselor the genealogy of the client or couple may be investigated. This is particularly helpful when a hereditary problem has been identified in a person's family, but the potential incidence of the defect is unknown. The investigation may include pedigree analysis and tissue studies to determine chromosomal patterns and biological constituents. Counseling by the service may also be of value in cases of possible alteration or damage of an individual's genetic components. (See also Chapter 19, p. 272.)

SUBFERTILITY OR INFERTILITY

In a world where population increase is a major problem it may seem inconsistent to be concerned about the inability of a man and wife to conceive. Yet the capacity to have children of one's own lineage is particularly desired by and meaningful to most persons even if they are not ruling monarchs or shahs! Some authorities have stated that a marriage may be regarded as infertile when pregnancy has not occurred after a year of periodic intercourse without the use of contraception.

Occasionally, instruction concerning the fertile period and the rhythm technique in reverse is all that is necessary. However, anatomical or physiological problems may exist. If infertility is present, it may be caused by problems associated with either or both sexual partners. Statistically when a definite cause is determined, the male is found to be the cause as often as the female. Alan Guttmacher, past President of Planned Parenthood Federation of America, estimated that one third to one half of childless couples could be helped to have children if they received "prompt investigation and treatment."*

This investigation usually begins with an evaluation of the reproductive capacity of the man. Recent semen samples are examined microscopically to detect abnormalities in the number, form, and motility of his sperm. If few or no sperm are found, a testicular biopsy and x-ray studies may determine whether the spermatozoa are being manufactured but lack transport because of a blockage of his reproductive system. If this is the case, surgery to relieve the obstacle is sometimes possible. If sperm are not being produced or are limited in quantity, hormonal therapy may be helpful. Attention to the general overall physical and emotional condition of the patient may also prove rewarding.

Evaluation of the capacity of the female to conceive is more complex because of the difference in anatomy. A complete physical examination is usually followed by a determination of the ability of the woman to ovulate. Several methods may be used; these include detection of a characteristic pattern of basal body temperature reading (see Fig. 14-2), microscopic examination of a biopsy of the endometrium, or lining of the uterus, and investigation of the viscosity of the cervical mucus. If ovulation is estab-

lished, examination of the patency of the fallopian tubes through dye and gas studies may be performed. The uterine cavity, the vaginal canal, and the type and action of cervical and vaginal secretions may also be investigated.

If ovulation does not occur, hormonal therapy as well as general measures to improve health may be helpful. One example of a hormonal product that stimulates ovarian function is follicle-stimulating hormone (Pergonal). Another medication that has been used to promote pregnancy is clomiphene citrate (Clomid). These medications have been known to promote the maturation of more than one ovum during the menstrual cycle, causing the development of multiple births (for example, quadruplets and quintuplets). Since these infants are usually of low birth weight and very fragile, multiple births are a mixed blessing to even the most eager parents.

The surgical intervention to open blocked passageways that must be traversed by the ascending sperm or the descending egg may also be performed with varying success depending on the area to be treated. Sometimes the diagnostic procedures used to detect fallopian tube obstruction also serve as therapy, causing the removal of minor blocks in the oviducts. Medical treatment of pelvic inflammatory disease may enable conception to occur.

How intensively solutions for infertility will be sought depends on the ages of the couple, their continued interest, cooperation, and financial resources. At times, persistent failure to conceive because of certain defects of the male can be circumvented through artificial insemination techniques using the husband's sperm. More rarely, semen from an anonymous healthy, normal male may be employed. Adoption or foster parenthood, although sometimes not available to couples and often involving long waiting periods, may be a satisfying alternative. There are certainly many children already on earth who need loving care.

---

*Guttmacher, A. F.: Birth control and love, New York, 1969, The Macmillan Co., p. 236.

• • •

Never before in the history of our world have the questions of population, ecology, and reproduction appeared more pressing than in this last half of the twentieth century. It behooves all our citizenry to be informed concerning the problems to be faced and their possible solutions. All those engaged in the provision of maternal and child health, whether within or outside the hospital setting, need to be especially involved in striving to increase the possibility that a newborn boy or girl will not only be well and well-formed, but also welcome.

unit six
Suggested selected readings and references

Abortion—one year after Supreme Court decision, Contemp. OB/GYN 3:26-46, Jan., 1974.

Almound, A. M.: Is breast feeding right for you? Parents' Magazine and Better Homemaking 49:29-31, April, 1974.

Anonymous: Personal experience at a legal abortion center, Am. J. Nurs. 72:110-112, Jan., 1972.

Ausubel, F., Beckwith, J., and Janssen, K.: Stimulus/response: the politics of genetic engineering: who decides who's defective? Psychology Today 8:30-43, June, 1974.

Bauman, K., and Udry, J. R.: Evaluation of the five-year family planning plan: five million poor women and unwanted births, Health Services Reports 88:814-817, Nov., 1973.

Berk, H.: Complications of intrauterine instillation of saline for abortion, Contemp. OB/GYN 2:11-13, Dec., 1973.

Blake, J.: The teenage birth control dilemma and public opinion, Nurs. Digest 1:67-71, Oct., 1973.

Branson, H.: Nurses talk about abortion, Am. J. Nurs. 72:106-109, Jan., 1972.

Calderone, M. S.: Sex and social responsibility, J. Home Economics 57:499-502, Sept., 1965.

Calderone, M. S.: Education in human sexuality for health professionals, Nurs. Digest 1:48-54, Dec., 1973. Condensed from Am. Rev. World Health 18:25-29, Winter-Spring-Summer, 1970.

Catz, C. S., and Giacoia, G. P.: Drugs and breast milk, Pediatr. Clin. North Am. 19:151-164, Feb., 1972.

Clark, A. L., and Hale, R. W.: Sex during and after pregnancy, Am. J. Nurs. 74:1430-1431, Aug., 1974.

Clausen, J.: Efficient postpartum checks, Nurs. '72 2:24-25, Oct., 1972.

Connell, E. B.: The pill and the problems, Am. J. Nurs. 71:326-332, Feb., 1971.

Countryman, B. A.: Breast care in the early puerperium, J. Obstet. Gynecol. Neonatal Nurs. 2:36-40, Sept.-Oct., 1973.

Crist, T.: Assistance for the sexually active female, J. Obstet. Gynecol. Neonatal Nurs. 2:36-40, March-April, 1973.

Cronenwett, L. R., and Choyce, J. M.: Saline abortion, Am. J. Nurs. 71:1754-1757, Sept., 1971.

The crucial math of motherhood, Life 72:46-52B, May 19, 1972.

Davis, J. E.: Vasectomy, Am. J. Nurs. 72:509-513, March, 1972.

DeBell, G., editor: The environmental handbook, New York, 1970, Ballantine Books, Inc.

DeMarest, R. J., and Sciarra, J. J.: Conception, birth, and contraception, New York, 1969, McGraw-Hill Book Co., Inc.

Edwards, J.: Wrong and right approaches in maternal care, RN 33:65-81, Jan., 1970.

Edwards, J.: When the baby is stillborn, RN 34:44+, Nov., 1971.

Ehrlich, P. R.: The population bomb, New York, 1968, Ballantine Books, Inc.

Estok, P. J.: What do nurses know about breast-feeding problems? J. Obstet. Gynecol. Neonatal Nurs. 2:36-39, Nov.-Dec., 1973.

Gardner, R. F. R.: Christian choices in a liberal abortion climate, Christianity Today 14:766-768, May 22, 1970.

Guttmacher, A. F.: Birth control and love (wholly revised and greatly expanded edition of the complete book of birth control, Ballantine Books, Inc., 1961), New York, 1969, Macmillan Publishing Co., Inc.

Holt, L. F., and others: A study of premature infants fed cold formula, J. Pediatr. 61:556-561, 1962.

Houghton, B.: Vasectomies affect women, too, Am. J. Nurs. 73:821, May, 1973.

Hubbard, E.: How we solve breast feeding problems, RN 33:46+, March, 1970.

Iffrig, M. C.: Nursing care and success in breast feeding, Nurs. Clin. North Am. 3:345-354, June, 1968.

Johnson, J. M.: Stillbirth—a personal experience, Am. J. Nurs. 72:1595-1596, Sept., 1972.

Johnson, L. B., Burket, R. L., and Rauh, J. L.: Problems with contraception in adolescents, Clin. Pediatr. 10:315-319, June, 1971.

Keller, C., and Copeland, P.: Counseling the abortion patient is more than talk, Am. J. Nurs. 72:102-106, Jan., 1972.

Kilker, R., and Wilkerson, B.: 8-point postpartum assessment, Nurs. '73 3:56, May, 1973.

Ledger, W. J.: The new face of puerperal sepsis, J. Obstet. Gynecol. Neonatal Nurs. 3:36-32, March-April, 1974.

Lerch, C.: Maternity nursing, ed. 2, St. Louis, 1974, The C. V. Mosby Co., pp. 20-44, 270-277.

Lipkin, G. B.: Psychosocial aspects of maternal-child nursing, St. Louis, 1974, The C. V. Mosby Co.

Manisoff, M. T.: Intrauterine devices, Am. J. Nurs. **73:**1188-1191, July, 1973.

Masters, W., and Johnson, V.: Human sexual response, Boston, 1966, Little, Brown and Co.

McCalister, D. V., Thiessen, V., and McDermott, M.: Readings in family planning, St. Louis, 1973, The C. V. Mosby Co.

Meadows, D. H., and others: The limits to growth, New York, 1972, Universe Books.

Moore, F. I.: Influence of postpartum home visits on postpartum clinic attendance, Public Health Reports **89:**360, July-Aug., 1974.

Newcomb, R. F., and Nader, A. F.: Children: to have or not, RN **36:**23, April, 1973.

Newton, N.: Maternal emotions, New York, 1955, Paul B. Hoeber, Inc.

Newton, N., and Newton, M.: Relation of the let-down reflex to the ability to breast feed, Pediatrics **5:**726, May, 1950.

Noonan, J. T., Jr.: The church and contraception: the issues at stake, New York, 1967, Paulist Press.

Paulshock, B. Z.: Birth control: "What I want my daughter to know," Today's Health **53:**20-23+, Feb., 1975.

Pomerance, J.: Steroid contraception and its effects on lactation are a public health dilemma, Health Services Reports **87:**611-616, Aug.-Sept., 1972.

Robinson, A. M.: Sterilization of women, RN **36:**33-35+, April, 1973.

Robinson, A. M.: Vasectomy: advantages and limitations, RN **36:**30-33, April, 1973.

Seward, E. M.: Preventing postpartum psychosis, Am. J. Nurs. **72:**520-523, March, 1972.

Smith, E. D. I.: Group conference for postpartum patients, Am. J. Nurs. **71:**112-113, Jan., 1971.

Stiegler, A. M.: Principles and practice: a review of tubal sterilization, J. Obstet. Gynecol. Neonatal Nurs. **1:**23-28, July-Aug., 1972.

Tyrer, L. B., and Granzig, W. A.: The new morality, ethics, and nursing, J. Obstet. Gynecol. Neonatal Nurs. **2:**54-55, Sept.-Oct., 1973.

Von Hildebrand, D.: The encyclical humanae: a sign of contradiction, Chicago, 1969, Franciscan Herald Press.

Warrick, L. H.: Family-centered care in the premature nursery, Am. J. Nurs. **71:**2134-2138, Nov., 1971.

Whitley, N. N.: Breast feeding the premature, Am. J. Nurs. **70:**1909, Sept., 1970.

Whitley, N. N.: Second trimester abortion: a program of counseling and teaching, J. Obstet. Gynecol. Neonatal Nurs. **2:**15-21, Sept.-Oct., 1973.

Yates, S. A.: Stillbirth—what staff can do, Am. J. Nurs. **72:**1592-1594, Sept., 1972.

unit seven
The newborn infant

15

The normal newborn infant

The newborn infant is a marvelous creation, the results of approximately 40 weeks of intensive growth and development never to be equaled at any future period during his life. A passive participant in the drama of birth, his present and near future is almost totally dependent on the physical care, emotional support, and mental stimulus given his inborn potential by his immediate environment. The human newborn does little for himself. In his egocentric way he waits impatiently for his needs to be met by others as if no other needs exist, and indeed as far as he knows they do not.

Although newborn infants have shared similar environments during their approximately 9 months of prenatal life, even this basic experience is not identical. True, all lived in the warm, watery environment of the amniotic sac, but not all infants receive identical portions of nourishment or oxygen. Their genetic backgrounds, greatly influencing basic body strengths and weaknesses, are very unlike. The stresses and strains of each delivery are not always duplicated. Babies are individuals; each is different, and there is a wide range of shapes, sizes, and behavior patterns that despite their variations must still be labeled "normal." So although we often speak of the typical newborn infant, we must realize that in reality he exists only within the pages of some text.

QUALIFICATIONS OF NURSERY PERSONNEL

The nursery nurse caring for the newborn infant has a tremendous responsibility.

Her observational capacity must be keen because these little persons cannot express themselves in the same ways as the older child or adult. Her technique and skills should be based on scientific principles, precise yet gentle. Her health must be frequently evaluated to be certain that she is not a source of infection to her susceptible charges. Her ethics must be above question as she cares for these small future citizens.

THE TYPICAL NEWBORN INFANT

Having explained that a baby is really an individual, we will now describe the general appearance, anatomy, and physiology of the "representative" newborn infant. First some statistics are in order. For unknown reasons there are approximately 106 male infants born to every 100 female infants. It can be said, however, that the male newborn infant appears to be more fragile than the female, having a higher mortality. The average male newborn infant weighs about 7½ pounds, or 3.400 kg., whereas the average female weighs about half a pound less, or 3.180 kg. The average male length is 20 inches, half an inch longer than his female counterpart. Of course, these figures are just averages, and much depends on the hereditary background of the child. Negroes and Orientals usually have smaller babies, whereas Caucasians tend to have larger children.

When uninitiated persons see a newborn infant for the first time, certain reactions are fairly standard: "He seems to be all head." "Where is his chin?" "Nurse, my baby has flat feet!" "Boy! He sure is red." "Will his skull always be that shape?"

The head

The head of a newborn infant represents one fourth of his total length (Fig. 15-1), but in adulthood the head equals only one eighth of the individual's total height. The newborn infant's head circumference equals or exceeds that of his chest or abdomen, and the normal limits of his head size are from 33 to 37 cm., or 13.2 to 14.8 inches. No wonder its relative size causes comment!

The shape of baby's head can also cause a mother or father needless concern. Cesarean section babies and even breech babies usually have quite rounded "normal appearing" heads. But infants who are delivered vaginally in cephalic presentations, particularly those who are firstborn, usually

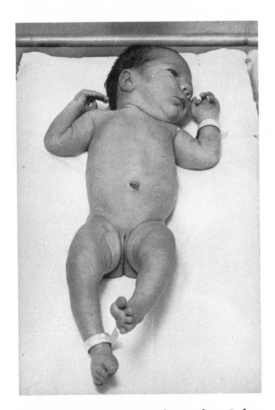

Fig. 15-1. Representative newborn infant, 3 days old. Note the size of the head relative to total length. (Courtesy Grossmont Hospital, La Mesa, Calif.)

undergo considerable head sculpture, or *molding.* This molding is caused by the compression of the head in the pelvic canal during labor. The infant skull, because of the soft membranous seams separating the skull bones, has the possibility of becoming shaped in its journey through the canal. In response to the pressure of the cervix and bony pelvis, the head usually elongates, and the skull bones may even overlap in places. This phenomenon is called *overriding;* the molding lasts for only about a week or less.

The fontanels, or soft spots, where sutures cross or meet are particularly noteworthy. There are two that are easily felt and identified: the anterior diamond-shaped fontanel through which a pulse is sometimes visible, hence the name fontanel, or "little fountain," and the smaller posterior fontanel just in front of the occiput. The larger fontanel closes at 9 to 18 months of age. Occasionally it is the site of "cradle cap," or "milk crust," also called seborrhea. This occurs when the mother or nurse is fearful of cleaning this soft area, and secretions from the oil glands and cellular debris build up. Actually the cartilage covering the fontanels is quite tough; the mother should be assured that no harm will come from shampooing the area well. The posterior fontanel is so small that it is closed at 2 to 3 months of age.

There are two other temporary conditions involving the head that may manifest themselves and cause parental anxiety. These are usually caused by the continued pressure of the undelivered head against the partially dilated cervix. The first and less important is called *caput succedaneum,* or caput. Caput is an abnormal collection of fluid under the scalp on top of the skull that may or may not cross suture lines, depending on its size. It is usually absorbed over a period of days and requires no treatment. The second condition is *cephalhematoma* (Fig. 15-2), caused by a collection of bloody fluid under the first covering layer (the periosteum) of a flat cranial bone. Since cephalhematoma is located within the bone struc-

The newborn infant

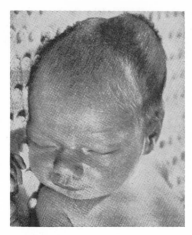

Fig. 15-2. Cephalhematoma over the parietal bone. (From Davis, M. E., and Rubin, R.: DeLee's obstetrics for nurses, ed. 17, Philadelphia, 1962, W. B. Saunders Co.)

ture, it cannot cross suture lines. It usually develops when labor is particularly prolonged and the passageway is tight in relation to the needs of the passenger, causing bruising against the pelvis. As a result of the trauma, small blood vessels under the periosteum break. A cephalhematoma may not be apparent at the time of birth because of the presence of a more inclusive caput. Like caput, cephalhematoma, although temporarily disfiguring, is not harmful and requires no treatment. In fact, many believe that aspiration of the swelling should not be attempted because of the danger of infection.

General body proportions

Parents are often amazed to see the small size of the child's face compared with his total head size. The facial bones are underdeveloped, and the chin is almost nonexistent. The baby's neck is usually short and creased and difficult to clean unless the head is tipped backward and unsupported while the child is held at his shoulders. The torso of the normal newborn infant displays a relatively small thorax and a soft, rather protuberant abdomen. The genitalia are small but may be swollen. The extremities are quite short in relation to body length. The feet are always flat because of the pres-

ence of a fatty pad that normally disappears as the child begins to exercise and purposefully use his feet.

Ears and eyes

The ears may be folded and creased and seem out of shape because they contain little hardened cartilage. The infant usually responds to sound within hours after birth. The eyes may not track properly and may cross (strabismus) or twitch (nystagmus). These symptoms are usually not considered significant unless persistent beyond the age of 6 months. The irises are slate blue, and true eye color is usually not determined until 3 to 6 months of age. It is difficult to tell what a baby is able to see. We do know that the pupils react to light and that he is able to focus on objects (for example, on another person's eyes) held about 8 inches away. Blinking is an inborn protective reflex. The lacrimal glands evidently function only minimally at birth, and the newborn infant's cries are characteristically tearless. Occasionally, an eye discharge that is caused by eye irritation initiated by the prophylactic against *ophthalmia neonatorum* (a condition that results from a gonorrheal infection in the mother) is apparent. The prophylactic, which is required by most states, is usually silver nitrate, 1%. Because of sensitivity problems, penicillin is not often used for this purpose. The reason for the eye irritation should be explained to the parents.

Skin

The skin of the newborn infant is subject to numerous conditions and manifestations that always elicit questions.

Vernix caseosa. The skin of the fetus is protected from its watery environment by a soft, yellowish cream named *vernix caseosa*, or "cheesy varnish." This is an accumulation of old cutaneous cells mixed with an early secretion from the oil glands. Sometimes the baby is thickly covered with vernix at birth. Sometimes it is found in abundance only in the body creases. Many nursery units believe that vernix is a good culture medium for bacterial growth and now meticulously remove all of it from their newborn patients.

The skin of the newborn infant is quite thin. The more immature he is the less developed will be his layer of subcutaneous fat. For this reason, babies not many hours after birth, when oxygenation is optimal, tend to be quite red. The smaller the baby, the more tomato colored he will tend to be —especially when upset and crying. Nurses should be aware that Negro babies are quite fair at birth and darken gradually.

Lanugo. A relatively long, soft growth of fine hair is often observed on the shoulders, back, and forehead of the newborn infant. In fact, the infant at times may seem to have sideburns. The more premature the infant the more conspicuous this extra growth of hair tends to be. It is called *lanugo* and falls away and disappears early in postnatal life.

Toxic erythema. Another skin manifestation that can be quite puzzling but is altogether harmless is a condition known to the nursery staff as "newborn rash," *toxic erythema.* The adjective "toxic" perhaps should not be used, since there has never been any poison proved to be associated with the cause. In fact, the cause is unknown. Some authors list it as a possible allergic response and call it instead *erythema allergicum.* The lesions consist of red blotches that quickly develop hivelike elevations, which may later become blisters containing clear fluid. These may appear on the day of birth and persist for days or weeks. They are most often seen on the trunk but may appear elsewhere. They are not contagious and are most often seen on vigorous, healthy babies. No treatment is needed.

Mongolian spots. Babies of Negro, Indian, Mongolian, or "Mediterranean" ancestry often exhibit blue-black colorations on their lower backs, buttocks, anterior trunks, and rarely, fingers or feet. These are not bruise marks or signals of ill treatment, nor are they associated with mental retardation. These so-called *Mongolian,* or *Asiatic, spots* disappear in early childhood.

Jaundice. The skin of the infant on about the third day may begin to take on a yellow cast. This icterus, or jaundice, is not in most cases considered to be pathological but is thought to be associated with the destruction of red blood cells that are no longer needed in as great a number as when external respiration via the lungs was impossible in utero. However, if jaundice is present before 36 hours of age, the possibility of Rh factor or main blood group incompatibility (AB-O) most certainly should be recognized and determined. Indeed, no matter what the age of the baby, the fact that the baby is jaundiced should be reported and evaluated because there is nothing magical about the number 36, and although it is not common, difficulty could occur later. The jaundice caused by the expected erythrocyte destruction is seen to some extent in almost all newborn infants and has been termed *physiological jaundice.*

Petechiae. Another possible signal of trouble associated with the skin that usually turns out to be a false alarm is the presence of petechiae, or small blue-red dots on the body, the result of the breakage of minute capillaries. If present, these dots are usually seen on the face as a result of the pressure exerted on the head during birth. Nevertheless, if petechiae are accompanied by jaundice or begin to increase measurably after birth, one may consider a diagnosis of blood disease.

Milia. Small pinpoint white or yellow dots are common on the nose, forehead, and cheeks of the newborn infant. They are clogged sweat and oil glands that have not yet begun to function normally and are called *milia.* They will disappear with time and under no circumstances should they be expressed.

Birthmarks. Small reddened areas are sometimes present on the eyelids, midforehead, and nape of the neck. They are probably the result of a local dilatation of skin capillaries and abnormal thinness of the skin. Because of the frequent involvement of the nape of the neck they are sometimes called "stork bites," but another name often heard is *telangiectasia* (Fig. 15-3). Some writers term such an area *nevus flammeus,* an unfortunate choice since this term is also used for the so-called port-wine stain, which is disfiguring and difficult to treat. Whatever the choice of terms, however, the parents should be told that in most cases these small areas fade and disappear altogether. Some are noticeable only when the person blushes or becomes excited.

Other birthmarks are sometimes seen. The so-called strawberry mark may not be present at birth but may develop days or weeks later. It is characterized by a dark or bright red raised, rough surface, and since it is formed by a collection of capillaries at the skin's surface it may be classed as a blood vessel tumor, or *hemangioma.* The

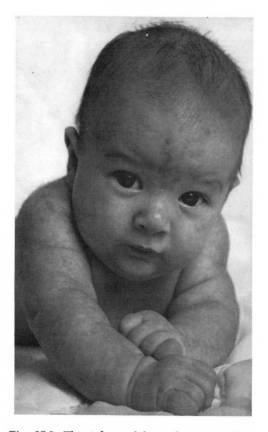

Fig. 15-3. This infant exhibits telangiectasia between the eyes and on the lower forehead. The skin of the arms also shows a slight amount of "mottling," a circulatory pattern common during periods of inactivity and exposure.

first signs of a strawberry mark may be a grouping of red dots that eventually coalesce, forming the clear-cut raised lesion. Many times this mark will disappear spontaneously in early childhood without treatment. However, some such hemangiomas tend to increase in size rather than subside, and some seem so disfiguring to the parents that efforts to remove the lesion are made at an early age. The application of dry ice at brief intervals or actual surgical excision, depending on the location of the strawberry mark, are methods of removal. A "wait-and-see" attitude is advocated, since many such lesions regress spontaneously.

Additional birthmarks that may sometimes cause concern are various flat or raised, frequently pigmented irregularities of the skin that are generally termed moles or *nevi* (singular, *nevus*). For the most part, these lesions are benign, causing only occasional cosmetic difficulties. Nevertheless, there is a type of blue-black mole that is considered precancerous, and any such lesion must be evaluated by the physician to ascertain its true character.

Vital signs in the newborn infant

Temperature. The newborn infant's body temperature drops immediately after birth from a reading about 1° F. higher than that of his mother to a subnormal range. His heat-regulating center and circulatory system have not yet matured, and his body temperature rapidly reflects that of its environment. When he is placed in a warm incubator or wrapped in warm blankets, his temperature usually reaches "normal" (98.6° F. or above, rectally) within 8 to 12 hours. Maintaining body warmth as much as possible in the immediate postnatal period may be critical to the well-being of an infant; therefore, special efforts have been initiated to provide warmth to newborns in many delivery rooms. A newborn infant's feet and hands are bluish (acrocyanosis) and circulation is particularly poor in his extremities. For this reason one should not attempt to judge an infant's temperature by feeling his feet or hands. Evaluating the warmth of his trunk is more accurate. Newborn infants are sometimes overheated by overzealous nurses or mothers who put too much clothing or bedding on or around them. Since the newborn infant is not yet able to perspire effectively (his sweat glands are not functioning adequately), he breaks out in a pinpoint reddish rash. This is sometimes called *prickly heat* or *miliaria*.

Pulse. It is very difficult to take a radial pulse on an infant. For this reason all "pulse" readings are routinely taken with a stethoscope over the heart region, either through the chest or back. The reading is called an *apical pulse*. Newborn infants' pulse rates usually range between 120 and 160 per minute (the same as the fetal heart tone range).

Respirations. Newborn infants' respirations are irregular and usually abdominal or diaphragmatic in character, typically ranging from 30 to 80 breathes per minute depending on the baby's activity. If respirations at rest are persistently 50 or more per minute, the rate is usually considered abnormal, and further respiratory evaluation is required. At no time are costal or sternal retractions considered normal in the new-

born infant. Retraction, or a sucking in of the chest wall in the rib or sternal area on inspiration, is an indication of respiratory distress.

A nurse is seldom called on to take the blood pressure of a normal newborn. However, occasionally such orders are written. With a cuff 1 inch wide, the average blood pressure at birth is 80/46 mm. Hg. Such a blood pressure is often difficult to determine and many times is inaudible. If it is unheard, the nurse is allowed to record the systolic reading at the point indicated on the sphygmomanometer when she palpates the return to the brachial pulse. Students should know that as a person grows older, pulse and respiratory rates decrease, whereas blood pressure readings rise.

Survey of the newborn infant's body systems
Gastrointestinal system

Mouth. The newborn infant's mouth is of great interest to parent and physician and should be carefully examined for gross abnormalities such as cleft lip and palate. However, certain small structural differences in the normal newborn infant may need to be explained to the first-time parent to alleviate anxiety. Near the center of the hard palate little, white, glistening spots may be occasionally observed. These are called *Epstein's pearls*. They mark the fusion of the halves of the palate and will disappear in time.

Sometimes the mother has heard of an oral infection called *thrush* and thinks that Epstein's pearls are an indication of this infection. Thrush, or oral moniliasis, caused by a fungus called *Candida (Monilia) albicans*, is a coating on the tongue and cheeks that looks something like milk curds (Fig. 15-4). But it does not disappear when water is given to the infant as do true milk curds. The white patches adhere to the mucous membrane, but when they are forcibly lifted by an applicator, a raw, red, sore surface is revealed. These sore lesions may discourage appetite. The organism causing thrush is found frequently in the vaginal canal of

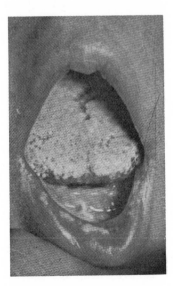

Fig. 15-4. Thrush. (From Potter, E. L.: Pathology of the fetus and the newborn, Chicago, 1952, Year Book Medical Publishers, Inc.)

women where it may or may not cause symptoms. The child may contact the fungus during his passage down the pelvic canal or while nursing if the mother's nipples or the nursing bottles are contaminated. The organism is very prevalent and may be especially troublesome in the debilitated patient. The use of broad-spectrum antibiotics kills off much normal intestinal flora but allows *Candida albicans* to abnormally multiply. Babies receiving such therapy may develop thrush. The fungus can involve other parts of the gastrointestinal or respiratory tract as well as the mouth and occasionally may cause a diaper rash. Treatment of thrush, the oral form of infection, is usually quite simple. Nystatin (Mycostatin) is most often prescribed.

The gums of the newborn infant may at times appear quite jagged, and the rear gums may be whitish. Although the deciduous teeth are semiformed, they are not erupted. If a tooth is present at birth, it usually is an "extra," which has little root. These so-called rice teeth are sometimes pulled to prevent aspiration when they loosen.

The cheeks of the newborn infant have quite a chubby appearance because of the development of fatty sucking pads that persist until food is obtained in other ways.

Mothers are often quite worried about the possibility of tonguetie or a restrictively short frenulum at the base of the tongue. Actually problems in food manipulation or speech are rare because of this condition.

Stomach and intestines. The fetus has no need for a digestive system of its own. All its food is provided predigested via the placental circulation. A good share of the waste products created are eliminated through the same circulation. After birth, however, digestion is a different story.

The capacity of the newborn infant's stomach at birth probably varies from 1 to 2 ounces and increases rapidly. The feeding usually begins to leave the stomach before the total taken is completed. It is common for the infant to swallow air as he feeds, especially when bottle fed. Swallowed air in the stomach may cause difficulty in continuing the feeding, or it may cause vomiting later. Air passing into the intestines may cause colic (abdominal cramping). Bottle-fed babies need to be bubbled frequently. Newborn infants are usually bubbled after every ounce of formula. The older infant is bubbled once halfway through the feeding and again at the end of the feeding. Nursing babies are usually bubbled once or twice during a feeding. Immediately after the feeding, a little milk may come up with a bubble. This is termed a "wet burp" or small regurgitation and is not significant.

The first stool of the newborn infant is meconium, a greenish black, tarry, odorless, but very tenacious material. It consists of old lining cells of the gastrointestinal tract, swallowed amniotic fluid debris, and early tract secretions. The first stool should appear in a maximum of 24 hours. If it does not, malformation of the gastrointestinal tract is strongly suspected. Meconium continues to be the normal stool for about 2 days, then the products of digestion of the offered milk begin to change the color of the stool. It becomes first brown and then yellow-green and more loose in consistency. These are the *transitional* stools. Later the stool will become yellow as more milk product digestion takes place. The stools of formula-fed babies are characteristically lemon-yellow and curdy. The stools of breast-fed babies have a more yellow-orange color, are usually softer, and during the first few weeks are more frequent.

Circulatory system

In fetal life the circulatory system serves also as a modified respiratory system, since oxygen is not obtained through the breathing of air into the lungs of the baby but through the successive pulsations of the vein in the umbilical cord leading from the placenta attached to the uterine wall. Carbon dioxide is also eliminated through this attachment via the two umbilical arteries.

At birth, of course, this type of respiratory function is not continued, since the cord is cut and/or the placenta soon becomes detached. The fetal circulation, which is designed to channel blood flow to functioning organs and largely avoid the lung fields, is rerouted after birth. (See discussion of fetal circulation, p. 34.) The two fetal shunts that direct blood flow away from the pulmonary circulation normally close, apparently because of changes in internal pressures and vascular reflexes resulting from loss of the maternal oxygen source and subsequent lung expansion. The opening between the two atria of the heart, the *foramen ovale,* shuts, closing off the blood flow to the left atrium from the right heart and forcing more blood into the right ventricle. The *ductus arteriosus,* the fetal vessel between the pulmonary artery and aorta, collapses, obliging the pulmonary artery to send its total contents on to the lungs.

The circulation of blood in the baby at birth is not at the same stage of development throughout the body. The hands and feet are typically blue. At times the entire body of a baby at delivery may be quite blue because the fetal blood has a relatively low oxygen content, and a momentary disturbance of the placental circulation may occur before expansion of the lungs is possible. However, as soon as the airway is cleared and a healthy cry is elicited, the skin "pinks up" dramatically. Although significant, color is the least important of the characteristics or vital signs to be considered when using the Apgar scoring method in evaluating a newborn infant's need for resuscitation aid (Fig. 9-20). If a newborn infant is chilled or inactive for a period of time, a mottled pattern may be seen on the skin—particularly on the extremities. This purplish mottling called *cutis marmorata* is transitory in nature and soon disappears.

Newborn infants' blood pressure readings and pulse rates have been mentioned in previous paragraphs.

Vitamin K is routinely given to newborn infants in many nurseries to prevent hemorrhage because of the natural low prothrombin level in this period of life. It is especially recommended for those suffering from hemorrhagic disease of the newborn, infants born of complicated deliveries, or premature infants. However, it has been found that too high a dosage (usually over 5 mg.) may be accompanied by an increase in jaundice and in some cases kernicterus (the yellow staining of the basal ganglia of the brain, causing possible cerebral damage).

There are three blood vessels in the umbilical cord—one vein and two arteries. These are fairly easily seen in the cut umbilical stump. Recently, considerable interest has developed in counting these vessels at the time of the nursery admission, since if only two vessels are found, there seems to be a significant incidence of internal congenital defects (malformed kidneys, heart, etc.).

The vessels of the umbilical cord are fairly soon occluded through the formation of a clot and contraction of the vessels at its end. However, if the cord is manipulated often, the clot may become dislodged, and bleeding through the cord stump may occur if the ligature or cord clamp is loose. Large cords that contain a great amount of gelatinous connective tissue, called *Wharton's jelly,* must be especially watched for bleeding, since the cord will shrink in diameter and the clamp or ligature may become ineffective. There are no sensory nerves in the cord. The baby does not feel it when the cord is clamped or cut. The umbilical cord drops off, and the place of attachment heals in about 1 week.

Respiratory system

Although the fetus may make some occasional shallow lung movements in utero, the lungs serve no respiratory function, since the oxygen supply is secured through the placental circulatory system from the mother. Until the first breath of air is taken, the air sacs (alveoli) in the lungs are in an almost total state of collapse, or *atelectasis.* This is as it should be, however, because we would not want the lungs to fill with amniotic fluid or other liquids. In fact, one of the physician's main concerns at delivery is

193

the possible aspiration by the baby of thick secretions before the airway can be cleared, thereby plugging or irritating the respiratory tree. Newborn respiratory rates and patterns have been previously discussed on p. 191.

Babies normally are nose breathers and do not breathe through open mouths. Cyanosis of other than the hands and feet, costal or substernal retractions, flaring nostrils, and expiratory grunts heard with or without a stethoscope are all possible signs of respiratory distress.

The most frequent cause of respiratory difficulty in the first few minutes or hours of birth in the United States has been the too liberal use of sedatives, tranquilizers, analgesics, and anesthetics that not only affect the mother but also pass over the placenta to the baby, making him sleepy and disinclined to take his first breath. Because of this, there has been a real effort to reduce the use of these agents in the last few years.

We do not know exactly why a baby takes his first breath, but we believe the following are significant factors:

1. The buildup of carbon dioxide in the fetal bloodstream caused by the beginning separation of the placenta from the uterine wall and the pressure of the uterine contractions
2. The decrease of oxygen in the fetal bloodstream
3. The rapid change in the baby's environment at the moment of birth
4. The direct handling of the baby for the first time in his life

Urinary system

The newborn infant's renal system does not have the ability to concentrate urine to the degree of the older child or adult. Water is not reabsorbed as freely by the nephrons, and a newborn infant may become dehydrated rather easily. A newborn infant with profuse diarrhea or vomiting is in imminent danger of dehydration.

Uric acid is found in relatively large amounts in the urine of the newborn infant. Occasionally this substance may "crystal-

lize out" as it cools in the diaper, leaving a pink stain like "brick dust."

It is important to record all infant voidings in the delivery room or nursery. Although the newborn infant may not void a large amount or often at first, it is very important to note the fact that he is able to void normally.

Endocrine system and genital area

The endocrine system of the newborn infant is supplemented by maternal hormones that have crossed the placental barrier. These maternal contributions, presumably the estrogenic hormone, luteal hormone, and lactogenic hormone, when withdrawn from the baby through the act of birth, bring about certain phenomena that may cause parents concern and should be explained. The maternal hormones crossing to the fetus may affect the breasts of both male and female infants, causing swelling, which is particularly noticeable about the third day of life. This condition is usually called *gynecomastia*. The breast secretion sometimes seen has been given the interesting name of *witch's milk*. The breasts may continue to be swollen for about 2 or 3 weeks, but gradually the congestion subsides without treatment. The breasts should not be squeezed; this only increases the possibility of infection and injures the tender tissue.

Maternal hormones acting on the miniature uterus of the female newborn infant may set the stage for *infantile menstruation*. The hormones help thicken the infant's tiny endometrial lining. Withdrawn at the time of birth, they no longer maintain this thickened uterine lining, and a tiny menstrual flow may be observed. Usually only a few blood spots are seen on the diapers. The entire process may terminate in one or two days. This bleeding should not be profuse, and any considerable blood loss may be an indication of hemorrhagic disease. White mucoid vaginal discharge in the newborn infant is also thought to be stimulated by maternal endocrine secretions. The genitalia of both the male and female may be swollen. Hymenal tags that regress spontaneously may be seen on the female. Breech infants may have particularly swollen genitalia because of the prolonged pressure on the area. In male infants the scrotum most often contains the testes, although sometimes the descent of one or both is delayed. The foreskin may adhere to the glans penis (phimosis). Circumcision may be advised.

At birth, the thymus gland, located under the sternum and above the heart, is larger than a baby's fist. The thymus, long a mysterious lymphoid tissue difficult to classify, has recently been reevaluated as an endocrine gland. It seems that a hormone, thymosin, has been identified, which in cases of thymus lack, can be administered to help prevent or control infection. It is now thought to initiate the body's complex immunity reactions by producing special defensive cells that are distributed to the spleen, bone marrow, and lymph nodes. After puberty, however, the thymus atrophies, and the change in the gland's size is thought to either stimulate or reflect the development of sexual maturity. Pressure on the respiratory tract from a large thymus has, in the past, been cited as the cause of occasional infant suffocation. This has not been adequately substantiated. The primary cause of so-called crib-death or sudden infant death syndrome (SIDS), is still unknown.

Neuromuscular system

The nervous system of the normal newborn infant is very immature. Essential activites for maintenance of life and protection are largely reflex in character—inborn reactions making life possible until the nervous system and associated muscles can "grow up" to the demands of more complex living. Inborn reflexes that normal newborn infants possess include the rooting, sucking, and swallowing reflexes employed in eating and the protective reflexes, such as coughing, sneezing, gagging, blinking, and perhaps crying. Other muscular reactions in newborn infants are also reflex.

The most commonly tested muscular reflex is a total body response known as the Moro reflex, normally present during the first 3 months of life. It is elicited when the baby is startled, usually by a sudden jarring of his support such as occurs when the physician abruptly pounds on the examining table with his fist. The infant responds symmetrically, throwing out his arms sideways and drawing up his legs with the soles of his feet in opposition. The absence of the Moro reflex in the newborn infant may indicate brain damage (Fig. 15-5).

Another often-seen reflex position is called the tonic neck reflex. The child assumes a modified fencer's position while on his back. The arm and leg on one side of the body are extended while the opposing arm and leg are flexed. The fists are shut and the toes curled. The head is turned toward the extended arm, which incidentally is usually the dominant side. This reflex position may be seen quite commonly until about 4 months of age (see Fig. 20-1, *B*). Grasping is also an inborn reflex.

The immaturity of the nervous system is demonstrated by the unstable temperature regulation of the newborn infant and his limited ability to pursue purposeful activity. He sees but probably is unable to interpret much of what he sees. He may turn his head, blink, or grimace in response to sound but be unable to sort out the sound and make it meaningful. The sense of taste is quite well developed. The sense of smell is rather hard to evaluate, but evidently some newborn infants can detect the smell of breast milk. Cutaneous sensation is highly developed. Pressure, temperature, and pain are increasingly felt by the infant. The newborn reacts to cuddling, caresses, and skillful, gentle handling with greater relaxation and acceptance of care.

The newborn infant at first sleeps about 20 hours per day, waking to be fed, bathed, changed, repositioned, and briefly entertained. Usually he stays in the position in which he is placed, since he seldom has the ability to turn himself. However, no baby should be left alone on an unguarded table or bed. Accidents can happen! The order

195

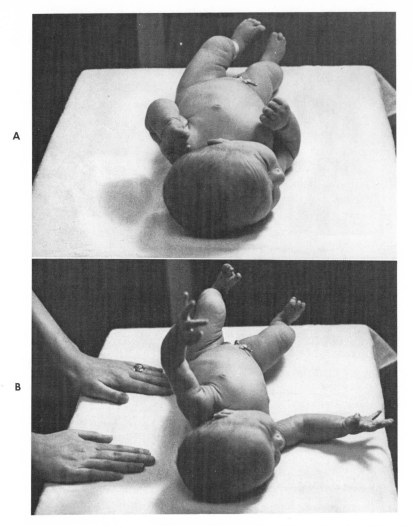

Fig. 15-5. **A**, Infant at rest. **B**, Typical Moro reflex, stimulated by jarring the table. (Courtesy Mead Johnson Laboratories, Evansville, Ind.)

of peripheral nervous system development and muscular coordination proceeds from the head region to the arms and then the legs. Later, the finer activities of the hands and feet are perfected.

Intellectual development is difficult to assess in the newborn infant, but we are reassured when all the normally present reflexes are active. We are concerned when a baby fails to suck well, lacks good muscle tone, or is lethargic and unresponsive to care.

• • •

All in all, the newborn infant is quite an invention, and the succeeding months of his life will include some of the most perplexing, exasperating, and wonderful hours ever experienced by any family lucky enough to welcome him into their home.

16

Care of the normal newborn infant

UNIVERSAL NEEDS

Today, in the United States the trend in the care of the newborn is toward specialization, particularly in centers that serve a large high-risk maternity or infant population. One encounters recovery or transition nurseries devoted to the care of the infant less than 24 hours old or the newborn surgical patient; special care nurseries designed for care of the small premature or sick infants (see Chapter 18), and intermediate or progressive care units for those infants whose nursing needs are not as intensive. Such care opportunities now enable us to save many babies who formerly would have died or suffered severe damage. But no matter what the circumstances or locale of his birth or the type of care facilities available, every newborn infant has certain needs that must be met for him to thrive and take his place in society. Some of these needs take priority; some can be met simultaneously; and still others are important but need not be rushed. Following are listed nine universal needs of the newborn infant; the first two must be met in order:

1. A clear airway
2. Established respiration
3. Warmth
4. Protection from hemorrhage
5. Protection from infection
6. Identification and observation
7. Nourishment and fluids
8. Rest
9. Love

A *clear airway*

The first two needs must be met immediately or the baby will not survive, and no amount of oxygen, mouth-to-mouth resuscitation, or intermittent positive pressure will stimulate a newborn infant to breathe if his airway is not open. Conversely, if his airway is not clear but filled with amniotic fluid, meconium particles, blood, etc., and he does try to take a breath and inhale, he may plug, irritate, or contaminate his respiratory tree. The airway may be cleared by:

1. Wiping off the child's face at birth of the head
2. Gently suctioning first the mouth and then the nose with a small, soft, short bulb aspirator or a soft catheter attached to a trap before delivery is complete
3. Holding the child's head down to drain immediately after birth, while gently compressing the throat toward the mouth to milk out secretions
4. Visualizing the larynx with a laryngoscope and suctioning the trachea by trained personnel in unresponsive cases

Established respiration

With the introduction of closed-chest cardiac massage techniques and appliances to electrically stimulate heartbeat, perhaps "established respiration" should read "established respiration *and* heartbeat." However, for this discussion it will be assumed that heart action is present and adequate. (For cardiopulmonary resuscitation of the newborn infant see p. 259.) If respiration does not occur spontaneously after the airway is clear, the child should be stimulated to cry. This may be done by slapping the heels, lightly spanking the buttocks, rubbing the back gently, or gently suctioning the nose with a soft catheter. Any rough treatment or such procedures as alternating hot and cold baths is now considered to add to the child's problems rather than offer a solution. If breathing is not initiated soon, methods of breathing for the infant must be employed. Sometimes this means the use of intermittent positive pressure via orotracheal tube or mask and bag. Sometimes the operator will blow directly through a patent endotracheal tube. Also, the much publicized mouth-to-mouth resuscitation may be attempted. No matter what method is used, it must be emphasized that an airway must be maintained through proper head positioning or the use of a small oropharyngeal airway to keep the tongue from falling back and obstructing the pharynx.

When a child is being resuscitated, is breathing poorly on his own, has generalized cyanosis, or a heart rate under 100 beats per minute he should receive supplementary oxygen.

Warmth

Heat is provided for the infant in most delivery room settings through the use of unenclosed infant warmers that provide easy accessibility for care by utilizing overhead radiant heat panels. The baby should be dried immediately after birth with a warm towel or blanket to decrease heat loss. In emergency situations, placing the baby against the mother's body will provide considerable warmth.

Recently the importance of maintaining an infant's body heat immediately after delivery and in the extended neonatal period has been emphasized. The temperature of the infant affects the amount of calories he must burn to keep warm, his oxygen consumption, the incidenec of apnea, and the acid-base balance of his blood. In the instance of a sick infant, the provision of appropriate heat may be critical.

The way in which the baby is dressed will depend on the temperature of the nursery or rooming-in area. It is now recommended that nursery air temperature be 28° to 30° C. (82.4° to 86° F.) with a relative humidity lower than 50% for personnel comfort. Some babies are perfectly warm in only a cotton shirt and diaper, covered by a light cotton blanket. Premature infants in a controlled environment, such as that provided by the Isolette, may wear no clothing. In some models of incubators the temperature of the artificial environment may be automatically controlled by the baby's own skin temperature through the use of a heat-sensitive probe taped to the baby. This is advantageous in maintaining body temperature. Abdominal skin sensor temperatures within a range of 97° to 99° F. taken in such an automatically controlled incubator probably indicate a reasonable environmental temperature. However, an early abnormal rise in an infant's temperature may be masked unless the simultaneous records of the temperature of the incubator and the skin of the infant are compared because as the infant's temperature rises, the heat source will not be activated and the incubator temperature will decrease The temperature setting of other appliances is adjusted manually, depending on the results of intermittent temperature readings. Except for an initial reading when a check is made for imperforate anus, axillary temperature determinations, rather than rectal, are now advocated more often in the nursery. An electronic thermometer may be employed.

Protection from hemorrhage

Today, most babies born in hospitals have their cords clamped with a type of compressive metal band rather than tied with the woven cotton umbilical tape used for so many years. These commercial clamps have proved to be quite satisfactory, and although the cord must still be frequently observed for bleeding, incidences of difficulty are extremely rare. When a ligature of any kind is being used, it is usually tied approximately 1 inch from the abdominal wall in a depression in the cord made by a previously placed hemostat, if one is available. The tie is secured by a square knot for stability and checked frequently during the first few hours to detect any loosening or bleeding.

Protection from hemorrhage in the newborn infant also becomes important when caring for the male infant after circumcision, to be discussed later in this chapter. In an effort to decrease the possibility of abnormal cerebral pressure and subsequent intracranial bleeding, newborn infants in their beds are not placed in as steep a head-down position as was popular several years ago when it was quite common to tilt the nursery bassinet on a steep incline for the first 12 hours to aid in the drainage of mucus from the respiratory tree. Vitamin K to decrease coagulation time is routinely administered in many hospitals.

Protection from infection

Protection of the newborn infant from infection is a constant challenge to the delivery room and nursery nurses. It involves the entire environment of the baby and the techniques used in handling and nourishing him. It even can be said to reach back to the prenatal period when we strive to prevent any contamination of the fetus by organisms that are able to pass over the placental barrier (viruses, spirochetes). The baby, while in the hands of the delivering physician, is considered and maintained sterile. The physician clamps and cuts the cord aseptically. Then the baby is usually handed to a circulating nurse who, having carefully washed her hands and put on a clean overgown, receives him for further care without contaminating the physician's sterile gloves.

In most states of the United States, protection of the infant from infection involves the use of some prophylactic against ophthalmia neonatorum caused by the gonorrheal organism. Usually this prophylactic (silver nitrate, 1%, rather than penicillin ophthalmic ointment) is instilled in the delivery room, unless the child's condition or delivery circumstances dictate a more rapid transfer of the child to the nursery. Care must be taken in administering the drops or ointment; no pressure should be put on

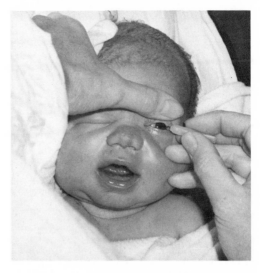

Fig. 16-1. The nurse stabilizes the head with one hand and pulls down on the conjunctival sac with one finger of the other hand while dropping in the silver nitrate. (Courtesy Grossmont Hospital, La Mesa, Calif.)

the eyeball itself. Occasionally, if the eye area has not been previously touched, shading the baby's eyes from the light will cause them to open spontaneously, making instillation comparatively easy. If this helpful reaction does not occur, the nurse pulls down on the lower lid to instill the $AgNO_3$ into the conjunctival sac (Fig. 16-1). This instillation is usually followed by a brief irrigation with sterile physiological saline or distilled water (see footnote, p. 108). All the while the nurse guards the child from cold and continues to observe his color and respiration patterns.

In the nursery the infant has his own individual bassinet and should also have his own bath equipment, supply of linen, and layette (Fig. 16-2). He should be bathed in his own bed and not on a common bathing table. The scale used for determining weight should be protected and balanced and handled in such a way that no cross infection could take place. Technique papers may be used if necessary. Any instruments or appliances that must be used for more than one infant because it is not feasible to supply individual equipment must

199

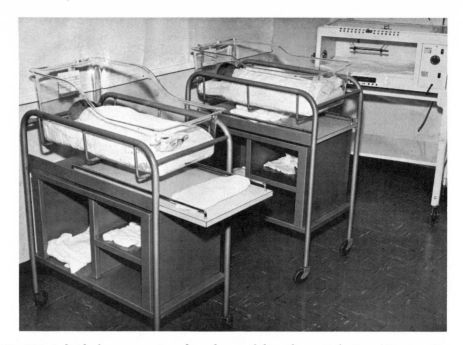

Fig. 16-2. Individual nursery units reduce the possibility of cross infection. (Courtesy Grossmont Hospital, La Mesa, Calif.)

be carefully disinfected or sterilized after use. This would apply to stethoscopes, circumcision boards and instruments, resuscitators, etc.

Staff members should wear simple, hospital supplied and laundered scrub gowns on duty, keep their fingernails short, restrict jewelry, and evaluate their own health. No personnel should assume responsibility in a nursery if suffering from a contagious respiratory condition, a skin infection, or diarrhea. Some hospitals require that nursery staff have periodic or irregular nose and throat cultures. However, since the flora of the human respiratory tract is so changeable, this measure has not been carried out with any sense of having proved anything conclusive in relation to the future safety of the nursery.

Personnel entering the nursery should wash their hands and arms above the elbow with an antibacterial product such as Betadine before starting patient care. Hand washing is mandatory after the care of each baby or his unit and in the care of the same baby after changing a soiled diaper and proceeding with further needs. The hands should always be washed before treating the cord. The cord can become the site of serious infection. It should be observed for signs of inflammation and drainage. A nurse who leaves the nursery area should wear a cover gown to protect her clean nursery gown. If her gown should become soiled in the nursery with urine, regurgitation, or stool at any time, it should be changed. Unless wrapped in a protective blanket or on a protective cover, the infant should be held away from the nurse's gown during care and feedings to protect the nurse's dress from becoming a source of cross contamination to other infants. Precautions not necessary at home are a must when many infants from many backgrounds and family units are being cared for in a small area, such as the hospital nursery.

To help protect our youngest citizens, professional organizations such as the American Academy of Pediatrics, hospital accreditation boards, and local public health and safety officials take an active part in making recommendations and requirements governing the construction, maintenance, and operation of the nursery as well as other parts of the hospital. They are concerned about the floor space available, the distance between bassinets, the type of ventilation, the control of temperature and humidity, the provision for adequate lighting, the safety of electrical appliances, the elimination of possible fire hazards, appropriate dressing and hand-washing facilities, and safe formula preparation as well as optimum techniques. The maternity floor should be separated from other hospital services, and personnel should not be borrowed from other services where infectious sources may exist.

Identification and observation

Identification of the infant may be accomplished in various ways, but it should always be done beyond doubt before the baby leaves the delivery room. In case of multiple births, the infants should be identified immediately after birth so that no confusion will result. Identification that can be easily counterchecked, such as the use of double or triple bands, is recommended.

Admission bath

Although some newborn infants receive their first bath in the delivery room or its annex, most infants have their "admission bath" in the nursery after being checked in, identified, weighed, and measured. Many infants are not bathed completely until several hours after birth when the body temperature is higher. Newborn infants are covered with varying amounts of vernix and blood. They may also be soiled with meconium. During the admission bath the nurse usually seeks to remove this soil, reaffirm identification, inspect the infant more carefully than was possible in the delivery room, take his temperature, dress him appropriately, and tuck him into bed. An admission bath may make use of a mild soap solution, an antibacterial product, or oil. Mineral oil is used relatively infrequently for total cleansing purposes now,

since it is thought that it may interfere with the proper functioning of the skin by suppressing the action of the oil glands, it has no antibacterial action, and it temporarily stains clothing. The following description tells what may occur during the admission bath, although details may differ from hospital to hospital. The nurse's hands are freshly washed before she starts.

ADMISSION BATH

Materials:
1. Basin of warm water
2. Mild soap or antibacterial product
3. Paper mesh squares
4. Sterile cotton balls
5. Alcohol, 70%, or other antiseptic for cord care
6. Applicators for cord care
7. Two towels or soft diapers for covering and drying
8. Individual thermometer
9. Small plastic comb
10. Laundry hamper
11. Appropriate clothing, diaper, shirt, and receiving blanket

Procedure:
1. The newborn infant is usually wrapped partially with a towel or coverlet to prevent chilling.
2. The eyes may be wiped with cotton balls moistened with sterile water if necessary.
   a. Irrigation or wiping starts at the nose and proceeds outward to try to prevent unwanted drainage from the inner canthus of the eye down the lacrimal duct to the nose. (One cotton ball is used for each wipe.)
3. The face is cleaned with a paper mesh square or cotton balls dipped in clear water. No soap is necessary, as it may be drying to the skin.
   a. If necessary, the opening of the nose is cleared with water-moistened, firmly twisted wisps of cotton (remember, babies are nose breathers).
   b. The external ears may be gently wiped with water-moistened cotton balls, but the canal is never probed.
4. The head is gently but efficiently sudsed and rinsed over the wash basin.
   a. A football hold on the baby is best.
   b. A small comb, gently used, helps to lift out particles of vernix that are difficult to dislodge.
5. The bath is continued, washing, rinsing, and drying the neck, chest, arms, hands, abdomen, and back.

a. The recently clamped cord and its base are usually avoided until later when an antiseptic is applied. Many nurseries today put no gauze dressing on the cord whatsoever and have found that it dries much faster and has no greater incidence of infection for having been left exposed.

b. Most nurseries now remove all vernix found in skin folds as well as all blood and meconium at the time of the initial bath. Special attention should be paid to the neck creases.

c. After turning the baby on his side to wash, rinse, and dry, a clean, dry, partially folded towel may be placed under the washed portion of the infant to be completely unfolded when his "bottom half" is clean.

d. A small undershirt may be put on at this time, rolled up away from the cord to conserve warmth until the bath is complete.

6. The temperature is taken.

a. If a rectal temperature is to be taken, it should be completed before bathing the buttocks and genitalia, since the stubby rectal thermometer used often initiates a stool.

b. Usual time is 3 minutes or until the mercury stops rising.

7. The bath is continued, washing the legs, feet, and then the buttocks and perianal region.

8. The nurse's hands are again washed and any ordered antiseptic is applied with an applicator to the cord end and the inner rim of the skin cuff surrounding the base of the cord. The vessels in the cord may be counted at this time.

9. The genitalia are inspected and cleansed with cotton balls previously moistened with clear water.

a. In the case of a baby girl the cotton balls may be wiped gently from front to back between the labia, never using a ball more than once.

b. In the case of a baby boy the foreskin may be retracted gently if possible and the glans carefully wiped. It should never be forced and if retracted should be immediately replaced.

10. The diaper is put on and the infant is tucked into bed. The crib identification card is checked against his own personal identification.

a. Newborn infants are frequently propped on their right sides with a rolled blanket. In the older infant a right-side position is supposed to be better because of the aid gravity gives to the flow of food from the stomach and because any air or bubble remaining will rest near the entrance of the stomach and be more easily expelled.

b. No newborn infant should be placed on his back because of the danger of aspiration.

c. In some hospitals the newborn infant is not dressed until shown to the parents and waiting relatives through a nursery window.

11. Notations regarding voidings, stool, or any pertinent observations should be appropriately recorded.

All during the bath procedure the nurse is inspecting and evaluating the infant. As she cleans the eyes, she watches for discharge, conjunctival hemorrhage, or areas of opacity. As she feels the head, she checks the contour, the relative size of the fontanels, and the presence of areas of swelling. Pushing down on the chin, she peers into the mouth. Continuing in her bath procedure, she evaluates respirations, counts and separates fingers, and judges skin turgor and muscle tone. As she washes each part, she inspects. She is not trying to diagnose, but she wants to be able to report significant findings so that the pediatrician or general practitioner may be called if necessary. Every new baby should be completely examined by a physician within 24 hours of birth, and the condition of some may necessitate a much earlier examination.

Inspection bath

On the following days, the bath of the newborn infant serves two main purposes—inspection and stimulation. An example of this procedure follows.

DAILY INSPECTION BATH

Materials:
1. Each infant should have his own individual unit including:
   a. Thermometer
   b. Diapers, shirts
   c. Linen supply
   d. Blankets
2. Paper mesh squares or two washcloths
3. Mild soap
4. Alcohol, 70%, or other cord antiseptic
5. Applicators for cord care
6. Scales and scale paper, technique paper

7. Scratch paper and pencil
8. Laundry hamper
9. Amphyl solution, 2%, or other disinfectant for equipment cleanup

Procedure:

1. Wash your hands; check crib for materials needed.
2. Identify the baby.
3. Undress the infant as necessary to take temperature and drop clothing into hamper.
4. Take the temperature (axillary or rectal) following appropriate technique.
5. Place the baby on a clean paper mesh square on scale; weigh, using technique papers to handle scale weights and pencil.
6. Apply alcohol or other ordered antiseptic to the cord at the base by the skin margin and at the tip.
7. Replace the baby in the crib on the scale paper and wash his face with a paper mesh square and clear water. Wash the rest of the baby with mild soap and water solution in the following order: external ears, head, neck, arms, front of body (avoiding the cord), back, legs and feet, lower back and anus. Pat dry. (Genitalia are cleansed as necessary with newly washed hands and a separate paper mesh square or cotton ball.)
8. Dress the infant and change the bed as necessary.
9. Place the baby on his abdomen, head to one side. Tuck one blanket over the infant.
10. Record weight, temperature, general condition, stool, and urine on work paper. Loose, watery stools should be reported.
11. Hands should be washed before and after each baby's care and after caring for the anal-genital area before proceeding with additional tasks with the same child. Hands should also be washed before removing a cord clamp.
12. Avoid chilling the baby during the procedure.
13. All equipment that becomes contaminated while weighing should be washed with disinfectant before it is reused. Scales, cart, and all equipment are washed with disinfectant at the end of daily care.
14. As you bathe the infant, inspect for the following:
    a. Color—jaundice
    b. Rash
    c. Petechiae
    d. Bruise marks
    e. Swellings on the head
    f. Condition of the mouth—excess salivation
    g. Condition of the eyes (cleaned only if a discharge is present)
    h. Condition of genitalia
    i. Condition of the cord (signs of inflammation, discharge, bleeding)
    j. Signs of possible paralysis or spasticity
    k. General level of alertness and activity
    l. Indications of respiratory distress
    m. Possible congenital malformations

Lifting and holding

The positioning, handling, and transporting of young babies can sometimes be very frightening to new mothers or beginning student nurses. It is almost as if they expect to see sawdust leaking out of a tiny joint after touching the child. Both need to be reassured of their ability to learn to care for their charges and to learn comfortable and safe methods of handling a baby. A baby does not break, and knowledge of certain principles will help to give him greater support and confidence.

The newborn infant usually tries to maintain his fetal position. With a little coaxing —a pat here, a little pressure there—he usually readily assumes his unborn posture. This is sometimes useful to the pediatrician trying to evaluate the placement of a foot or the line of a mandible.

The newborn infant has one continuous anteroposterior spinal curve and no real control of his head movements, although in prone position he may raise his head slightly and briefly. Whenever the baby is lifted or transported, his head, being so large and heavy in relation to the rest of his body, must be supported for comfort and to prevent muscle strain. For safety, all lifts must have at least two contact points so that if one fails, another is still available. Babies, even small ones, can be wriggly and sometimes slippery. Following is one of the most common methods of lifting an infant on his back from his bed.

1. Facing the soles of his feet, lift his legs and buttocks slightly with one hand by grasping the feet, ankles separated by a finger.
2. Slide the opposite hand, palm up, under the full length of the baby until finally the entire back and head are supported.

A second method follows (Fig. 16-3):

1. Facing the baby's side, slide one

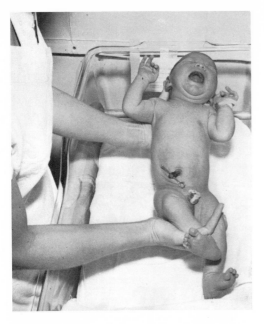

Fig. 16-3. One method of lifting a baby, starting from a side position. The head and upper back are supported by one hand, the legs by the other. Note that the baby is gently grasped. (Courtesy Grossmont Hospital, La Mesa, Calif.)

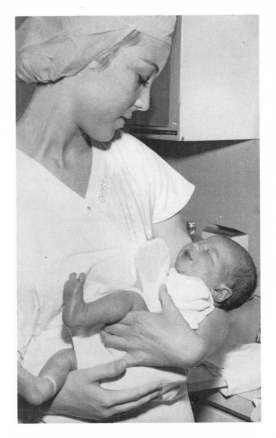

Fig. 16-4. Traditional cradle hold. This baby was a wriggler! (Courtesy Grossmont Hospital, La Mesa, Calif.)

hand from the side under the head and neck to grasp the farther arm. The head is supported by the forearm, or the head and neck may be supported by the grasping hand.

2. With the other hand reach under the legs to grasp the farther thigh or grasp the feet holding one finger between the ankles. This is a good lift for weighing the baby or putting him into a tub.

A baby should not be lifted by his arms. When head stability is attained at about 3 months of age, the child may be lifted by grasping his trunk with both hands below the arms. A newborn infant should not be left alone flat on his back. He may be propped with a rolled blanket along his back to maintain a side position or may be placed on his abdomen with his head turned to one side. Some newborn infants, when placed in this position for protracted periods, seem to object and rub their knees up and down on the linen, causing red-

dened shins. Baby beds should have firm mattresses regardless of the style. No pillow should be used. A child should not always be placed in the same position, since this can distort the shape of his head or chest or cause localized baldness.

There are many ways that babies have been carried. Some ways are more comfortable for the one who carries and give the baby a greater sense of safety and support. Three ways are common in the United States and are recommended:

1. The traditional cradle hold (Fig. 16-4): The child's head is cradled in the bend of the elbow; the forearm reaches around the outside of his body to grasp the outer leg with the fingers. The nurse's opposite hand and forearm helps support the back

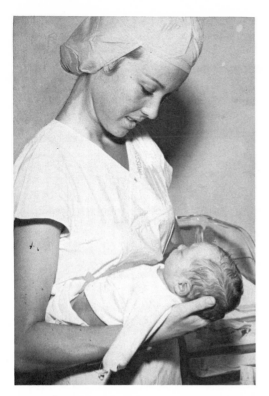

Fig. 16-5. Football hold. (Courtesy Grossmont Hospital, La Mesa, Calif.)

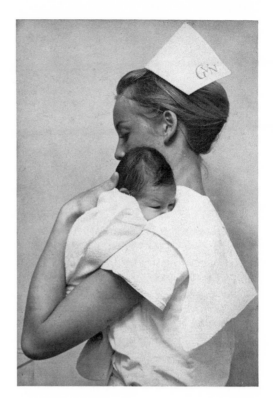

Fig. 16-6. Shoulder hold. (Courtesy Grossmont Hospital, La Mesa, Calif.)

and buttocks. This additional support may be momentarily withdrawn if the hand is needed for a task.

2. The football hold (Fig. 16-5): About half the length of the baby's body is supported by the nurse's forearm with his head and neck resting in her palm. The rest of baby's body, legs, and buttocks are firmly wedged between the nurse's elbow and hip. This is a fine secure hold, and it was definitely designed to provide the mother or nurse with a free hand.

3. The shoulder hold (Fig. 16-6): The baby is held up against the chest and shoulder. The palm of one hand supports the baby's buttocks. The other hand keeps the head and back from sagging. Two hands are needed to support the baby's back correctly. This is the old hold used often for bubbling the baby.

Newborn infants love to be cuddled, and the way they are handled, touched, and fed are ways we can show love and respect for them as individuals and as very important members of humanity.

Nourishment

Nourishment is the least pressing of a newborn infant's needs, but eventually it becomes paramount. In modern society there are two ways of meeting this need—breast feeding and formula feeding.

Breast feeding

Breast feeding, of course, has an ancient biological basis and is still the most universally recommended way of providing infant nourishment. A mother should carefully consider its advantages when deciding how she will feed her infant.

Advantages. Putting the baby to breast contributes to the mother's well-being in

205

that the stimulation of the infant nursing causes the recently emptied uterus to contract and helps in the return of this organ to its proper size and position, a process called involution. Many investigators believe that the baby receives certain immune factors through the breast milk that help protect the baby against diseases to which the mother may have been previously exposed. However, this has not been proved. It is agreed that as a general rule breast-fed babies have fewer respiratory tract infections and alimentary tract disturbances. Certainly, when environmental hygiene is poor, breast feeding is to be preferred over the great possibility of the contamination of artifically prepared feedings.

The observation that cow's milk was first designed for calves, whereas mother's milk is specifically designed for babies is indisputable. The curd of human milk is softer than that of cow's milk and is easier for a baby to digest. Breast-fed babies have fewer allergy problems. At first, breast-fed babies have more frequent stools than formula-fed youngsters. The stools are yellow-orange and aromatic but not necessarily offensive. Later on they may have fewer stools than their formula-fed counterparts. There is no prolonged preparation time necessary except that of washing the breasts, and in the long run, successful nursing is less expensive. If the mother nurses her baby, the return of menstruation will probably be delayed until 6 to 8 months after the birth of the baby, but nursing is no guarantee that pregnancy will not occur. However, the nursing mother may experience such a sense of fulfillment and motherliness in her role that this becomes the primary reason she continues to nurse.

Problems. But there are other considerations, and to say that breast feeding has all the advantages and no negative aspects would be unfair and untrue. The nursing mother must have a good diet to maintain her resources and provide sufficient nourishment for her infant. She produces approximately 30 ounces of milk per day when lactation is fully established. She needs more calories (1,000 more than the usual daily adult allowance) and increased fluid intake to maintain her milk production. Her diet should also include at least 1½ quarts of skimmed or whole milk in liquid form or cooking mixtures per day to protect her personal calcium supply and avoid possible *osteoporosis,* or weakening of the bony skeleton. Calcium in the form of medication can be supplied if necessary, but a balanced diet containing calcium-rich foods would give her other healthful nutrients, benefit the whole family unit, and eliminate the need for pills. Some foods eaten by the mother have been said to cause the nursing baby abdominal distress such as cramping or diarrhea, but no one food seems to affect every baby. Probabilities are chocolate and "strong" vegetables such as cabbage, Brussel sprouts, and asparagus. Other notorious "gas formers" should be approached with an attitude of caution, but some babies do not seem aware of any deviation in diet. Certain drugs taken by the mother may pass through the milk to the baby and cause difficulty; however, most must be taken in considerable quantity to cause symptoms. One exception is the drug thiouracil used in treating hyperthyroidism. It actually becomes more concentrated in the maternal milk and may affect the infant severely. Certain laxatives are equally as effective on baby as on his mother and should be avoided or used only very judiciously. Common medications to be avoided include cascara, milk of magnesia, Epsom salt, and Ex-lax, but not inert mineral oil. It is wise to counsel mothers to remind their physicians that they are nursing when receiving new prescriptions. Concern has been expressed regarding the amount of DDT found in some human milk samples. This is part of the general environmental problem of our time.

Some cultures teach that an intake of low-percentage beer or, for those more affluent, the addition of champaign to the diet increases milk production. We are convinced that it is not the beer or champagne as such that may produce results, but the fact that they come in liquid form and for some people produce a feeling of relaxation and ease. It is true that a tense, worried mother may have difficulty in maintaining an adequate milk supply.

Mothers who must or who prefer to work outside the home may find it difficult to maintain breast feeding, depending on the demands of their employment. To maintain a milk supply the breasts must be stimulated and emptied at fairly frequent intervals. A nursing mother may manually empty her breasts when unable to feed her infant because of separation, but this procedure may not always be convenient. The nursing mother needs good breast support. The typical nursing bra, with the lift-down cup, is usually efficient and easily used. Many mothers use freshly laundered handkerchiefs or soft-cellulose pads strategically placed, to prevent soiling.

To be completely successful most nursing mothers must really want to nurse, be convinced of its advantages, and receive instruction in the prenatal period regarding the care and normal function of their breasts as well as encouragement and assistance in the postpartum period. If a woman has flattened or inverted nipples, they should be treated during this period of preparation by massage and possibly suction as directed by her physician. In some localities groups of mothers particularly interested in promoting nursing have formed organizations to help the new mother or mother-to-be. La Leche League International, founded in Illinois in 1956, is an organization that is very dedicated and active in this field. The League's address is 9616 Minneapolis Avenue, Franklin Park, Illinois, 60131.

Contraindications. Even though some mothers may want to nurse, occasionally the condition of the mother or baby makes it inadvisable. Maternal illness that is particularly protracted, severe, or contagious in nature may preclude any breast feeding. A mother who had tuberculosis is usually not allowed to nurse because of the drain on her own resources and the possibility of reactivating the disease and infecting the very susceptible infant. Likewise, a woman with cardiac disease or established renal disease may be discouraged from nursing. Mentally disturbed mothers would probably not be allowed the close contact needed for feeding their infants either artificially or by breast unless closely supervised. A mother with severely cracked nipples or breast abscess may find it best to terminate nursing. With proper initial management such conditions are increasingly uncommon.

The condition of the baby may influence the decision of whether or not to nurse. Small premature infants usually do not have the strength to suckle at breast, but they may benefit from the expressed maternal milk. For this reason, mothers of premature infants may wish to maintain their milk supply for the immediate use of the baby in the hospital (to be given per gavage) and for later use when the baby goes home. Other babies, unable to suckle, may benefit from maternal milk—for example, the child with a cleft lip or palate whose defect is too large to allow suction and who is in danger of aspiration. In a few communities maternal milk banks have been established for the benefit of babies with special feeding problems. Milk that is expressed for use of a baby must be carefully handled to safeguard its purity, and a mother expressing milk to be used by her baby needs to be instructed meticulously to prevent contamination. If household freezing techniques are used, maternal milk may be stored for 2 weeks. Longer storage necessitates quick freezing and deep-freezer storage.

Techniques. The breast-feeding mother and her baby should be comfortably positioned. The mother may lie on her side with her lower arm raised to shoulder level, helping support the baby. Sitting up in bed, she usually finds it more comfortable to place the baby on a pillow in her lap. This brings the infant closer to the breast with less strain. Because soaps, detergents, and antiseptics used routinely are drying to the nipples and may cause fissures or cracking, many hospitals have changed their breast care procedures. Often the nipples are wiped with cotton balls saturated only with water and then gently dried prior to nursing. The mother's hands should be previously washed. In her own home she will probably find that a clear water wash to the nipple and breast area once a day is sufficient unless a protective cream or ointment used on the nipples requires removal before nursing.

When putting the baby to breast, the nurse and mother have some powerful allies—inborn reflexes and hunger. If it is the first time at breast or a relatively new procedure for the baby, gently expressing a drop of milk on the tip of the nipple will serve as an appetizer and help give him the basic idea. If the breasts are engorged, expressing some milk before beginning to nurse will relieve the tension of the breast and make it easier for baby to grasp the nipple. Most babies resent having their mouth shoved at the breast to begin nurs-

ing and protest. It is infinitely better to rely on the rooting reflex. When the baby's cheek is touched to the breast, he almost invariably turns his open lips to seek the nipple. The mother should compress the breast with her thumb and forefingers while the baby nurses to regulate flow and draw the breast away from his nose, making it easier for him to breathe. The baby must nurse with the nipple plus almost the entire areola in his mouth in order to suck successfully and preserve the good condition of the nipple. Cracked or fissured nipples may originate by allowing the baby to chew on the end of the nipple or to nurse too long at one time, by routinely using drying soaps and antiseptics, or by allowing the nipples to stay covered and damp for extended periods. Different maternity services have different nursing schedules, but most do not advocate allowing the baby to nurse more than 3 to 5 minutes at a time the first day. Each succeeding day the nursing time is gradually increased to 5 or 10 minutes or longer, depending on the state of the nipples and the baby's desires.

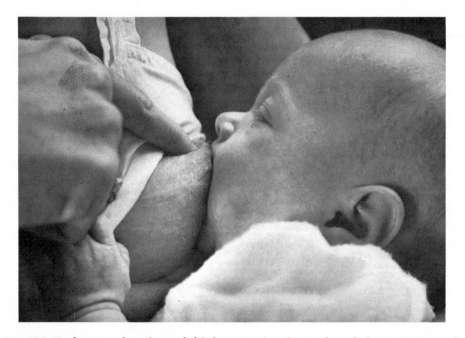

Fig. 16-7. Feeding time for a breast-fed baby. Note that the nipple and almost all the areola are within the baby's mouth.

Fair-skinned, blonde, and redheaded mothers should be especially careful about nursing too long because their delicate skin may need greater protection. Once nursing has been established the infant gets most of his nourishment the first 10 minutes at breast. The rest of the time he spends satisfying his sucking reflex and enjoying the whole procedure. Twenty minutes is usually the maximum time allowed. The first few days the baby obtains an "introductory milk" called colostrum, which has a laxative effect and supposedly contains protective antibodies. Maternal milk becomes "complete," that is, possessing its characteristic content, several weeks later.

When removing the baby from the breast, remember that he is capable of considerable tenacity. To convince him that it is best to let go, pull down on the chin, the corner of the mouth or cheek, or press the

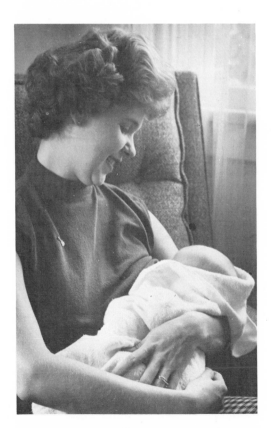

Fig. 16-8. It is possible to nurse an infant unobtrusively.

breast away from the baby's mouth, but please do not just pull!

It must be emphasized that the greatest aid to milk production is frequent stimulation and emptying of the breasts. If the breasts are not emptied, milk production may dwindle. Probably the ideal maternity accommodations for a nursing mother, particularly if the child involved is her first, is the rooming-in plan or a modification of rooming-in. In this setting the baby may be put to breast as desired and is not limited to 4-hour feeding schedules followed by most hospitals. Breast-feeding methods also differ in various hospitals. Some alternate breasts, emptying one side for one feeding, emptying the other for the next. Other maternity services advocate putting a child to breast on one side, allowing him to empty the breast, and changing him to the other breast for a few minutes to stimulate milk production. Perhaps the most important consideration is that the breast be emptied. If it is not emptied by baby, the mother should empty it manually or with the aid of a pump to maintain milk production. For a brief presentation of breast anatomy and more details of breast care, see the section on postpartal care (p. 159).

Breast-fed babies, like formula-fed babies, must be bubbled to get rid of swallowed air. Sitting the infant up or holding him over a protected shoulder while gently rubbing his back, plus patience, produces results for both breast and bottle babies.

Artificial feeding

Today, with our knowledge of nutrition and our increased understanding of food processing and preservation, it is no tragedy if a child is not breast-fed. He need not be threatened with malnutrition or disease. While mothers should be told the advantages of breast feeding, they should not be considered or made to feel like maternal failures if they cannot or choose not to nurse. To assume such a position is unrealistic and unkind. To force a mother to nurse against her will may cause an unhappy cycle of rebellion, failure, and regret and make those few mothers who cannot or should not nurse feel lacking in maternal virtue. Some have schedules difficult to combine with nursing; some are concerned that their youngsters get enough to eat; and some have felt like failures nursing in the past. For others the process of nursing is physically unattractive. Many are the healthy children who have been formula fed in our society. A loving mother cuddling her baby while tilting a milk-filled bottle need not consider herself to be a "poor mother."

Comparison of cow's milk and human milk. A comparison of the components of cow's milk and human milk gives a clue to formula preparation in the event that breast feeding is not undertaken.

	Cow's milk	Human milk
Protein	3.3%	1.25%
Fat	3.5 to 4%	3.8%
Carbohydrate	4 to 5%	7.0%
Salts (calcium, phosphorus, and potassium principally)	0.75%	0.20%

Most formulas seek to modify cow's milk to make it as much as possible like human milk. To do this, cow's milk is usually diluted to decrease the protein, and more carbohydrate is added. The most commonly used formula has an evaporated milk base. Remember, evaporated milk is twice the strength of whole cow's milk. Formula composition and amount is determined by the infant's body weight, growth, activity, and specific dietary needs. (See Fig. 21-1 for relative calorie requirements of children.)

A sample 17-calorie-per-ounce formula would be:

8 ounces evaporated milk
16 ounces water
2 tablespoons Dextri-Maltose No. 1 or 1 tablespoon Karo syrup

Human milk, when "complete," has approximately the same caloric count as whole cow's milk, 20 calories per ounce. However, some young babies do not tolerate the proportions of ingredients found in whole cow's milk and must have a modification. A so-called full-strength, 20-calorie-per-ounce formula would be as follows:

13 ounces evaporated milk
19 ounces water
4 tablespoons Dextri-Maltose No. 1 or 2 tablespoons Karo syrup

The general practitioner or pediatrician is the one to guide the use of infant formulas. There are now a wide variety of possibilities available. In addition to the different strengths of evaporated milk formulas with a variety of possible carbohydrates—Dextri-Maltose, Karo syrup, table sugar (sucrose), etc.—there is a shelfful of the so-called proprietary formulas premixed to various specifications. These may come in liquid or powder form and are usually constituted by the addition of warm, sterile water. Their use saves some preparation time and bother, but they are more expensive. (See Table 16-1.) A number of companies are manufacturing disposable prefilled nursing units. Most hospitals use commercial baby formula services.

Preparation of the formula. If the more expensive prepared bottle formula is not purchased, there are three ways of preparing infant formula: the standard or aseptic method, the terminal sterilization method, and the tap water method. Most hospitals use a combination of the first two because of their increased exposure and greater responsibility. They may assemble the entire formula supply aseptically and then sterilize it at the end of the procedure. Such precautions are not necessary in the home.

The aseptic method involves an initial 10-minute disinfection of all the bottles and apparatus needed to assemble and mix the formula and careful handling of all the equipment and formula ingredients thereafter to prevent contamination. This is difficult for many parents to do properly. However, it is the method of choice if the infant is on prescribed formulas that should not be heated for long periods (for example, acidified or cultured milks or special

Table 16-1. Composition of milk and of various infant formulas

Product	Calories/ 100 ml	Protein (gm/100 ml)	Carbohydrate (gm/100 ml)	Fat (gm/100 ml)	Minerals (gm/100 ml)	Sodium (mEq/L)	Potassium (mEq/L)	Calcium (mEq/L)	Phosphorus (mEq/L)	Iron (mg/L)
Whole cow's milk	67	3.3	4.8 (lactose)	3.7	0.72	25	35	60	62	1.0
Human milk	67	1.2	7.0 (lactose)	3.8	0.21	7	14	17	9	1.5
Similac with iron	67	1.8	7.1 (lactose)	3.4	0.4	12	20	30	26	12.0
Similac PM 60/40	67	1.5	7.2 (lactose)	3.4	0.2	7	14	17	10	2.6
SMA	67	1.5	7.2 (lactose)	3.6	0.25	7	14	21	21	12.7
Enfamil	67	1.5	7.0 (lactose)	3.7	0.3	11	19	32	32	12.7
ProSobee	67	2.5	6.8 (glucose, sucrose)	3.4	0.5	24	23	47	42	12.7
Probana	67	3.9	7.3 (lactose)	2.0	0.6	26	31	58	58	1.5
Premature	67-100	2.8	9.0 (sucrose, lactose)	3.7	0.6			49	49	trace
Cho-Free	67	1.8	(13% solution added)	3.5	0.5	17	25	47	47	8.4
Pregestimil	67	2.2 (hydrolysate)	8.8 (glucose)	2.8 (MCT)	0.6	18	48	48	47	12.7
Nutramigen	67	2.2 (hydrolysate)	8.5 (sucrose)	2.6	0.6	14	27	48	43	12.7
Portagen	67	2.7	7.7 (sucrose, maltodextrins)	3.2 (MCT)	0.7	17	27	35	36	12.7
Lambase	67	2.4	7.9 (maltose, dextrose, starch)	2.4	0.3	11	11	37	32	7.8
Isomil	67	2.0	6.8 (corn sugar, sucrose)	3.6	0.38	13	18	35	29	12.0
Advance	56	3.6	6.6 (sucrose)	1.6	0.7	17	32	50	47	18.0

From Fitzgerald, J. F.: Postgrad. Medicine **56**:49, 1974.
MCT, medium-chain triglycerides.

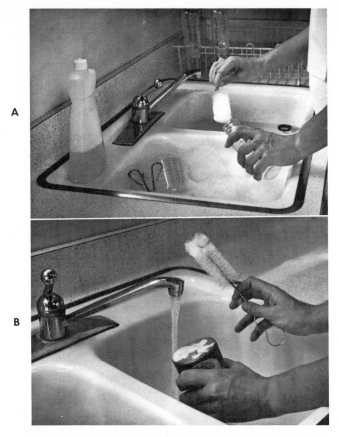

Fig. 16-9. Formula preparation—terminal method. *Procedure:* **A** and **B**, Washing. Wash all the equipment to be used, including the top of any can to be opened; rinse everything with hot water and drain dry.

vitamin-reinforced formulas). Because of its much greater popularity, only the terminal method will be pictured in detail (Fig. 16-9, *A* to *H*). It is simpler and, for most families' use, equally effective.

Materials for terminal method:
Small bottle "sterilizer" or container with a tight lid large enough for bottles
Quart-sized measuring pitcher
Large mixing spoons
Measuring spoons
Knife (if powdered carbohydrate is used)
Funnel
Six or seven formula bottles (an extra is handy for an additional supply of formula or sterile water)
Can opener
Eight nipples, rings, and discs, if appropriate
Watch, clock, or timer
Formula ingredients as ordered by the physician

Bottle brush
Soap or detergent

TAP WATER METHOD—FORMULA PREPARATION

This method of formula is to be recommended only to intelligent parents who understand its limitations and who will not abuse its simplicity. It is a good method to know in emergencies.

Materials:

Capped formula bottle	Saucepan
Nipple	Can opener
Bottle brush	Spoon
Soap or detergent	

Procedure: (Not illustrated.) Using canned milk.

1. Boil the nipple in the saucepan for 5 minutes.
2. Add enough carbohydrate (if ordered), canned milk, and warm water from the tap if water is approved (otherwise boil the

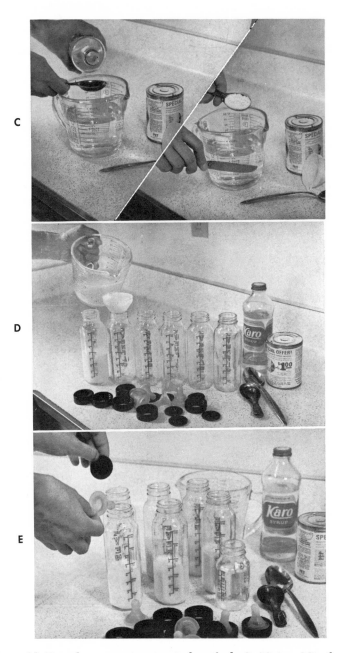

Fig. 16-9, cont'd. Formula preparation—terminal method. **C,** Mixing. Mix the formula with clean, not "sterile," equipment. Add the correct amount of clean, warm water to the pitcher and measure out the ordered carbohydrate and canned milk; stir. **D** and **E,** Assembly. Pour the formula into the clean bottles and place the clean nipples on the bottles; cap loosely.

Continued.

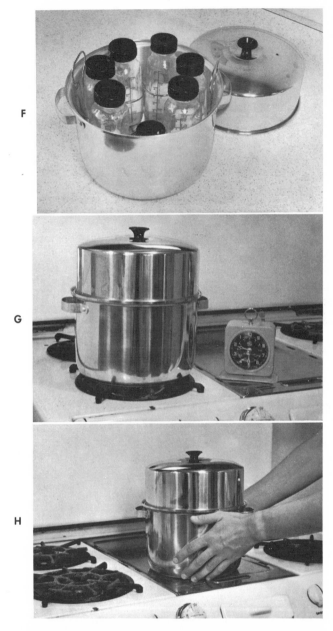

Fig. 16-9, cont'd. Formula preparation—terminal method. **F,** Preparation for disinfection. Place bottles in sterilizer on rack or washcloth. Pour 2 to 3 inches of water in the bottom of the container. **G,** Disinfection. Time the heating phase for terminal sterilization for 25 minutes after the steam appears. **H,** Cooling. Move the container from the burner to cool without lifting the lid. When the sides of the sterilizer are cool enough to be comfortable to the hands, the lid may be lifted, the caps on the bottles tightened, and the formula refrigerated.

water) to a meticulously clean formula bottle for one feeding. Mix with a clean spoon.
3. Place nipple on bottle.
4. Feed *immediately*; do not save formula from one feeding to the next or for more than an hour.

Sterilization of formula is necessary because milk is such an ideal medium for the nourishment and growth of other living things besides human babies. Microorganisms not at all compatible with the baby's digestive system may multiply rapidly in milk if it is improperly "sterilized" or is left open to air and warmed for an extended period. Once a bottle has been opened, it should be used fairly soon and under most circumstances should not be saved to use over again. The typhoid organisms used to be fairly common contaminants of milk and milk products before pasteurization became widespread. Because of the baby's susceptibility, sterilization is carried out in most households until he is about 6 months old or is drinking milk from a cup and putting all kinds of things unbidden into his mouth. If there is any question about the purity of the milk or water supply, sterilization should be continued longer.

Techniques of feeding. Feeding an infant his formula can be a very enjoyable experience. The hands should be clean; the milk should be tepid (no sensation of hot or cold, just slightly warm) falling on the inside of the nurse's wrist.

Experiments using cold formula for feeding the newborn have demonstrated no un-toward effects even on premature babies. However, personally we find it psychologically difficult to give a young infant a *cold* meal. Many nurseries are discarding formula warmers because of problems with elevated bacterial count on the equipment. They are offering feedings at room temperature. The rate of nipple flow should be almost one drop per second when the bottle is inverted. Nipple holes may be enlarged by a hot needle mounted on a cork. Vigorously sucking babies should be given a resistant nipple. Babies who tire easily and premature babies do better on a soft, pliable nipple. Be sure the nipple is on top of the tongue, and do not push it too far back —it may stimulate the gag reflex (Fig. 16-10). Babies seem to drink best when held on a definite incline. Studies have indicated that such positioning minimizes the possibility of retrograde infection through the eustachian tubes to the middle ear as well as helps prevent aspiration. The neck of the bottle should always be tipped so that it is full of milk. Air in the baby's stomach may cause pain, decrease appetite, or promote regurgitation. Bubbles may be expelled by rubbing the baby's back in an upright position. This may be done after each ounce with very small babies or halfway through and at the end of the feeding for larger babies. Some babies, particularly finger suckers, may be best bubbled before feedings as well. Newborns should be carefully observed before and during feedings for indications of any abnormality in the

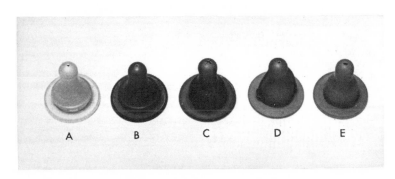

Fig. 16-10. Various types of nipples. *A,* Regular; *B,* soft rubber, for premature infants; *C,* crosscut; *D,* winged; *E,* cereal (with large hole).

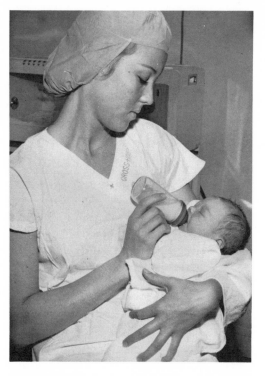 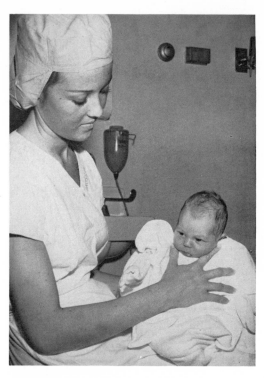

Fig. 16-11. The "en face" position. The nipple should always be full of formula and the infant preferably upright. (Courtesy Grossmont Hospital, La Mesa, Calif.)

Fig. 16-12. Let's hear a "thank you!" (Courtesy Grossmont Hospital, La Mesa, Calif.)

Table 16-2. Suggested schedule on an approximate 4-hour basis

Age	Ounces per feeding	Number of feedings	Time of feedings
First week	2 to 3	6	6, 10, 2, 6, 10, 2
Two to four weeks	3 to 5	6	6, 10, 2, 6, 10, 2
Second to third months	4 to 6	5	6, 10, 2, 6, 10
Fourth and fifth months	5 to 7	5	6, 10, 2, 6, 10
Sixth and seventh months	7 to 8	4	6, 10, 2, 6
Eighth to twelfth months	8*	3	7, 12, 6

From Williams, S. R.: Nutrition and diet therapy, St. Louis, 1969, The C. V. Mosby Co., p. 384.
*4 oz. milk may be given midafternoon.

digestive or respiratory tracts. Prefeeding coughing, cyanosis, and excessive mucus may be associated with anatomical abnormalities. Regurgitation of a feeding through the nose and mouth should be reported at once. Most babies are offered water before they are put to breast or fed formula to evaluate their ability to drink without difficulty.

After feeding, the infant should have his diaper changed if needed and be placed on his right side or abdomen to sleep. The amount taken should be recorded in nursery records. The newborn infant may take only 1 ounce the first day and 2 to 3 ounces per feeding on the second and third days. See Table 16-2 for usual formula amounts and number of feedings.

Evaluation of nutritional status

There are numerous ways of judging if a newborn infant, whether formula- or breast-fed, is receiving enough to eat.

1. Observing his behavior; does he seem content, or is he a short sleeper and irritable? (Note that babies cry for reasons other than hunger pangs; for example if they are wet, too tightly bundled, too warm, or have gas pains.)
2. Watching for signs of dehydration from poor fluid intake.
   a. Dark, concentrated urine; dry, hard stools.
   b. Dry skin with little "bounce."
   c. Low-grade fever. (Note that the most common cause of low-grade fever is dehydration, although the nurse does not want to overlook the possibility of infection.)
   d. In severe cases, sunken fontanels.
3. Measuring intake.
   a. This is routinely done on bottle babies.
   b. If measuring is ordered, breast-fed babies are weighed directly before the feeding and directly after the feeding, before any diapers are changed.
   c. Intake should be evaluated in terms of a 24-hour period and not individual feedings.
4. Measuring weight gain.
   a. This method is of little use in the nursery because of the short hospital stays of most newborn infants in the United States (approximately 3 days).
   b. All babies lose weight directly after birth, and we are not concerned unless the weight loss approaches 10% of the birth weight. Babies may not begin to gain again until the fourth or fifth day of life.
   c. After weight gain is reestablished, a gain of about an ounce a day is average, equalling about 6 ounces a week; at the end of 5 months

most babies have doubled their birth weight.

Rest and love

The birthday of a child is certainly a special occasion, and, although the child needs to be protected against infection and overexposure, the way that the child is introduced to the parents is of great importance. Both the father and the mother should have an opportunity to see the infant without hurry directly after birth.

The importance of this period directly following birth to the formation of positive mother-child and mother-father-child relationships is now being explored attentively. The newborn has been reported to be often more alert during the first hour following delivery than in the immediate subsequent hours.[*] If the mother is also alert and willing and the circumstances of the labor and delivery are conducive, an early parent-child interaction followed by frequent visits would appear to help young parents develop gratifying maternal-paternal identities.

Long-term studies of maternal attachment to normal and high-risk infants in the early postpartum period, its manifestations, and long term influence on the child are now underway.[†] Numerous investigators have described the typical initial exploratory behavior of human mothers and fathers. Gentle fingertip touching of the hands and feet progresses to massagelike motions of the palm on the baby's trunk. Eye-to-eye contact is remarkable, and a characteristic "en face" position is often demonstrated (the mother's face poised directly in front of and in line with that of her infant). These observations appear to be particularly significant because there has been some indication already that increased maternal attention seems to facilitate later exploratory behavior in infants. Could the

[*]Rising, S. S.: Fourth stage of labor: family integration, Am. J. Nurs. 74:870-872, May, 1974.
[†]Klaus, M. H., and Fanaroff, A. A.: Care of the high risk neonate, Philadelphia, 1973, W. B. Saunders Co., pp. 101-103.

early postdelivery interval be a possible critical period in the growth and development of the human offspring as it is in the case of some other species?

If grandparents and adult aunts and uncles visit, they should be able to see baby through a glass window, too. If the viewing area is outside the actual maternity area, smaller members of the family should also be invited to see little brother or sister. Some new nurseries have a covered walk outside the nursery windows that is ideal for this adventure. The newborn infant may receive all other things, but if he does not receive true love, he will not thrive.

SPECIAL NEEDS
Baptism

Sometimes other occasions of special meaning and deep significance occur in the nursery. Catholic parents and occasionally Protestant families may request the baptism of their child while he is in the nursery. When the child is in no immediate danger, a member of the clergy involved should always be called. Most hospitals have appropriate utensils available. If doubt exists concerning what should be in readiness, the clergy may always be consulted. Some will bring their own articles. Most require only a pitcher of pure water. If the child is a member of a Catholic family and appears to be in immediate danger of death, a nurse may baptize the baby. It is preferable that a nurse of the Catholic faith should do so, but any adult may do so. In performing the baptism, she should pour water on the head or face of the child while saying, "I baptize thee in the name of the Father, and of the Son, and of the Holy Spirit." A record of the baptism should be made in the nurse's notes and the parents notified. This simple but deeply meaningful act can be of great comfort to the family.

Circumcision

Circumcision entails the slitting or surgical removal of all or part of the foreskin, or prepuce, of the penis. Advocates of the procedure believe that it makes hygiene easier and decreases irritation of the area from an accumulation of cellular debris (smegma) under the foreskin and may help avoid cancer. Other practitioners declare that circumcision is unnecessary and a possible source of infection, hemorrhage, and meatal stenosis. The outcome of this ancient surgery would seem to be frequently dependent on the skill and technique of the operator. The American Academy of Pediatrics has stated that there are no valid medical indications for circumcision in the newborn period. Routine circumcision of all male infants appears to be decreasing.

The circumcision of a Jewish infant has religious import as well. Among Orthodox Jews it is undertaken by an ordained circumciser called a "mohel." This ceremony is usually performed after the child leaves the hospital on the eighth day of life. The child is then officially named.

Each physician usually has his own preferences regarding the technique used, but the following setup list and procedure may help in anticipating his wants.

CIRCUMCISION PROCEDURE

Materials:
1. Sterile setup including:
   a. One circumcision drape
   b. Two 4 × 4 squares (flats or gauze compresses)
   c. Two cotton balls
   d. Three small hemostats (mosquito clamps)
   e. One Yellen (Gomco) clamp, 1.3 to 1.1 cm. in diameter
   f. One scalpel handle and added blade
   g. Possibly needle holder, needle, and suture materials (chromic 000)
   h. One grooved director and probe
   i. One thumb forceps
2. Sterile gloves, appropriately sized
3. Ordered antiseptic for skin preparation
   a. Tincture of benzalkonium chloride (Zephiran), 1:750
   b. Tincture of thimerosal (Merthiolate)
4. Dressing materials
   a. Petrolatum-impregnated gauze
   b. Tincture of benzoin application
5. A circumcision board, diapers, pins, or special restraining halter that ties over the board

Procedure:
1. Preliminary
   a. Obtain a signed permit from parent before procedure.
   b. Properly identify the baby. Check for possible reasons for not proceeding with the operation (presence of inflammation, tendency to bleed). Clean diaper area.
   c. Restrain the baby gently but firmly on a padded or plastic circumcision board.
   d. Assure good light. A stool or chair may be appreciated by the operator.
   e. Use of a pacifier may comfort the baby during the procedure.
2. Technique.
   a. The technique of circumcision differs considerably from physician to physician. Rarely local anesthetic will be given, but most physicians seem to feel it may cause more problems than it solves (distortion of tissues) and consider the operation of such short duration, performed in an area which, at this age, has a low level of sensitivity, that it is not truly necessary.
   b. The Yellen (Gomco) clamp may be used to cut off circulation, and the foreskin excised. Sutures may or may not be used.
   c. The foreskin may be freed from the glans with probe, cut away, bleeders controlled and sutured.
   d. A nonconstrictive dressing is applied.
3. Aftercare.
   a. Notice of the recent circumcision should be attached to the crib.
   b. Frequent checks should be made to determine possible swelling and bleeding.
   c. Voidings, especially the first after the procedure, should be carefully charted. There is a danger of urinary retention.
   d. The area should be kept clean; soiled or displaced dressings should be replaced with clean materials.
   e. The infant is positioned on his side.

Rarely, circumcisions are performed in the delivery room, but most are performed the second or third day of life. Sometimes

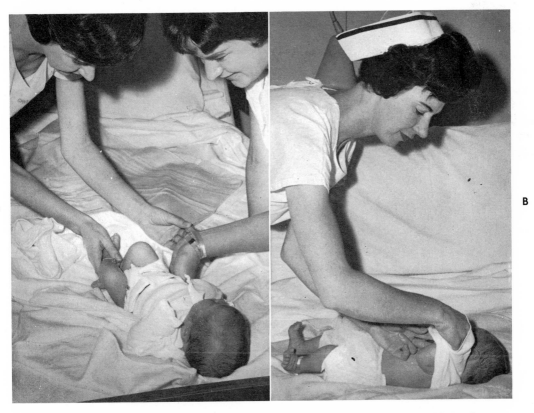

Fig. 16-13. **A,** Identification of the baby before hospital discharge using the double-banding technique. **B,** Dressing the baby in his own clothes for discharge. (Note the method of placing the sleeve over the infant's hand and arm.) (Courtesy Grossmont Hospital, La Mesa, Calif.)

they are performed not long before the baby's discharge home. In this event, the mother should be carefully instructed regarding observation and care of the area.

DISCHARGE PROCEDURE

Discharge is an exciting, trying time for most mothers. It is strongly advised that first-time mothers do not depend on the brief period of their hospitalization to learn all about baby and his needs. Many new mothers know very little about the child they are taking home and need much more instruction and reassurance than the nursery or postpartum nurse is able to provide or the patient is able to assimilate in so brief a time. This is one reason why prenatal courses in child care and preparation for motherhood are so important and should be emphasized during her antepartum period. Perhaps better yet, courses in child care and "parenting" are also being included in some high school curricula. Another assist that may be available to the new mother is the home guidance of the visiting nurse who, in cooperation with her physician, helps the mother feel confident doing such things as preparing formula, sponge bathing a new baby, or, after the umbilicus heals, putting him into a tub for the first time. Many times a grandmother, other relative, or neighbor can help.

Before the actual time of departure, the physician's order for discharge is checked, and home orders are reviewed. The mother's belongings are packed, and clothes are put out for the infant. Mothers should have ready at least two diapers, pins, a baby shirt, kimono, and receiving blanket or comparable wardrobe. The baby is usually brought in from the nursery wrapped only in a blanket and dressed at the bedside. Identification should be established, the discharge of the baby signed and witnessed, the baby unwrapped, viewed, and dressed in his own clothes (Fig. 16-13). If the mother wishes it, a supply of formula may be available to take home to tide her over until formula can be made. Before saying goodbye to the family, the nurse should make sure discharge instructions are understood and preferably written out. Before leaving the infant, she should take one last peek at his face to assure herself of his condition. Then, no matter what she may desire, she must let him go.

17

Infants with special needs: prematurity and abnormality

This chapter is included to help the student appreciate some of the more common abnormalities or conditions encountered during her practical experience and to help her more intelligently assist in the care of infants who have these conditions. Some of the conditions discussed are found and treated in the nursery and pose few or no problems later. Other anomalies by their very nature call for prolonged therapy and correction long after the neonatal period, infancy, or, indeed, childhood has passed.

THE PREMATURE INFANT
(Figs. 17-1 and 17-2)

Among those babies with special needs the first to be discussed are the premature infants. The most common definition of prematurity is based on weight. Usually, babies having a birth weight under 5½ pounds or 2,500 grams are considered premature. However, in reality some of these babies have completed a term gestation and are underweight because of genetic or intrauterine factors. When this is the case, the terms "low birth weight" or "small for gestational age" are more accurately applied rather than "premature." The survival rate of these infants depends on their general condition as well as weight. Some of them are quite vigorous, whereas others of the same weight are feeble. However, certain broad predictions can be made. (See Fig. 17-3 depicting neonatal mortality based on birth weight and gestational age.)

It would be much more scientific if the prenatal period were included in the total months considered when computing the age of a child. To compare a 1-month-old, small, premature infant with a 1-month-old child of normal gestation is grossly unfair. The premature infant is indeed born too soon. Just how much too soon is many times difficult to determine. As a general rule, assuming that the estimated normal birth date is fairly accurate, babies are considered premature if born before the end of the thirty-seventh week of gestation. Indeed, the World Health Organization suggests that the definition of the premature infant be based on this calendar calculation, regardless of birth weight. Infants of less than 28 weeks' gestation have been known to survive, but this is rare. Actually, in determining the status of the small infant, birth weight, heredity, possible length of gestation, clinical appearance, and behavior all must be considered. Although some babies cannot be classified premature by the scale or calendar, they are judged underdeveloped and treated as "premies."

Role of the nurse

The student nurse who wishes to work with premature babies should seek more supervised advanced training than is possible in her basic course. The nursery care of these infants must be very gentle, deft, and precise, and the ability to properly evaluate their behavior and reactions takes an extended period of time to acquire. However, although as a student she may not have the opportunity to be involved in the direct nursing of many premature infants, she should understand the nature of the problems encountered in such nursing.

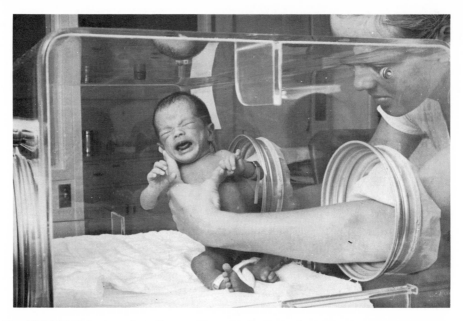

Fig. 17-1. This baby is technically premature if only his birth weight is considered. However, his Oriental ancestry influenced his size; he is probably a "finished product," although he weighs less than 5½ pounds. (Courtesy Grossmont Hospital, La Mesa, Calif.)

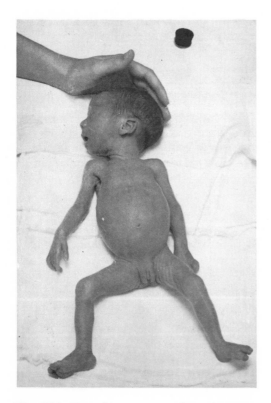

Fig. 17-2. Typical premature infant. (Courtesy Grossmont Hospital, La Mesa, Calif.)

Some of these babies will be cared for in an ICU setting, others in the pediatric area. The first cause of infant mortality, remember, is prematurity.

Causes

The causes of prematurity or low birth weight infants are not always known. However, it is recognized that there is a higher incidence of these infants born to mothers of lower socioeconomic status. This may be related to the extent of medical supervision available, the obstetrical complications encountered, nutrition, and general health practices. Young teen-age mothers have a higher rate of low birth weight babies. Multiple births are almost always associated with prematurity. Heavy smoking seems to be an etiological factor. Approximately 10% of all deliveries in the United States are premature.

Appearance and activity

The typical premature infant has a "wrinkled old man" appearance resulting from lack of subcutaneous fat. He has a

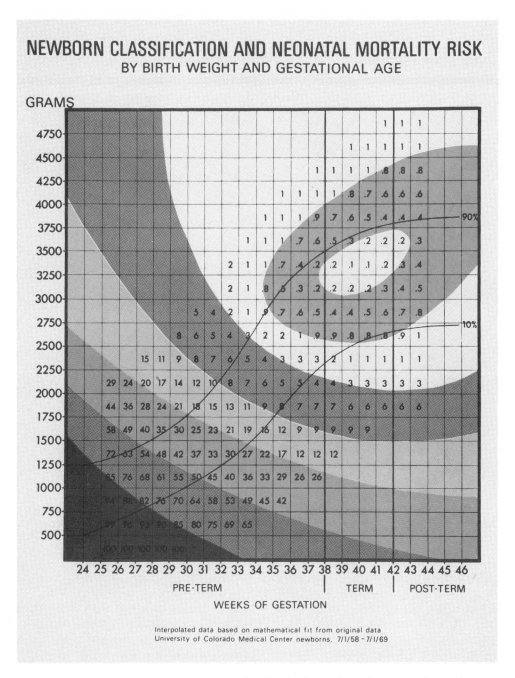

Fig. 17-3. Neonatal mortality percentages related to birth weight and gestational age. (From Lubchenco, L. O., Searls, D. T., and Brazie, J. V.: J. Pediatr. **81**:814-822, 1972.)

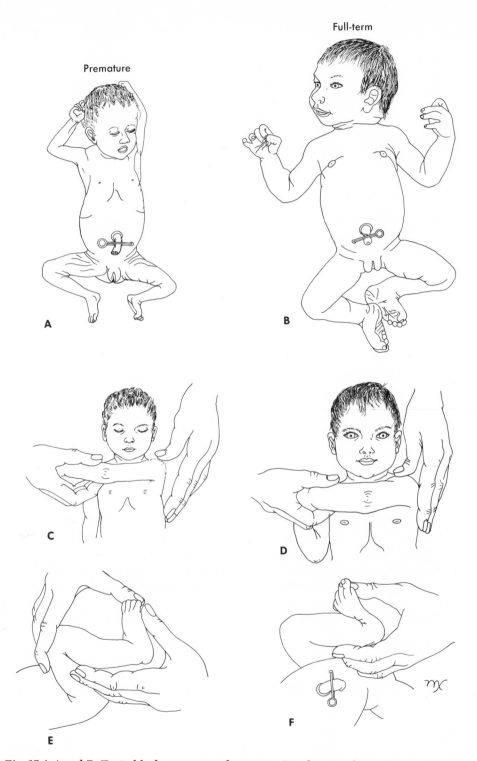

Fig. 17-4. **A** and **B**, Typical body contours and postures. **C** and **D**, Scarf sign: immaturity seen when elbow passes midline. Lanugo more prominent on premature. **E** and **F**, Prematurity seen when heel cord is short and sole crease is scanty.

good supply of long, soft body hair called "lanugo"; his head and abdomen are relatively large; and his thorax is small. There is little molding of the skull. His respirations are usually quite irregular, and he may be surprisingly active.

Nutrition

Sucking and swallowing reflexes may be weak or absent in very small infants, necessitating feedings by gavage (the insertion of a stomach tube) or by intravenous feedings. Intravenous feedings are now quite commonly given especially to infants weighing less than 1200 grams or classified as "sick" prematures. These feedings may be given by umbilical catheter or peripheral veins. Stronger "premies" may do well fed with a soft rubber nipple.

The subject of premature feeding schedules and techniques is controversial at the present time. However, after a period of evaluation of feeding tolerances for glucose water, oral feedings generally progress to formulas richer in calories than those normally fed to full-term infants because of the premature infant's lack of nutritional reserves and his great need for rapid growth. Later his diet is supplemented by iron administration.

Most premature infants are put on a 2- or 3-hour feeding schedule. Nourishment is offered in extremely small amounts of 3 to 5 ml. at a time since the danger of overfeeding the premie is very real. Overfeeding may increase abdominal distention, cause respiratory embarrassment, and trigger vomiting, which may involve aspiration. The infant must be bubbled frequently. After a feeding, the baby's head and chest are elevated by tilting the incubator mattress tray, and the infant is positioned on his side to discourage emesis and aspiration.

Special needs

The maintenance of body temperature is a real challenge in the care of premature infants. Because of the immaturity of the temperature-regulating center in the brain, little stability is seen. The baby must be specially assisted in his efforts to keep warm. This aid may be provided by the open-type infant warmer or an enclosed plastic incubator.

Oxygen levels above that of room air (21%) may be required to meet the infant's metabolic needs. The most accurate way to evaluate a baby's oxygen status is through the use of intermittent arterial blood gas determinations. Although some babies may approach oxygen toxicity levels when the environmental oxygen reaches 40%, others with diminished respiratory function will need higher levels of environmental oxygen to achieve correct blood concentrations. Environmental oxygen concentrations together with blood gas analysis are very important. They are monitored to evaluate the infant's general condition in response to therapy and to prevent the blindness or visual loss called *retrolental fibroplasia,* which can be produced by prolonged exposure to a high-oxygen environment. The veins in the retinas of the eyes dilate and hemorrhage. The retinas partially or completely detach from the inner surfaces of the posterior chambers of the eyes. They become fibrous masses behind the lenses, unable to receive visual stimuli.

The premature infant is especially susceptible to injury and must be handled with extreme gentleness and discretion. (He needs his rest to grow!) He is particularly prone to injury at the time of birth and may suffer from intracranial hemorrhage and brain damage. A large percentage of cerebral palsied children, who exhibit some form of spastictiy, or lack of muscle control, were premature. Lack of muscular coordination and mental retardation may stem from brain injury, prolonged lack of oxygen caused by delayed or interrupted breathing at the time of or subsequent to birth, or bilirubin deposits in the brain tissue due to the inability of the immature liver to handle red blood cell breakdown satisfactorily. Jaundice is a significant finding.

"Premies," because of their abrupt debut,

are said to be deprived of antibody protection given by mothers to full-term infants. They are also less prepared to manufacture their own antibodies. They are easy victims of infection and must be scrupulously guarded.

Significant immaturity of the respiratory system is an often encountered finding. Failure of lung tissue to expand, or atelectasis, is frequently reported. *Hyaline membrane disease,* or *developmental respiratory distress syndrome,* is found in a high percentage of premature babies, particularly those delivered by cesarean section, and in children of diabetic mothers. (These babies, although large, appear to be physiologically immature and should be treated similarly to premature infants.) This disease is the commonest cause of death in premature infants and is discussed on p. 256.

• • •

The care of the premature infant is a heavy responsibility; life is enclosed in a fragile package. Yet some of the celebrated figures of history, who have made vast contributions to mankind, entered the world in just such an unfinished state—such men as Sir Isaac Newton and Sir Winston Churchill. Do not underestimate the "premie"!

ABNORMALITIES OF THE NEWBORN INFANT

One would wish that each baby born would be perfect in every detail—physically, intellectually, and emotionally ready to meet the challenge of life without an initial obstacle or defect. Sadly, such is not the case. Approximately one in sixteen of all children born have some kind of serious abnormality, causing disfigurement or resulting in physical or mental handicaps or a shortened life.

The birth of a handicapped or ill child is always a distressing time for the family. Feelings of anxiety, guilt, frustration, and exhaustion are common. Parents at first may be unable to believe that their child is abnormal, and when the realization comes,

grief may be intense. Problems in organizing the family to meet the unexpected demands created by the necessary trips to the hospital, doctor, and therapist and the extra financial burden it all entails can seem almost without end to the often perplexed and unprepared parents.

Although the vocational nurse is not in a position to give professional guidance to people to mobilize the total resources of the family and community to meet the needs involved, she should recognize the pressures under which they are operating. She should know how much has been told the mother regarding her child and be extremely discreet in her conversations. She should be supportive in allowing the parents to express themselves and in relaying any problems that seem to be causing worry to the charge nurse or physician. It is *very important* that the parents not feel isolated in their attempt to adjust to the reality of their child's imperfection. In an attempt to prevent isolation the nurse can be a vital liason between the family, medical staff, clergy, and community resource personnel.

Birth injuries

Cerebral hemorrhage. The most common type of birth injury is *intracranial hemorrhage.* As noted previously, it is most often seen in premature infants but can be diagnosed in full-term babies as well, particularly those who had a traumatic passage to this external world. Symptoms or signs of hemorrhage within the skull may manifest themselves suddenly or gradually. They may include irritability, listlessness or cyanosis, marked irregular respiration, varying degree of paralysis, lack of appetite or poor sucking reflex, tremors, convulsions, projectile vomiting, unequally dilated pupils, tense or bulging fontanels, and a high, shrill cry. These kinds of symptoms could arise from other causes, such as intracranial abscess, cerebral edema, tumor, or developing hydrocephalus—in fact, from anything that would increase the pressure within the skull. Diagnosis is usually made through the history and observation of the infant. Sometimes the bleeding is mild and stops of itself, and the child recovers with little or no effects. Sometimes pressure is so intense it must be relieved by aspiration of the subdural space or by surgery. Sometimes brain damage is permanent, or death results from the condition.

The infant is usually placed in an incubator with the head slightly elevated in an attempt to relieve pressure. Rarely, a spinal tap may be done for the same reason or as a diagnostic aid. Vitamin K to relieve bleeding tendencies may be prescribed. Sedatives such as phenobarbital may be ordered in case of tremor. It is very important for the nurse observing the infant to be able to accurately describe the type of tremor, convulsion, or abnormal behavior pattern seen; her description of the part of the body affected—one or both sides—how long it lasted, and what, if anything apparent, occurred just beforehand may be able to help the physician localize the area of bleeding. The child is kept as quiet as possible.

Fractures. Fractures may occur at birth. The most frequently broken bone is the clavicle, or collarbone. It usually heals without treatment. Fractures of long bones are uncommon; they may be splinted. All broken bones normally heal rapidly during infancy.

Facial paralysis. Temporary or even permanent paralysis occasionally results from nerve injury during delivery. Facial paralysis may be caused by forceps pressure. The side of the face affected does not move, and the eye may remain open. This condition usually disappears gradually.

Erb's palsy. Injury to the brachial plexus, the network of nerves that branches to supply the nervous control of the upper extremities, may cause the arm on the affected side to hang limply from the shoulder and rotate internally. With this condition, the Moro reflex is asymmetrical. The infant cannot raise his arm. This injury, called Erb's palsy, is usually not permanent. Treatment consists of immobilizing the arm in an abducted, externally rotated position with flexion at the elbow.

Hydrocephalus

Hydrocephalus is a defect that results from the accumulation of abnormally large

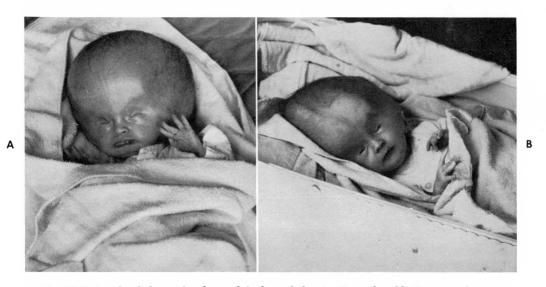

Fig. 17-5. **A,** This baby with advanced hydrocephalus is 4½ weeks old. However, he was delivered 7 weeks early per cesarean section. **B,** The same child at 3 months of age. The cranium has collapsed. He died at 5½ months of age.

amounts of cerebrospinal fluid within the cranium, causing abnormal enlargement of the immature skull (Fig. 17-5).

Types. There are a variety of causes of hydrocephalus. A congenital structural defect may exist in the cerebrospinal fluid drainage system, preventing the flow of the fluid from the ventricles of the brain into the subarachnoid space and into the venous system. Such blockage may also occur as the result of developing brain tumor or abscess. This type of blockage produces noncommunicating hydrocephalus. Occasionally, the flow of cerebrospinal fluid from the ventricles to the subarachnoid space is normal, but the absorption of the fluid into the venous system is abnormal and inadequate because of an obscure developmental defect. This situation, described as communicating hydrocephalus, may occur as a sequela to meningitis or subarachnoid hemorrhage. It sometimes coexists with a congenital defect called *myelomeningocele*, a herniation of a part

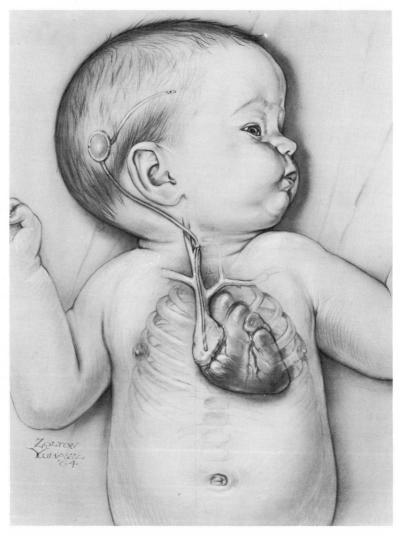

Fig. 17-6. Pudenz valve—one type of shunting device that drains cerebrospinal fluid from the ventricles of the brain into the right atrium. (Courtesy R. H. Pudenz, M.D., and the Heyer-Schulte Corp., Santa Barbara, Calif.)

of the spinal cord elements and its coverings through an abnormal opening in the back of the bony spine. The hydrocephalus usually becomes more evident after the myelomeningocele is surgically repaired. Circulation pathways outside the brain for the cerebrospinal fluid that had previously been available may be disturbed or unavailable.

Early recognition and treatment. The infant responds to mounting cerebrospinal fluid pressure by a progressive symmetrical increase in head size. Other manifestations noted shortly after birth include bulging of the fontanels, separation of sutures, distended scalp veins, irritability, and vomiting. A downward displacement of the eyes and skin tension giving the pupils a "setting-sun" appearance is a late symptom.

Early reduction in ventricular size is essential if the child is to have the best chance of becoming a useful individual. The treatment of hydrocephalus is influenced by the degree of intracranial pressure, the level of obstruction, and any associated major congenital defects found. Spontaneous arrest occurs in 30% to 40% of children affected but usually does not occur until the hydrocephalus is well advanced. By this time a useful existence may be impossible.

Hydrocephalus is usually treated by insertion of a tube or shunt that drains the ventricular fluid into a body space outside the skull. The well-being of the child depends on the continuous functioning of the shunt. Ventriculoatrial and ventriculoperitoneal shunt systems are the most effective.

VENTRICULOATRIAL SHUNT. The insertion of Silastic tubes and valves that allow one-way flow of fluid has led to the successful shunting of cerebrospinal fluid into the jugular vein and right atrium (Fig. 17-6). A burr hole is made in the skull, and a small tube is directed into the lateral ventricle of the brain. Through a small neck incision the cardiac tube is inserted into the right atrium via the internal jugular vein. The ventricular and cardiac tubes are then connected to the flushing device situated

beneath the skin and behind the ear. The flushing device is shaped to fit into the burr hole with its flange overlying the surrounding skull. Under normal operating conditions cerebrospinal fluid flow is unobstructed. The flushing devices differ on the various tubes used. In the Pudenz-Mishler double-lumen device, the ventricular cardiac catheters are flushed when the reservoir is compressed. Pumping the functioning shunt permits highly effective flushing in both directions. Obstruction of the ventricular tube, the commonest cause of shunt malfunctions, may be cleared by occluding the easily felt atrial catheter with finger pressure and compressing the reservoir. Thus the flushing device serves a dual purpose; it flushes and checks the operation of the entire system. In postoperative care, a daily check by manually depressing the

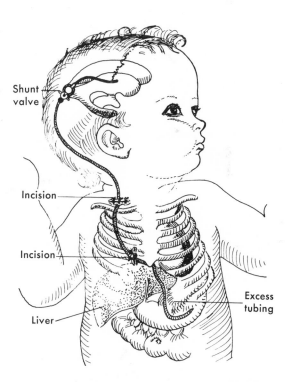

Fig. 17-7. Ventriculoperitoneal shunt with the multipurpose valve designed by the Heyer-Schulte Corp. Provides a sophisticated system for the control of hydrocephalus. Can be used with any of the various Heyer-Schulte ventricular and distal catheters.

229

skin (pumping) over the reservoir of the flushing device and watching for refill will determine if the shunt is functioning properly.

VENTRICULOPERITONEAL SHUNT. The ventricular catheter is inserted into the lateral ventricle through a small burr hole. The distal catheter is passed beneath the skin down the neck and may tunnel across the front of the chest to enter the abdomen over the liver or may be passed subcutaneously down the back and around the flank to enter the peritoneal cavity in the area of the right lower abdominal quadrant. Several inches of coiled catheter are left in the peritoneal cavity, hopefully to provide needed increased length automatically as growth proceeds. The ventriculoperitoneal shunt is commonly inserted in infants because of the ease with which it can be surgically revised, if necessary, to compensate for the growth of the child.

VOLUME-CONTROL SYSTEM. To eliminate dependence on shunts in the care of hydrocephalus, a system for intermittent ventricular drainage via a manually controlled on and off valve has been devised. Hopefully, more transventricular absorption of cerebrospinal fluid will be achieved, and active hydrocephalus can be converted to arrested hydrocephalus with the aid of the Multi-Purpose-Valve (Fig. 17-8).

POSTOPERATIVE CARE. When the infant is wide awake, dextrose in water is offered by mouth. If it is tolerated, formula may be given. It is important that the nurse observe the baby before the shunting procedure to compare and evaluate his postoperative condition. To avoid respiratory complications the child must have his position changed at least every 2 hours. The head should be placed carefully to avoid pressure on the cranial wound, which might predispose the skin to break down. The fontanel should be less tense and slightly depressed. If the fontanels are sunken, the child is kept flat. If the fontanels are full or bulging, his head is elevated. Pulse and respiration determinations and pupil equality checks are done frequently. The nurse

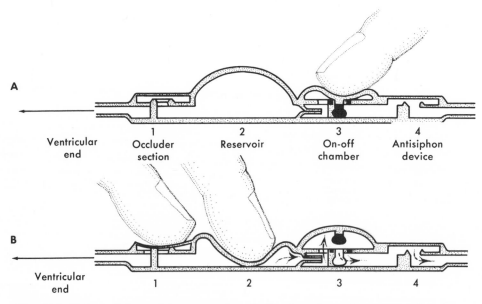

Fig. 17-8. Hydrocephalus multipurpose valve. **A,** To close the multipurpose valve, depress the on-off chamber, which is located between the reservoir and antisiphon device. **B,** To open the on-off chamber, compress the occluder section (1). While holding the occluder section closed, compress the reservoir (2), which will open the on-off chamber (3). The shunt will stay in the open position until force is reapplied to the on-off chamber.

must be constantly alert for any signs of increased intracranial pressure such as slowed pulse and respirations, lethargy, irritability, vomiting, and tense fontanels. Head circumference should be measured at the widest diameter daily. Any abnormalities detected by those observations, signs of faulty functioning of the flushing device, or an elevated temperature should be recorded carefully and immediately called to the attention of the physician.

COMPLICATIONS. Infections continue to be the major problem in both type of shunts. Despite all methods of parenteral antibiotic therapy, including injections into the spinal canal, bacteremia, a complication especially associated with ventriculoatrial shunts, can be cleared only by the replacement of a new shunt mechanism in a different site. Debilitated infants seem to be prone to infection. Other problems include obstruction of the shunt system due to plugged tubing by debris at the ventricular end, thrombus formation at the cardiac end, and adhesion formation at the peritoneal end. Although the new Multi-Purpose-Valve is a considerable advance in the treatment of hydrocephalus, improved methods of controlling this problem continue to be sought.

Continued care. When surgical intervention cannot be considered, nursing care of the child with advanced hydrocephalus takes considerable gentleness and patience. The head may be extremely large with widely separated cranial bones, broad sutures, and bulging fontanels. Despite the plasticity of the infant skull, pressure on the brain usually causes some degree of mental retardation. There may be wide swings in body temperature, tremors or convulsions, lack of appetite, or vomiting. The tension of fontanels and other signs of increasing intracranial pressure should be checked daily.

Attention must be given to preventing pressure sores on the scalp by frequent turning and soft pillow supports. When not being supervised directly, the child should be positioned on his side or abdomen with his head turned to the side to prevent aspiration. Support for the head must always be given during feedings, and the nurse may find it more comfortable for the baby and less tiring for herself to place a pillow on her arm for head support and to rest her elbow on the chair arm. After feeding and bubbling, the infant should be left as quiet as possible to prevent vomiting. Malnutrition and infection are frequent complications for these unfortunate babies.

Cranial stenosis and microcephaly

Other congenital deformities of the skull may be found, but happily they are rare. The sutures of the skull may prematurely close (cranial stenosis), causing abnormal pressure on the brain and possible mental retardation, as well as an asymmetrical distorted appearance of the head, if unrelieved. In another instance the brain may fail to continue growing, and a severely retarded, *microcephalic* individual may result. Very rarely, a child may be born without a developed brain and lack the usual cranial covering of the brain. This condition is called *anencephaly;* the infant soon dies.

Mental retardation

Mental retardation is an extremely common problem. It affects approximately 3% of the general population. Good prenatal and delivery care helps prevent some of the possible causes (birth injury, anoxia). Some types of mental retardation can be prevented or aided by dietary supervision, hormonal therapy, or genetic counseling.

Intelligence classifications. Because of the many problems that have been identified in trying to determine a person's intellectual capacity by testing devices, the concept of I.Q., or intelligence quotient, has lost much of its former significance. The mental age score attained by an individual in testing may be influenced by his motivation and environment, as well as the test presentation itself. Nevertheless, I.Q. scores are still often obtained. They repre-

Table 17-1. Intelligence classifications

Classification	Intelligence quotient	Performance level
Profound retardation	I.Q. 0 to 24	Unable to attend to personal needs; always requires supervision. 0- to 2-year-old behavior
Severe retardation	I.Q. 25 to 50	May be trained to meet personal needs but not self-sustaining. 3- to 7-year-old behavior
Moderately severe retardation	I.Q. 50 to 75	Self-sustaining in simple jobs with supervision
Mild retardation	I.Q. 75 to 90	
Average	I.Q. 90 to 110	What most of us are
Above average	I.Q. 110 to 130	What most of us would like to be
Gifted	I.Q. 130 to 150 ⎫	
Genius	I.Q. 150 and above ⎬	These people have problems in adjustment, too

sent a special testing score (mental age) divided by the individual's chronological age multiplied by 100. Table 17-1 shows certain ranges of I.Q., representing various degrees of intelligence.

Down's syndrome. A common (1 in 650 live births) type of mental retardation associated with certain physical characteristics that has undergone considerable investigation is that of Down's syndrome, or mongolism. The most common of the three types known is called "trisomy 21" because it is associated with an abnormal chromosome count in the baby's body cells. (See p. 266.) These children range from profoundly to mildly retarded.

Mongoloid children are usually identified in the nursery, but some are diagnosed later. Characteristically, infants with Down's syndrome are short; they have relatively small skulls, flattened from front to back; their birth weights are usually low; and their behavior is lethargic. The most reliable signs of mongolism are exaggerated epicanthic folds, which make the eyes slant up and out; short hands and fingers with the little finger bent in; a deep, horizontal crease across the palm; and a large space between the great and small toes. Physicians will examine the eyes in an effort to detect small white dots on the iris, which, when present, are helpful in making a diagnosis. Decreased muscle tone and excessive joint mobility are also significant findings (Figs. 17-9 and 17-10).

After the newborn period, other signs manifest themselves such as delayed eruption of teeth, fissured tongue, and retarded intellectual and physical development. These youngsters often have congenital heart malformations, umbilical hernias, and duodenal atresia. If they survive long enough, they usually possess rather affectionate, placid personalities. Many times, depending on home circumstances and the individual needs of the child, they can remain with the family, and care outside the home community is not necessary. No one knows for sure the true cause of this condition, but trisomy 21 is found most often in cases in which the mother is near the end of her reproductive life. The translocation type of Downs' syndrome may be hereditary.

Phenylketonuria. Another type of mental retardation that is much less common and has been publicized a great deal is that produced by an inherited error in metabolism of a certain amino acid, or protein, called *phenylalanine.* The disease is called PKU, a short way of saying phenylketonuria. It results when an enzyme normally produced by the liver is missing or inadequate. Unless appropriate measures are taken, poisons build up in the bloodstream that, after a few months, begin to produce noticeable damage to the brain. A high level of the potentially poisonous substance can be detected in the blood serum of the newborn infant, but a few weeks are usu-

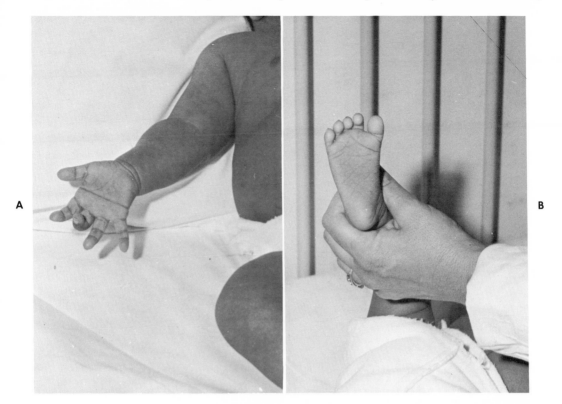

Fig. 17-9. **A,** Hand of an infant with Down's syndrome. Note the deep, straight palmar crease. **B,** Same infant's foot. Note the exaggerated space between the big and little toes. (Courtesy U. S. Naval Regional Medical Center, San Diego, Calif.)

ally needed before the offending chemical is found in the urine. Blood tests to detect the disease may be done the third day of life just before discharge from the hospital; urine examinations are not valid until later. Treatment consists of eliminating as much of the offending protein as possible from the diet for an indeterminate time. Since phenylalanine is found in many protein foods, the diet is extremely curtailed, and synthetic protein foods are necessary. Results of treatment have been highly gratifying.

Galactosemia. Galactosemia, another rare metabolic error that may produce mental retardation, involves the metabolism of galactose.

Cretinism. Cretinism, or infantile hypothyroidism, may also be a cause of mental retardation. The thyroid hormone is absent from the time of birth. Prenatally, the in-

fant is supplied with thyroid by his mother. The signs of hypothyroidism develop gradually.

The typically affected baby has a large tongue that, because of its size, may protrude from his mouth, causing problems in feeding. His cry is hoarse; his hair is coarse, and his skin is dry (no perspiration is observed); constipation is a continuous problem; and growth is retarded if the condition is untreated.

If cretinism is diagnosed early by studies of the thyroid gland or the iodine content of the blood and the child is given hormone replacement therapy, he usually progresses fairly normally, although slight intellectual retardation may persist.

Spina bifida

Spina bifida, a condition briefly noted in the discussion of hydrocephalus, may exist

233

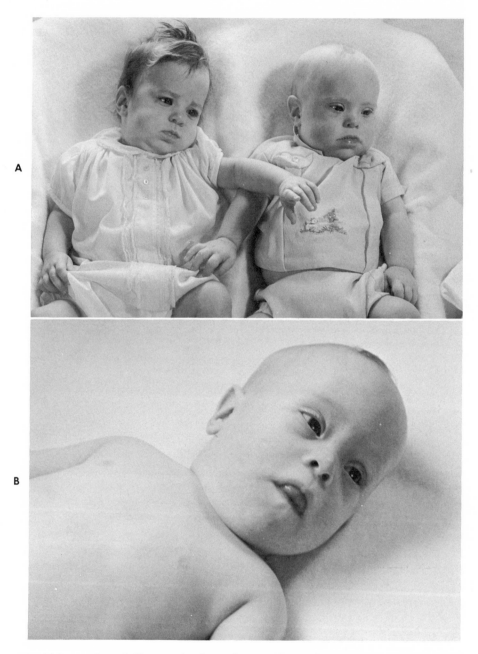

Fig. 17-10. **A,** These children are brother and sister (fraternal twins). The little boy manifests Down's syndrome; his sister is unaffected. **B,** Close-up of the male twin. Note the large tongue and typical eyes.

in several degrees of severity. The term "spina bifida" simply means "divided spine" or that a portion of the posterior wall of the spine is missing.

Types. The defect may be so small that it offers no difficulty and is discovered only when an x-ray examination of the spine is done for other reasons. This type of defect is called "spina bifida occulta," or "hidden divided spine." The second main type of spina bifida (meningocele) involves a protrusion of only the meninges of the spinal cord through the opening, usually causing a tumor on the lower back that contains cerebrospinal fluid. The child usually develops normal urinary and intestinal control and suffers from no paralysis, but the tumor, until removed, is a cosmetic problem, and its possible injury always poses the problem of infection of the meninges or brain. A third type of spina bifida has been called *myelomeningocele,* or meningomyelocele. In this condition the meninges protrude through the spinal opening, and nerve tissues are also found in the herniated sac. Children with this problem are often troubled with persistent incontinence, partial or complete lower extremity paralysis, and sensory disturbance. Hydrocephalus frequently accompanies this defect (Figs. 17-11 to 17-13).

Nursing care. The nursing care of the child with either meningocele or myelomeningocele is challenging. Before surgery, the sac, or tumor as it is sometimes called, must be protected from injury and infection. The child must be adequately nourished and should be assured of loving care. To protect the sac, the child is usually positioned on his abdomen or carefully propped on his side. Because of the usual position of the tumor, no diapers are pinned in place. To avoid putting strain or pressure on the sac, the nurse must be extremely careful in lifting the infant. Slipping her hands and forearms palms up under the leg and chest area to grasp the farther thigh, arm, and shoulder seems to be a safe, effective way of lifting and moving the smaller infants. Caution must be taken when putting these children in sitting position even if no direct pressure is exerted on the tumor. Sometimes the sac is so low on the spine that the sitting position puts too much tension on the area. A positioning device called a Bradford frame may be used. This consists of a metal framework that rests

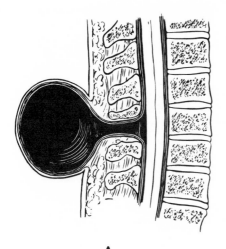 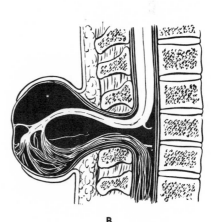

A   B

Fig. 17-11. **A,** Section of the spinal cord and vertebral column showing a meningocele. Note that no nervous tissue protrudes through the defect into the sac. **B,** Section of the spinal cord and vertebral column showing a myelomeningocele. Nervous tissue is found in the herniated meningeal sac. (From Benz, G. S.: Pediatric nursing, ed. 5, St. Louis, 1964, The C. V. Mosby Co.)

on the bed and elevates the baby on a divided, padded canvas support. The perineal area and sac are placed directly over splits in the canvas, and a bedpan is positioned directly underneath. Plastic strips hanging from the opening of the frame help direct urine and feces into the pan.

This device helps protect the area from soil and pressure.

When being fed, the infant may be propped on his side with his head elevated, held by one nurse with his head over her shoulder while fed by another nurse holding the bottle or, his condition permitting,

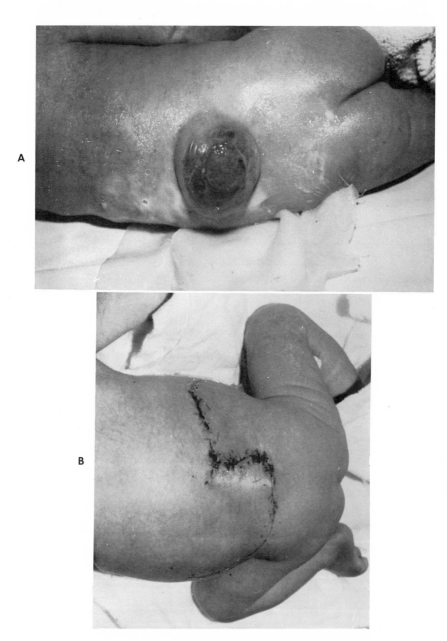

Fig. 17-12. **A,** Myelomeningocele before surgery. (An antibacterial dressing was used.) **B,** Repair of the same patient. (Courtesy M. C. Gleason, M.D., San Diego, Calif.)

held in a sitting position with no pressure on the sac.

Meticulous skin care must be observed and pressure areas prevented. Occasionally, to avoid infection, the tumor area will be irrigated periodically with a mild antiseptic. It may be covered by sterile petrolatum or medicated strips and gauze compresses. A foam rubber ring with a hole large enough to admit the tumor may be placed over the sterile compresses and wrapped in place with an elastic bandage. Treatment depends on the tumor's size, location, and condition. The sac should be observed for variance in size and tenseness as well as ulceration. The head of a child with any type of meningocele usually is regularly measured to try to detect developing hydrocephalus. The sensation and movement of the lower extremities are evaluated as care is given.

After surgery (usually a flap-type pro-

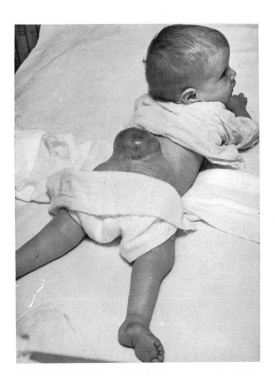

Fig. 17-13. This youngster's myelomeningocele was repaired shortly after this photograph was taken. (Courtesy Children's Health Center, San Diego, Calif.)

cedure done in stages), the prone position is maintained, at least until the sutures are removed. There may be no dressing over the incision, and a dry incision and body warmth may be maintained by a carefully positioned gooseneck lamp or the use of an incubator. Although surgery rarely improves function, it certainly improves the child's appearance and facilitates care. The care of a patient with spina bifida, complicated by a herniation of nerve tissue elements, continues for life. Many orthopedic procedures may have to be completed before the child achieves even the ability to walk with braces. Many spina bifida babies also have clubfeet. Urinary complications are the rule rather than the exception. To avoid the problems created by continued long-term use of indwelling catheters, a urinary diversion may be made from an excised part of the ileum into which the ureters have been placed. It drains continually through an opening on the abdominal wall. The prevention or treatment of decubiti is a real concern. The child needs constant psychological and emotional support, as well as physical assistance, to attain a healthy personality capable of giving to as well as receiving from his environment.

Cleft lip and cleft palate

Cleft lip and cleft palate are fairly common congenital malformations. They appear approximately once in every 500 to 1,000 births. They constitute a failure in the embryonic development of the child, and the hereditary factor is often found to be significant. Cleft lip is found more often in males, whereas females more often have cleft palates. Cleft lip, sometimes called harelip, may vary from a single notching of the border of the lip to a deep split extending through the lip to or into the nose. It may exist on only one side of center or be found on both sides. It may create a problem in feeding, dentition, and appearance but fortunately usually has an excellent prognosis. A cleft lip is usually repaired very early—as soon as the infant's

237

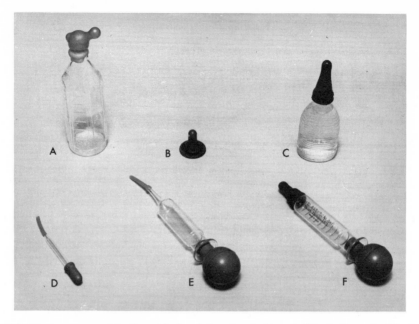

Fig. 17-14. Various types of feeding aids for cleft palate babies. *A,* "Ducky" nipple (the hump fits into the defect); *B,* soft "premie" nipple is often used; *C,* lamb's nipple; *D,* rubber-tipped medicine dropper; *E,* rubber-tipped Asepto syringe; *F,* Brecht feeder. (Courtesy Children's Health Center, San Diego, Calif.)

condition is sufficiently stable, at approximately 2 months of age or before. A cleft palate may involve lack of fusion of only part of the hard or soft palate or may extend along the entire roof of the mouth. Cleft palate is repaired later according to the child's individual needs.

Before taking their baby home to await surgery for cleft lip or palate, the parents must receive detailed instructions regarding his care and have several opportunities to feed the infant with supervision. The baby usually has difficulty sucking normally, since he cannot create the necessary vacuum in his mouth. He may be fed slowly with a rubber-tipped Asepto syringe, a rubber-tipped medicine dropper, or a Brecht feeder, no faster than his capacity to swallow (Fig. 17-14). Occasionally, the defect is so placed or is so small that a regularly shaped soft nipple with a large hole may be used. Rarely, a specially molded cleft-palate nipple with an extra built-in hump that fits the cleft in the palate and makes sucking possible is em-

ployed. Because of their shape, these are sometimes called "ducky nipples." Occasionally, soft, long lamb's nipples are tried, or the child may be fed off the end of a small spoon. Levin gavage is avoided if at all possible. The baby is fed in an upright position to help prevent aspiration and, in the case of cleft palate, to prevent regurgitation through the nose. The method of feeding that is most successful and closest to that used by a normal baby is the method of choice. Since these babies swallow more air than usual, they should be bubbled frequently. This will lessen the possibility of emesis or unattended "wet burps" and subsequent aspiration. Some children with cleft palate are fitted early with a prosthesis to help guard against nasal regurgitation, aid in the formation of speech patterns, and maintain anatomical relationships important to the final repair.

The success of plastic surgery depends on the extent of the defect, the developmental stage of the individual, the repair techniques available, the skill of the sur-

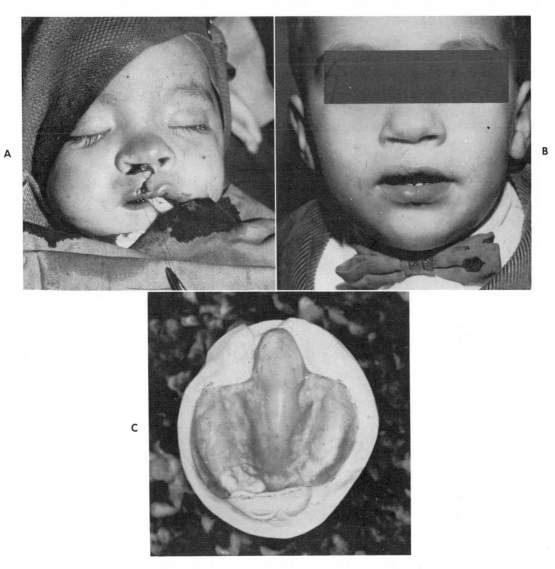

Fig. 17-15. A, Closure of a unilateral complete cleft lip. B, Same child 13 months later. C, Palate prosthesis resting in a plaster-of-Paris mold. The prosthesis is used until a child is old enough for optimal palate repair. (Courtesy M. C. Gleason, M.D., San Diego, Calif.)

geon, the standard of nursing care, and the cooperation of the parents. A cleft palate is much more difficult to repair, and the child may have to undergo several procedures at different ages (Fig. 17-15).

Nursing care of the patient with cleft lip. After surgery for a cleft lip the infant should have his arms restrained to prevent damage to the suture line or pulling on an indwelling gavage tube. Elbow or wrist restraints may be used. Very young infants may have their arms restrained adequately by pulling their long shirt sleeves past their hands and pinning the sleeves to their diaper. Periodically, these restraints should be removed one at a time to provide needed exercise and inspection of the arms. Infrequently an indwelling, nasal Levin tube is used to provide feedings for several days to lessen the lip motion that would take place if a nipple were placed in the mouth, thus helping to safeguard the suture line.

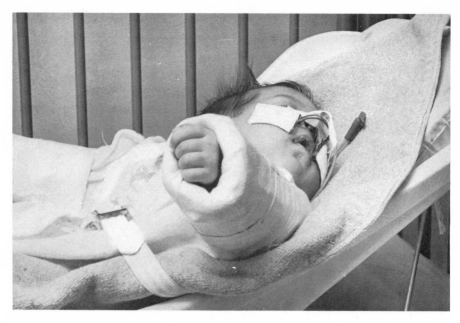

Fig. 17-16. Infant with a newly repaired cleft lip. Note the Logan bow, gavage tube, and elbow restraints. The child has a palate prosthesis in place. (Courtesy Children's Health Center, San Diego, Calif.)

A soft nasal packing may be in place in the opposite nostril to prevent bleeding of the operative site and help "mold" the nose properly. It is removed after approximately 2 days (Fig. 17-16).

The suture line should be kept clean, and no crust should be allowed to form because crusting enlarges the scar. Various solutions are used for cleaning, depending on the physician's preference; examples are hydrogen peroxide, warm sterile water, or physiological saline solution. Tightly wrapped, sterile cotton applicators or small gauze sponges mounted on forceps may be used to remove blood. Such maneuvers must be done gently but persistently. Soaking the area for a brief period with a saturated applicator or sponge before any motion over the area is attempted aids considerably. Afterward, the lip should be gently dried, and any protective covering ordered should be applied. Sometimes an antibiotic ointment is used, or a small "mustache" of petrolatum gauze may be left on the lip.

A Logan bow may be employed to prevent lateral tension on the suture line. This metal loop arches over the suture line and is held in place on both cheeks by pieces of adhesive tape. When a Logan bow is used, an indwelling gavage tube is usually taped to its arch to prevent tension on the nose and eliminate the use of more adhesive tape on the skin.

Every effort should be made to keep the child happy—not just because we want a child to be happy, which we do, but because a happy child cries less and puts less strain on his repair. The parents should be allowed to cuddle the infant and, as soon as feasible, participate in feedings under supervision. Usually, the tube is removed about the third postoperative day. The child may then be fed by Asepto syringe, Brecht feeder, or a rubber-tipped medicine dropper, and graduated to a soft nipple when sucking is allowed. The ability to suck is usually markedly improved by the repair.

Nursing care of the patient with cleft palate (Fig. 17-17). As stated before, repair of a cleft palate is usually more difficult than repair of a cleft lip. A series of opera-

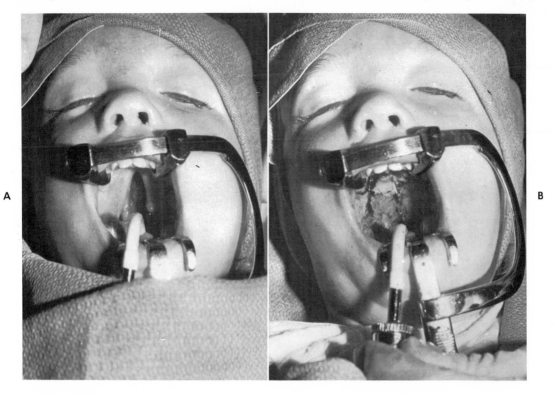

Fig. 17-17. A, Cleft palate just before survery. **B,** Closure of the cleft palate. (Courtesy M. C. Gleason, M.D., San Diego, Calif.)

tions may be needed. A cleft palate is also a more serious defect, considering the impairment of function it produces. Not only is feeding difficult, involving possible problems of aspiration and dental placement, but speech is often nasalized, and infections of the respiratory tract and middle ear are common. The child who has undergone palate surgery is usually fed from a cup or side of a spoon. Nothing is introduced into the mouth that may endanger the suture line, and, unless the child is old enough to understand and cooperate, arm restraints must be used. The diet progresses from clear liquid to full liquid to soft food over a period of approximately 1 week. The mouth should be rinsed with water at the end of a meal.

The problems of the child with cleft lip, cleft palate, or both are occasionally so complex that the combined therapy of a plastic surgeon, pediatrician, orthodontist, speech therapist, child psychiatrist, and medical social worker may be needed. For this reason, clinics for those with cleft lip and palate are found in most large cities.

Other digestive tract abnormalities

Other abnormalities of the digestive tract are found with enough frequency to at least merit mention, especially since they are so serious in nature.

Esophageal atresia and tracheoesophageal fistula
(Fig. 17-18)

Esophageal atresia refers to the congenital absence or closure of the esophagus at some point. The upper portion usually ends in a blind pouch. Tracheoesophageal fistula represents an open connection between the trachea and the esophagus. There is a frequent association between esophageal atresia and tracheoesophageal fistula due to the nature of embryonic development.

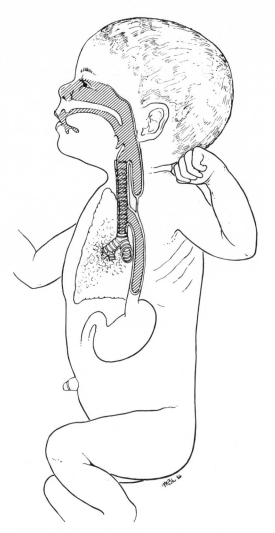

Fig. 17-18. The most common type of esophageal atresia involves an upper esophageal segment ending in a blind pouch and a lower tracheoesophageal fistula. There is great danger of aspiration.

Several varieties of these malformations are known, but the three major types are:
1. Tracheoesophageal fistula with esophageal atresia (80% to 95% of cases). The upper esophagus ends in a blind pouch, and the lower esophageal segment connects with the trachea.
2. Esophageal atresia alone.
3. Tracheoesophageal fistula alone.

These anomalies are relatively common. About 25% of the infants with digestive tract abnormalities are premature. An-

other 25% usually have associated defects (primarily other gastrointestinal malformations, such as imperforate anus). Maternal polyhydramnios is frequently noted in these infants due to the inability of the fetus to dispose of swallowed amniotic fluid. The malformations are slightly more common in the male.

Symptoms. The infant usually cries at birth, breathes well, and becomes a normal, pink color. Soon, however, saliva accumulates in the pharynx and mouth, and the infant is noted to be frothing or drooling. The mucus is thick and seems excessive, but it is actually a normal amount of mucus that simply cannot pass through to the stomach and therefore pools in the esophageal pouch. Respirations become noisy, gurgling, and rapid. The cry is hoarse. Respiratory difficulty increases, and cyanosis occurs. If the infant is fed, he will repeatedly cough, gag, and regurgitate. Feeding is usually followed by aspiration of formula into the lungs, which leads to pneumonia and often to atelectasis. All pulmonary symptoms are caused by the drainage of secretions into the lungs via the esophageal connection or overflow from the blind pouch.

Diagnosis. Diagnosis can be easily made in the delivery room or nursery by inability to pass a catheter into the stomach. X-ray films positively confirm the diagnosis.

Treatment. Surgical repair is the only method of treatment and should be instituted within 12 to 24 hours after birth. The chest is opened, and the tracheoesophageal fistula is tied off (ligated). Connection of the esophageal segments is also performed, if possible; otherwise, this is accomplished at 1 to 2 years of age. A gastrostomy is performed, and a chest tube is inserted.

Nursing care. Preoperative care is directed toward rapid stabilization of the infant. He is kept in a head-up position, given oxygen with humidification to thin the secretions, and constant gentle suction is applied to the esophageal pouch via a specialized (sump) tube. He is handled minimally and receives nothing orally. Fluids

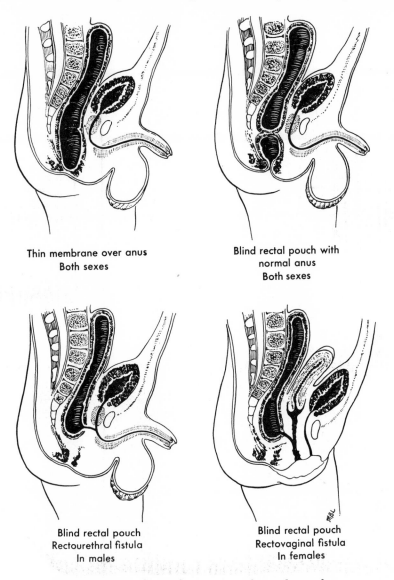

Thin membrane over anus
Both sexes

Blind rectal pouch with
normal anus
Both sexes

Blind rectal pouch
Rectourethral fistula
In males

Blind rectal pouch
Rectovaginal fistula
In females

Fig. 17-19. Types of imperforate anus in the newborn infant.

are administered intravenously by way of a peripheral vein or by umbilical catheter. Postoperative care is much the same, but includes proper care of the surgical incision, chest tube, gastrostomy, and frequent turning. Initially the gastrostomy is allowed to drain freely into a collection bag. When feedings are begun through the gastrostomy in 2 to 3 days, the tube is elevated and left open. An esophageal sump tube is not used postoperatively—suctioning is performed very gently only as needed.

Prognosis depends largely upon the initial condition of the infant at the time of diagnosis, the degree of prematurity, presence of other malformations, and whether or not feedings had been given. Once all surgical repair is complete and recovery has taken place, these infants usually develop normally. They do, however, have a higher incidence of pulmonary infections during their first year and usually a harsh cough for some time. Continued medical supervision is essential.

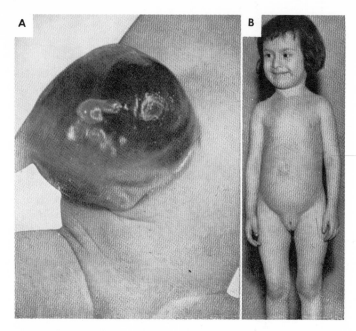

Fig. 17-20. A, Omphalocele before repair. B, After corrective surgery. (From Potter, E. L.: Pathology of the fetus and the newborn, Chicago, 1952, Year Book Medical Publishers, Inc.)

Imperforate anus

Occasionally the infant's rectum ends as a closed or blind pouch or connects to an adjacent canal (urethra, vagina) via a fistula (Fig. 17-19). The possibility of this defect is one reason observation of the stools of the newborn is so important. Many times a temporary colostomy, an abdominal exit for the contents of the colon, must be made. Later the creation of a normally placed functional rectal opening will be attempted surgically.

Omphalocele (Fig. 17-20) is an absence of the normal abdominal wall in the region of the umbilicus that may allow a portion of the intestinal contents to be clearly observed, virtually unprotected, and subject to herniation and strangulation. The defect may be small or exaggerated. Its repair is usually considered a surgical emergency. Another type of hernia, involving the abdominal contents and causing respiratory distress as well as digestive problems, is the *diaphragmatic hernia*. In this condition an abnormally large opening is present in the diaphragm that allows part of the con-

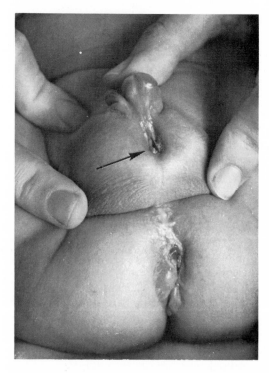

Fig. 17-21. This infant suffers from multiple congenital anomalies. The arrow indicates the opening of the urethra at the base of the penis (hypospadias). An imperforate anus was previously repaired.

tents of the abdominal cavity to displace upward into the chest. Sometimes the entire stomach, as well as portions of the intestine, is found in the thorax, crowding the heart and lungs. This situation, too, is a surgical emergency.

Hypospadias

A fairly common malformation of the urinary system that is found in male infants is hypospadias (Fig. 17-21). The urethra, instead of traveling the entire length of the penis, opens out on the underside of the penis, either at its base or at varying distances from the tip. Sometimes the presence of hypospadias, coupled with other irregularities of the external genital organs, leads to confusion in the determining the sex of the infant, and cell studies and exploratory operative procedures may be necessary. The repair of well-defined hypospadias by the extension of the urethral canal is usually accomplished by a series of operative procedures before the child is of school age. Minor positional deviations of the urethral meatus may not require treatment.

Congenital heart deformities

Congenital cardiac conditions many times stem from the persistence of some part of the fetal circulation pattern, so it would be of benefit to review the basic circulation present before birth (see Fig. 5-6). The foramen ovale may fail to close, resulting in an *atrial septal* defect. The *ductus arteriosus* may persist. However, real structural deviations may also exist in many different combinations. (See pp. 582 to 592 for more detail.) Open-heart surgery, with the use of the heart-lung machine, now gives more hope of survival and the possibility of a more normal life for victims of congenital heart defects.

Hemolytic disease of the newborn infant

A number of conditions can cause blood destruction in the fetus or newborn infant. Probably the most well-known cause is Rh factor incompatibility, which may initiate the condition *erythroblastosis fetalis*. The Rh factor is a protein that was first identified in the blood of Rhesus monkeys. It is found in approximately 85% of the Caucasian population and in higher percentages among the non-Caucasian population (Fig. 17-22).

Rh incompatibility

If a woman who lacks the Rh protein in her blood marries a man who also lacks it, no problem will exist because of the Rh factor for their offspring. However, if her husband is Rh positive and their child inherits Rh-positive blood from his father, trouble may occur.

Probable mechanism. Some of the baby's blood cells carrying the Rh protein may pass through a microscopic tear in the placental barrier and reach the mother's bloodstream. The mother's body automatically manufactures antibodies (protective substances) designed to destroy the foreign protein in her body. These antibodies may then find themselves in the fetal circulation. There, they do just what they were designed to do. They destroy the Rh protein, or factor, and, in so doing, also destroy the red blood cell to which it is attached. The fetus suffers from the effects of anemia. Making a valiant effort to supply more red cells, it forces out into its bloodstream immature, inadequate forms of red blood cells called erythroblasts. This is the reason that the resulting disease is termed *erythroblastosis fetalis*. In severe cases congestive heart failure associated with enlargement of the spleen and liver occurs. If the pregnancy is not successfully terminated before advanced damage results, the unborn child will die.

Shortly after birth, toxicity caused by the large amount of red blood cell breakdown products (chiefly bilirubin) circulating in the baby's body may lead to brain damage known as kernicterus. This condition causes neurological impairment, such as spasticity, deafness, or mental retardation, or may even lead to death.

245

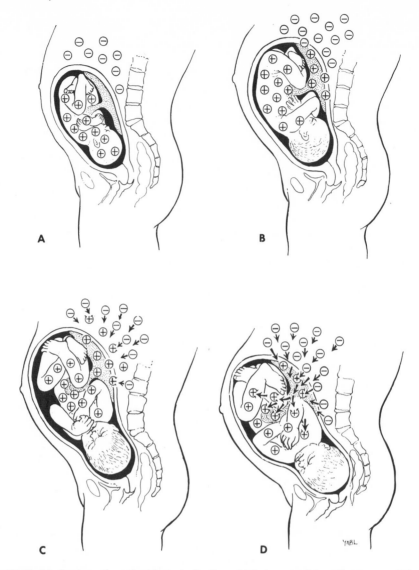

Fig. 17-22. Mechanism of erythroblastosis fetalis, which is caused by Rh incompatibility. **A,** Rh-positive child is carried by Rh-negative mother. **B,** Rh protein crosses the placental barrier and invades the mother's bloodstream. **C,** Mother's system manufactures antibodies to destroy the foreign Rh protein. **D,** Antibodies cross back over the placenta and destroy the baby's blood cells, which are intimately associated with his Rh protein.

One of the first clinical manifestations of Rh factor sensitivity in the infant is the appearance of jaundice within 24 to 36 hours. The baby with a more severe case may be lethargic, suck poorly, and manifest spasticity.

However, not all mothers with Rh-negative blood have such sick babies. Sometimes the baby is also Rh negative and no

such problem arises. Sometimes the number of antibodies the mother has produced in response to the baby's cells in her bloodstream is so small that no damage to the baby is detected. Usually, trouble is not encountered until the second or third infant. After several pregnancies, the titer of antibodies in the blood usually increases markedly. This titer may be measured during pregnancy; also the progress of the disease may be estimated by analyzing amniotic fluid aspirated from the sac surrounding the baby. These tests allow the physician to evaluate the health of the fetus and plan for the baby's delivery and care.

Often the question is asked, "Why doesn't an Rh-positive mother become ill when her unborn child is Rh negative?" The answer seems to be in the relative inability of the fetus to produce enough antibodies to attack the mother's blood cells in sufficient number.

Treatment. When the presence of erythroblastosis fetalis is determined in a newborn infant, exchange transfusion is carried out. The umbilical vein is used to achieve access to the baby's bloodstream per polyethylene catheter. A carefully measured amount of blood is slowly withdrawn and discarded by a syringe equipped with a complex of stopcocks. Then crossmatched, Rh-negative donor blood with a low Rh antibody titer warmed to room temperature is pushed slowly per syringe back into the baby's body as a replacement. This process is repeated many times until complete replacement is estimated to have occurred. During the procedure, close observation of the baby's vital signs and the blood volume exchange is essential. The baby must be kept warm, and oxygen may be administered. This treatment must occasionally be repeated, but the results are usually highly successful, and the child born in good condition and receiving prompt transfusion when needed has an excellent prognosis.

Recently, another method of treating erythroblastosis has been publicized; it is a new dramatic approach—intrauterine transfusion of those unborn infants that show signs of not being able to survive until viable. This procedure, now available at a few research centers, is not without risk but may be considered when no other real choice is possible.

The exposure of infants with elevated blood bilirubin levels to blue or fluorescent light to reduce the amount of circulating bilirubin is now being evaluated. The naked infant is positioned under the lamps with protective eye shields in place. He is turned periodically to increase body surface exposure. (See Chapter 18.)

Prevention. For the Rh-negative primipara who has never received Rh-positive blood in a transfusion or miscarried an Rh-positive infant, a fairly recent wonderful discovery will prove beneficial. It has been found that passive immunization or ready-made antibody protection, given at a certain time will destroy the invading foreign Rh protein and inhibit the natural formation of antibodies by the individual. If passive Rh_0D antibodies are injected intramuscularly into a previously unsensitized patient within 3 days after her delivery, the subsequent pregnancy has little risk of developing hemolytic problems because of the Rh factor. This special passive immunization has been marketed as Rh_0GAM. Unfortunately, it does not aid Rh-negative women who have already actively developed their own immunization against the Rh factor.

A mechanism similar to the Rh problem, but usually of a less serious nature, can operate when the mother has type O blood and the baby has type A, B, or AB. Such a situation is called "ABO incompatibility."

Orthopedic abnormalities

Orthopedic abnormalities are quite common in the newborn nursery. As a general rule, the earlier they are treated the better the prognosis.

Congenital dislocation of the hip (CDH)

There are two main types of congenital dislocations of the hip: (1) *teratologic,* which develops during life in utero and is commonly associated with other orthopedic problems; and (2) *typical,* which occur just before, during, or shortly after birth, probably due to the softening effects of the maternal hormone relaxin on the baby's ligaments and the stress of labor and delivery. The hip joints of every newborn should be examined within 24 hours of birth for congenital dislocation. They can usually be successfully treated by simple manipulation. There are 1.5 cases of CDH per 1,000 live births. It affects girls 8 times more frequently than boys. Dislocation, or luxation, is present when the femoral head is completely displaced from the socket, or acetabulum. Subluxation, or partial displacement, is more common, occurring in approximately 1 in 60 births. A subluxated hip may become completely dislocated during a baby's care unless certain types of maneuvers are avoided. These infants should never be lifted by their feet for diapering. Their legs should never be pulled nor should their hips be completely extended when wrapped in a blanket. Since one does not always know which child may have incipient hip problems, these cautions should apply to the care of all babies. Barring complications, the subluxated hips of 88% of the affected newborns become normal by 2 months of age.

Physical findings that the licensed practical or vocational nurse can detect include asymmetry of the thigh folds, limited abduction of the affected hip, and shortening of the femur when the knees and hips are flexed at right angles and when abduction is attempted with the child lying supine on a firm table. The diagnosis is usually confirmed by x-ray film. Since the socket becomes progressively more distorted if reduction is delayed, the goal of treatment is the immediate return of the femoral head to the acetabulum. A normal hip joint can be obtained when treatment is begun in the first few weeks of life. Reduction of the hip is not difficult and involves maintenance of the hip in a stable position of flexion and abduction. The Frejka pillow-splint allows some hip motion in a relatively "normal position" while at the same time maintaining flexion and abduction. Semirigid abduction devices are more practical and preferred by some orthopedists. The child's orthopedic condition is frequently evaluated on an outpatient basis. Early treatment may reduce therapy to about 3 months' duration. If the child's x-ray film indicates normal location of the hip at 2 years of

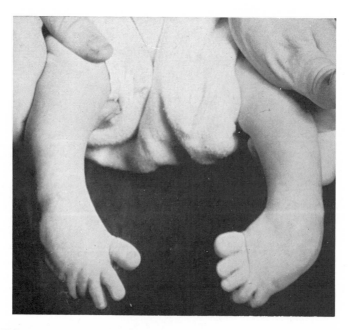

Fig. 17-23. Talipes equinovarus. (From Larson, C. B., and Gould, M.: Orthopedic nursing, ed. 8, St. Louis, 1974, The C. V. Mosby Co.)

age, he may be considered cured. Treatment after age 6 months varies. It may involve traction for a few weeks followed by casting and/or operative reduction. However, when one sees a child with CDH for the first time at age 2, the outcome is seldom optimal. In children over 8 years of age, even the most extensive operative procedures cannot produce a functionally satisfactory hip. About one third of the degenerative hip joint disease found in adults is caused by the residual effects of CDH. In adults such conditions may be helped by a total hip arthroplasty. For information regarding the nursing care of the child with congenital dislocation of the hips see

Chapter 30, Progressive abduction traction (Figs. 30-1 and 30-2).

Clubfoot (talipes)

Clubfoot, or *talipes,* is a fairly common orthopedic deformity. It is not always congenital, since it can be the result of neurological or muscle disorders in later life, but, of course, in the newborn nursery all cases would be classed as congenital; many are hereditary. A clubbing of the foot can mean many types of distortion. The foot may turn in (talipes varus), may turn outward (talipes valgus), may turn down forcing the heel off the walking surface (talipes equinus), may turn up forc-

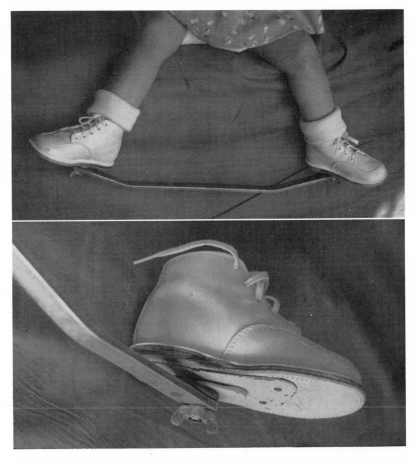

Fig. 17-24. Modified Denis Browne splint is often used to help maintain corrected positions of the feet. (From Larson, C. B., and Gould, M.: Orthopedic nursing, ed. 8, St. Louis, 1974, The C. V. Mosby Co.)

ing the toes off the walking surface (talipes calcaneus), or a combination of these types of defects may occur. One or both feet may be involved. The most common clubfoot is *talipes equinovarus* (Fig. 17-23).

The feet of the newborn infant must be carefully evaluated. Not all apparent deformities are true clubfoot. Some distortions are simply caused by intrauterine positions and not real structural differences. These feet can be corrected to neutral position in all elements of the deformity by manipulation during examination. A true clubfoot cannot.

The treatment of clubfoot depends on the individual case. Sometimes, simple exercises are prescribed, or foot braces, special shoes, or casts may be worn (even while the child is in the nursery) (Fig. 17-24). In some cases subsequent surgery may be necessary. A plantar stripping of the fibrous tissue of the foot and a lengthening of the heel cord or tendon of Achilles may be performed. Turco has developed an extensive operative procedure in which all the elements of talipes equinovarus are corrected at the same time.

Syndactyly and polydactylism

Syndactyly, or webbing of the fingers or toes, is a very interesting anomaly, usually responding well to surgical separation. Syndactyly may accompany another digital abnormality called *polydactylism*, or the presence of extra fingers or toes. At times, these extra digits have no bony connection with the hand or foot and, when a ligature is tied around the fleshy stalk, cutting off circulation, the digit soon drops off. When a bony connection exists, surgery is necessary if gloves are to be worn with ease in later years.

Effect of contagious diseases

The effect of contagious diseases on the fetus and newborn infant is discussed in Chapter 12. Those considered are syphilis, gonorrhea, tuberculosis, and rubella (German measles).

• • •

Many are the abnormalities possible in the newborn infant, but when one considers the intricacies of life, the miracle is that more of them do not occur.

18
Intensive care of the newborn

THE SPECIAL CARE NURSERY

Neonatology, the study and treatment of the sick newborn, has rapidly become a highly specialized area of pediatrics. Continuing advances in detection, prevention, and treatment of disorders of the newborn have led to the development of specialized neonatal units with highly trained personnel. Basic nursing courses do not attempt to equip the vocational nurse to work in these units. However, with further training and education, selected LV and LP nurses are being included in the staffing patterns of these specialized units, and students may have a period of observation and closely guided participation during their obstetrical or pediatric experiences. This chapter is designed to help these nursing students obtain a better understanding of the types of patients, conditions, and procedures the nurse encounters in the special care nursery (SCN) or neonatal intensive care unit.

The main objective of the SCN is to provide the earliest and maximum degree of medical and nursing care for the infant at risk, so that each infant attains his best possible outcome. As neonatal mortality is reduced, continuing efforts must also be made to decrease the incidence of such long-term problems as chronic lung disease, intestinal disorders, and, most important, neurological sequelae, such as mental deficit, blindness, and deafness. Thus an awareness of the causes and prevention of residual damage is necessary for the SCN nurse.

Ideally, the facility that provides the SCN should also have a high-risk obstetrics department, with both specialized areas providing regional care for a determined geographic area. Thus comprehensive care of the high-risk mother and infant becomes centralized, and unnecessary and costly duplication of equipment and premium personnel is avoided. Medical and nursing teaching programs and continuing research in perinatology are added benefits of such a facility.

Regionalization requires an emergency transport team composed of highly skilled, specially equipped medical and nursing personnel (RN or LVN) who travel to area hospitals at a moment's notice to provide expert evaluation, stabilization, and ultimately safe transfer of the high-risk neonate back to the SCN. This transport involves the use of an ambulance and/or helicopter and a specially designed transport incubator to provide the proper environment, such as warmth and oxygen, if necessary, for the infant en route to the SCN. This type of emergency system helps promote the critical continuity of care necessary for optimal outcome.

On such an assignment the nurse evaluates the infant, prepares him for transport, and assists the physician with any necessary procedures. She meets with the parents, establishing rapport with them and giving them a brief explanation of the SCN. She makes certain that they know its location and telephone number and explains the unit's visiting policy.

The concept of rigid visiting hours is fortunately becoming outdated. The mother's early and frequent contact with her new baby is important for the proper development of maternal-child attachment, which is the foundation of future interpersonal relationships. Many SCN's now have virtually unlimited visiting privileges, and

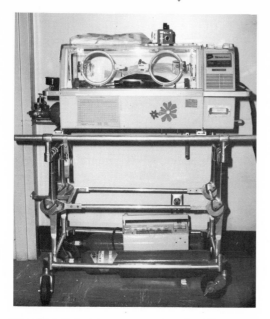

Fig. 18-1. Infant transport equipped with oxygen, resuscitation, and temperature control apparatus. (Courtesy Louis Gluck, M.D., University Hospital, San Diego, Calif.)

parents are asked to visit often when possible. They are taught to wash and gown properly, and physical contact with their baby is encouraged. As the infant's condition improves, the parents begin to hold and feed him and gradually assume more of his daily care, in preparation for his eventual discharge from the hospital. Equipment and procedures are explained in detail and questions readily answered. The critical nature of the situation is greatly eased when parents understand what is being done and are allowed to participate.

Parents have daily contact with the physicians and nurses and are kept well informed of their infant's condition. The infant often has a primary nurse, one who cares for him throughout his entire hospital stay. She is the primary resource person for the parents and works with the physicians, social worker, and other personnel in planning optimal care of the infant, counseling parents, and planning discharge. Thus continuity of care is again enhanced. The primary nurse is responsible

for beginning the nursing care plan as soon after admission as possible.

Staffing in the SCN

The SCN is an emergency room type of setting where emergencies may not only be met and handled immediately but may be anticipated and often prevented. The nurses work closely with the physicians, some of whom must be present on the unit at all times. Since potentially life-threatening conditions may be heralded by subtle changes in the patient's behavior or appearance, the SCN nurse must develop astute powers of observation. A clear understanding of each infant's disease process is imperative, and preparation must be made for any emergency situation that might result from the disease itself or from the treatment (for example, a pneumothorax that develops in an infant receiving mechanical ventilation). The nurse must also be familiar with the technical equipment (such as monitors and ventilators) that play such an important role in the SCN.

The nurse-patient ratio is 1:1 for infants who are critically ill or in an immediate postoperative phase. The average ratio is 1:2 for most sick infants and up to 1:4 during the convalescent phase. These ratios allow maximum efficiency in nursing care, which is of vital importance. Some hospital settings provide a separate progressive care unit where staffing ratio can be increased.

Nursery personnel wear scrub clothes and use a separate cover gown technique for each infant. Handwashing is of major importance; personnel wash meticulously before and after handling any infant or piece of equipment. Scrubbing with a brush is not necessary and may injure the skin, thereby increasing the chance for bacterial contamination. Caps and masks are not used. In some hospitals persons may freely enter the SCN without gowning or washing as long as no infant or equipment is touched. Scrub gowns are worn over street clothing by physicians, parents, and other personnel.

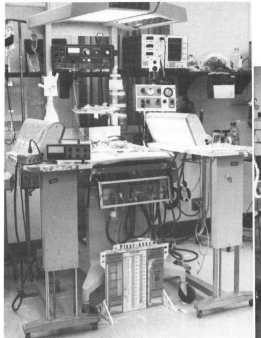
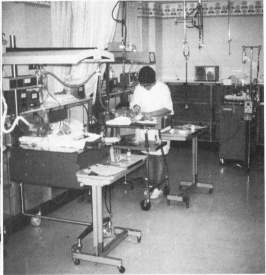

Fig. 18-2. A, This little infant of 1 lb. 10 oz. (750 gm.) is obscured by his equipment. He has recently undergone heart surgery. His most valuable monitor, his nurse, is standing to one side, just outside the picture. B, Another pediatric intensive care setting showing different types of equipment used. (A Courtesy Louis Gluck, M.D., University Hospital, San Diego, Calif.; B courtesy Alan Shumacher, M.D., Children's Health Center, San Diego, Calif.)

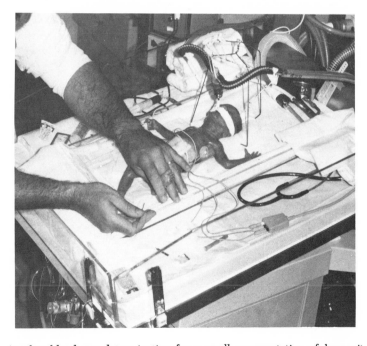

Fig. 18-3. Another blood gas determination for a small representative of humanity who has RDS. (Courtesy Louis Gluck, M.D., University Hospital, San Diego, Calif.)

253

THE CRITICALLY ILL NEONATE
Anticipation of the high-risk neonate

Prompt recognition and treatment of the sick infant is of utmost importance in obtaining the best possible outcome for each patient. The majority of SCN patients are the products of a relatively small number of so-called high-risk pregnancies; therefore, a knowledge of certain predisposing factors often allows anticipation and early treatment when appropriate. An increased incidence of neonatal disease is seen in infants whose mothers have any of the following risk factors: (1) lack of prenatal care, poor nutrition, or other socioeconomic problems; (2) previous history of obstetrical complications, such as abortion, stillbirth or neonatal death, premature delivery, prolonged infertility, toxemia, placenta previa, placental abruption, or blood group incompatibilities; and (3) medical illnesses, such as diabetes mellitus, hypertension, infection, and cardiac or renal disease. Complications of labor and delivery may also adversely affect the infant. These include premature rupture of membranes, abnormal presentation or fetal size, multiple births, meconium staining of amniotic fluid, and inappropriate maternal analgesia or anesthesia.

These infants deserve special attention, usually including the presence of the pediatrician at the delivery and frequently requiring a period of observation in the SCN.

Nursing care of the critically ill neonate

Close and continuous monitoring of the infant is a most important duty of the nurse. Vital signs (total pulse rate and blood pressure) are checked at least hourly. Axillary temperatures are usually taken with an electronic thermometer. In addition, a temperature sensor may be taped to the infant's abdomen to help prevent either cooling or overheating. The infant should be kept in the neutral thermal range, the temperature at which his normal body temperature can be maintained with the least expenditure of energy. This decreases the baby's requirements of oxygen, calories, and fluid and also reduces his production of carbon dioxide. It is an extremely important measure, particularly in the small premature infant with little reserve capacity.

Pulse and respirations are monitored continuously by one of the cardiac-respiratory monitors available. Blood pressure is measured by either the Doppler method, a standard infant blood pressure cuff, or by means of a pressure transducer connected to an indwelling arterial catheter (usually umbilical).

With each voiding, the infant's urine is measured and tested for blood, glucose, protein, pH, and specific gravity. Some type of automatic infusion pump should be used for regulating the IV flow. The IVAC infusion pump is capable of delivering a rate ranging from 1 to 99 ml. per hour and is invaluable for the accuracy and slow rates needed. Accurate intake and output charts must be maintained and must include blood withdrawn for diagnostic tests. Daily weights should also be recorded.

Open radiant heaters provide easy accessibility to the infant who requires frequent intervention and close observation. Treatments, x-ray films, procedures, and nursing care can be easily performed without moving the infant. The bed can be tilted up or down. Special enclosed infant care units such as the Isolette are important for the infant at risk who needs to be isolated or does not require such frequent direct contact.

The oxygen content of the inspired gas ideally should be monitored continuously or at least checked hourly. In patients receiving either continuous positive airway pressure (CPAP) or mechanical ventilation, the nurse must also check the ventilator pressure settings, endotracheal tube position, and the infant's respirations and listen to his breath sounds. Equipment failure or malfunction occasionally occurs and must be detected and corrected quickly.

While all the sophisticated equipment being used today in the SCN is a great asset, *the nurse is the most important and accurate monitor* of the infant's condition, and the tendency to rely on mechanical devices must be avoided.

Fluid therapy and feeding

The fluid requirements of the newborn are highly variable and dependent on many factors. In the healthy full-term infant an intake of 75 to 90 ml./kg. per 24 hours is usually adequate. The premature infant, however, has increased insensible water losses and may normally require 140 to 160 ml./kg. per 24 hours. Water losses are also increased by tachypnea, abnormal gastrointestinal losses, administration of a concentrated solution (either orally or intravenously), and fever. The frequently used overhead radiant heater further increases evaporative loss of water, as does the use of phototherapy for hyperbilirubinemia. Thus a small infant in whom several of these factors are operative may need 200 ml./kg. per day or even more. The most important aspect of fluid therapy management is constant monitoring of the infant's state of hydration and appropriate readjustment of fluid intake. This can be done simply and accurately by following daily weights and intake and output charts. Urine specific gravity (normal range 1.004 to 1.008) is also useful as an indicator of hydration.

Caloric requirements are also somewhat variable and are higher in the low birth weight infant (120 to 150 calories/kg. per 24 hours) than in the full-term infant (110 to 130 calories/kg. per 24 hours). Increased metabolic rate, for any reason, increases caloric requirements. The presence of disease, environmental temperature above or below the neutral thermal environment, and increased physical activity all increase the baby's needs.

Fluids are administered to the patient either orally, by nipple or gavage, or intravenously. Intravenous fluids may be given through a peripheral vein, an umbilical artery catheter (if one is needed for blood gas sampling), or a central venous line. The use of an umbilical venous catheter for routine fluid maintenance should be avoided. In gavage feeding, the stomach must be aspirated before each feeding to check for residual contents from the previous feeding. The amount per feeding is gradually advanced as tolerated; care must be taken not to exceed the capacity of the stomach because an excess may cause regurgitation and possible aspiration. Nipple feedings may be attempted in the vigorous infant with intact gag and suck reflexes. The breast-feeding mother is encouraged to begin nursing as soon as the baby's condition permits. Previous to this, she is asked to manually express milk and bring it to the nursery, where it is then fed to her baby by gavage.

Special techniques for administering fluid and calories include continuous infusion into the stomach or, more recently, into the jejunum and parenteral IV hyperalimentation. The latter can be given peripherally but is usually infused through a central venous catheter. Hyperalimentation fluid may provide most or all of the nutritional requirements for an infant who is unable to tolerate oral feedings for an extended period of time, such as after bowel surgery. Complications, primarily infection and metabolic imbalance, are frequent, and a team effort involving the pharmacist, nurse, pediatrician, and surgeon is necessary for success.

Chest physiotherapy and postural drainage

Chest physiotherapy (CPT), another important responsibility of the nurse, is assisting the infant in clearing secretions from his airway when he is not able to do so himself. CPT is indicated in any infant with respiratory distress syndrome (RDS), aspiration of meconium, pneumonia, atelectasis, or other pulmonary disorders. It is usually done every 2 hours, more often if required, and only as the infant tolerates it. (He is already weak and often very small and has a poor tolerance to handling.) Postural drainage includes 1 or 2 minutes of percussion and then vibration during expiration. This can be done manually or mechanically using either an electric toothbrush covered with foam rubber or a small portable vibrator. Suctioning (oropharyngeal, nasopharyngeal, and endotracheal) must be gentle; no more than 5 to 10 seconds of intermittent suction is applied as the catheter is withdrawn. Sterile technique must be observed during suctioning through an endotracheal tube (either oral or nasal) but is unnecessary for the mouth, nose, and pharynx. Sterile normal saline solution (0.5 ml.) may be instilled into the endotracheal tube before suctioning to thin the secretions if necessary. The infant should be hand ventilated with an Ambu or anesthesia bag for a few breaths before and after suctioning to prevent drastically lowering the Po_2 (blood oxygen level).

The infant with pulmonary disease should have his position changed approximately hourly from side to side and from back to abdomen. This helps prevent the pooling of secretions in any one area of the lungs. Even with an umbilical catheter in place, the infant may be placed on his abdomen. When CPAP is delivered by a mask, gentle massage of the face is routinely done whenever the mask is removed for suctioning.

Care of the umbilical catheter

Umbilical arterial catheters are frequently used in the SCN, usually for frequent monitoring of arterial blood gases and aortic blood pressure. Umbilical venous catheters are used only on rare occasions in most SCN's, primarily for exchange transfusions, emergency administration of fluids or blood, or for monitoring of central venous pressure. Either type of catheter may lead to serious complications if proper precautions are not observed. Hypovolemic shock or death may result from sudden blood loss if the catheter is accidentally removed or if loose connections at the stop-

cock or extension tubing allow leakage. Infection or emboli (air or blood clots) may be introduced with careless withdrawal of blood samples, administration of medications, or changing of tubing. Finally, clot formation in the aorta or other major arteries may lead to infarction of the kidneys, intestines, or lower extremities. The nurse should watch for discoloration of the legs and should never allow the catheter to be opened directly to room air. The physician must be informed of any difficulty in the withdrawal of blood or in the infusion of fluid.

Respiratory distress syndrome

Respiratory distress syndrome (RDS), or hyaline membrane disease, is the most common problem in the SCN and the leading cause of neonatal mortality. It is most frequently seen in premature infants (less than 37 weeks' gestation) although an occasional full-term baby is affected.

The onset of symptoms often occurs in the delivery room where the baby has low Apgar scores and requires assistance in establishing respirations. In other cases the infant may appear normal initially but begin to have expiratory grunting and nasal flaring in the first few hours of life (usually less than 6 hours). Respiratory distress becomes increasingly obvious with the onset of tachypnea, retractions, and cyanosis in room air. A chest x-ray film is diagnostic, revealing a characteristic granular appearing air bronchogram and diminished lung volume. Arterial blood gases show hypoxia and usually a combined metabolic and respiratory acidosis.

Etiology. The cause of RDS is a subject of some controversy, but the most widely believed theory is that it results from a deficiency of surfactant in the lungs. Surfactant is actually the collective term for a group of surface-active phospholipids, most important of which is lecithin. These substances, normally present at birth, oppose the natural tendency of the alveoli to collapse with each expiration and thereby keep the lung partially expanded at all times. Infants in whom these substances are deficient or absent must completely re-expand their lungs with each breath, thereby greatly increasing the work of breathing. Extreme stiffness of the lungs (decreased compliance) and progressive atelectasis (collapse of alveoli) lead to hypoxia, fatigue, and decreased ventilation, and a vicious cycle is started.

The presence of lecithin in the lungs depends on enzyme systems that normally become active at approximately 33 to 34 weeks' gestation. Certain factors, such as chronic abruptio placentae, prolonged rupture of membranes, maternal hypertension, and possibly maternal narcotic drug usage, induce a much earlier activation of these enzymes and, therefore, mature the lungs and protect the infant from RDS. On the other hand, maternal diabetes and erythroblastosis fetalis appear to delay lung maturation.

Treatment. The treatment of RDS is aimed at supporting the infant by assisting his oxygenation and ventilation until his lungs begin to produce surfactant (usually within 2 or 3 days). The measures utilized depend on the severity of the disease. Mild to moderate cases are treated with increased concentration of environmental oxygen, usually given via a hood. If the infant is unable to oxygenate adequately while breathing 60% oxygen, some form of continuous positive airway pressure (CPAP) is usually applied to his airways. The purpose of this is to prevent the atelectasis (collapse of the alveoli), which occurs at the end of expiration. This in turn improves oxygenation and decreases the work of breathing. There are several methods of applying this pressure. The infant may be intubated intratracheally or may have the pressure applied to his mouth and/or nose by means of a face mask, nasal prongs, or a head hood (a plastic chamber with a loosely fitted seal around the neck). Alternatively, the same purpose may be accomplished by applying negative pressure to the infant's body, leaving his head open to atmospheric pressure. This is done with the negative pressure respirator and is referred to as continuous negative airway pressure (CNAP).

If the infant develops hypoxia, respiratory failure, or recurrent apnea despite continuous positive airway pressure (CPAP), mechanical ventilation is instituted with any of several infant respirators. The machine then takes over essentially all ventilatory functions for the baby. Appropriate adjustments must be made for respiratory rate, expiratory pressure, inspiratory pressure, and concentration of oxygen. Positive end expiratory pressure (PEEP) can be maintained with such mechanical ventilation as needed. The timing of the breathing cycle can also be adjusted.

It must be remembered that all of these forms of treatment carry certain risks to the baby. High concentrations of inspired oxygen are known to be toxic to lungs, whereas high arterial Po_2 (exact critical levels are unknown) in the retinal arteries can cause blindness in premature infants due to retrolental fibroplasia. Infants receiving increased pressure therapy (CPAP or mechanical ventilators) are at risk for pneumothorax and cardiovascular disturbances. Endotracheal intubation predis-

---

ARTERIAL BLOOD GASES (ABG)

Indications
   To monitor oxygenation, ventilation, and acid-base balance

Methods of obtaining
   1. Umbilical arterial catheter
   2. Arterial puncture (radial, temporal)
   3. Arterialized heelstick capillary blood sample (Extremity is first warmed for 5 to 10 minutes.)

The ABG can be determined from as little as 0.3 ml. of blood drawn into a heparinized tuberculin syringe and placed on ice.

Normal values for arterial blood in newborns

pH	7.35 to 7.45
Po_2	50 to 100 mm. Hg
Pco_2	35 to 45 mm. Hg

poses the infant to infection, or the tube itself may become totally occluded with secretions. Because of these potential complications, the infant with RDS must be carefully evaluated, and the risks of therapy balanced against the benefit.

General supportive measures, such as proper regulation of fluids, acid-base status, and thermal environment, are of great importance in the infant with RDS. An umbilical artery catheter is often used for frequent arterial blood gas sampling as well as administration of parenteral fluids, medications, and transfusions (blood drawn for samples must be replaced periodically). Antibiotics are not effective against the disease itself but are often used as a prophylactic measure.

Complications. Aside from the risks of therapy mentioned above, the complications of RDS include hypoglycemia, hypocalcemia, hyperbilirubinemia, intracranial hemorrhage, and patent ductus arteriosus (PDA). Intracranial hemorrhage is more common in infants of less than 32 weeks' gestation and is becoming a major cause of death as newer therapeutic measures improve the prognosis of RDS. The onset of symptoms due to PDA usually coincides with the recovery phase of RDS. Typical congestive heart failure may occur with enlarged heart and liver and tachycardia. More often, however, an infant who has been improving clinically simply stops making progress and becomes dependent on oxygen, CPAP, or a respirator. A trial of medical therapy with digitalization is usually attempted. If this is unsuccessful, surgical ligation of the ductus should be performed.

Amniocentesis for lecithin/sphinomyelin ratio. Analysis of the amniotic fluid for the presence of lung phospholipids has been developed recently as an index of lung maturity. Expressed as a ratio of lecithin to sphingomyelin (another lung phospholipid), this method has been extremely accurate in identifying the infant who will develop RDS. Fluid is obtained by transabdominal amniocentesis, and the lecithin/sphingomyelin (L/S) ratio is measured on infants for whom elective delivery is contemplated. (See p. 417.)

The development and widespread clinical use of amniocentesis for L/S ratio, newer methods of ventilatory assistance (such as CPAP and respirators), and refinement of supportive care in the SCN's have combined to greatly improve the outlook for RDS. Both mortality and morbidity have been markedly reduced.

Aspiration of meconium

Staining of the amniotic fluid with meconium, the stool of the newborn infant, occurs in approximately 10% of all deliveries. It may indicate intrauterine distress, and in some instances the infant may make gasping respiration before the head is delivered and thus aspirate the meconium into his lungs. While normal amniotic fluid is virtually harmless to the lungs, the particles of meconium produce obstruction of the airways and cause respiratory difficulty. The infant may be vigorous and breathe easily, but if intrauterine asphyxia has occurred, he may be depressed and require assistance in establishing respirations. In the latter case, intubation and direct tracheal suction must be performed prior to the use of positive pressure ventilation. This will hopefully prevent the forcing of meconium into more distal airways and reduce the severity of the disease. Symptoms of respiratory distress occur in about 15% of meconium-stained infants and vary from mild to very severe. In most cases symptoms resolve by 48 hours of life, but occasionally respiratory assistance must be continued for much longer periods. Treatment consists of oxygen, CPT and suction, and general supportive measures. Antibiotics may be used, and mechanical ventilation is sometimes necessary for severe cases. Pneumothorax is a common complication.

Pneumothorax

Approximately 1% of all newborns develop pneumothorax (free air in the pleu-

CARDIOPULMONARY RESUSCITATION IN THE SCN

If the depressed infant is not resuscitated within his first few minutes of extrauterine life, severe metabolic and respiratory acidosis occurs.

Severely depressed infant with cardiac arrest

A. Signs
1. Apgar 0 to 2
2. HR 20 to 30 beats per minute, or absent
B. Care
1. Immediate intubation needed
2. Orotracheal tube for emergency use (may use nasotracheal tube later)
3. Pencil-handled laryngoscope with premature infant, blade used
4. External cardiac massage begun

Important points with CPR

1. Infant supine and on flat surface
2. Index and middle finger placed over heart to left of lower sternal border
3. Chest wall compressed ½ inch
4. Ratio 3:1 (3 compressions to 1 ventilation)
5. Ventilation with 100% oxygen
6. Continuous EKG monitoring
7. Palpate femoral pulses for effectiveness of the CPR

Complications

1. Pneumothorax and pneumomediastinum—*never* perform compression and ventilation simultaneously!
2. Rib fractures
3. Damage to liver or other organs

Emergency medications must be available

1. Sodium bicarbonate
2. Epinephrine
3. Calcium gluconate
4. Isoproterenol (Isuprel) hydrochloride
5. Antiarrhythmic drug (lidocaine)
6. A narcotic antagonist, naloxone hydrochloride (Narcan) or nalorphine (Nalline), to be used for respiratory distress due to maternal medication with narcotic drugs

ral space), but the great majority of them remain asymptomatic, and the condition resolves without treatment. Most cases occur spontaneously as a result of the high intrathoracic pressures that infants generate when expanding their lungs with the first few breaths. In other cases, aspiration of meconium or blood or positive pressure ventilation can be causative. Premature infants are more susceptible to spontaneous pneumothorax. Clinical signs include respiratory difficulty, tachypnea, cyanosis, shifting of the cardiac impulse, and irritability. Diagnosis is confirmed by chest x-ray film.

Treatment of the infant with pneumothorax depends on the severity of the symptoms. The infant with mild or no symptoms needs only careful observation or may be placed in 100% oxygen to speed absorption of the free air. If severe distress is present, the pneumothorax should be aspirated (best done with an Intracath or Medicut needle) and a chest tube inserted into the pleural space. Follow-up x-ray films are indicated to determine the position of the chest tube and reexpansion of lung. Patency of the tube must be maintained by preventing kinking, clotting, and looping. The chest tube can usually be removed within 24 to 48 hours.

Hyperbilirubinemia

Hyperbilirubinemia occurs to some degree in normal newborns and is often exaggerated in the premature or sick neonate. Bilirubin, the majority of which is formed from the breakdown of hemoglobin, is taken up by liver cells, where it is modified and excreted through the bile ducts into the intestine. The so-called physiological hyperbilirubinemia that occurs in normal newborns is due to several factors: (1) increased destruction of red blood cells, (2) decreased blood flow to the liver, (3) decreased uptake of bilirubin into the liver cells, and (4) increased absorption of bilirubin from the intestine (enterohepatic circulation).

Hyperbilirubinemia is considered pathological if the serum bilirubin level exceeds 12 mg. per 100 ml. or if obvious jaundice appears in the first 24 hours. The most common cause is hemolytic disease (Rh or ABO blood group incompatibility). Other frequently encountered causes are polycythemia, excessive bruising, hemolytic anemias, sepsis, intrauterine viral infection, or metabolic disorders.

The treatment of hyperbilirubinemia, in addition to treatment of the underlying cause, is the use of phototherapy and exchange transfusions. The effect of phototherapy (cool white or blue lamps) is apparently the breakdown of bilirubin pigments in the skin. In an exchange transfusion, the infant's blood is simply replaced, hopefully removing much bilirubin from the baby. The objective of treatment is the prevention of kernicterus, a neurological condition caused by deposition of bilirubin in the basal ganglia of the brain. The exact level at which this can occur varies widely depending on the maturity and clinical condition of the infant. Hypoxia, acidosis, hypoalbuminemia, and certain drugs lower the threshold as does prematurity. All of these factors must be considered in the treatment of the baby with hyperbilirubinemia.

Neonatal sepsis

The newborn infant has incompletely developed immunological responses and, therefore, has increased susceptibility to infection—bacterial, viral, and other types. Once an infection is acquired, it may quickly invade the bloodstream (neonatal sepsis or septicemia) and lead to meningitis, pneumonia, urinary tract infection, osteomyelitis, or other infections. They are more frequently associated with prematurity, prolonged rupture of membranes, maternal infection (chorioamnionitis, urinary tract infection, etc.), difficult labor with fetal distress, and with babies requiring special procedures, such as resuscitation and umbilical catheterization. Presenting symptoms include respiratory distress with grunting and tachypnea, poor feeding, vomiting, lethargy, temperature instability, unexplained jaundice, and apnea.

Early treatment is of extreme importance in obtaining a favorable outcome. Once the diagnosis of infection is suspected, cultures should be taken promptly of blood, urine, spinal fluid, stool, tracheal aspirate, and additional sites as indicated. Antibiotic therapy with two drugs, one for gram-negative and one for gram-positive organisms, should be instituted immediately. Subsequent choice of antibiotics is determined by identification of the offending organism and its sensitivity patterns.

Infants born to diabetic mothers

Infants born to diabetic mothers (IDM) are predisposed to a number of neonatal disorders and are frequently encountered in the SCN. First of all, because there is an increased incidence of fetal death late in pregnancy, these pregnancies must be monitored carefully by the obstetrician. Amniocentesis is usually performed at weekly intervals after about 36 weeks' gestation, and the baby is delivered as soon as the L/S ratio indicates lung maturity. Lung maturity is often delayed in these infants, and if the L/S ratio is not performed, an infant may be delivered who will have severe RDS. If delivered at term, the infants may be very large (10 to 12 pounds) and, therefore, prone to birth injury unless a cesarean section is done.

Once delivered there is a high incidence of hypoglycemia in these babies, usually occurring during the first 12 hours. Dextrostix determinations or blood glucose levels should be done at intervals and the infants fed early to hopefully prevent its occurrence. Glucagon injections may relieve the hypoglycemia, but glucose water administered intravenously is usually necessary. IDM's are also susceptible to hypocalcemia, hyperbilirubinemia, polycythemia, congenital anomalies, and renal vein thrombosis.

Infants born to mothers with severe or long-standing diabetes suffer intrauterine growth retardation and are usually very small rather than large for their gestational age. Their lungs mature early, and they almost never have RDS.

Necrotizing enterocolitis

This acute, often lethal, intestinal disorder in the newborn is most common in the premature. Clinical symptoms include abdominal distention, vomiting, diarrhea with blood in the stool, apnea, lethargy, hypothermia, and shock. Positive diagnosis is established by abdominal x-ray film, which may show pneumatosis intestinalis (air in the intestinal wall) or free air in the peritoneum.

Initial treatment consists of nasogastric suction, intravenous fluids, antibiotics, and transfusions. Serial abdominal x-ray films are obtained at frequent intervals to ascertain the progression of the disease or perforation of the bowel, either of which is an indication for surgery. At surgery, the areas of necrotic bowel are resected and a colostomy is usually performed. Anastomosis of the intestine is then done as an elective procedure after the infant has recovered.

The cause of necrotizing enterocolitis is unknown, but lack of oxygen supply to the intestinal mucosa and bacterial infection are two possible factors. The use of breast milk for feeding of premature infants has been introduced recently in the hopes of decreasing the incidence of the disease.

Postmaturity

The postmature infant is one who is born after 42 weeks' gestation. He has dry, parchmentlike skin, long fingernails and a wide-eyed, alert expression. Meconium staining of the skin is not uncommon. Mortality of the postmature infant is nearly twice as high as that of the term infant. The postmature infant has diminished glycogen stores and is, therefore, susceptible to hypoglycemia. He should be fed early (at 3 to 4 hours) and have periodic blood glucose determinations with Dextrostix.

• • •

It is important to remember that the material presented here represents only some of the highlights of neonatal intensive care nursing. The student interested in this area should refer to one of the many books now available on the subject.

unit seven
Suggested selected readings and references

Agrafiotis, P. C.: Teaching parents about Pierre Robin syndrome, Am. J. Nurs. 72:2040-2041, Nov., 1972.

Almound, A. M.: Is breast-feeding right for you? Parents' Magazine and Better Homemaking 49:29-31, April, 1974.

Atkinson, H. C.: Care of the child with cleft lip and palate, Am. J. Nurs. 67:1889, Sept., 1967.

Auld, P.: Resuscitation of the newborn infant, Am. J. Nurs. 74:68-70, Jan., 1974.

Behrman, R. E., editor: The newborn, Pediatr. Clin. North Am. 17:entire volume, 1970.

Blake, F. G., Wright, F. H., and Waechter, E. H.: Nursing care of children, ed. 8, Philadelphia, 1970, J. B. Lippincott Co.

Braney, M. L.: The child with hydrocephalus, Am. J. Nurs. 73:828-831, May, 1973.

Caldwell, J. G.: Congenital syphilis: a nonvenereal disease, Am. J. Nurs. 71:1768-1772, Sept., 1971.

Davis, A. R.: Billy has a tracheo-esophageal fistula, Am. J. Nurs. 70:326-329, Feb., 1970.

Donnes, J. J., and others: Respiratory distress syndrome of newborn infants, Clin. Pediatr. 9:325-330, 1970.

Epstein, F., and others: A volume control system for the treatment of hydrocephalus, J. Neurosurg. 38:282-287, March, 1973.

Estok, P. J.: What do nurses know about breast-feeding problems? J. Obstet. Gynecol. Neonatal Nurs. 2:36-39, Nov.-Dec., 1973.

Faber, M. M.: Circumcision revisited, Birth and Fam. J. 1:19-21, Spring, 1974.

Finnegan, L. P., and Macnew, B. A.: Care of the addicted infant, Am. J. Nurs. 74:685-693, April, 1974.

Fitzpatrick, E. N., and others: Maternity nursing, ed. 12, Philadelphia, 1971, J. B. Lippincott Co.

Galloway, K.: Early detection of congenital anomalies, J. Obstet. Gynecol. Neonatal Nurs. 2:37-38, July-Aug., 1973.

Gluck, L., editor: Symposium on respiratory disorders in the newborn, Pediatr. Clin. North Am. 20:entire volume, May, 1973.

Irwin, E. C., and McWilliams, B. J.: Play therapy for children with cleft palates, Children Today 3:18-22, May-June, 1974.

Johnson, C. F.: What is the best age to discontinue the low phenylalanine diet in phenylketonuria, Clin. Pediatr. 11:148-156, March, 1972.

Johnson and Johnson: Review your knowledge of narcotic addiction in the newborn, J. Obstet. Gynecol. Neonatal Nurs. 2:72-73, Jan.-Feb., 1973.

Kallop, F.: Working with parents through a devastating experience: the birth of a mongoloid child, J. Obstet. Gynecol. Neonatal Nurs. 2:36-41, May-June, 1973.

Klaus, M. H., and Fanaroff, A. A.: Care of the high-risk neonate, Philadelphia, 1973, W. B. Saunders Co.

Korones, S. B.: High-risk newborn infants: the basis for intensive nursing care, St. Louis, 1972, The C. V. Mosby Co.

Lee, L. G., and Jackson, J. F.: Diagnosis of Down's syndrome: clinical vs. laboratory, Clin. Pediatr. 11:353-356, June, 1972.

Lerch, C.: Maternity nursing, ed. 2, St. Louis, 1974, The C. V. Mosby Co.

Lipkin, G. B.: Psychosocial aspects of maternal-child nursing, St. Louis, 1974, The C. V. Mosby Co.

Marlow, D. R.: Textbook of pediatric nursing, ed. 4, Philadelphia, 1973, W. B. Saunders Co.

Miezio, P.: Care of the child with myelomeningocele, Nurs. Digest 1:45-51, Nov., 1973.

Mori, W.: My child has Down's syndrome, Am. J. Nurs. 73:1386-1387, Aug., 1973.

O'Brien, J. S.: The high-risk pregnancy: Tay-Sachs disease, prenatal diagnosis, Contemp. OB/GYN 3:73-76, Feb., 1974.

O'Grady, R. S.: Nursing care of infants with esophageal anomalies, Am. J. Nurs. 71:736-739, April, 1971.

O'Regan, G. W.: Foster family care for children with mental retardation, Children Today 3:20-24+, Jan.-Feb., 1974.

Paradise, J. L.: Pediatric and otologic aspects of clinical research in cleft palate, Clin. Pediatr. 13:587, July, 1974.

Penfold, K. M.: Supporting mother love, Am. J. Nurs. 74:464-467, March, 1974.

Persaud, T. V. N., and Moore, K. L.: Causes and prenatal diagnosis of congenital abnormalities, J. Obstet. Gynecol. Neonatal Nurs. 3:50-55, July-Aug., 1974.

Pierog, S. H., and Ferrara, A.: Approach to the medical care of the sick newborn, St. Louis, 1971, The C. V. Mosby Co.

Shanklin, D. R.: On the treatment of the idiopathic respiratory distress syndrome, Clin. Pediatr. 10:434-438, Aug., 1971.

Shapiro, C. S., Johnson, J., Vincent, M., and Fleury, A. F.: Nursing care of the cleft-lip/cleft-palate child, RN 36:46-60, Aug., 1973.

Specht, E. E.: Congenital dislocation of the hip, Am. Fam. Physician 9:88-96, Feb., 1974.

Stutz, S. D.: When the baby isn't normal, RN 34:40-43, Nov., 1971.

Whitley, N. N.: Breast feeding the premature, Am. J. Nurs. 70:1909, Sept., 1970.

Wiley, R.: Spina bifida: immediate concern . . . long-term goals, Nurs. '73 3:42-47, Oct., 1973.

Wolman, I. J.: Further recommendations for PKU management. Part I, II, Clin. Pediatr. 10:16B, Aug.-Sept., 1971.

Yasunaga, S., and Rivera, R.: Cephalhematoma in the newborn, Clin. Pediatr. 13:256-260, March, 1974.

Young, D. G., and Weller, B. F.: Baby surgery, nursing management and care, Baltimore, 1971, University Park Press.

Zachary, R. B.: The improving prognosis in spina bifida, Clin. Pediatr. 11:11-14, Jan., 1972.

19

Structural, functional, and psychological changes in the child

CONCEPTS OF GROWTH AND DEVELOPMENT

As the child grows up he is constantly changing physically and functionally. This is the main factor that distinguishes the child from the adult. Growth is exhibited by all healthy children, although it may be impaired by malnutrition and disease. Growth is the one feature that sets apart pediatrics as a specialty.

Every nurse interested in the care of children needs to have a basic understanding of human growth and development. Such an understanding will be of great help in evaluating the physical, intellectual, emotional, and social behavior of the dynamic child patient.

Terminology

The terms "growth" and "development" are closely bound together and sometimes used interchangeably. Increases in structure (growth) are accompanied by increases in function (development). As a child grows in size he grows up or matures mentally, emotionally, and socially. Differences in the way a child thinks, feels, or acts are just as real as changes in size.

As growth and development proceed, various levels of maturity are observable. *Maturation* is the process whereby inherited tendencies begin to unfold, independent of any special practice or training. Each child has his own built-in growth pattern. Some children have patterns that allow them to mature very rapidly; other children are very slow physically, mentally, and emotionally and are called late maturers. There can be a wide range in the growth and development rates of normal children. Mary enjoyed walking at 12 months of age; her sister was 15 months old when she took her first steps. The child will advance physiologically toward maturity at his own rate.

Because of similarities in children, cultures, learning methods, and child-rearing practices, generalizations can be made concerning growth and development. Although these generalizations are not applicable in every case, they do provide valuable points of departure in understanding and dealing with groups. This discussion of growth and development follows the child through an orderly sequence beginning with the prenatal phase and continuing through babyhood, childhood, and adolescence.

Principles

The normal growth and development of a child through the successive periods of babyhood, childhood, and adolescence are guided by certain basic principles, five of which follow. Growth and development: (1) occur in an orderly sequence; (2) although continuous, are characterized by spurts of growth and periods of relative rest; (3) progress at highly individualized rates from child to child; (4) vary at different ages

Table 19-1. Progressive stages of development

Stages of life	Divisions of life stages	Chronological age
Prenatal		
Conception to birth	Germinal	Conception to 10 days' gestation
	Embryonic	10 days to 2 months' gestation
	Fetal	2 months' gestation to birth
Babyhood		
Birth to 1 year	Newborn (neonate)	Birth to 1 month
	Infancy	1 month to 1 year
Childhood		
1 to 12 years	Toddler	1 to 3 years
	Preschool	3 to 6 years
	School	6 to 10 years
	Preadolescence	10 to 12 years
Adolescence		
12 to 19 years	Early adolescence	12 to 16 years
	Late adolescence	16 to 19 years

for specific structures; and (5) represent a total process involving the whole child.

Orderly sequence. Growth and development occur in an orderly sequence and are continuous. The sequence of development is the same for all children, even though some children do things earlier than others. Children generally creep before they stand and stand alone before they walk. The *average* child talks before he reads and usually reads before he can write. One child will read at 4 years of age, and another will read at 6 years of age. What happens at one stage influences what happens in the next stage; each stage in the development of the individual is an outgrowth of an earlier stage. During the first year the baby babbles; as he grows, he begins to say simple words. The toddler uses words in phrases, and the preschooler uses words in short sentences. No child speaks clearly before babbling, and each stage in the sequence can surely be anticipated.

Continuity. Growth and development continue from the moment of conception until the individual reaches maturity, but at no time is growth even and regular. There are spurts and rest periods within the same child even though there are no real interruptions until growth is completed. Growth is greatest during the prenatal period and is still rapid during babyhood (infancy) and early childhood. It is slow but constant in middle childhood. It shows a spurt during early puberty and then tapers off in the latter part of puberty.

Differences in growth rates. Each child has his own unique growth timetable. A child who develops rapidly at first will continue to do so. Jimmy sat alone at 6 months of age and walked alone at 9 months of age. His brother John sat alone at 8 months and walked alone at 15 months. Even in the same family no two children grow at the same rate.

Variation of growth rates for different body structures. Not all parts of the body mature at the same time. The brain attains its adult size when the child is about 6 or 7 years of age, but it certainly does not attain organization until many years later. Different phases of physical and mental growth occur at their own individual rates and reach maturity at different times.

Growth and development as a total process. The child does not grow physically one day and mentally the next day. He grows physically, mentally, socially, and emotionally at the same time. The child develops as a whole being. Changes in interest and mental growth are closely related to growth in walking and talking. Growth is a total process involving the whole child, not just his body, his mind, or his emotions. Each child passes slowly and almost imperceptibly from stage to stage, preserving a patterned integration of behavior throughout his life.

GENETIC AND ENVIRONMENTAL INFLUENCES AND LIMITATIONS

Every child's growth and development (pattern, rate, rhythm, and extent) are governed by genetic and environmental forces. Within the broad categories of genetic and environmental influences may be found such overlapping and diverse factors as sex differences, endocrine gland function, racial ancestry, cellular mutations, other inherited strengths and weaknesses; psychological and cultural milieu, nutritional and physical advantages or disadvantages; intercurrent malformation or disease. For many years controversy raged regarding the respective importance of genetics and environment, or "nature versus nurture." Today this interest has been somewhat tempered, and most writers in the field contend that both are important and try to determine ways that both can be improved to enhance the individual and his society. The first main category to be discussed is that of genetics.

Genetic influences

A child's cellular inheritance and early embryonic growth may be a lifetime asset or a continuing liability. About one quarter of all hospitalized children have diseases or defects with genetic components. The science of genetics is based on principles of inheritance first described in the mid-1880's by the Augustinian monk scientist, Gregor Mendel. Mendel's law explains certain aspects of gene activity in humans during the formation of gametes (eggs and sperm) and during fertilization (the union of an egg and spermatozoon).

Genes, the ultimate and, as yet, invisible particles of inheritance are strands of deoxyribonucleic acid (DNA) in structures called chromosomes, which are found in every cell's nucleus. Twenty-three chromosomes from each parent, combining to make a total of 46, endow the offspring at fertilization. Each of 22 chromosomes donated by one parent has a microscopically similar counterpart that is donated by the other parent. These chromosomic counterparts can be paired whether the developing individual is a boy or a girl. They are called *autosomes*. Two other, different chromosomes, labeled X and Y, determine sex.

They are called *sex chromosomes*. Each parent donates only one. The mother is able to contribute only an X chromosome, while the father may give to his child either an X or a Y chromosome. Babies having an XX inheritance are girls; those with XY are boys.

Genetic problems are of three main types: (1) chromosomal, gross genetic defects involving innumerable genes located on the specific defective chromosome; (2) limited gene defects, involving one or two abnormal genes; and (3) polygenic or multifactorial defects, involving many unspecified genes and environmental influences. Defects in chromosomal structure or numbers can be considered *"packaging" defects*. The chromosomes are the "packages" that carry the genes from generation to generation. Defects in individual genes, *the contents* of these packages, are not evident upon inspection of the chromosomes themselves but are evidenced by disease and abnormalities in the affected person.

First, let us briefly discuss chromosomal analysis and some sample problems. *Cytogenetics* is the study of the structure, number, and relationships of the various chromosomes. Chromosomes for analysis are obtained from white blood cells or less often from skin biopsies, which can be grown as tissue cultures in the laboratory. A *karyotype* is an orderly arrangement of an individual's autosomal and sex chromosomes according to size, shape, and staining peculiarities as they appear in cutouts of photographic enlargements (Fig. 19-1). Until very recently the chromosomes were usually grouped as pairs into categories A through G. Now most are only numbered in pairs 1 to 22 plus the sex chromosomes XX or XY, according to international agreement.

Chromosomal abnormalities in some cases may be passed on to future generations, but more often they occur only sporadically and are not inherited. When a chromosomal pattern is abnormal, a gain or loss of numerous genes is usually involved; therefore, chromosomal changes usually cause multiple congenital malformations or abortions.

265

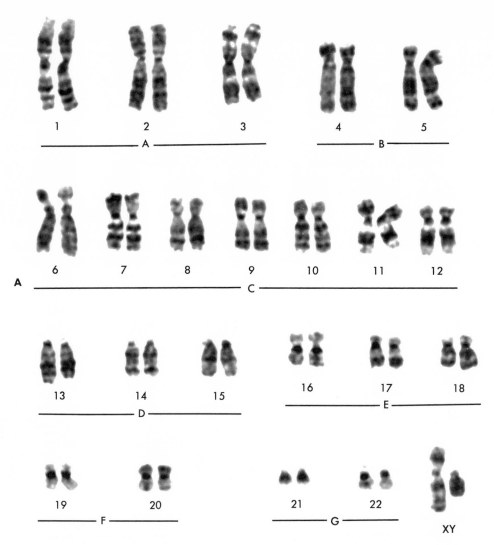

Fig. 19-1. **A,** Normal male karytoype (46 XY); **B,** normal female karyotype (46XX).

Chromosomal defects

Numerous factors have been implicated in the genesis of chromosomal defects. Maternal age is significant because the human eggs, or ova, have been present in the ovary since birth and may undergo change with passing time. Even aging in the male may be related to new autosomal dominant mutations such as dwarfism. Radiation, certain drugs, viral infections, and possibly chronic diseases may contribute to chromosomal abnormalities.

Sometimes the normal chromosome num-

ber of a cell is altered. Alteration may occur when a cell is being formed in the testes or ovaries where the chromosome count in the sex cell is ordinarily reduced to half in preparation for fertilization. As a result, gametes may contain different chromosome counts. For example, one sex cell may receive 24 chromosomes instead of 23, while another may have only 22.

Down's syndrome. The presence of one additional chromosome (a condition called trisomy) frequently involves the triplication of chromosome number 21. The fertilization

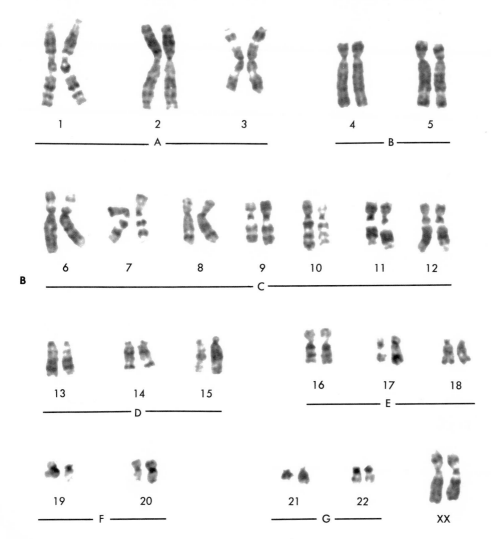

1   2   3   4   5
———————— A ————————   ——— B ———

6   7   8   9   10   11   12
B
———————————————— C ————————————

13   14   15   16   17   18
———————— D ————————   ——————— E ———————

19   20   21   22   XX
——— F ———   ——— G ———

Fig. 19-1, cont'd. For legend see opposite page.

of a gamete having two number 21 chromosomes by a normal sex cell having only one number 21 chromosome results in an abnormality known as trisomy 21, which is the kind of Down's syndrome, or mongolism, most often occurring in children of older women (Fig. 19-2, *A*).

In a small number of cases, Down's syndrome is due to *translocation,* in which the extra number 21 chromosome becomes attached to a number 13, 14, 15, another 21, or 22. In this instance the total chromosome *count* is considered normal (that is, 46)

even though the genetic material from an extra number 21 has become part of another chromosome. This type of mongolism is possibly inherited, and maternal age is not significant (Fig. 19-2, *B*).

As long as the chromosomes involved in translocation are balanced, that is, no material is lost or added, there will be no evident effects. There is a risk that a carrier of a translocated chromosome will produce a genetically "unbalanced" and thus defective child. Each translocation risk has to be determined for the particular family and can

267

Standard Trisomy
1:600 Births/Rarely Familial

A

The most common chromosomal abnormality in Down's syndrome (Mongolism) is trisomy of chromosome 21. The total chromosome count is 47 instead of the normal 46. Failure of the two chromosomes of pair 21 to separate during gametogenesis in the mother produces an abnormal ovum and thus a child with trisomy 21. This usually occurs in children born to older women.

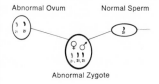

Abnormal Ovum   Normal Sperm

Abnormal Zygote

The abnormal zygote has an overdose of chromosome 21 which causes Down's syndrome.

Translocation
Rare/Familial

B

The abnormally large chromosome in pair 15 shown at left is the result of the translocation of extra chromosome 21 material producing Down's syndrome. The actual chromosome count is the normal 46. In spite of this normal count these individuals have the same overdose of chromosome 21 as those with standard trisomy.

Down's syndrome translocation	Down's syndrome standard trisomy
15 15/21 & 21 21	15 15 & 21 21 21
chromosome count 46	chromosome count 47

Children with translocation type Down's syndrome are usually born to younger parents, one of whom carries the 15/21 translocation. The carrier has a chromosome count of 45 instead of 46 but has the same amount of chromosome 21 material as the normal.

Carrier Parent	Normal Parent
15, 15/21 & O, 21	15, 15 & 21, 21
observed offspring	

Down's Syndrome	Normal Appearing Carrier	Normal
15/21, 15 & 21, 21	15/21, 15 & O, 21	15, 15 & 21, 21
chromosome count 46	chromosome count 45	chromosome count 46

(Theoretically possible: 15, 15, 21, O; non-viable; chromosome count 45.)

Mosaicism
Very rare/not familial

C

Mosaicism in Down's syndrome is the co-existence in one individual of cells with different chromosome counts. For example, cultures of skin cells may show 46 chromosomes, blood cells 47. The abnormalities may be less in this type. Mosaicism is the result of an error in division of an early embryonic cell.

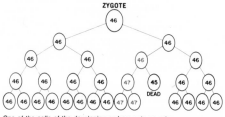

One of the cells of the developing embryo gets an extra chromosome 21 and passes it on to its descendants. Thus there are two cell lines with different chromosome counts.

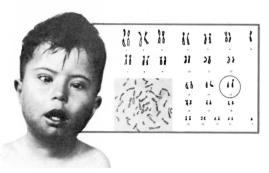

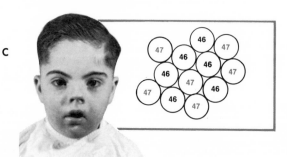

Fig. 19-2. Down's syndrome. (Courtesy the National Foundation, March of Dimes.)

be accurately assessed only by chromosomal analysis of both parents.

Occasionally a child with Down's syndrome will display both trisomic and normal cells. As the embryonic body cells of the child divide, part of the tissues receives 47 (an extra chromosome 21) and part receives 46. This mixture of cells is called *mosaicism* (Fig. 19-2, *C*).

The genetic problem known as Down's syndrome, involving aberrations in the number or location of chromosome 21 in the cell, is quite common, affecting about 1 in 650 births. Similar abnormalities (trisomy, translocation, and mosaicism) of chromosomes other than number 21, although rare, are also possible. For example, severe and lethal defects are associated with trisomies of the 13 and 18 chromosomes (from groups D and E, respectively).

Sex chromosome aberrations. Numerical disorders of the sex chromosomes may also be present. The only condition characterized by chromosome loss (45 instead of 46) that supports life is Turner's syndrome, coded as 45 X0 to show that one X chromosome is missing. Abnormal ovarian development, sexual immaturity, sterility, short stature, and an increased incidence of mental retardation characterize these females. Persons having Klinefelter's syndrome (XXY) are anatomically male though they have two XX chromosomes. They are sterile and may be mentally retarded. Since the Y chromosome is male determining, a duplication of this chromosome (XYY) has been accused of causing overaggresive or criminal behavior. This conclusion is questionable since it has been found that XYY males are half as frequent in the population as children with Down's syndrome; therefore, there must be many who exhibit normal behavior and go undetected.

Genic influences

The characteristics or traits of an individual also depend on the individual genes in the chromosomes that he receives, or the *contents of the chromosomal package.* Each gene located at a specific place on an individual chromosome has the potential of producing a specific outcome in the offspring. The structure and activity of the ductless, or endocrine, glands (thyroid, isles of Langerhans of the pancreas, pituitary, etc.), which may influence so much of body metabolism and behavior, may also be determined at least in part by genes. Certain racial and familial characteristics (such as hair and skin color, bony structure) have a genic basis.

Certain genes have more influence than others and are expressed regardless of the complementary, or counterpart, genes contributed by the other parent. They are called *dominant* genes. Those specific genes that are not expressed unless they exist in pairs are called *recessive*. For example, if the paired genes controlling numbers of digits differ and one produces 6 fingers and the other, 5 fingers, the child will have 6 fingers, since this is the dominant trait. The unexpressed gene for 5 fingers is called a recessive trait. (See Figs. 19-3 and 19-4 for an explanation of the statistical potential for each type of inheritance.) When neither gene is dominant, the resulting effect is a mixture as in the case of a person with type AB blood. The gene producing A antigen is *codominant* with that producing B antigen, and both are expressed. When an individual inherits either two dominant genes or two recessive genes controlling a certain characteristic from his parents, he is *homozygous* for that characteristic. If he inherits a recessive gene from one parent and a dominant gene from the other, he is called *heterozygous.* (Which parent is heterozygous in Fig. 19-3?)

Genic defects. Some inherited autosomal dominant diseases or malformations are Huntington's chorea, Marfan's syndrome, neurofibromatosis, and certain types of osteogenesis imperfecta. Some inherited autosomal recessive problems include albinism, cystic fibrosis, galactosemia, thalassemia, phenylketonuria, and sickle cell anemia.

Gross abnormalities may result from a single gene defect, yet they may also be due to a combination of genic differences.

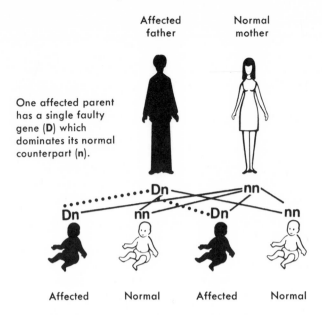

One affected parent
has a single faulty
gene (**D**) which
dominates its normal
counterpart (**n**).

Each child's chances of inheriting either the **D** or the **n**
from the affected parent are 50%.

Fig. 19-3. Dominant inheritance. (Courtesy the National Foundation, March of Dimes.)

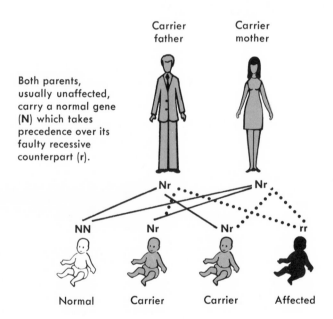

Both parents,
usually unaffected,
carry a normal gene
(**N**) which takes
precedence over its
faulty recessive
counterpart (r).

The odds for each child are:
1. A 25% risk of inheriting a "double dose" of **r** genes
   which may cause a serious birth defect
2. A 25% chance of inheriting two **N**s, thus being unaffected
3. A 50% chance of being a carrier as both parents are

Fig. 19-4. Recessive inheritance. (Courtesy the National Foundation, March of Dimes.)

Some polygenic, or multifactorially, inherited defects demonstrated are cleft lip with or without cleft palate, congenital dislocated hip, spina bifida cystica, anencephaly, pyloric stenosis, club foot, diabetes, and certain types of congenital heart disease. The change in the structure of a gene that results in the transmission of a different trait is called a *mutation*. Only mutations in the reproductive cells may be transmitted to individual offspring.

X-linked (sex-linked) inheritance (Fig. 19-5). The term refers to transmission of those genes located on the X chromosome. The male can contribute only one X chromosome, which he derived from his mother. Therefore, a male may not transfer X-linked genes to his sons, but all of his daughters will be recipients. The female, receiving two X chromosomes, one from her father and one from her mother, can be either homozygous or heterozygous for genes located on the X chromosome. If she is heterozygous, she may transmit a gene for either a normal or an abnormal characteristic. Females transmit X-linked genes to both male and female offspring. This X-linked inheritance process may involve either dominant or recessive genes.

X-LINKED RECESSIVE DISORDERS. More is known concerning the transmission of X-linked recessive disorders than other types of X-linked problems. Heterozygous females are seldom affected by the recessive gene they carry. Every male child of a female carrier has a chance of inheriting the recessive gene from his mother and, therefore, a 50% chance of being affected, since

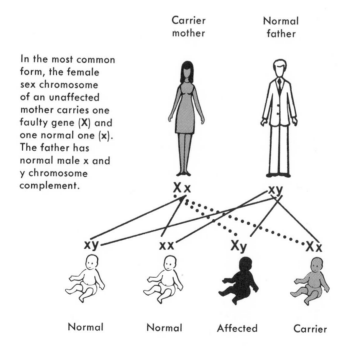

Carrier mother   Normal father

In the most common form, the female sex chromosome of an unaffected mother carries one faulty gene (X) and one normal one (x). The father has normal male x and y chromosome complement.

X x   x y

xy   xx   Xy   Xx

Normal   Normal   Affected   Carrier

The odds for each *male* child are 50/50:
1. A 50% risk of inheriting the faulty X and the disorder
2. A 50% chance of inheriting normal x and y chromosomes
For each *female* child, the odds are:
1. A 50% risk of inheriting one faulty X, to be a carrier like mother
2. A 50% chance of inheriting no faulty gene

Fig. 19-5. X-linked inheritance. (Courtesy the National Foundation, March of Dimes.)

there is no paired gene on the Y chromosome from his father to block out the effect of the recessive gene. The family pedigree will show that there is no male-to-male transmission in this type of inheritance. Daughters born to a carrier mother and an unaffected father will not be affected, but 50% of them may be carriers. Females who are homozygous for recessive X-linked conditions are very rare. They are the product of the mating of an affected male and a mother who is a carrier. These women will show symptoms of the disease in as severe a form as the men with only the single gene. (The cause may also be due to a fresh mutation if the family history is negative.) Some serious X-linked recessively inherited diseases are Aldrich syndrome, Duchenne's dystrophy, hemophilia A and B, one form of hydrocephalus, and agammaglobulinemia.

Genetic counseling

Although individual birth defects may seem to be relatively rare (2% of all births), the total number of families affected is well into the millions. About 250,000 American babies are born each year with mild to severe physical or mental defects. These defects may not become apparent until months or years later. Using pedigree studies, modern laboratory detection techniques (such as blood tests, enzyme assays, amniocentesis, and chromosome analysis), knowledge of basic laws of heredity, and incidence statistics, the genetic counselor can often predict the probability of recurrence of a given abnormality in a family. The primary aim is to prevent genetic defects, or when that is impossible, at least to reduce their damaging effects to the minimum. Genetic counseling is a form of preventive medicine. The National Foundation March of Dimes is dedicated to finding a means of preventing or treating birth defects. A list of genetic counseling units throughout the United States is sent to physicians or to the general public free upon request to the Professional Educational Department of the National Foundation. (See also p. 182.)

Environmental influences

Although the impact of a child's genetic background is great, there is another modifying force that exerts an important influence on growth and development—environment. Examples of environmental factors include the family composition, interrelationships, culture and life styles, the degree and type of assessibility and stimulation offered by the primary caretakers to the inquisitive infant and young child, health habits, nutrition, and the presence of malformation or disease. A child not only interprets his environment in terms of his inherited tendencies and mental ability but also in terms of his health and emotional balance. A strong, happy child will make the best use of his environment and will be most able to deal with obstacles or defects in his surroundings.

Home and family. To develop naturally and wholesomely, the child needs devoted care and a family setting that is loving, accepting, and understanding. Such a home ideally supplies the growing child with more than the physical necessities. It provides positive, helpful, broad maternal and paternal role models. It fosters respect for the individual not on the basis of his beauty or intelligence (over which he may have little control) but according to his attitudes, behavior, and willingness to accept and complete appropriate responsibilities. It increases the child's sense of personal esteem in ways that allow him to seek experience and enjoy new opportunities and challenges. The psychological nurture given by the home is as important as its physical support. Lack of real affection alone will result in little or no smiling, loss of appetite, poor sleep, failure to gain weight, and persistent respiratory tract infections. Numerous studies indicate that children deprived of love and the kindly stimulation of the home fail to thrive.*

Nutrition. The growing child is vulnerable to many nutritional inadequacies. Dis-

---

*Brady, S.: Patterns of mothering, New York, 1956, International Universities Press, Inc., p. 97.

turbed patterns of skeletal development caused by the lack or overabundance of one nutrient exemplify the need for "balance." Lack of protein during the prenatal period and early infancy may limit the number and size of brain cells. A well-balanced diet is essential for the development of bones and teeth, good skin, resistance to disease caused by dietary deficiency and infections, and general physical well-being. Clarification of the nutritional needs of children and the general abundance of high-quality foods available have simplified the feeding of infants and children. Despite this, nutritional inadequacies may occur in the midst of plenty through faulty dietary habits, food fads, or psychic tensions centering around mealtime and the feeding situation.

Overnutrition rather than undernutrition seems to present more problems in the United States. However, a severe form of protein deprivation, kwashiorkor, is common in underdeveloped countries of South America and Africa. Kwashiorkor is found among children under 4 years of age. It typically manifests itself after a child is weaned because of the birth of a younger sibling. Characteristically, these children lag in growth and in skeletal development. (For more information regarding nutritional needs see p. 315.)

Disease. Illness is both a physical and a psychological hazard for the young child. Arrested growth is the obvious effect of fever and anorexia. Prolonged illness causes a definite decrease in the rate of growth and height as well as decreased ability to function. Any disease that interferes with physical activity and metabolic processes over a long period will deter normal progress.

Although there may be some growth loss during a minor illness, a subsequent growth spurt will compensate for the temporary setback.

Uncontrolled diabetes always results in retarded growth in both height and weight. Chronic heart disability associated with hypoxia hampers growth as do malabsorp-

tion syndromes such as cystic fibrosis and celiac disease.

Growth and development depend on each other and represent a continuous process of interactions between genetic potential on one hand and environment on the other. The kind of environment a child lives in will determine whether or not he will realize all his inborn capacities for physical, social, mental, and emotional growth. Although nothing can make a child do more than his inborn capacities permit, he must have a favorable environment to develop and learn as fast as his growth patterns allow.

PHYSICAL GROWTH

Although all phases of growth are continuous and take place concurrently, for convenience and clarity discussions of the main aspects of growth and development will be presented separately. Since physical growth is most obvious, it shall be discussed first.

Physical growth may be divided into four well-defined periods:
1. The period of very rapid growth during babyhood
2. The period of slow, steady growth during childhood years
3. The period of the growth spurt during puberty
4. The period of decreasing growth and attainment of maximum height

The greatest increase in extrauterine growth occurs during the early part of babyhood. Small, steady gains continue during the slow periods. This general pattern of growth is characteristic of all the body systems with two exceptions. The nervous system grows rapidly during infancy, then decelerates, and after puberty ceases growing; the reproductive organs, however, grow very slowly until sexual maturation, which occurs during the pubertal spurt.

Tables of average height and weight are commonly used to show that a boy or girl of a particular age should approximate a certain height and weigh within a certain number of pounds. In the course of devel-

Text continued on p. 278.

INFANT GIRLS

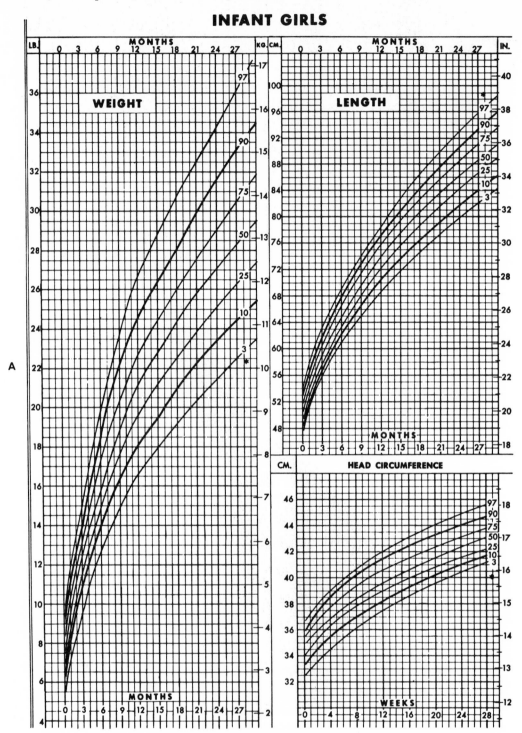

Fig. 19-6. **A** to **D,** The percentiles on these charts are based on repeated measurements of children under comprehensive studies of health and development by Harold C. Stuart, M.D., and associates, Department of Maternal and Child Health, Harvard School of Public Health, Boston, Mass. The charts were constructed by the staff of the department for use at the Infant's Hospital. (Reproduced with permission of the Children's Hospital Medical Center, Boston, Mass.)

INFANT BOYS

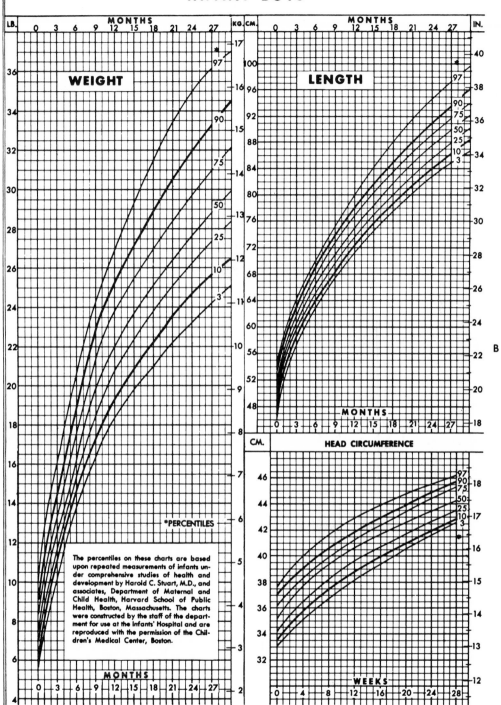

Fig. 19-6, cont'd. For legend see opposite page.   *Continued.*

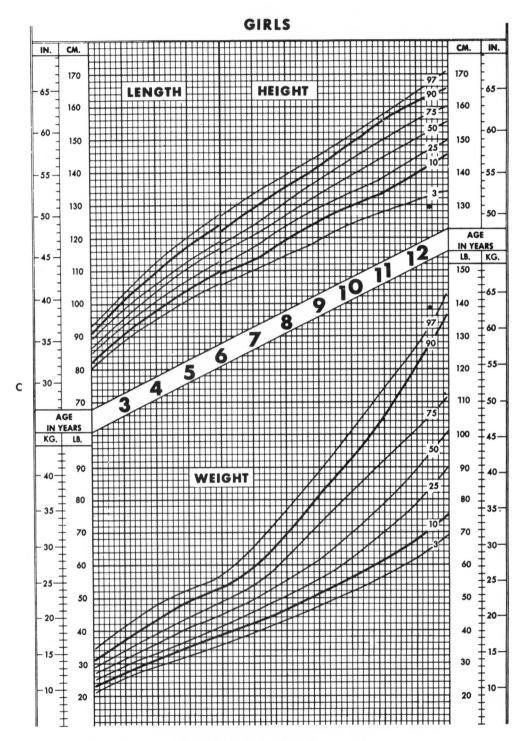

Fig. 19-6, cont'd. For legend see p. 274.

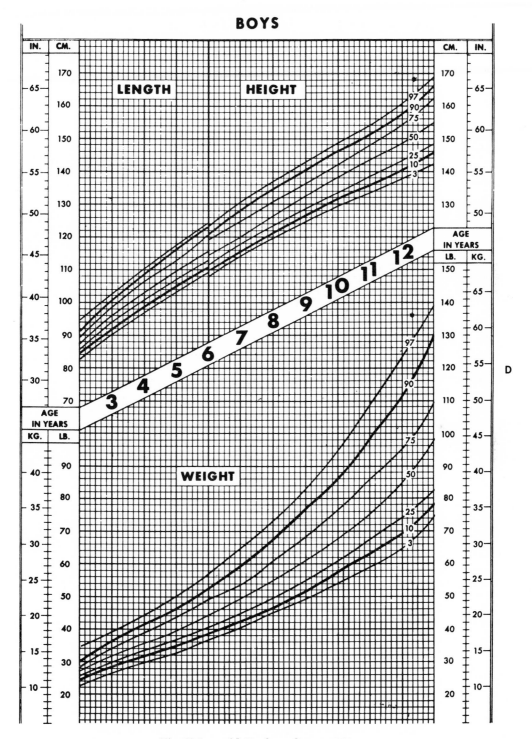

Fig. 19-6, cont'd. For legend see p. 274.

opment, observable trends in height and weight imply that one can draw certain conclusions regarding these aspects of growth. In connection with growth, norms can be successfully determined for a group of children and may serve as a point of reference for making comparisons. However, any table of averages should be interpreted with caution. Although these tables may accurately state averages, they do not necessarily state what is desirable for individuals. It should also be noted that the particular charts reproduced as Figs. 19-6, *A* to *D*, were devised almost 20 years ago, and undoubtedly norms in height and weight have increased since that time. However, these charts are still the ones most commonly employed.

The best method of evaluating a child's general growth progress is by comparing the child with himself from time to time. A large number of observations and measurements recorded periodically demonstrates the individuality of the child's own progress. The grid, a special graph devised by Wetzel,* has become a common instrument for evaluating the individual's progress.

Height

Infants average about 20 inches in length at birth. During the first year of life the child grows about 10 inches. Five inches are added during the second year, and the child grows 3 inches per annum during the preschool period. From the sixth to the tenth year of life the annual gain is reduced to approximately 2 inches. The maximum growth in height occurs during the pubertal period at the approximate time of sexual maturity. Growth in height reaches a peak for boys at about 14 years of age and a year or so earlier for girls. It ceases sometime before the twenties.

Puberty occurs at widely different ages. An early pubertal growth spurt is associated with an early cessation of growth. In-

dividuals who mature late tend to grow for a longer period of time and ultimately become tall adults.

Weight

At birth the infant weighs about 7½ pounds. This weight doubles by the end of the fifth month of life, and by 1 year the birth weight has approximately tripled. A sharp drop in the rate of gain occurs after the first year. The child characteristically appears lanky and even skinny. During the preschool years the weight rises slowly, averaging about 5 pounds each year.

During the school years the weight gain is slightly increased. Weight varies more than height, since it is readily susceptible to external factors such as dietary intake.

Generally, boys are taller and heavier than girls except in the years preceding puberty. A rapid gain in weight usually occurs in both sexes during puberty, corresponding closely with the gain in height. Girls begin their preadolescent growth spurt at about 10 to 12 years of age, 2 years earlier than boys. Girls also reach their adult proportions sooner than boys.

Body proportions (Fig. 19-7)

There are distinct changes in body proportions between birth and maturity. The small child not only differs from the adult in size but also in body form. At birth the head is relatively large, about one fourth of the total body length, whereas in the adult it is about one eighth to one tenth of the body length. The arms and legs are relatively short. During infancy the trunk is longer than the extremities. The midpoint of the total length of the infant is at the umbilicus, whereas in the adult it is at the symphysis pubis.

During puberty, adult proportions are attained, and the characteristic mature body shape for each sex becomes differentiated. The straight leg lines of the young girl become curved by 15 years of age. Her hips grow wider, but her shoulders remain narrow. The boy's shoulders become broader, whereas his hips remain narrow.

Body proportion and build, or physique,

---

*Wetzel, N. C.: The baby grid. An application of the grid technique to growth and development in infants, J. Pediatr. 29:439-454, 1946.

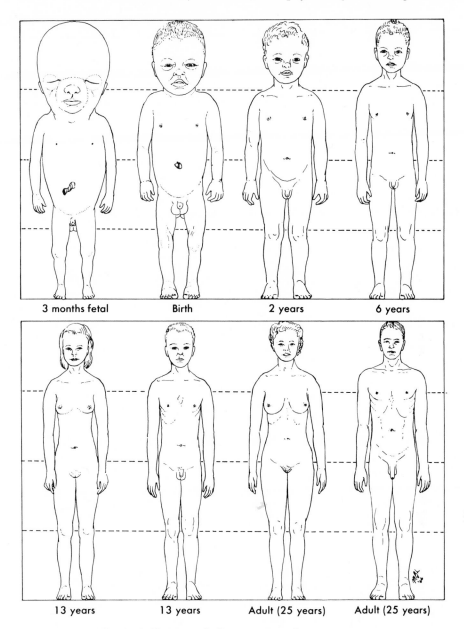

Fig. 19-7. Changes in body proportions, fetus to maturity.

is unique to the individual. Within his own general pattern—slender, stocky, muscular—the child's body build seems to be constant.

Bone formation

During the early days of fetal development, bones begin as simple connective tissue. Later, this tissue becomes cartilage. By the end of the fifth month of gestation, certain mineral salts, especially calcium phos-phate, are deposited in the cartilage, causing it to harden. Cartilage is gradually replaced by bone; this process is called *ossification*. During the early years of life, cartilage per-sists between the diaphysis (shaft) and epiphyses (ends) of long bones. Bones grow in length by a continual thickening of the epiphyseal cartilage.

As the child grows, changes occur in the texture, size, and shape of the "old" bones,

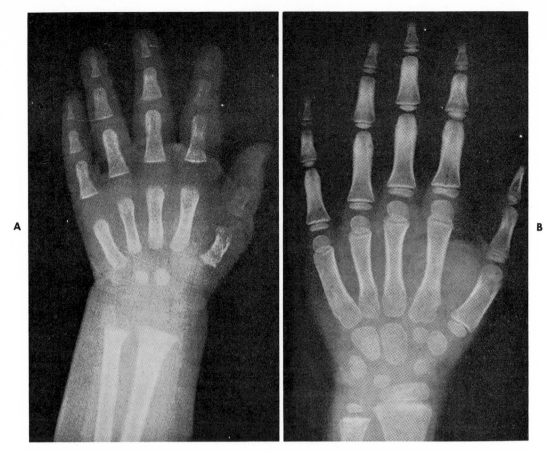

Fig. 19-8. Progessive ossification of the hand of a white female. **A,** Age 3 months. **B,** Age 6 years 3 months. (From Todd, T. W.: Atlas of skeletal maturation, St. Louis, 1937, The C. V. Mosby Co.)

and new bones appear. The process of skeletal maturation is perhaps the best evidence of general growth. Bone development continues in an orderly sequence and is completed by the third decade of life.

Bone age can be determined by x-ray examination of certain joints. The information gained is compared with a standard. The x-ray films are studied to detect the following:

1. The appearance of new bones
2. Changes in the contour of the ends of bones
3. The union of the epiphyses with the bone shaft

Growth of the long bones is complete when the epiphyses and diaphysis are fused.

Bone development of the hand and wrist is a good index of the individual's progress in skeletal growth. Since boys lag behind girls in bone development at all ages, separate standards are used.

At birth the ends of the arm bones (epiphyses) are not developed, and the carpal bones are not present (Fig. 19-8). Shortly thereafter, the carpal bones and epiphyses gradually appear, and changes in the size and contour of the ends of bones continue through the school years. Bone development of the wrist and hand is complete at the seventeenth year of life for girls and 2 years later for boys.

Tooth formation (Fig. 19-9)

The foundation of a child's tooth structure is formed early in fetal life. At birth, all the temporary (deciduous or baby) teeth

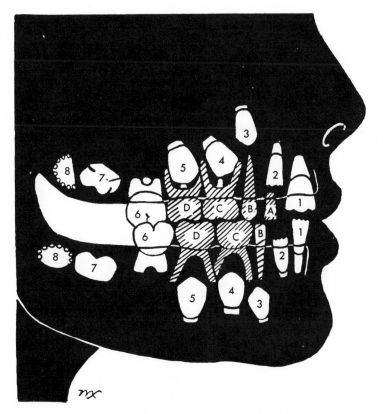

Fig. 19-9. Illustration of 7-year-old child with good occlusion. Deciduous teeth: *A*, lateral incisors; *B*, cuspids; *C*, first molars; *D*, second molars. Permanent teeth: *1*, central incisors; *2*, lateral incisors; *3*, cuspids; *4*, first bicuspids; *5*, second bicuspids; *6*, first molars; *7*, second molars; *8*, site of wisdom teeth.

Table 19-2. Usual pattern of dentition

Teeth	Lower (mandibular) appear at age	Upper (maxillary) appear at age
Deciduous		
Central incisors	5 to 7 months	6 to 8 months
Lateral incisors	12 to 15 months	8 to 11 months
Cuspids (canines)	16 to 20 months	16 to 20 months
First molars	10 to 16 months	10 to 16 months
Second molars	20 to 30 months	20 to 30 months
Total per jaw—10		
Total set—20		
Permanent		
Central incisors	6 to 7 years	6 to 7 years
Lateral incisors	7 to 9 years	8 to 9 years
Cuspids (canines)	8 to 11 years	11 to 12 years
First bicuspids	10 to 12 years	10 to 11 years
Second bicuspids	11 to 13 years	10 to 12 years
First molars (6-year molars)	6 to 7 years	6 to 7 years
Second molars (12-year molars)	12 to 13 years	12 to 13 years
Third molars (wisdom teeth)	17 to 22 years	17 to 22 years
Total per jaw—16		
Total set—32		

and the first permanent teeth (6-year molars) are developing in the child's jaw. Dentition is characterized by wide variation.

It is not always possible to predict exactly when the first tooth will erupt, but it is possible to predict with some accuracy which teeth will erupt first. The two lower central incisors usually appear first, between 5 and 7 months. The upper central incisors appear next. Most children have six teeth at 1 year of age and all twenty deciduous teeth by 2½ years of age.

There is a wide variation in the pattern of temporary tooth shedding and permanent tooth eruption. Before the appearance of the first molars (6-year molars), all the permanent teeth are growing and maturing.

During this time the roots of the temporary teeth are disappearing by the process of resorption. Only the crown of the temporary tooth is left when the permanent tooth below is ready to erupt. The loose tooth then drops out. The care and preservation of the temporary teeth are important. Unless they are beyond repair, temporary teeth should not be pulled out. They contribute in large measure to proper alignment and good health of the permanent teeth.

Tetracycline antibiotics have an adverse effect on newly formed bones. The drug stains developing teeth with a yellow-brown material. Tetracyclines also cross the placenta. After the sixth month of gestation, the deciduous teeth of the developing fetus

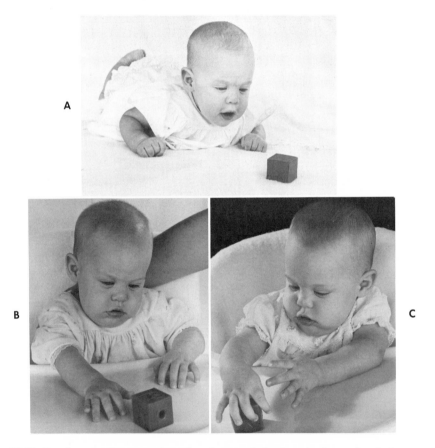

Fig. 19-10. Developmental progression of prehensory behavior: **A,** 3 months, looks at cube; **B,** 5 months, looks and approaches; **C,** 6 months, looks and crudely grasps with whole hand; **D,** 9 months, looks and deftly grasps with fingers; **E,** 12 months, looks, grasps with forefinger and thumb, and deftly releases; **F,** 15 months, looks, grasps, and releases to build a tower of two blocks.

are also affected. Such discoloration of the teeth may be avoided by *not using* the drugs during pregnancy and the first 8 years of life.

MOTOR DEVELOPMENT

As the child's body grows he acquires the ability to function in increasingly complex ways. Motor changes accompany physical growth. Motor abilities involve various types of body movements that result from the coordinated activity of nerves and muscles. Maturation of the nervous system and learning are interrelated in the acquisition of motor abilities.

Motor development is the process of learning, controlling, and integrating muscular responses. Great advances in body control and locomotion are accomplished during the first 2 years of life. At first an uncoordinated, helpless infant, the child is soon able to sit, stand, walk, reach, and grasp.

Like other phases of growth, motor development unfolds in an orderly sequence that is closely related to the maturation of the nervous system. It follows a definite sequence. Characteristically, motor development begins in the head region of the individual and moves downward toward the feet (cephalocaudal). Development also tends to proceed from the center of the body toward the extremities (proximodistal). At first motor response to stimulation (such as an ice cube touching the foot) is diffuse, involving the whole body. As maturation proceeds, the response becomes more specific and may involve only the withdrawal of the foot. The sequence of motor development is similar for all children, but the rate at which the development progresses varies with each individual child.

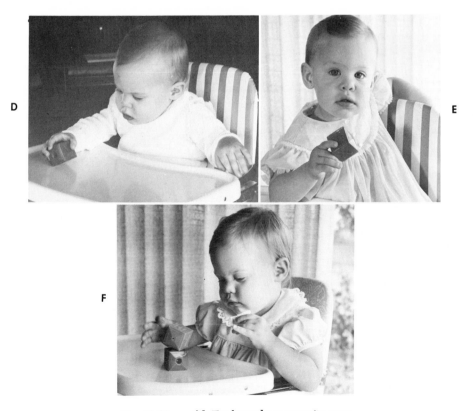

Fig. 19-10, cont'd. For legend see opposite page.

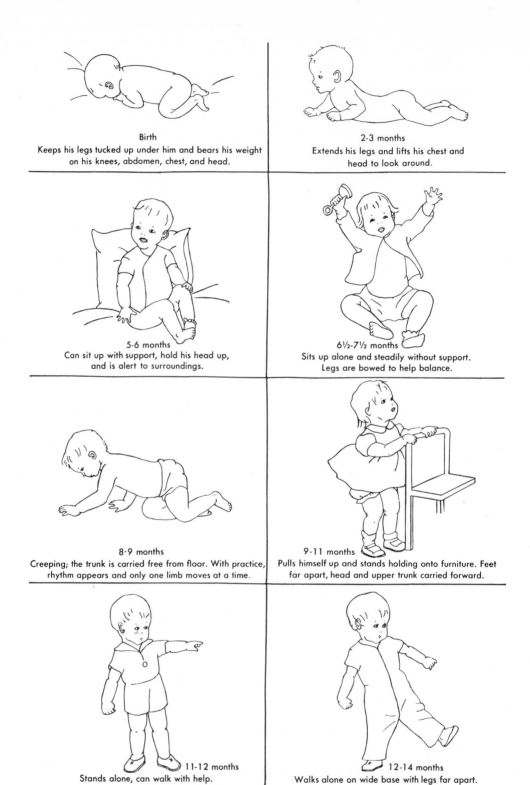

Birth
Keeps his legs tucked up under him and bears his weight
on his knees, abdomen, chest, and head.

2-3 months
Extends his legs and lifts his chest and
head to look around.

5-6 months
Can sit up with support, hold his head up,
and is alert to surroundings.

6½-7½ months
Sits up alone and steadily without support.
Legs are bowed to help balance.

8-9 months
Creeping; the trunk is carried free from floor. With practice,
rhythm appears and only one limb moves at a time.

9-11 months
Pulls himself up and stands holding onto furniture. Feet
far apart, head and upper trunk carried forward.

11-12 months
Stands alone, can walk with help.

12-14 months
Walks alone on wide base with legs far apart.

Fig. 19-11. Guideposts in motor development, emphasizing the average child.

Prehension and locomotion provide examples of the usual sequences in the course of motor development.

Prehension

The development of the ability to oppose the thumb to the fingers in picking up an object is preceded by reaching, grasping, and raking movements. Early attempts in reaching also involve eye-hand coordination. Effective use of the hands for picking up small objects or for grasping is called prehension. The developmental sequence proceeds from eye-hand coordination in grasping to reaching without looking, from large muscle activity of the arms and shoulders to fine muscle activity of the fingers, and from a crude pawing closure to a closure of the fingertips in a refined fashion.

Gesell tested prehension by placing a little red cube before a baby. He described the grasping sequence as follows (Fig. 19-10):

Development progression in grasping

12 weeks	Looks at cube
20 weeks	Looks and approaches
24 weeks	Looks and crudely grasps with whole hand
36 weeks	Looks and deftly grasps with fingers
52 weeks	Looks, grasps with forefinger and thumb, and deftly releases
15 months	Looks, grasps, and releases to build a tower of two cubes*

Locomotion

The ability to walk alone is also attained gradually after a sequence of developments that can be traced back to the first days of life. Moving from place to place and walking are examples of gross motor skills. Complete establishment of this control usually takes most of the first year for early walkers and about 15 months for those who mature later.

The walking sequence begins when the

---

*From Gesell, A., and Ilg, L. B.: The child from five to ten, New York, 1946, Harper & Row, Publishers.

baby is able to hold his head up, and it is half accomplished when he can sit alone. When an infant is able to change from a prone to a sitting position, he tends to begin to creep. He usually creeps to an object or person, where he pulls himself to a standing position. Gradually he stands alone and finally walks independently.

The motor sequence (Fig. 19-11)

½ to 1 month	Lifts head
2 to 3 months	Raises chest
3 to 4 months	Turns from side to back
5 to 6 months	Sits with support
6 to 7 months	Rolls from back to abdomen
6½ to 7½ months	Sits alone
8 to 9 months	Creeps
9 to 11 months	Pulls self up
11 to 12 months	Walks with help
12 to 14 months	Walks alone

Prehension and locomotion develop independently of any teaching. Knowledge of these motor abilities "just comes." Each skill follows an orderly sequential course whose rate may be affected by environmental factors.

As each skill develops, opportunity to use it and practice it is necessary. This means that the child needs plenty of space for walking, objects to pick up and handle, and, most of all, he needs health, vigor, freedom, and encouragement to venture. The nurse who understands the development of motor skills will not restrict the child to his crib but encourage his full capacity for motor growth.

INTELLECTUAL DEVELOPMENT

Of all the factors influencing the overall development of the child, his intelligence seems to be the most important. Superior intelligence is associated with superior development, whereas inferior intelligence is associated with retarded development.

A child's intelligence, defined as the ability to solve problems or achieve a goal, will affect his observation, thought, and understanding. It strongly influences the level of difficulty at which the child is able to function efficiently and the scope of his activities.

Many changes take place in the intellectual life of the child as he develops from infancy to adulthood. At birth the centers of higher intellectual activity in the brain are not fully developed. Furthermore, the sensory acuity necessary for these higher intellectual functions is likewise immature. The mental world of the newborn infant seems to consist primarily of experiences arising through direct physical contact with the environment and through the sensations that originate within his own body. New experiences expand his mental world and are interpreted in the light of previous learning. Though it is not readily detected by casual observers, the length of a behavior labeled "habituation" has been said to be predictive of an infant's intelligence. Habituation is defined as the period of time that elapses between the infant's initial response and the cessation of that response to a repeated stimulus. The duration of his response is measured by skin electrode and an assessment of motor activity. The shorter his habituation, the higher his intellectual potential. Do infants demonstrating rapid habituation investigate more? We don't know. Watching intently is an important primary skill.

Beginning very early, children exhibit the ability to imagine and to engage in make-believe activities. Such make-believe activities aid in exploring the real world, organizing experiences, and solving problems. Through make-believe, the child is able to participate in a wider range of experiences and partially overcome his own limitations. Such fantasies are a necessary and normal part of learning.

As growth proceeds, the ability to concentrate develops. The child's span of attention is likely to be longer during activities that he has chosen or that are at least related to his own desires.

The development of a child's ability to reason is gradual and continuous. The young child is concerned with events related to his own immediate experience and well-being. As he grows, he becomes increasingly able to occupy himself with more remote issues and deal with abstractions. Such changes can be noted in connection with the enlargement of the meanings associated with various terms in the language he uses, the interest and ability he eventually displays in facing social issues, and his ability to relate to events in the world beyond his immediate experience.

EMOTIONAL GROWTH

Every infant, child, and adult possesses the drive to express himself in some way. The reaction that accompanies either the satisfaction or frustration of a basic need may be termed an "emotion." Another way of describing an emotional response is to define it as a psychological reaction caused by internal or external stimuli. Although emotions are not identical to basic drives, they are related. The basic drives can be physical, social, intellectual, or personal. Emotional experience includes feelings, impulses, and physical and physiological reactions. For example, if a baby's needs are fulfilled, he is happy, joyful, contented, or loving; if a baby's drives are frustrated, he is anxious, fretful, frightened, or angry. Physiological changes initiated by emotions may stimulate a person to violent action.

All emotions cause a physical response. But just as no two persons think or act alike, no two react to the same emotion in the same way. For example, because of fear one person may feel belligerent, another anxious, or still another depressed. As soon as one begins to experience emotion, physiological changes take place. Manifestations of these changes include facial expressions, laughter, and crying.

Emotions appear early in life. Even during the first days of life the infant's need to satisfy his physical needs is accompanied by emotional response. The infant usually reacts by crying or kicking. Soon the baby finds a given stimulation pleasant or unpleasant. When the infant is hungry or uncomfortable, an unpleasant state results, which he makes known by crying or restlessness. When his wants are satisfied, a pleasant state of well-being ensues, which is evidenced by cooing, gurgling, or sleep. Thus the emotional responses of the infant are initially stimulated by physiological needs.

Through a combination of maturation and learning, more specialized responses soon occur. By the end of the first year, emotions of fear, rage, excitement, anger, and joy become recognizable; and facial expression, vocalization, and body movement become part of the child's emotional equipment. Changes in the expression of the emotions continue progressively throughout the childhood years.

Love. Love is the most important of all the emotions because it is the foundation on which all positive relationships are built. The child's first love is centered on his mother, since she is the one who initially loves and serves him. The child's capacity for affection and love develops gradually from his early association. During the normal course of development the child transfers a part of his affection to other individuals who share his pleasures and achievements. Eventually this love will grow to form the nucleus of another family—his own. A child who receives loving and considerate care is prepared to give as well as receive love. His security is not simply a passive thing but a safe feeling that allows him to be venturesome in the belief that people will be good to him.

Fear. Fear is aroused naturally when the infant experiences any startling, sudden occurrence such as a loud noise, an unexpected jar, or a fall. He characteristically responds to these threats to his security with crying and general body distress. The young child acquires other fears that are associated with objects and persons in his immediate environment. As children become older, fearful responses become increasingly specific; they are expressed by withdrawal from the fearful situation. Later, children learn to avoid situations that cause anxiety.

Once a child becomes afraid in a certain situation, any repetition of the same or similar situation will reproduce fear. However, if the boy or girl learns that the situ-ation is not truly hazardous, the fear diminishes or disappears. Parents and other adults should not laugh at or ridicule a child's fears—identified or unnamed as they may be—but help the child to understand the situation or thing that is frightening him. Reasonable fear is a valuable safeguard against many dangers. Fear acts as a check on behavior. A person may be driven to action by anger, hate, or jealousy, but his conduct is held within reasonable bounds through the fear of consequences. In other words, fear may act as a negative guide to more orderly behavior.

Anger. Anger denotes a variety of emotional states that range from turbulent rage to milder forms of resentment. In infancy, anger arises primarily through interference with body movement or gratification of basic needs such as feeding. Crying, screaming, biting, hitting, and kicking are expressions of anger. In early childhood, anger may take the form of numerous acts of disobedience and resistance. When the child learns to talk, he gains command of new ways to express his anger. Children may find outbursts of anger useful for attracting attention to themselves and for obtaining a desired end. Children are even more likely to give vent to anger when suffering from lack of sleep, hunger, or fatigue.

Anger may be controlled in small children by guarding the child's general health and physical condition and by providing regular meals, sleep, and time with his mother and father for pleasurable experiences. Feelings of anger may be very frightening. A young child needs to be reassured that these feelings are very common. However, he also needs to be guided toward more appropriate means for expressing anger. He is likely to feel more secure when behavior such as "acting out," hitting, and biting are firmly limited by adults. Parents can also aid by maintaining poise and self-control, refusing to be manipulated by theatrical displays of emotion (temper tantrums), and encouraging a friendly home atmosphere.

Jealousy. Jealousy is an emotional response compounded of anger, fear, and love. It is an emotion that, in general, seems to arise when persons or objects threaten to take away something, share something, or interfere with that which is felt to belong to oneself. In the young child, jealousy tends to develop when the child is threatened by possible loss of love as a result of the presence of a newborn brother or sister. Because of the mother's preoccupation with the infant, the older child may equate loss of time and attention with loss of love. He sees the younger sibling as a rival and becomes jealous. The reaction of the child may be positive and result in either aggression toward or competition with the new baby. Thus the jealous child may resort to hitting the baby or may turn to infantile habits to gain the attention he desires. A negative reaction may consist of withdrawal from competition or repression. For example, a child may sulk or refuse meals. The expression of jealousy varies with age. Behavior caused by such personal envy gradually becomes less direct and less openly violent; it is more subtle but no less real.

The factors precipitating emotions and the reaction patterns they initiate have typical stages of development and can be traced just as the other stages of growth and development. The emotional responses of individuals not only vary in form and intensity from person to person but also from age to age. The emotions identified and the reactions they stimulate are closely related to the individual's maturity and life experience. Emotions always find an outlet; if the most desired expression is blocked, another, perhaps less desirable, is substituted. This observation has many practical applications and is basic to the understanding of many behavior problems and the concept of psychosomatic illness. Talking out problems and learning to communicate rather than "acting out" one's feelings or burying them in the subconscious, where they can cause physical and emotional problems, is extremely important.

SOCIAL BEHAVIOR AND MORAL VALUES

An individual's characteristic response to social situations is a useful way of describing personal-social behavior. Personal-social behavior includes all the modes of behavior that characterize the child's own individuality.

The dynamic interaction of a child's thoughts and feelings that produces his characteristic responses to his environment is what we call "personality." Personality includes one's intelligence, physique, habits, and appeal to others. As a child grows older, his ways of responding become more and more characteristic of himself. The first social group for a child is his family, a group that plays an important role in establishing his attitudes and habits.

The major source of personality growth for the child resides in the maturity and harmony of his parents. The parents provide the models that the child consciously and unconsciously emulates. Home is the place where the child learns, even as a tiny infant, what people and life are like. At home he learns friendliness, confidence, security, belonging, loving, and sharing as these are reflected in the people in his immediate environment.

The awakening of social behavior manifests itself as the baby grows alert to his surroundings and is able to distinguish between persons and objects. During the first weeks of life the infant reacts instinctively to his immediate surroundings and those persons, particularly his mother, who care for him. The infant, who is primarily concerned with satisfying his basic needs, does not readily make distinctions between people and things. Soon, however, he begins to respond to the presence of others and their behavior toward him. The baby's awareness of persons around him grows out of the simple responses he gives as they care for him and supply his wants. For example, if a baby is handled gently and lovingly, his natural response will be a happy one such as cooing, smiling, or tranquil rest. If a baby is treated roughly with impatience, agitation, and frustration, he will respond accordingly, perhaps with fretful crying, kicking, or enraged screaming. Thus certain forms of social behavior begin to develop as the child responds to those in contact with him.

Early in babyhood the child learns to imitate adults, children, and other babies around him in order to become a part of the family or social group. At about 3 months of age the baby first imitates facial expressions, such as smiling and wincing. Gestures and movements such as waving "bye-bye," shaking the head, or throwing a kiss develop at approximately 6 months of age.

A happy, smiling child is a good indication that his social development is progressing well; and the framework for this positive, outgoing nature is built most firmly by parents who have made their child feel loved in the early months and years of life. The way people work and play, their ability to enjoy other people, and how they feel about tackling new things (even the foods they prefer or will not touch) have had beginnings early in life's experience. People can change, but the effects of early childhood experiences are likely to persist.

Probably the most important medium of socialization is language. Socrates said, "Speak that I may see thee." The early vocalizations of the infant quickly develop from throaty noises at 4 weeks of age to three-word sentences at 2 years of age. The young baby rapidly recognizes the urgency to verbalize as he becomes part of the social group. Although language at first consists of object naming and identification, it soon becomes a vehicle for the transportation of ideas. Hence hand in hand with language development goes the development of understanding.

In the first few weeks of life the infant has no understanding of his environment. Gradually, as language ability increases as a result of maturation and learning, the child becomes more able to understand what he observes. It is important to note,

however, that no two children can be expected to have the same understanding of an object or situation, since no one has exactly the same intellectual abilities or experiences. If an infant is handicapped in sensory development through deafness or blindness, he will be handicapped in language growth and understanding. To the extent that a child is deprived of such sensory stimulation, his personal and social behavior is proportionately delayed or impaired.

The child learns the values and expectations of his culture through the examples and teachings that are provided by the key adults in his life. One of the important functions of the family is to help provide the appropriate learning experiences for the child during his first few years, whereby the primary drives will bring forth socially acceptable behavior. The child must learn to satisfy his needs in a culturally conforming manner. The hazards involved in this learning are great. Effective training helps build secure personalities whose capacities for adjustment to the needs of others is sufficient to assure wholesome and mutually satisfying relationships throughout life. The style of social interaction, guidance, and discipline displayed by the parents does not appear to be as important as its consistency or reliability.

It is largely in the home that the child's basic moral and spiritual concepts are developed. Community agencies, school, and church make significant contributions, but they do not usually occupy the primary position in the child's esteem. It is the parents' behavior and not their words that influences the child. To reword an old saying, "What they are speaks so loud that the child does not hear what they say."

Physical growth, psychological development, and moral sensitivity should not proceed independently of one another. They are like branches of the same tree, which, when mature, provide strength, protection, meaning, and beauty to both the individual and his community.

20

Ages and stages of childhood and youth

In caring for children, one must have an awareness of the approximate ages at which the child is capable of various activities and functions and the different types of behavior that are likely to emerge at each stage of development. This information will assist the nurse in fostering the child's growth and development while caring for him in illness and in health. Many books have been written to describe the physical, motor, and psychological changes that take place as an individual goes through the process we call "growing up." The sections that follow are designed to aid the student in the rapid identification of some of the outstanding characteristics of certain ages and the basic psychosocial challenges of that stage of development as identified by Erik Erikson. The performance times noted are averages only, and allowance must always be made for individual differences.

At the end of the chapter is a description of the Denver Developmental Screening Test, a device that is commonly used to detect developmental delays in young children. This standardized test is easily administered and evaluates the child's functioning in four areas of development: gross motor, fine motor-adaptive, language, and personal-social.

NEWBORN

Physical growth. Average weight, 7½ pounds, gains 1 ounce per day during first 6 months; average height, 20 inches, grows 10 inches during first year.

Motor development. Readily assumes fetal position; palmar grasp; asymmetrical tonic neck, Moro, rooting, and sucking reflexes present; raises head but not stable, can turn head from side to side.

Language development. Vocalizes small, throaty, undifferentiated noises.

Common behavior. Sleeps about 20 hours a day; cries when hungry; displays impassive face; regards face of another.

Nutrition. Formula (2½ to 3 ounces per pound divided into 6 feedings daily) or breast milk supplemented with vitamins;

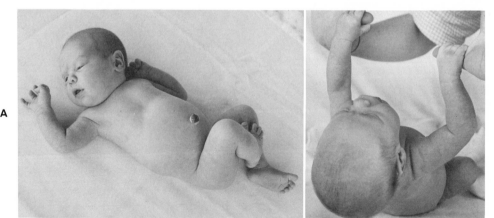

Fig. 20-1. Newborn infant: **A,** tonic neck posture is readily assumed; **B,** grasp reflex is strong.

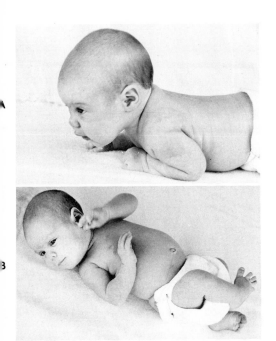

Fig. 20-2. Infant at 1 month: **A,** lifts and turns head when supine; **B,** activity is diffuse and random.

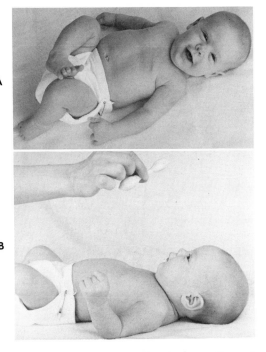

Fig. 20-3. Infant at 2 months: **A,** a sociable smile appears; **B,** eyes follow objects.

water; schedule for introduction of semi-solid foods depends on infant and physician; small amounts of thin pabulum offered at 3 to 4 weeks.

INFANT (ONE MONTH TO ONE YEAR)

The basic psychosocial challenge of infancy is trust versus mistrust.* As the infant grows older he acquires an increasing awareness of himself as an individual who can be happy and satisfied or frustrated and anxious. When he senses he is loved (that is, when his needs are grati-

---

*All material on psychosocial challenges is adapted from Erikson, E. H.: Childhood and society, ed. 2, New York, 1963, W. W. Norton & Co., Inc.

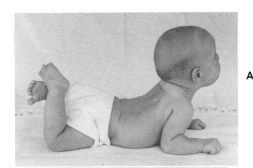

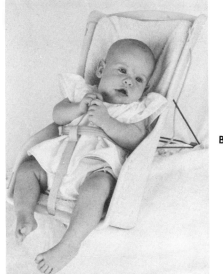

Fig. 20-4. Infant at 3 months: **A,** raises head when prone, supported on forearms; **B,** sits for short period when supported.

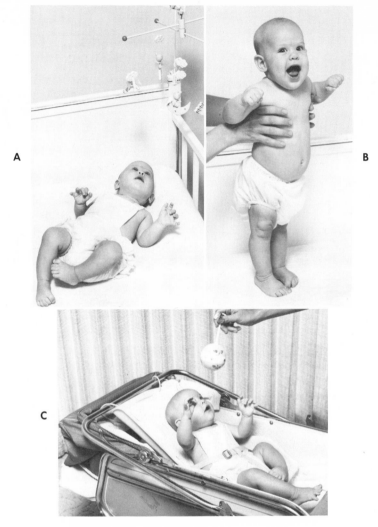

Fig. 20-5. Infant at 4 months: **A**, gazes straight up, symmetrical posture predominates; **B**, pushes with feet when held erect; **C**, reaches and grasps at objects.

fied), he is happy, content; he begins to develop a basic sense of trust, which is fostered by a warm and loving mother-child relationship. Discontinuities in care bring frustration and pain; the child may then develop basic mistrust that may last throughout life.

One to three months

Physical growth. Posterior fontanel closed at 2 to 3 months.

Motor development. Pulse, 110 to 150 beats per minute; respirations, 30 to 50 per minute; activity, diffuse and random; specific activities limited to reflexes; cries with tears; raises chest at 3 months; Moro reflex absent at 3 months.

Language development. Coos at 2 months.

Nutrition. Pureed fruits and vegetables offered at 4 to 6 weeks; pureed meats at 3 months.

Common behavior. May have periods of colic; responsive social smile; attentive to voices and light; eyes can follow moving object to 180 degrees.

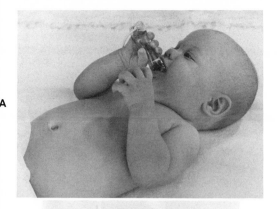

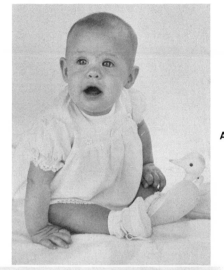

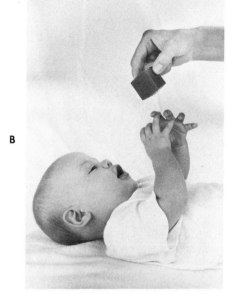

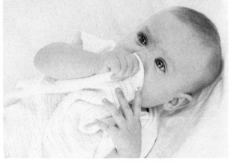

Fig. 20-6. Infant at 5 months; **A**, manipulates and chews small objects; **B**, alert to surroundings.

Fig. 20-7. Infant at 6 months: **A**, sits alone, leaning forward on one hand; **B**, sleeps with favorite blanket and thumb in mouth.

Four to six months

Physical growth. Birth weight doubled at 5 months; teething, lower central incisors appear at 5 to 7 months.

Motor development. Turns from side to back at 3 to 4 months; reaches out at objects; rooting reflex absent at 4 months (awake); rolls over at 5 months; asymmetrical tonic neck absent at 5 months; sits with support at 6 months; palmar grasp absent at 6 months.

Language development. Laughs aloud; babbles vowellike sounds at 5 months.

Nutrition. Egg yolks offered.

Common behavior. Sleeps through the night, 8 to 12 hours; recognizes mother; puts things into mouth.

Seven to eleven months

Physical growth. Has first deciduous teeth.

Motor development. Sits alone between 6½ and 7½ months; crawls, creeps at 9 months, and pulls self to standing position at 10 months; crude pincer grasp picks up small object using part of thumb and fingers in opposition.

293

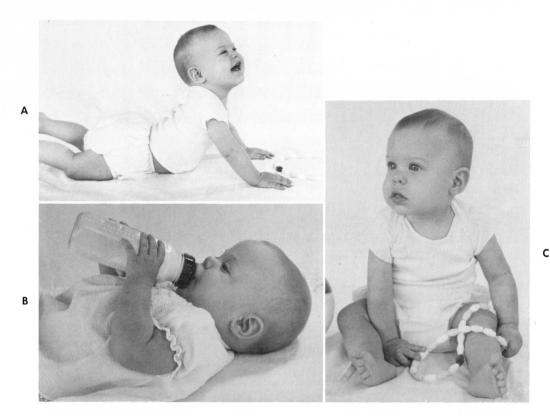

Fig. 20-8. Infant at 7 months: **A,** propels self forward on belly (crawling); **B,** can hold bottle; **C,** sits alone without support.

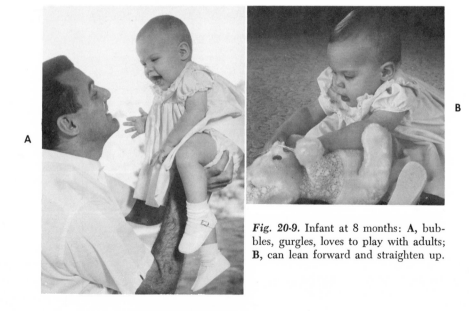

Fig. 20-9. Infant at 8 months: **A,** bubbles, gurgles, loves to play with adults; **B,** can lean forward and straighten up.

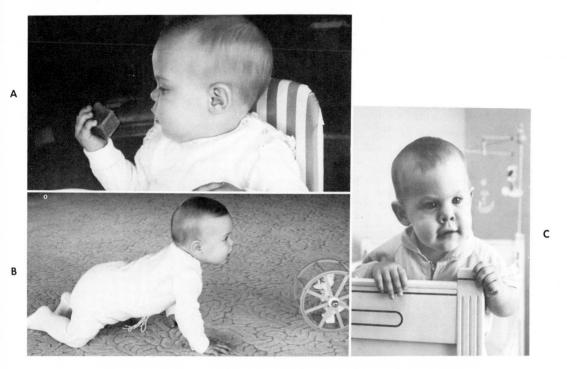

Fig. 20-10. Infant at 9 months: **A,** hand preference appears; **B,** propels self forward on all fours, trunk above and parallel to floor (creeping); **C,** can pull self to standing position.

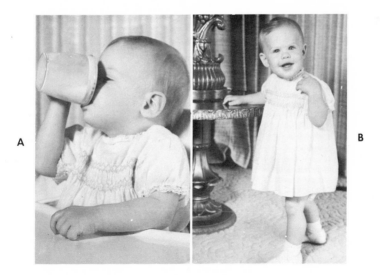

Fig. 20-11. Infant at 10 to 11 months: **A,** drinks from a cup with ease; **B,** cruises around, holding on to furniture.

Language development. Vocalizes "m-m-m" when crying; says "da-da" or "ma-ma" at 10 months.

Nutrition. Gradual substitution of home mashed cooked vegetables and junior foods, depending on dentition; eats 3 meals a day.

Common behavior. Recognizes and avoids strangers at 7 to 8 months; responds to name; holds bottle at 7 months; has well-defined pattern of sleep; has special blanket or cuddly toy; begins to feed self at 10 months; plays spontaneously.

Twelve months

Physical growth. Birth weight tripled; height, 29 to 30 inches; has 6 teeth.

Motor development. Walks alone with wide stance and short steps; picks up small objects with forefinger and thumb; drinks from a cup with ease.

Language development. Says "mama" and "dada" plus 2 other small words, such as "no-no" and "bye-bye."

Nutrition. Eats 3 meals a day.

Common behavior. Takes one nap per day; cooperates in dressing; plays spontaneously; can give a kiss.

TODDLER (ONE TO THREE YEARS)

Trust, the cornerstone of a healthy personality, is usually established by end of the first year. The basic psychosocial challenge of the toddler is self-esteem (auton-

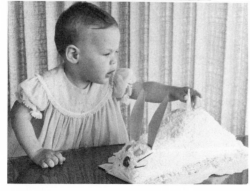

Fig. 20-12. Infant at 12 months; **A,** stands alone on wide base; **B,** good finger-thumb opposition.

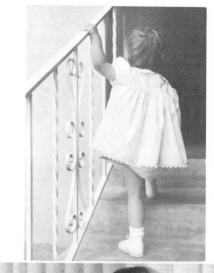
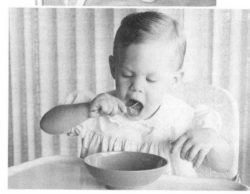

Fig. 20-13. Toddler at 15 months: **A,** climbs up stairs, holding rail; **B,** uses spoon to feed self.

omy) versus shame and doubt. The child's energies are now centered around asserting that he is an individual with his own mind and will; he has to have the right to choose; he wants to do more and more for himself. Feelings of self-esteem, pride, and independence develop. With guidance from his parents and others, he learns to make decisions and to become more self-reliant. Those who guide the growing child wisely will be firm and tolerant of him and will avoid shaming him and causing him to doubt his sense of worth.

Fifteen months

Physical growth. Growth rate slows down; has 8 teeth.

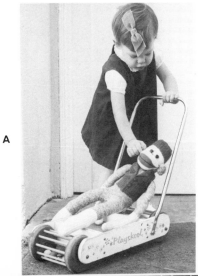

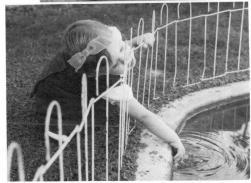

Fig. 20-14. Toddler at 18 months: **A,** loves to push and pull toys; **B,** needs independence but supervision, too.

Motor development. Walks well without support; can build a tower of two blocks; uses spoon but spills; can throw object.

Language development. Vocabulary of 6 words.

Nutrition. Enjoys finger foods; appetite normally decreases.

Common behavior. One nap per day; co-operates in dressing; very active, assertive, and independent; beginning to be negativistic; becomes angry when frustrated.

Eighteen months

Physical growth. Anterior fontanel closed; abdomen protrudes; has 12 teeth.

Motor development. Plateau of motor development; runs, seldom falls, increasingly mobile.

Language development. May say 10 words; follows simple commands.

Nutrition. Small attractive servings desired; feeds self with little spilling.

Common behavior. Gets into everything; accident hazard high; pulls toys, carries special toy or blanket; takes off shoes and socks.

Twenty-four months (2 years)

Physical growth. Pulse, 90 to 120 beats per minute; respirations, 20 to 35 per minute; has 16 teeth; weighs 26 to 28 pounds; grows 3 to 4 inches in second year; gains 5 pounds in second year.

Motor development. Walks up and down stairs alone. Runs without falling. Opens door. Can kick ball. Throws ball overhand.

Language development. Names familiar objects; says simple phrases; has vocabulary of 300 words.

Nutrition. Do not insist that child eat but prevent snacking to sharpen appetite.

Common behavior. Parallel play is characteristic; has difficulty playing with others and sharing; bedtime ritual, enjoys stories; is bowel trained; points to eye, nose, and mouth.

Thirty months (2½ years)

Physical growth. Has complete set of deciduous teeth (20).

Motor development. Builds tower of 8 blocks; jumps with both feet; walks on tiptoes.

Language development. Can say full name; sings; begins to express his needs.

Nutrition. Has definite likes and dislikes.

Common behavior. Washes and dries hands; likes to be with mother; has short attention span.

PRESCHOOLER (THREE TO SIX YEARS)

The basic psychosocial challenge of the preschooler is initiative versus guilt. Knowing that he is a person in his own right, the child of 4 or 5 wants to find out what kind of person he can be; he imagines what it is like to be grown up. Little girls want to be like "mamma" and boys like "daddy." The

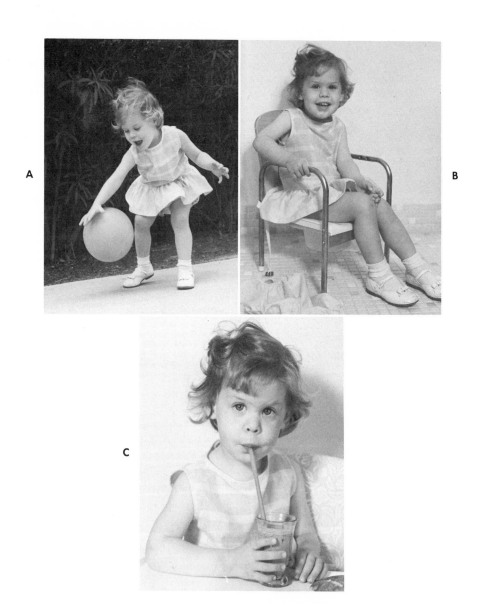

Fig. 20-15. Toddler at 24 months: **A,** muscular coordination greatly advanced; **B,** verbalizes toilet needs; **C,** drinks from straw.

preschooler imitates his parents and yearns to share in their activities. By this age, conscience has developed. This is an age of avid curiosity and consuming fantasies, which lead to feelings of guilt and anxiety; initiative must be fostered and care taken to prevent the young child from feeling guilty because he dared to dream.

Three years

Physical growth. Period of relatively slow growth; gains about 5 pounds; height increase an average of 3 inches per year.

Motor development. Uses stairs with al-

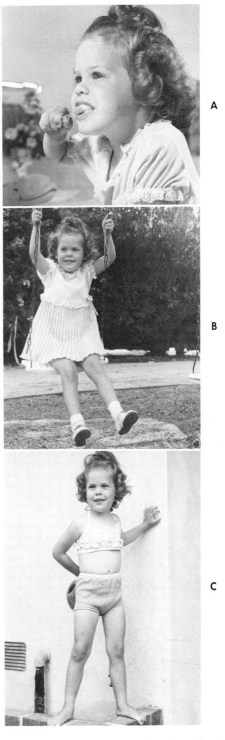

Fig. 20-17. Preschooler at 36 months: **A,** can brush teeth and wash hands; **B,** can pump swing with legs; **C,** knows own age and sex and has good balance.

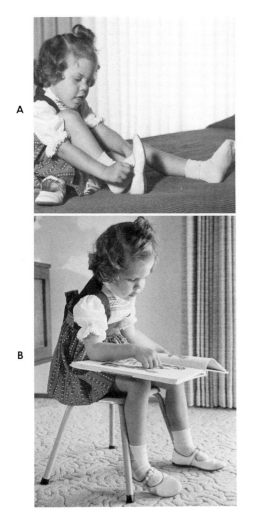

Fig. 20-16. Toddler at 30 months: **A,** can put shoes on; **B,** enjoys looking at animal picture book.

ternate feet; strings large beads; hops on one foot; rides tricycle.

Language development. Has vocabulary of 900 words or more; knows two colors; talks with an imaginary playmate.

Nutrition. In hospital toddlers and preschoolers often eat well together with supervision.

Common behavior. Can brush teeth; helps dress self; may display sibling rivalry; sensitive observation of sex differences and parental attitudes toward sex; has daytime bladder control; asks questions; enjoys preschool experience.

Four years

Physical growth. Height, 39 to 41 inches; weight, 35 to 37 pounds; continued relative slow growth; gains 5 pounds per year; height increases 3 inches per year.

Motor development. Uses one foot per step when going down stairs; climbs and jumps well; increasing finger dexterity; can button and unbutton clothes.

Language development. Vocabulary of 1500 words; tells what he has drawn; knows several colors; can repeat rhymes and songs; asks many questions.

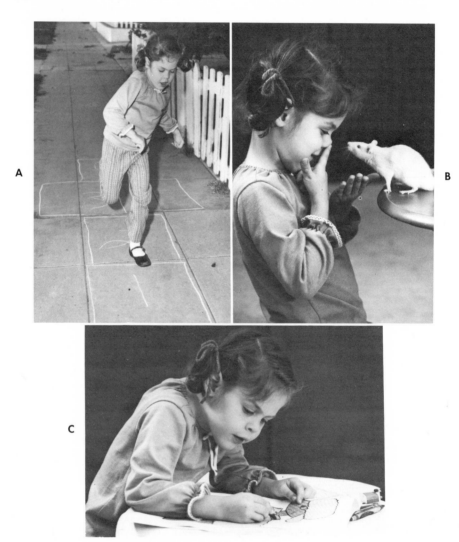

Fig. 20-18. Preschooler at 4 years: **A,** hops on one leg; **B,** enjoys playing with animals; **C,** increasing finger dexterity with crayons.

Nutrition. Habitual good nutrition brings current and future benefits.

Common behavior. Relatively unstable age; imaginative play with doll (for example, playing nurse); attends to toilet needs; cooperative play is enjoyed; draws a man with four parts; knows how old he is.

Five years

Physical growth. Height, 43 to 44 inches; weight, 40 pounds; may lose lower central incisors.

Motor development. Good muscular coordination; can hop, skip, run, and catch ball; climbs on jungle gym.

Language development. Names all the primary colors and coins; talks in sentences.

Nutrition. Variety of fruits and vegetables should be provided to ensure vitamin A and C requirement; likes food that he can eat with fingers.

Common behavior. Talks constantly; tells tales; enjoys group activities and conformity; enjoys kindergarten experience; prints first name; dresses and undresses without help.

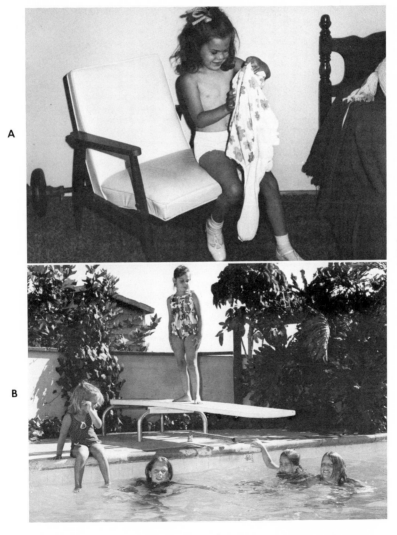

Fig. 20-19. Preschooler at 5 years: **A,** dresses and undresses without help; **B,** enjoys group activities.

THE SCHOOL YEARS (SIX TO TEN)

The basic psychosocial challenge of the school-age child is industry versus inferiority. Preoccupation with fantasy subsides; the child wants to be engaged in real tasks that he can carry through. In learning to accept instruction and win recognition by producing "things," he develops a sense of adequacy and accomplishment. When the child does not receive recognition for his efforts, he develops a sense of inadequacy and inferiority.

Six years

Physical growth. Six-year molars; first permanent teeth; annual growth of 2 inches.

Motor development. Good balance; increased dexterity, advanced throwing; roller skates, swims.

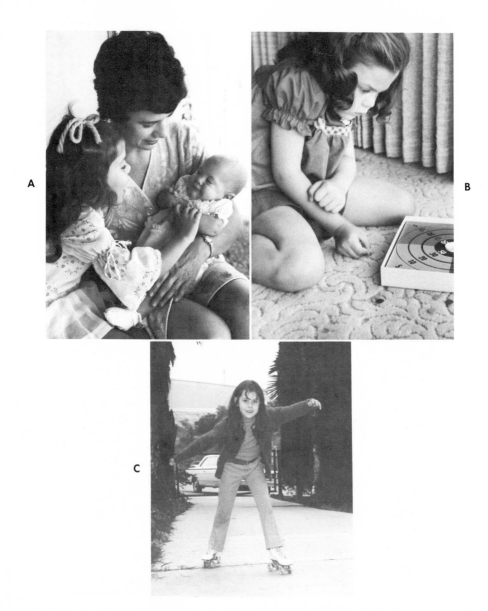

Fig. 20-20. School-age child at 6 years: **A**, likes to help with younger children; **B**, increased interest in games; **C**, can roller skate.

Language development. Vocabulary of 2500 words; skillful with language; can read and sound out simple words; can count.

Nutrition. Home schedules must allow time for adequate breakfast before school; supervision of lunch habits needed; to preserve appetite and protect teeth, avoid sugar and rich foods.

Common behavior. Period of transition from home to school; can tie shoes; prints first and last name; religious interest increases; has favorite T.V. shows; enjoys babies and helps with younger siblings; enjoys storytime.

Seven years

Physical growth. Height, 47 to 48 inches; weight, 50 to 51 pounds; loses upper central incisors.

Motor development. Enjoys outdoor sports; can ride bicycle, swim, and jump rope; can walk straight line.

Language development. Can read and write; learning to read clock.

Nutrition. Midafternoon snacking is common.

Common behavior. Usually stable age; enjoys solitary or group play; begins to prefer own sex; can bathe self and goes to bed when told; modest.

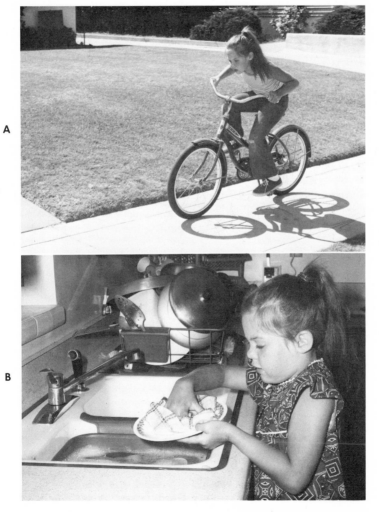

Fig. 20-21. School-age child at 7 years: **A,** can ride a bicycle; **B,** mother's helper.

Eight and nine years

Physical growth. Slow, gradual increase in size; permanent upper incisors present; may have 6 to 8 permanent teeth.

Motor development. Movements more graceful; manual skills more complex.

Language development. Can tell days of week at 8 years; can tell months of year at 9 years.

Nutrition. Manners and punctuality at meals may present problems; increasing interest and participation in other activities that compete with mealtime.

Common behavior. Eager, curious age; many projects, not always completed; begins to write rather than print. At 9 years, peer group very important; clubs, gangs, hero worship pronounced; competitive sports valued.

PREADOLESCENCE OR PUBERTY (TEN TO TWELVE YEARS)

Physical growth. Appearance and development of secondary sexual characteristics; growth spurt 2 years earlier for girls. Girls may show widening of hips, budding breasts, pubic hair, and occasionally menses. Boys ahead of girls in physical strength and endurance; boys increase in muscle mass and bone size especially shoulder girdle and ribs; penis and scrotum enlarge.

Nutrition. Huge appetite; may satisfy hunger with carbohydrate foods; need protein foods and minerals, especially calcium and iron.

Common behavior. Group activities intensify; sociable and sensitive to power of suggestion; has high aspirations; critical of parent and self.

ADOLESCENCE (TWELVE TO NINETEEN YEARS)

Early adolescence (twelve to sixteen years)

The basic psychosocial challenge of early adolescence is identity versus diffusion. The adolescent seeks to establish a sense of identity. If a good foundation has been laid (including the building blocks of trust,

autonomy, sexual identification, initiative, and learning), he will be able to integrate childhood identifications, basic biological drives, native endowment, and opportunities offered in social roles and feel secure regarding his part in society. Self-diffusion, or lack of a feeling of identity, may be temporarily unavoidable because of the physiological changes and psychological upheavals in this period.

Physical growth. Slow, continuous growth; secondary sex characteristics appear; girls mature earlier than boys.

Motor development. Hands and feet out of proportion; self-conscious, awkward.

Nutrition. Search for independence may be reflected by nutritional rebellion and fad diets.

Common behavior, activities, and problems. Participation in organizations may continue; interest in opposite sex increases; boys involved in sports; constantly challenges existing society; emotionally unstable, alternately depressed and exuberant; problems in self-knowledge, adjustment, and relations with opposite sex; ambivalence toward parents; activities reflect preparation for adult roles of citizen, homemaker, wage earner, and parent; increasing concern with philosophical and religious questions.

Late adolescence (sixteen to nineteen years)

The basic psychosocial challenge of late adolescence is intimacy versus isolation. When a young person feels secure in his identity, he is then able to establish warm, meaningful, constructive relationships with others and eventually a love-based, mutually satisfying sexual relationship with a member of the opposite sex; when the adolescent is unable to relate to others, he may develop a deep sense of isolation.

Physical growth. Adult size and proportions usually attained.

Motor development. Male physical strength and athletic ability highly prized.

Nutrition. Boys have tremendous, unwise appetites; girls are weight conscious and have erratic habits of food consumption. Good nutrition still requires parental encouragement and provision.

Common behavior. Need for acceptable self-image and self-respect; age of many problems, difficult decisions: school expenses, continuing education, work, or military service, courtship, and marriage plans; responsibilities of citizenship and of political and religious affiliations.

DENVER DEVELOPMENTAL SCREENING TEST (REVISED)*

The Denver Developmental Screening Test (DDST), a device for detecting developmental delays in infancy and the preschool years, has been standardized on a large cross section of the Denver population. The test is administered with ease and speed and lends itself to serial evaluations on the same test sheet.

Test materials

Skein of red wool, box of raisins, rattle with a narrow handle, Abbott aspirin bottle (Abbott—50 children's aluminum), bell, tennis ball, test form, pencil, eight 1-in. cubical counting blocks.

General administration instructions

The mother should be told that this is a developmental screening device to obtain an estimate of the child's level of development. This test relies on observations of what the child can do and on report by a parent who knows the child. Direct observation should be used whenever possible. Since the test requires active participation by the child, every effort should be made to put the child at ease. The child above 6 months of age may be tested while sitting on the mother's lap. This should be done in such a way that he can comfortably reach the test materials on the table. The test should [not] be administered before

---

*Prepared by William K. Frankenburg and Josiah B. Dodds, University of Colorado Medical Center, Denver, Colorado; reprinted with permission of the authors.

any frightening or painful procedures. A child will often withdraw if the examiner rushes demands on the child. One may start by laying out one or two test items in front of the child while asking the mother whether he performs some of the personal-social items. It is best to administer the first few test items well below the child's age level in order to assure him an initial successful experience. It is best to remove all test materials from the table, except the one that is being administered, to avoid distractions.

Steps in administering the test

1. Draw a vertical line on the examination sheet through the four sectors (Gross Motor, Fine Motor-Adaptive, Language, and Personal-Social) to represent the child's chronological age. Place the date of the examination at the top of the age line. For premature children, subtract the months prematurity from the chronological age. After 2 years of age it is no longer necessary to compensate for prematurity.

2. The items to be administered are those through which the child's chronological age line passes unless there are obvious deviations. In each sector one should establish the area where the child passes all of the items and the point at which he fails all of the items.

3. In the event that a child refuses to do some of the items requested by the examiner, it is suggested that the parent administer the item, provided she does so in the prescribed manner.

4. If a child passes an item, a large letter "P" is written on the bar at the 50% passing point. "F" designates a failure, and "R" designates a refusal.

5. Note how the child adjusted to the examination, that is, his cooperation, attention span, self-confidence, and how he related to his mother, the examiner and the test materials.

6. Ask the parent if the child's performance was typical of his performance at other times.

7. To retest the child on the same form,

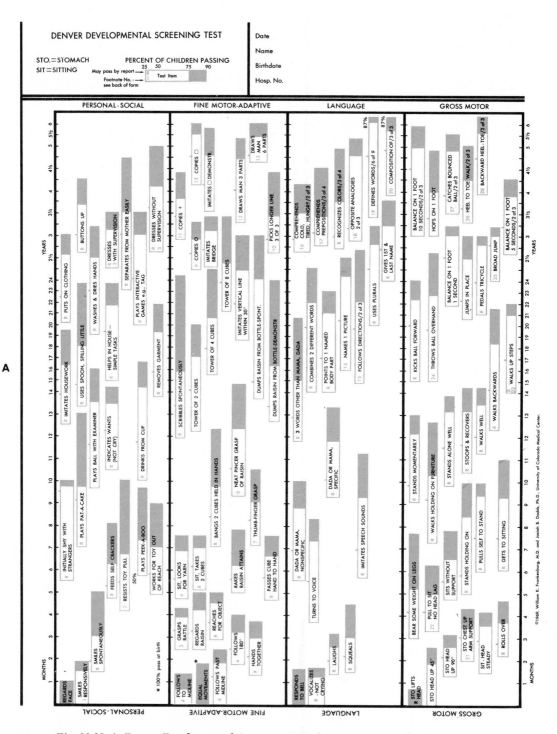

Fig. 20-22. A, Denver Developmental Screening Test sheet; **B,** reverse side of Denver Developmental Screening Test sheet. Footnotes correspond to numbered tasks on other side of test sheet.

```
                              DATE
                              NAME
        DIRECTIONS            BIRTHDATE
                              HOSP. NO.
```

1. Try to get child to smile by smiling, talking or waving to him. Do not touch him.
2. When child is playing with toy, pull it away from him. Pass if he resists.
3. Child does not have to be able to tie shoes or button in the back.
4. Move yarn slowly in an arc from one side to the other, about 6" above child's face.
   Pass if eyes follow 90° to midline. (Past midline; 180°)
5. Pass if child grasps rattle when it is touched to the backs or tips of fingers.
6. Pass if child continues to look where yarn disappeared or tries to see where it went. Yarn
   should be dropped quickly from sight from tester's hand without arm movement.
7. Pass if child picks up raisin with any part of thumb and a finger.
8. Pass if child picks up raisin with the ends of thumb and index finger using an over hand
   approach.

9. Pass any en-
   closed form.
   Fail continuous
   round motions.

10. Which line is longer?
    (Not bigger.) Turn
    paper upside down and
    repeat. (3/3 or 5/6)

11. Pass any
    crossing
    lines.

12. Have child copy
    first. If failed,
    demonstrate

   When giving items 9, 11 and 12, do not name the forms. Do not demonstrate 9 and 11.

13. When scoring, each pair (2 arms, 2 legs, etc.) counts as one part.
14. Point to picture and have child name it. (No credit is given for sounds only.)

B

    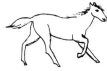

15. Tell child to: Give block to Mommie; put block on table; put block on floor. Pass 2 of 3.
    (Do not help child by pointing, moving head or eyes.)
16. Ask child: What do you do when you are cold? ..hungry? ..tired? Pass 2 of 3.
17. Tell child to: Put block on table; under table; in front of chair, behind chair.
    Pass 3 of 4. (Do not help child by pointing, moving head or eyes.)
18. Ask child: If fire is hot, ice is ?; Mother is a woman, Dad is a ?; a horse is big, a
    mouse is ?. Pass 2 of 3.
19. Ask child: What is a ball? ..lake? ..desk? ..house? ..banana? ..curtain? ..ceiling?
    ..hedge? ..pavement? Pass if defined in terms of use, shape, what it is made of or general
    category (such as banana is fruit, not just yellow). Pass 6 of 9.
20. Ask child: What is a spoon made of? ..a shoe made of? ..a door made of? (No other objects
    may be substituted.) Pass 3 of 3.
21. When placed on stomach, child lifts chest off table with support of forearms and/or hands.
22. When child is on back, grasp his hands and pull him to sitting. Pass if head does not hang back.
23. Child may use wall or rail only, not person. May not crawl.
24. Child must throw ball overhand 3 feet to within arm's reach of tester.
25. Child must perform standing broad jump over width of test sheet. (8-1/2 inches)
26. Tell child to walk forward, ⌐○⌐○⌐○⌐○→   heel within 1 inch of toe.
    Tester may demonstrate. Child must walk 4 consecutive steps, 2 out of 3 trials.
27. Bounce ball to child who should stand 3 feet away from tester. Child must catch ball with
    hands, not arms, 2 out of 3 trials.
28. Tell child to walk backward, ←○⌐○⌐○⌐○ toe within 1 inch of heel.
    Tester may demonstrate. Child must walk 4 consecutive steps, 2 out of 3 trials.

DATE AND BEHAVIORAL OBSERVATIONS (how child feels at time of test, relation to tester, attention
span, verbal behavior, self-confidence, etc,):

Fig. 20-22, cont'd. For legend see opposite page.

use a different color pencil for the scoring and age line.

8. Instructions for administering foot-noted items are on the back of the test form.

Interpretations

The test items are placed in four categories: Gross Motor, Fine Motor-Adaptive, Language, and Personal-Social. Each of the test items is designated by a bar which is so located under the age scale as to indicate clearly the ages at which 25%, 50%, 75%, and 90% of the standardization population could perform the particular test item. The left end of the bar designates the age at which 25% of the standardization population could perform the item; the hatch mark at the top of the bar, 50%; the left end of the shaded area, 75%; and the right end of the bar the age at which 90% of the standardization population could perform the items.

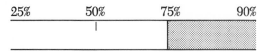

Failure to pass an item passed by 90% of children should be considered significant. Such a failure may be emphasized by coloring the right end of the bar of the failed item. Several failures in one sector are considered to be developmental delays. These delays may be due to:

1. the unwillingness of the child to use his ability

a. due to temporary phenomena, such as fatigue, illness, hospitalization, separation from the parent, fear, and so forth,

b. general unwillingness to do most things that are asked of him—such a condition may be just as detrimental as an inability to perform;

2. an inabiltiy to perform the item due to

a. general retardation,

b. pathological factors such as deafness or neurological impairment,

c. familial pattern of slow development in one or more areas.

If unexplained developmental delays are noted and are a valid reflection of a child's abilities, he should be rescreened one month later. If the delays persist, he should be further evaluated with more detailed diagnostic studies.

Caution:

1. [Fig. 20-22] is an overview of the test and is not complete.

2. The DDST is not an intelligence test. It is intended as a screening instrument for use in clinical practice to note whether the development of a particular child is within the normal range.

3. The training materials and test materials are available through LADOCA Foundation, East 51st Avenue and Lincoln Street, Denver, Colorado 80216.

21
Preventive pediatrics

The valuable "ounce of prevention" that we all have heard mentioned so often is frequently measured in milliliters, drops, or minutes spent with the physician and nurse for regular health supervision. The maintenance of an individual's optimal physical and mental health is a major goal of the physician and nurse.

Child health supervision is an extension of the prenatal care received by the mother and the developing fetus. Such supervision is designed to detect the presence of deformity or disease, to provide help in interpreting nutritional requirements and assuring proper food intake, to protect against certain preventable infectious diseases, and to offer appropriate counseling regarding child-rearing practices and commonly encountered child behavior patterns. Records of the child's individual health history are maintained, and his personal growth and development are often plotted in graph form. Health supervision may be carried on by the private physician, a public facility, or a child health conference.

The infant is usually scheduled to visit his physician monthly for the first 6 months and then every other month until his first birthday. Two to four visits should be made during the second year, and visits should be at least yearly thereafter. Special attention should be directed toward detection of any hearing impairment, visual defect, or orthopedic difficulty. Professional dental supervision should be started before any real problem is apparent, at about 3 years of age.

The school-age child in our society, because of his multiple community contacts and the activities of public health nurses in many schools, usually receives more consistent health supervision than the preschool child. Even so, the school-age child should have an annual physical examination and appropriate help and counseling as his growth and development level require.

The following topics of study are fundamental to the consideration of preventive pediatrics. It is hoped that these introductory discussions of basic nutrition, immunization, and child safety will encourage the student to continue investigation of the positive approach to health with increasing interest and reward.

SELF-FEEDING AND BASIC NUTRITION

Feeding and eating can be very natural. It is well to remember that a number of studies have indicated that infants and children select food of the right type at the right time and in the right amounts if it is available to them from the beginning of the self-feeding process. Babies accept solid foods and feed themselves when their neuromuscular progress permits them to do so.

Physiological guides
Hunger vs. appetite

Babies have a rhythmical pattern of hunger contractions characterized by discomfort, restlessness, and crying. The rhythm of hunger contractions differs in each baby, but they usually reappear every 3 to 4 hours. Babies should be fed according to their hunger rhythms, since rigidly prescribed feeding schedules ignore these hunger patterns. The normal young infant's nutritional needs can be met adequately the first 3 months by breast feeding or formula plus vitamins. The amount of milk or formula consumed varies from day to day, but in general most infants take 2 to 3 ounces of formula per pound of body weight, distributed over a 24-hour period. When sucking stops and the healthy infant falls asleep, the hunger-appetite mechanism has been satisfied. The infant should not be coaxed or forced to take more milk, regardless of the amount remaining in the bottle.

During infancy, hunger prompted by physiological needs chiefly controls food intake. Before 6 months, an infant will take almost any liquid consistently. However, in the latter half of the first year, preferences related to taste, appearance, and custom (that is, appetite) become important. Maternal diet, likes, and dislikes begin to condition the child's eating habits. By 1 year the baby shows definite preferences and dislikes. If the conditioning process has not been adverse, appetite may be trusted as a physiological index of the infant's nutritional needs. In this happy situation it is believed that if a baby refuses an essential food, he should not be forced to take it, since he will accept it later when he needs it.

Developmental guides
Protrusion reflex

The protrusion reflex manifests itself when the infant pushes out solid food placed on the anterior third of his tongue. This response, common during the first 9 weeks, disappears by the fourth month of life. It does not interfere with the baby's bottle or breast feeding because any nipple empties into the back of the mouth. However, it makes early feeding of solids difficult. The disappearance of the protrusion reflex is the neuromuscular indication for the introduction of semisolid food. A number of investigators believe that the practice of giving pureed food before 2½ or 3 months of age produces neither beneficial nor harmful results, but rather attests to the remarkable adaptability of the infant to whims of his caretakers.

Getting the baby to accept the spoon willingly is an important learning process that proceeds slowly. Usually, new food should be offered first, while the baby is hungry. However, a *very* hungry baby may refuse a new food because of his urgent desire for milk and his low frustration tolerance.

Place a small amount of food on the baby's lips to get him accustomed to the taste. The first solid food introduced is usually cereal and should be almost as thin as milk. Solid food may be introduced as early as 3 weeks but need not be stressed until the protrusion reflex has disappeared.

Self-feeding

Hand-to-mouth self-feeding begins before 1 year of age. If the baby is prevented from feeding himself when he is neuromuscularly ready, the acquisition of this skill may be delayed for weeks or months. A 6-month-old child can usually put his hands around a supported bottle and guide it to his lips. If permitted, the 7-month-old may hold the bottle by himself. At 8 months he can feed himself a cookie. Chewing motions appear at about 8 or 9 months and are the neuromuscular indications that lumpy foods can be introduced whether the teeth are present or not. Chopped foods should be introduced gradually. If undigested food appears in the stool, one should wait a week and try again. By 9 months, an empty plastic or metal cup may be placed on the baby's tray for practice. At 10 months of age he can begin practice with a spoon. Shortly after 12 months he can use a cup well, and by 18 months he can use a spoon skillfully. Self-feeding is usually accomplished between 12 and 18 months and consists of a combination of feeding skills using the spoon, hand, or cup.

Basic nutrition concepts

A happy child with good health reflects good eating habits. Good nutrition is like a good insurance policy. During the course of a lifetime it pays dividends in the form of a well-developed body with good muscles, smooth skin, glossy hair, and clear, bright eyes. As the dividends accumulate, one

Table 21-1. Clinical signs of nutritional status

	Good	*Poor*
General appearance	Alert, responsive	Listless, apathetic, cachexic
Hair	Shiny, lustrous; healthy scalp	Stringy, dull, brittle, dry, depigmented
Neck (glands)	No enlargement	Thyroid enlarged
Skin (face and neck)	Smooth, slightly moist; good color, reddish pink mucous membranes	Greasy, discolored, scaly
Eyes	Bright, clear; no fatigue circles beneath	Dryness, signs of infection, increased vascularity, glassiness, thickened conjunctiva
Lips	Good color, moist	Dry, scaly, swollen; angular lesions (stomatitis)
Tongue	Good pink color, surface papillae present, no lesions	Papillary atrophy, smooth appearance; swollen, red, beefy (glossitis)
Gums	Good pink color; no swelling or bleeding, firm	Marginal redness or swelling, receding, spongy
Teeth	Straight, no crowding, well-shaped jaw, clean, no discoloration	Unfilled caries, absent teeth, worn surfaces, mottled, malposition
Skin (general)	Smooth, slightly moist, good color	Rough, dry, scaly, pale, pigmented, irritated, petechiae, bruises
Abdomen	Flat	Swollen
Legs, feet	No tenderness, weakness, or swelling; good color	Edema, tender calf, tingling, weakness
Skeleton	No malformations	Bowlegs, knock-knees, chest deformity at diaphragm, beaded ribs, prominent scapulae
Weight	Normal for height, age, body build	Overweight or underweight
Posture	Erect, arms and legs straight, abdomen in, chest out	Sagging shoulders, sunken chest, humped back
Muscles	Well developed, firm	Flaccid, poor tone; undeveloped, tender
Nervous control	Good attention span for age; does not cry easily, not irritable or restless	Inattentive, irritable
Gastrointestinal function	Good appetite and digestion; normal, regular elimination	Anorexia, indigestion, constipation, or diarrhea
General vitality	Endurance, energetic, sleeps well at night; vigorous	Easily fatigued, no energy, falls asleep in school, looks tired, apathetic

From Williams, S. R.: Nutrition and diet therapy, ed. 2, St. Louis, 1973, The C. V. Mosby Co., p. 380.

finds that appetite, digestion, and elimination are good. Finally, the policy (good nutrition) matures as one enjoys a high level of health in old age.

All systems and tissues in the body depend on proper nourishment for their existence and maintenance; this nourishment is obtained from the foods we eat and drink. Our food must perform three functions within the body:

1. Provide heat and energy
2. Build and repair the tissues of the body
3. Regulate the body processes

Substances essential to perform these vital functions are the following:

1. Oxygen
2. Water
3. Carbohydrates
4. Proteins
5. Fats
6. Minerals
7. Vitamins

Oxygen

Oxygen is so vital to the activity of the body cells that without it, life would cease immediately. The natural source of oxygen is fresh air. Through the activity of the respiratory system, oxygen enters the circulating blood, which carries it to every living cell. An abundance of fresh air is desirable at all ages.

Water

Second only to oxygen, water is necessary for life. Without water, death ensues in just a few days. Water comprises about 70% of the body weight. It is a basic constituent of all cells and is a major component in blood, lymph, spinal fluid, and the various body excretions such as urine and sweat. During infancy, considerable water is lost through the kidneys and skin. To keep pace with normal fluid losses, the infant must receive a daily intake of at least 150 ml. per kilogram (2¼ ounces per pound). The infant is subject to conditions causing water loss, notably fever, vomiting, and diarrhea. Unless water intake is increased during these abnormal states, symptoms of dehydration and its grave consequences appear rapidly.

Carbohydrates

Carbohydrates serve as the body's primary source of heat and energy. Examples of carbohydrate-rich foods include grains, fruits, vegetables, and sweets. (Pure sugar is 100% carbohydrate.) Carbohydrates not utilized for heat and energy are stored in many of the body's organs (especially in the liver and muscles as glycogen), or they are converted to fatty tissue. Glycogen is readily converted in the liver to glucose when carbohydrate is not available in the food consumed. Since immediate heat and energy requirements have priority over tissue growth and repair, the body is also capable of utilizing tissue fat and protein to furnish its energy needs. It is therefore important to have sufficient carbohydrates in the diet to meet these needs adequately, thus sparing protein for its primary use of building and maintaining tissues.

The waste products of carbohydrate metabolism are excreted from the body in the form of carbon dioxide and water.

Protein

Every living cell and almost all body fluids contain protein. Protein is necessary for the growth, repair, and maintenance of all body tissues. Immune bodies, which help the body resist infection, contain protein. Enzymes and hormones also include protein in their composition.

The end products of protein digestion are amino acids—small units, which, when properly reassembled, form the needed body protein. Of the many amino acids known, nine are essential for normal growth and body maintenance. Amino acids are found in varying amounts in various forms in foods.

Proteins are divided into three groups: complete, partially complete, and incomplete. The complete proteins contain all nine essential amino acids. A dietary supply of these amino acids is necessary because they cannot be synthesized by the body. Proteins from animal sources such as meats, poultry, fresh eggs, milk, and cheese provide the essential amino acids. Gelatin is 100% protein from an animal source but is not a complete protein.

Partially complete proteins are found in cereal products and vegetables. They contain many amino acids but not all the essential ones. When protein intake is not sufficient, the result is a slow rate of growth and increased susceptibility to bacterial infections.

Incomplete proteins such as corn and gelatin are incapable of either maintaining or supporting life. When an incomplete protein is the only source of protein, malnutrition, or marasmus, results.

Children will receive adequate amounts of protein in meat, milk, and eggs. The overall protein value may be improved when both animal and vegetable protein are eaten together. Since there is no storage of amino acids in the body, it is essential that food contain sufficient amounts. Amino acids not needed by the body tissues are returned to the liver, where approximately half are converted into urea, a waste product excreted by the kidney, and half are changed into glycogen or fatty tissue and stored to meet future energy requirements.

Finally, it is important to note that all nine essential amino acids work together. New tissue cannot be formed unless all the essential amino acids are present in the bloodstream simultaneously. Therefore it is imperative that some form of complete protein be included at each meal.

Fats

Certain fatty acids found in dietary fats are necessary to maintain good nutrition. These essential fatty acids permit normal growth and the health and maintenance of normal skin. Fat also provides the vehicle of absorption of the fat-soluble vitamins, A, D, E, and K. Unless dissolved in fats, these vitamins cannot be retained in the body in adequate amounts.

Fats are found in both animal and vegetable foods. Egg yolks, butter, meat, soybean oil, cottonseed oil, corn oil, and olive oil are good sources of the essential fatty acids. It is important that one of these sources be included in the daily diet, since the essential fatty acids cannot be synthe-

sized from other fats. The waste products of fat metabolism, like those of carbohydrate metabolism, are carbon dioxide and water.

If fat intake is inadequate, the child may not receive the essential fatty acids required to prevent the formation of certain types of skin lesions. The rapidly growing young infant is highly susceptible to this deficiency and will develop dryness and thickening of the skin with chafing and desquamation if the cause is unrelieved.

Energy requirements

Whenever work is to be performed by the body, energy is needed. The body must be supplied with fuel in the form of food in sufficient amounts to meet the energy requirements of that individual. To determine how much food a child needs, it is necessary to know the child's metabolic rate, or "rate of heat production." The unit of heat in metabolism is called a *Calorie*. (It may be defined as the amount of heat needed to raise the temperature of 1 liter of water 1° C.) A person's *basal* metabolic rate (BMR) is described as the minimal amount of heat produced by body cells

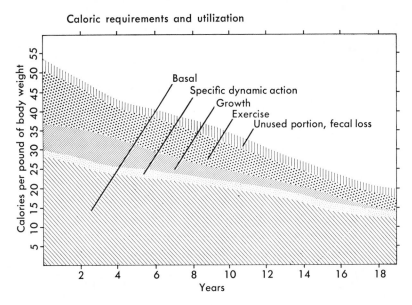

Fig. 21-1. To determine the total caloric requirements of a child, multiply his weight in pounds by the number of calories for his age.

when the body is at rest with only vital processes such as circulation and respiration functioning. Several factors—size, age, sex, hormonal levels, and body temperature—influence the BMR. The *total* metabolic rate of a person represents the total amount of heat produced by the body in a given time (usually 24 hours) under normal conditions. The total metabolic rate of a child represents the amount of food his body must burn not only to keep alive and awake but also to continue his physical activity, to support growth, to supply specific dynamic action (ingestion and assimilation of his food), and to replace calories lost (Fig. 21-1).

Total energy expended determines the need for calories. The fuel values of energy-producing foods are as follows:

Carbohydrates	4 calories per gram
Protein	4 calories per gram
Fats	9 calories per gram

Table 21-2. Significant vitamins

Vitamin	Function	Effects of deficiency
A	Promotes good eyesight	Night blindness
	Aids in maintaining resistance to infections	Frequent infections
	Maintains skin integrity	Dry, rough skin; papular eruptions
	Helps form and maintain mucous membrane	Burning, itching eyes
	Helps in formation of bone and teeth	Retarded growth; thin and defective tooth enamel
B complex		
B₁ (thiamine)	Aids in maintenance and function of nervous system	Beriberi
		Listlessness, fatigue, and irritability
	Regulates appetite; normal digestion	Anorexia, vomiting, and diarrhea
	Promotes a feeling of general well-being	Generalized weakness; gross symptoms of neuromuscular, digestive, and cardiovascular impairment
B₂ (riboflavin)	Aids in eye adaptation to light	Photophobia; impairment of visual acuity; cataracts
	Provides essentials for metabolism of carbohydrate, fat, and protein	Impaired formation of blood cells
	Necessary for normal growth	Anemia
Niacin (nicotinic acid)	Essential for normal function of digestive tract and nervous system	General poor health
		Gastrointestinal changes—loss of appetite, nausea, vomiting, abdominal pain, red tongue, ulcers and fissures of tongue
		Dermatitis
		Nervous system manifestations—headaches and dizziness, impairment of memory, and neurotic symptoms
C (ascorbic acid)	Important role in formation, maintenance, and repair of teeth, bones, and blood vessels	Scurvy
		Loose teeth; faulty bones; slow growth
	Facilitates absorption of dietary iron	Weakness and irritability
	Maintenance of normal blood hemoglobin levels	Delayed healing of wounds
		Cutaneous hemorrhages
D	Enhances absorption of calcium and phosphorus	Rickets
		Retarded growth and lack of vigor
	Plays a vital role in formation of normal bone	Variety of bone deformities—large head, pigeon chest, kyphosis, and curved long bones
	Promotes tooth development	Teeth erupt late and decay early

Table 21-3. Food intake for good nutrition according to food groups and the average size of servings at different age levels

Food group	Servings per day	Average size of servings					
		1 yr.	2-3 yr.	4-5 yr.	6-9 yr.	10-12 yr.	13-15 yr.
Milk and cheese (1½ oz. cheese = 1 cup milk)	4	½ cup	½-¾ cup	¾ cup	¾-1 cup	1 cup	1 cup
Meat group (protein foods)	At least 3						
Egg		1 egg	1 egg	1 egg	1 egg	1 egg	1 or more
Lean meat, fish, poultry (liver once a week)		2 tbsp.	2 tbsp.	4 tbsp.	2-3 oz. (4-6 tbsp.)	3-4 oz.	4 oz. or more
Peanut butter			1 tbsp.	2 tbsp.	2-3 tbsp.	3 tbsp.	3 tbsp.
Fruits and vegetables	At least 4, including:						
Vitamin C source (citrus fruits, berries, tomato, cabbage, cantaloupe)	1 or more (twice as much tomato as citrus)	⅓ cup citrus	½ cup	½ cup	1 medium orange	1 medium orange	1 medium orange
Vitamin A source (green or yellow fruits and vegetables)	1 or more	2 tbsp.	3 tbsp.	4 tbsp. (¼ cup)	¼ cup	⅓ cup	½ cup
Other vegetables (potato, legumes, etc.) *or*	2 or more	2 tbsp.	3 tbsp.	4 tbsp. (¼ cup)	⅓ cup	½ cup	¾ cup
Other fruits (apple, banana, etc.)		¼ cup	⅓ cup	½ cup	1 medium	1 medium	1 medium
Cereals (whole grain or enriched)	At least 4						
Bread		½ slice	1 slice	1½ slices	1-2 slices	2 slices	2 slices
Ready-to-eat cereals		½ oz.	¾ oz.	1 oz.	1 oz.	1 oz.	1 oz.
Cooked cereal (including macaroni, spaghetti, rice, etc.)		¼ cup	⅓ cup	½ cup	½ cup	¾ cup	1 cup or more
Fats and carbohydrates	To meet caloric needs						
Butter, margarine, mayonnaise, oils: 1 tbsp. = 100 calories		1 tbsp.	1 tbsp.	1 tbsp.	2 tbsp.	2 tbsp.	2-4 tbsp.
Desserts and sweets: 100-calorie portions as follows: ⅓ cup pudding or ice cream, 2 to 3 in. cookies, 1 oz. cake, 1⅓ oz. pie, 2 tbsp. jelly, jam, honey, sugar		1 portion	1½ portions	1½ portions	3 portions	3 portions	3-6 portions

Adapted by Bennett, M. J., and Hansen, A. E., from Four groups of the daily food guide, Institute of Home Economics, United States Department of Agriculture, Publication No. 30, Children's Bureau, United States Department of Health, Education, and Welfare, Washington, D. C., 1945.

The average distribution of calories in a well-balanced diet is as follows:

Carbohydrates	50%
Protein	15%
Fats	35% (or less)

If the number of grams of carbohydrate, protein, and fat in a food is known, the caloric value can be determined by multiplying each by the appropriate fuel value.

When food is not available, the body's nutritional reserves and tissues are consumed to meet its need for caloric energy. Carbohydrates stored as glycogen in different body organs are consumed first; fat deposits are consumed next. Usually, fat in the extremities is consumed before fat located in the trunk. Fat in the cheek pads is consumed last. Recessed cheeks in young children usually indicates severe malnutrition.

Minerals

Calcium	Phosphorus
Magnesium	Manganese
Sodium	Chloride
Potassium	Molybdenum
Iron	Selenium
Iodine	Fluoride
Copper	Arsenic
Zinc	Cobalt

The preceding list indicates minerals that are essential to many body structures and functions. The action of minerals are interrelated in the body, and often one mineral is combined with another to complete the reaction. (For example, in the bones, calcium and phosphorus function together, and sufficient vitamin D is necessary for the proper utilization of calcium.) Most of these minerals are readily obtained from a well-balanced diet. Two minerals, calcium and iron, require special attention. Deficits of the other minerals do not ordinarily arise from inadequate intake. However, large amounts of minerals may be lost through vomiting and diarrhea.

Iron. One of the most vital elements in the body is iron. It is a component of hemoglobin, the oxygen-bearing element in the blood. Iron is required for growth, and

Table 21-4. Recommended daily dietary allowances,[a] revised 1974

	Age (years)	Weight (kg)	Weight (lbs)	Height (cm)	Height (in)	Energy (kcal)[b]	Protein (g)	Vitamin A activity (RE)[c]	Vitamin A activity (IU)	Vitamin D (IU)	Vitamin E activity[e] (IU)	Ascorbic acid (mg)	Fola. (µg
								Fat-soluble vitamins					
Infants	0.0-0.5	6	14	60	24	kg × 117	kg × 2.2	420[d]	1400	400	4	35	5
	0.5-1.0	9	20	71	28	kg × 108	kg × 2.0	400	2000	400	5	35	5
Children	1-3	13	28	86	34	1300	23	400	2000	400	7	40	10
	4-6	20	44	110	44	1800	30	500	2500	400	9	40	20
	7-10	30	66	135	54	2400	36	700	3300	400	10	40	30
Males	11-14	44	97	158	63	2800	44	1000	5000	400	12	45	40
	15-18	61	134	172	69	3000	54	1000	5000	400	15	45	40
	19-22	67	147	172	69	3000	54	1000	5000	400	15	45	40
Females	11-14	44	97	155	62	2400	44	800	4000	400	12	45	40
	15-18	54	119	162	65	2100	48	800	4000	400	12	45	40
	19-22	58	128	162	65	2100	46	800	4000	400	12	45	40

Adapted from Recommended dietary allowances, ed. 8, Publication ISBN 0-309-02216-9, Food Nutrition Boa
[a]The allowances are intended to provide for individual variations among most normal persons as they live in provide other nutrients for which human requirements have been less well defined.
[b]Kilojoules (kJ) = 4.2 × kcal
[c]Retinol equivalents
[d]Assumed to be all as retinol in milk during the first six months of life. All subsequent intakes are assumed to be h as retinol and one fourth as β-carotene.
[e]Total vitamin E activity, estimated to be 80 percent as α-tocopherol and 20 percent other tocopherols.
[f]The folacin allowances refer to dietary sources as determined by *Lactobacillus casei* assay. Pure forms of folacin n
[g]Although allowances are expressed as niacin, it is recognized that on the average 1 mg of niacin is derived from ea

the need for iron varies with the rapidity of growth at different periods of infancy and childhood.

Iron deficiency leads to the development of anemia, or insufficient hemoglobin for the needs of the body. Anemia causes few deaths, but contributes seriously to the weakness, ill health, and substandard performance of many children throughout the world. The greatest incidence of iron-deficiency anemia occurs in infants and young children. Both cow's milk and breast milk contain insufficient iron. When the stores present at birth become depleted (at about 3 months of age), iron-deficiency anemia develops unless a supplement is given. The addition of iron-containing pabulum or cereal offered at about 3 weeks of age prevents this anemia and the need for additional iron supplements. Foods rich in iron are liver, meat, and egg yolk.

Calcium. Relatively large amounts of calcium are required to perform many vital functions in the body. Calcium is essential for normal heart action and is an important

element in the blood-clotting mechanism. Calcium builds bones and teeth and is necessary for normal muscular-skeletal action. When there is insufficient calcium in the diet, the blood will use the calcium in the bones to maintain the normal composition of the blood. Bowed legs and rickets may result. Hypocalcemia may cause neonatal tetany, crying, muscle twitching, and convulsions. Unrelieved, it may end in death. Milk and milk products are good sources of calcium.

Vitamins

Fat-soluble vitamins	Water-soluble vitamins
A	C
D	B complex
E	Thiamin (B_1)
K	Riboflavin (B_2)
	Niacin
	Folic acid
	Pyridoxine (B_6)
	Biotin
	Pantothenic acid
	Cyanocobalamin (B_{12})

Water-soluble vitamins					Minerals					
Niacin^g (mg)	Riboflavin (B_2) (mg)	Thiamin (B_1) (mg)	Vitamin B_6 (mg)	Vitamin B_{12} (μg)	Calcium (mg)	Phosphorus (mg)	Iodine (μg)	Iron (mg)	Magnesium (mg)	Zinc (mg)
5	0.4	0.3	0.3	0.3	360	240	35	10	60	3
8	0.6	0.5	0.4	0.3	540	400	45	15	70	5
9	0.8	0.7	0.6	1.0	800	800	60	15	150	10
12	1.1	0.9	0.9	1.5	800	800	80	10	200	10
16	1.2	1.2	1.2	2.0	800	800	110	10	250	10
18	1.5	1.4	1.6	3.0	1200	1200	130	18	350	15
20	1.8	1.5	2.0	3.0	1200	1200	150	18	400	15
20	1.8	1.5	2.0	3.0	800	800	140	10	350	15
16	1.3	1.2	1.6	3.0	1200	1200	115	18	300	15
14	1.4	1.1	2.0	3.0	1200	1200	115	18	300	15
14	1.4	1.1	2.0	3.0	800	800	100	18	300	15

tional Academy of Sciences, National Research Council, Washington, D. C., 1974.

ited States under usual environmental stresses. Diets should be based on a variety of common foods in order to

retinol and half as β-carotene when calculated from international units. As retinol equivalents, three fourths are

effective in doses less than one fourth of the recommended dietary allowance.

mg of dietary tryptophan.

Vitamins are organic compounds found in minute quantities in foods. They participate as catalysts in almost all metabolic processes and are vital to growth and good health. Vitamins A and D are the only two vitamins stored in the body. Excessive intake of these two vitamins will result in toxic manifestations such as skin lesions, liver enlargement, and bone spurs. Any vitamin may be lacking, causing disturbances in the pattern of growth, metabolism, and development of the child.

The best sources of vitamins are found in the natural foods. A well-balanced diet containing the Basic Four Food Groups (see Fig. 7-2, p. 54) will assure an adequate supply of vitamins. Six vitamins merit special consideration (Table 21-2). The foods that supply these vitamins also supply all other vitamin needs.

Summary

Digestion refers to those processes that prepare food for assimilation into the bloodstream or lymphatics of the body, but metabolism refers to all the changes that occur in the utilization of those nutrients by the cells and the generation of heat and energy. Amino acids, essential fatty acids, vitamins, and minerals are utilized primarily for cell growth and repair. They are also utilized in the formation of enzymes, hormones, and other body substances. Carbohydrates and fats are utilized primarily for caloric energy (that is, to supply fuel to keep the body warm) and mechanical energy for performing the body's work. When caloric needs are not met by fats and carbohydrates, protein is then utilized for energy. Adequate intake of carbohydrates and fats will spare protein for cell growth. Therefore it is necessary that the diet contain a balance of all six substances—carbohydrate, fat, protein, vitamins, minerals, and water—as each one plays its own vital role in the processes of growth and development.

IMMUNIZATION

The brilliant success achieved in conquering the classic contagious diseases of childhood is attributed to immunization. Through immunization a person is able to build up defenses against certain infectious diseases. When a person is able to resist a certain disease, he is said to be immune. He is immune because antibodies are present that injure or destroy the disease-producing agent or neutralize its toxins. Active immunization (artificial) is achieved when certain substances called *antigens* are injected into the body to stimulate the production of antibodies. Immunization is the best and cheapest method of preventing illness. In fact, it is the most routine procedure in preventive pediatrics.

Because the mechanisms for developing immunity are immature in the young infant, he is very susceptible to some infections. The protection he has against infection is obtained from his mother, if she is immune. Any passive immunity acquired from the mother lasts about 4 to 6 months and may protect the child against diphtheria, tetanus, measles, and poliomyelitis. Since there is great variability in such passive protection in the young infant and no passive immunity against pertussis (whooping cough), immunization should be initiated as early as possible. Combined antigens reduce the number of injections, enhance the action of each, and establish a desired immunity within the first 6 months of life.

Current practice begins immunization when the infant is between 8 and 12 weeks of age. A "triple toxoid" of diphtheria, pertussis, and tetanus antigens in one injection and a concurrent feeding of oral polio vaccine are given. The "triple toxoid" DTP is repeated three times at intervals of not less than 1 month. The necessity to prevent the high mortality from pertussis (whooping cough) in infancy is the main reason for the early start in basic DTP immunization. However, pertussis vaccine is not considered to be as satisfactory as diphtheria and tetanus toxoids. It does not provide absolute protection.

After the initial series of immunizations, "recall" or "booster" doses are given to stimulate high antibody levels and maintain

Table 21-5. Recommended schedule for active immunization of normal infants and children

2 mo	DTP[1]	TOPV[2]
4 mo	DTP	TOPV
6 mo	DTP	TOPV
1 yr	Measles[3]	Tuberculin Test[4]
	Rubella[3]	Mumps[3]
1½ yr	DTP	TOPV
4-6 yr	DTP	TOPV
14-16 yr	Td[5]	and thereafter every 10 years

From Report of the Committee on the Control of Infectious Diseases, Red Book, Evanston, Ill., 1974, American Academy of Pediatrics, p. 3. Readers must consult the publication to obtain details of immunization procedures.
[1]DTP—diphtheria and tetanus toxoids combined with pertussis vaccine.
[2]TOPV—trivalent oral poliovirus vaccine. This recommendation is suitable for breast-fed as well as bottle-fed infants.
[3]May be given at 1 year as measles-rubella or measles-mumps-rubella combined vaccines.
[4]Frequency of repeated tuberculin tests depends on risk of exposure of the child and on the prevalence of tuberculosis in the population group. The initial test should be at the time of, or preceding, the measles immunization.
[5]Td—combined tetanus and diphtheria toxoids (adult type) for those more than 6 years of age in contrast to diphtheria and tetanus (DT) which contains a larger amount of diphtheria antigen. *Tetanus toxoid at time of injury:* For clean, minor wounds, no booster dose is needed by a fully immunized child unless more than 10 years have elapsed since the last dose. For contaminated wounds, a booster dose should be given if more than 5 years have elapsed since the last dose.

Storage of vaccines

Because biologics are of varying stability, the manufacturers' recommendations for optimal storage conditions (e.g., temperature, light) should be carefully followed. Failure to observe these precautions may significantly reduce the potency and effectiveness of the vaccines.

maximum immunity. Children who have received three doses of "triple toxoid" (DPT) and oral polio vaccine (OPV) should be given a booster dose at 18 months of age. Subsequent booster doses are recommended between 4 and 6 years of age. Active, up-to-date immunization produces a degree of resistance in children comparable to that which follows the natural infection.

Precautions

1. Needles and syringes must be sterile before use.
2. Injection site and rubber stopper should be cleaned with an antiseptic solution such as 2% tincture of iodine.
3. Toxoids and vaccines (antigens) containing alum are given intramuscularly, preferably into the midlateral thigh or deltoid muscles.
4. Systemic and severe local reactions after an injection call for a delay or decrease in succeeding doses.
5. Aspirin, 1 grain per year of age (up to 5 grains), may be given 2 hours after the injection. This dosage may be repeated as needed *not more than five times at 4-hour intervals* without medical consultation.

Contraindications

1. When acute febrile illness and other infections are present, the interval between injections may be prolonged and does not interfere with final immunity.
2. Pertussis immunization should not be repeated if any symptoms of central nervous system disorders or platelet destruction (such as petechiae or bruising) develop after a DPT injection. DT should be used instead.
3. Neurological disorders *do not* constitute a valid reason for deferring or withholding routine immunization. However, if a convulsion or coma occurs, immunization may be delayed until after infancy and then begun cautiously.
4. Immunization procedures are deferred during the administration of steroids, irradiation, and anticancer drug therapy because antibody response is depressed or abnormal.
5. Live attenuated vaccines against measles, rubella, and mumps are *not* given to pregnant women, patients with generalized malignancy, or those

who have recently received immune serum globulin, plasma, or blood.

Rubella virus vaccine

The principal objective of rubella (German measles) control is preventing infection of the fetus. This can best be achieved by eliminating the transmission of the virus among children, who are the major source of infection for pregnant women. All children between 1 year of age and puberty should receive the *live rubella virus* vaccine. The primary target is children in kindergarten and the early grades. Pregnant women *should not* be given live rubella virus vaccine because it may cause damage to the fetus.

Mumps virus vaccine

The principal objective is prevention of mumps in preadolescent males and young male adults. Live attenuated mumps virus vaccine is recommended for all susceptible children and especially for preadolescent males and men who have not had the disease.

Measles (rubeola) vaccine

One successful inoculation with the live attenuated measles (rubeola) vaccine confers lifelong protection against the disease. The vaccine should be given to all children over 1 year of age unless documented evidence of the disease exists. It should also be given to children who have already been immunized against measles with either gamma globulin or vaccine made from killed organisms.

Smallpox vaccine

Smallpox immunization is no longer recommended since the risk of complications outweighs the risk of acquiring the disease. The last case of smallpox in the United States was recorded in 1949. In the years since 1949, it has been estimated that more than 160 vaccine-associated deaths have occurred. In addition, significant neurological and dermal complications have occurred at the rate of approximately 8,000 per year.

Smallpox vaccination is required only of individuals at special risk: travelers to and from endemic areas, such as India, Pakistan, Nepal, Sudan, and Ethiopia, and health service personnel who may contact affected patients. These individuals should be revaccinated every 3 years.

Passive immunity

Immune serum globulin (ISG), commonly known as gamma globulin, is an antibody-rich fraction of pooled plasma from normal donors. It confers temporary immunity that is attained in approximately 2 days and lasts from 2 to 6 weeks. The large, viscous dose should be divided and given intramuscularly in two different sites with an 18- or 20-gauge needle. ISG is limited in supply and has been clearly documented to be helpful in (1) prevention or modification of measles and hepatitis A (infectious) and (2) treatment of certain antibody deficiencies.

Nursing responsibilities

The office nurse can do a great deal by her efficient, yet kindly manner to help parents realize the importance of continuing the immunization program. She should be sure that the parent knows what type of injections the child is receiving. She should be aware of any allergies that the child has demonstrated and learn if there have been any noteworthy reactions to previous immunizations. A continuous written record of the type of protection the child has received and the dates of administration should be given the parents. The date and time of the next appointment should be clearly understood (Fig. 21-2).

The nurse's good-humored recognition that the medicine does sting a bit and that a sincere "ouch" is not out of place may help wary youngsters. A matter-of-fact, positive attitude rather than an overly solicitous manner seems to offer more support to the parent and child.

Sometimes it is worthwhile to inquire about the current status of the parents' immunizations. The proverbial daily apple really is not too successful in preventing

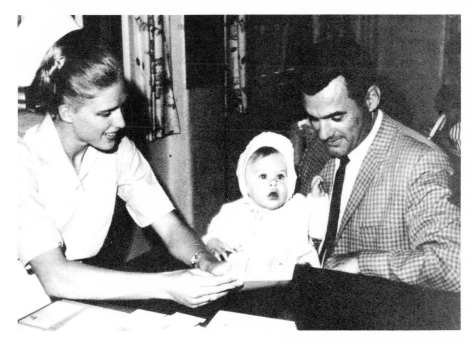

Fig. 21-2. Immunizations should not be given without follow-up instructions to the parents. This nurse is explaining the World Health Organization immunization record and what to do if certain signs and symptoms develop after Mary Ann's inoculation. (Courtesy U. S. Naval Regional Medical Center, San Diego, Calif.)

illness, but regular immunization is a proved and necessary protection for both young and old.

• • •

Immunization is so important that information about the procedure should be given in prenatal classes. New parents are very concerned about "doing what is right" for their child. Before going home from the hospital, the mother and father should be reminded again about the immunization program. Although immunizations are usually given by the private practitioner or his nurse as part of the baby's regular health checkups, parents of modest means should be told of community resources where free immunization services are available.

CHILD SAFETY

Successful prevention and treatment of infectious diseases and nutritional disorders have resulted in a marked decrease in child mortality. The greatest threat to the health and well-being of the child today is

the accident. An estimated 15,000 to 16,000 children under 15 years of age die annually in the United States from accidents.

Accidents kill more children than the next six leading causes of childhood death combined.

	Death rates* *Ages 1 to 14*
Accidents	23.0
Cancer	6.4
Congenital anomalies	4.1
Pneumonia	3.0
Homicide	1.1
Heart disease	1.1
Stroke	0.7

The magnitude of the accident problem is further stressed by the fact that 17 million children suffer nonfatal injuries every year. Many of these children are crippled or permanently disabled for life. Of course, not all childhood accidents are brought to the attention of medical personnel. Perhaps an additional 25% of children up to 14

*Deaths per 100,000 population, National Center for Health Statistics, 1970.

321

years of age have significant but unreported injuries. Thus the conservative figure of 17 million childhood injuries emphasizes a serious national problem.

Accidents

An accident is defined as "an unpremeditated event resulting in a recognizable injury." The most common accidents that injure children consist mainly of cuts, piercings with instruments, blows from objects, animal bites, and injuries related to motor vehicles. Motor vehicles are the major cause of accidental death. Also ranked among the leading causes of fatal accidents are drownings, fires, and falls (Fig. 21-3).

Certain factors seem to be influential in causing childhood accidents: (1) approximately half of all the fatalities occur in children under 5 years of age; (2) boys at all ages have more accidents than girls; (3) the nonwhite population has a considerably higher incidence of accidents than

does the white population; (4) most accidents occur during the spring and summer months; (5) a higher percentage of accidents occur in the home, especially during the preschool period; (6) the child between 1 and 2 years of age is most vulnerable to accidents of all sorts; (7) some children are accident-prone. Combinations of certain personality characteristics and environmental influences predispose a child toward repetitive accidents.

Prevention. Accidents do not just happen; there is always a cause. Good safety habits could eliminate many of these causes. Gains in safeguarding the lives of children depend on accident prevention.

In the past, much emphasis has been placed on two particular approaches to accident prevention: (1) elimination of specific environmental hazards peculiar to different age groups and (2) alterations of the child's behavior through safety education. A glance at the data of the past years

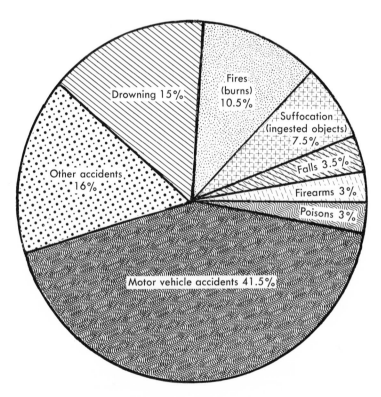

Fig. 21-3. Major causes of accidental death in children from birth to 14 years of age. (Data from Vital Statistics Division, National Center for Health Statistics, 1972.)

shows a continued increase in the actual number of accidents.

Our vital statistics indicate the number of children injured and the kinds of accidents causing the injuries. However, they do not provide sufficient detail about each individual case to fully describe the complete situation of each accident. This prevents the making of valid conclusions concerning accident causation and prevention in childhood. Often, vital information is not recorded. This is undoubtedly why specific recommendations for the prevention of certain injuries have not always been effective.

To date, there is no single approach to accident prevention. "Accidents" are the result of a large number of complex mechanisms. Like other illnesses, they can be conquered only through systematic investigation. To understand the nature and cause of accidents, several factors must be considered simultaneously: the host (the child who is affected), the agent (the object that is the direct cause), and the environment (the situation in which the accident takes place). This is known as the epidemiological approach to the study of accidents.

Although a great deal remains to be learned about the interaction of these major factors, the existing knowledge has led to the following new principles aimed at accident prevention:

1. Control of the agent whenever possible (for example, use of child-protective caps on medicine bottles and household products)

Table 21-6. Accidents common at various stages of development

Typical behavior	Type of accident	Precaution and safety education
Infant		
Sleeps most of time	Suffocation	Use a firm mattress, no pillow; destroy plastic covers and filmy bags
Wiggles and rolls	Falls	Never leave child unattended on a table, sofa, etc.; keep crib bars up
Helpless in water	Drowning	Never leave alone in bathtub or near pools
Sucks on objects	Choking; ingestion of foreign objects	Keep small objects out of reach, especially pins or other sharp objects; buy toys too large to swallow
	Poisoning	Keep medicines and poisons in a locked cabinet
Toddler		
Roams all over house Climbs into things	Falls	Use gates on stairways; keep windows and doors locked; fence yard
Takes things apart	Cuts	Provide large, sturdy toys without sharp edges or small removable parts; keep sharp instruments and knives out of reach
Curious about everything	Burns	Needs constant supervision; never leave hot coffeepot or running water unattended; turn pot handles inward; keep matches locked up; treat flimsy clothing with fire-retardant (7 oz. borax, 3 oz. boric acid, 2 qt. hot water)
Pokes and probes with fingers	Electric shock	Keep electrical appliances out of reach; cap unused light sockets with safety plugs
Chews everything	Poisoning	Keep medicines, cosmetics, and household poisons out of reach
	Ingestion of foreign objects and aspiration	Keep small objects such as coins, beans, needles, pins, jewelry, and doll's eyes out of reach
Enjoys playing in water	Drowning	Keep away from unattended pools, ponds, etc.; stay with child while in bathtub; fence in bodies of water

Continued.

Table 21-6. Accidents common at various stages of development—cont'd

Typical behavior	Type of accident	Precaution and safety education
Rides tricycle	Motor vehicle accidents	Be firm and instruct child to keep clear of driveways and out of streets
Likes to ride in car and wants to go everywhere with mother		Instruct child in proper car safety; keep car doors locked and use safety belts; never allow child to sit or stand in front seat of a car or allow him to put hands or head out of window
Preschooler		
Ventures out into neighborhood		Teach child safety rules and demonstrate principles by good example; enforce obedience
		Do not overprotect—the preschooler can begin to protect himself, and overprotection deprives him of experience he needs in growing up and learning independence
Inquisitive	Burns	Teach him danger of open flames and hot objects
Rides bicycle	Motor vehicle accidents	Instruct him in proper traffic safety rules—look both ways before crossing street, walk, never run across street, go with traffic light and walk in crosswalk, and never dart into street to go after a ball
Plays ball		
Climbs trees and fences	Falls	Teach him good footing and proper handholds when climbing
Enjoys playing in water	Drowning	Begin swimming instruction; never let child play around unsupervised pools
Plays rough; runs up and down stairs	Blows; cuts	Check play areas for hazards
		Store dangerous tools and equipment in a locked cupboard
	Poisoning	Teach him not to taste unidentified foods, especially berries
		Lock up poisons; store in labeled bottles
		Discard old medicines down drain before putting containers in trash
Early school age, 6-9 yr.		
Adventurous	Motor vehicle accidents	Needs intensive instruction in safety rules
Will try anything	Drowning	Encourage swimming safety
Loyal to his friends	Falls	Point out importance of fun and not getting hurt
		Needs to know consequences for failing to follow rules
	Burns	Teach him to avoid smoldering fires; bottles and cans may explode and cause fatal injuries
		Teach him danger of matches and fires
		Teach proper use of chemistry sets
	Firearms	Point out serious consequences of playing with Dry Ice, fireworks, etc.
Late school age, 10-14 yr.		
Rides bicycle constantly	Motor vehicle accidents	Enforce safety rules; explain reasons for them
Plays away from home, often in hazardous places	Drowning; burns; explosions	Know where child is at all times
Has lots of energy and enjoys strenuous play	Sprains; contusions	Point out importance of fun and not getting injured
Enjoys working with father's tools	Lacerations	Show boys how to work around house safely (they should not use power tools unless tools are in good condition and they have knowledge of their use and safety); use proper equipment and keep it in good condition

2. Recognition and protection of a vulnerable host (young, inquisitive children, especially those with a past history of accidents)
3. Control of the environment, or milieu by offering consistent love and discipline

Alerting and instructing parents. All parents should be made aware of the dangers confronting the child at each stage of his development, particularly the toddler and preschooler (Table 21-6). Parents need to realize fully the normal child's search for adventure and his ignorance of consequences. They should know that fatigue, hunger, family discord, and anxiety increase the likelihood of an accident. A wise and loving parent will know that discipline is a fundamental prerequisite for accident prevention. Children should be taught that disobedience leads to unpleasant consequences that are not limited to punishment. This discipline of obedience rapidly becomes the only reliable method for ensuring protection of the school-age child.

All children and families should be instructed in safety. Community educational efforts aimed at accident prevention should include information on burns, water safety, road safety, and the use and proper storage of potentially toxic household chemicals, medicines, and tools and equipment. Individual responsibility and alertness multiplied to assure intelligent community involvement is needed.

Poison ingestion

The variety and number of toxic substances children have been known to swallow are fantastic. The most frequent poisons are found in the medicine cabinet and under the kitchen sink. Often parental negligence has been directly responsible for the loss of a child's life. The majority of accidental poisonings in childhood are preventable.

Each year approximately 500 children die as the result of accidental poisoning, and an estimated 500,000 to 2 million children are involved in poisoning accidents. The major number of accidental poisonings occur in children under 4 years of age. This is the "age of curiosity," and these children are not selective about what they ingest. A number of nonfatal poisoning victims are left with permanent disabilities such as

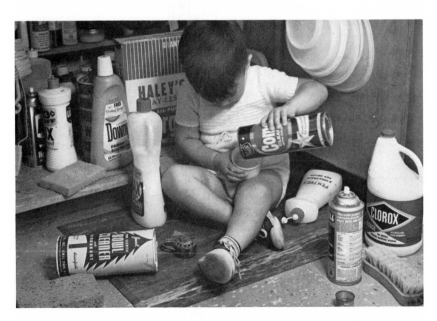

Fig. 21-4. Young children will eat and drink anything regardless of taste. Keep household poisons in a *locked* cupboard.

esophageal stricture or hepatic or renal damage.

Precautions. The following suggestions must be repeated until parents learn:

1. Keep all drugs, poisonous substances, and household chemicals in a locked cupboard out of the reach of little hands.
2. Do not transfer or store poisons or inflammable materials in food containers or bottles.
3. Never tell children that flavored medicine is candy (not even vitamins). Always refer to medicine as medicine!
4. Discard old medicines in drain before throwing away container.
5. Always read label before giving medicine.
6. Always return medicine to its proper place.
7. Do not underestimate the curiosity and abilities of children.

Emergency treatment. All accidental poisonings in young children are treated as an urgent emergency. Call the physician immediately and bring the child and the poisonous substance to a hospital emergency room. Supportive and symptomatic treatment should be initiated immediately, even though the specific poison substance may not be known.

Immediate management. The following immediate action should be taken in the case of poisoning:

1. Identify and remove the poison
2. Adminster the antidote
3. Administer other supportive treatment

REMOVAL OF POISON. In most cases the immediate necessity is to empty the child's stomach, even if hours have passed since the ingestion. *If not contraindicated,* emesis should be induced if possible. Removal (after prevention) is the most important aspect of poison management. However, emesis should not be induced in the event of the ingestion of corrosives (lye or strong acids), strychnine, or any hydrocarbons (kerosene, gasoline, fuel oil, paint thinner,

and cleaning fluid). Neither should it be initiated if the child is unconscious or convulsing.

1. To induce vomiting, first have the child drink a glass of milk or water, then stroke your finger on his posterior oral pharynx to stimulate the gag reflex. The child's head and shoulders should be lowered to prevent aspiration of the vomitus.
2. An emetic drug such as *syrup of ipecac* (never the fluid extract), 15 ml., may be used. If vomiting does not occur, administration should be repeated *once only* in 15 to 30 minutes. Packaged in 1 fluid ounce containers, syrup of ipecac may be sold without prescription for first-aid use. Gagging may also be helpful when syrup of ipecac fails to induce immediate vomiting. An apomorphine injection is used often in the hospital as an emetic.
3. Gastric lavage is usually reserved for the unconscious child, the child who has ingested large amounts of hydrocarbons (to prevent aspiration or chemical pneumonia), and the child who has not vomited after two doses of syrup of ipecac. Severe cardiac disturbances result from an overdose of syrup of ipecac. A gastric tube with a large lumen is inserted, and the stomach is irrigated with copious amounts of tap water. Because of the time lapse in getting to the hospital and because the stomach normally traps material inaccessible to the lumen of the tube, chemical emesis is now favored over gastric lavage.

Specific measures can be instituted as soon as the particular poison is identified. In most cases of acute poisoning, the physician can identify the agent by a quick history of the incident or by the label on the container. The poison container should always be brought to the hospital with the child.

POISON CONTROL CENTERS. Information

about poisons and emergency treatment of poison ingestion may be obtained immediately by telephoning the nearest Poison Control Center. Over 250,000 toxic or potentially toxic *trade name* products are on the consumer market. Federal law requires that the ingredients of drugs, pesticides, and caustic products be clearly stated on labels. However, many household products frequently involved in accidental ingestions are not required to be so labeled. To assist the physician with his very grave problem of identification, Poison Control Centers have been established in key areas of the United States. These centers are usually associated with medical schools or large hospitals equipped with laboratories, library, house staff, and faculty. They are available to dispense information 24 hours a day. They also serve as treatment centers and are actively engaged in programs of public education to prevent accidental poisoning. The Poison Control Centers give information to physicians only. Other persons calling receive first-aid instruction and are advised to call the physician at once.

ADMINISTRATION OF ANTIDOTES Antidotes should be given immediately after emesis or lavage to render any remaining poison inert or prevent its absorption. Specific antidotes are not available for all poisons. Among the few available antidotes is dimercaprol (BAL, British antilewisite). Dimercaprol is a good antidote for mercury, antimony, and lead poisoning. Activated charcoal is a powerful physical antidote that adsorbs most poisons to itself. It should *not* be used with other substances that may interfere with its adsorptive capacity or with which it may interfere (syrup of ipecac). Large doses of the adsorbent should be used, especially when a large dose of poison has been ingested.

An antidote should be put in the Levin tube before its removal from the stomach. The specific antidote is given if one is available. The so-called universal antidote (two parts burned toast, one part milk of magnesia, and one part strong tea) is neither universal nor an antidote. The three

ingredients "neutralize" each other—hence it is ineffective.

In the event of caustic ingestion, immediate administration of water or milk to dilute the poison has been advised. Both emesis and lavage are contraindicated because of possible further tissue injury.

SUPPORTIVE TREATMENT. Check the child's breathing immediately. Assure a clear airway and fresh air. Mouth-to-mouth resuscitation may be lifesaving. Overtreatment by emetics, sedatives, and stimulants is dangerous and should be avoided. Overtreatment may result in more harm than the ingestion of the poison. Keep the patient comfortable, warm, and dry.

Acute salicylate (aspirin) poisoning

More children die from accidental ingestion of salicylates (aspirin, sodium salicylate, oil of wintergreen) than from any other product. About 17% of all accidental

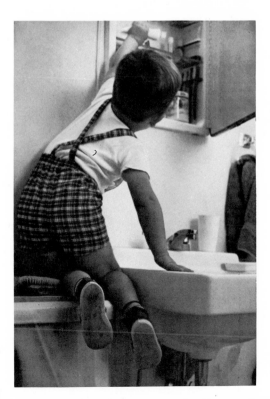

Fig. 21-5. Pink pills are *not* candy. Keep medicines in a locked cabinet.

deaths resulting from poisoning are attributed to salicylate intoxication.

The widespread use and availability of salicylates are prime factors in overdosage. The use of salicylates is so commonplace that parents and sometimes physicians underestimate the toxicity of the drug. Salicylates act rapidly but are excreted slowly. A small dose repeated frequently may accumulate to cause a severe state of salicylate poisoning.

Candy-flavored aspirin was invented to obtain an accurate, small dosage and improve the taste, but children should never be told that medicine is candy; flavored aspirin should *never* be left within a child's reach.

A common but grave error occurs when the parent mistakenly gives the child a teaspoon of oil of wintergreen instead of cough medicine. One teaspoon of oil of wintergreen contains as much salicylate as 60 grains of aspirin. It represents a *lethal* dose in most cases.

Clinical signs. There are many clinical signs of salicylate poisoning in children. In cases of acute poisoning the first manifestation is hyperpnea with an increase in respiration depth. Severe acidosis, electrolyte imbalance, and dehydration follow. Other common symptoms include restlessness, extreme thirst, fever (usually 103° F. or higher), profuse sweating, tremors, bleeding, delirium, convulsions, pulmonary edema, and coma. Cerebral hemorrhage may occur.

Treatment. The treatment of acute salicylate poisoning is always immediate emesis or lavage. Parents should attempt to induce vomiting as soon as the discovery is made. The physician or nearest Poison Control Center should be called for emergency instructions. The child is usually ordered to the hospital. The parents are requested to bring with the child any implicated container, loose pills, and sometimes the material vomited.

Gastric lavage is carried out in the hospital emergency room. A blood specimen is ordered immediately to determine the level of salicylate intoxication (30 mg./100 ml. invariably is associated with symptoms). Peak levels are usually reached about 90 minutes after ingestion. Treatment of salicylate intoxication is aimed at correcting electrolyte imbalance. Measures are instituted to promote the rapid excretion of salicylates in the urine. Parenteral fluids

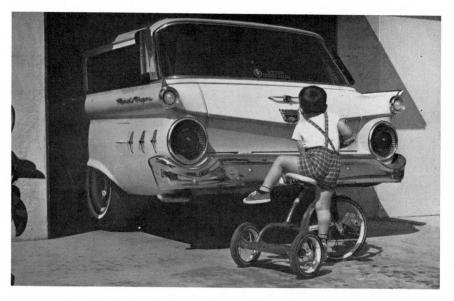

Fig. 21-6. Use firm discipline to keep child out of driveway and street.

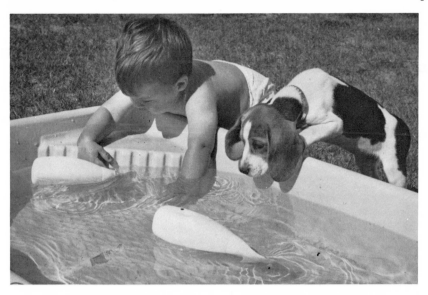

Fig. 21-7. Even shallow water is dangerous for the unattended child.

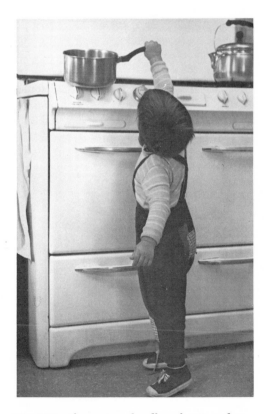

Fig. 21-8. Always turn handles of pots and pans to the back of stove.

are given both to combat dehydration and to facilitate prompt excretion of salicylates from the body. Salicylate excretion is greatly increased by small doses of acetazolamide (Diamox). Acetazolamide renders the urine alkaline moments after administration; this, in turn, favors the excretion of salicylates.

Nursing care. Nursing care for salicylate poisoning is supportive. Fever is reduced by cool sponges; hourly urinary output is recorded, and pH of the urine is tested with Nitrazine paper. Accurate hourly output notations will help determine amounts of parenteral fluids necessary. Temperature, pulse, and respiration are checked every 15 minutes until stable; oxygen is given as necessary. Exchange transfusions or dialysis may be considered in severe, life-threatening intoxication.

Poisoning is one of the most common pediatric emergencies. It is always difficult to treat. In more than half the cases the poisonous substances have been carelessly handled and stored by adults. The child often was improperly supervised. As part of the growing-up process, children investigate their environment. This investigation includes feeling and tasting, and these ac-

329

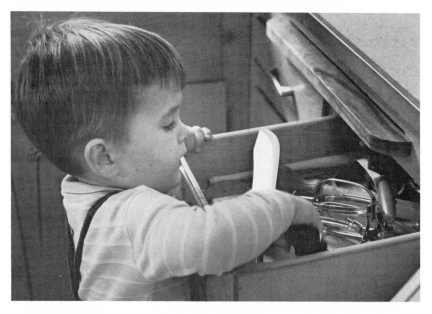

Fig. 21-9. Knives are highly dangerous. Keep them out of the toddler's reach.

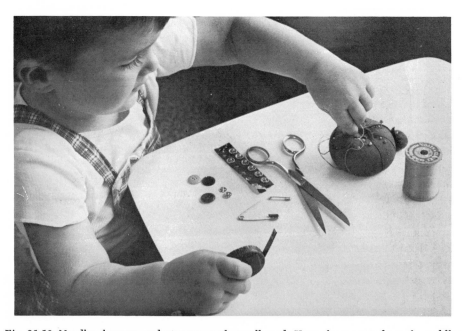

Fig. 21-10. Needles, buttons, and pins are easily swallowed. Keep them away from the toddler.

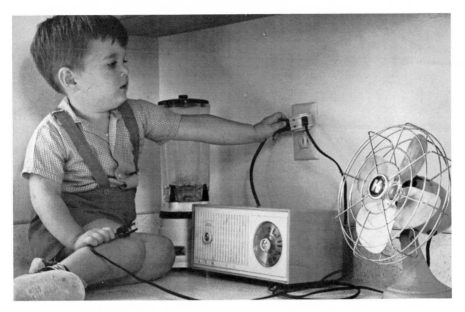

Fig. 21-11. Disconnect appliances not in use. Plug outlets and avoid hurts and burns.

tivities are always dangerous. However, opportunities for investigation must be available.

Parents must take time to answer questions, show their children how things work, and help them learn to do things safely for themselves. Patience and supervision will teach the child what he wants to know and show him the way to safety, too.

Misuse of drugs

The abuse of drugs by youth in our society is a major and growing social and personal problem. The average age level of drug users is dropping steadily. Many junior-high and grade-school children are now frequent offenders.

The magnitude of the problem is revealed by the fact that in New York City in 1970 more deaths in the 18 to 35 age group were caused by heroin use than by any other factor including accidents and disease. These statistics bode ill for the future if current trends continue.

The subject of drug abuse cannot be treated in any detail in this text, but students are encouraged to learn more about the causes, prevention, and treatment of

this problem. Because of the severity and widespread nature of the difficulty, it is likely that pediatric nurses will encounter a variety of different situations related to drug abuse. One usually thinks of teen-age involvement with hallucinogenic drugs, but recently two toddlers were admitted to a pediatric emergency room after ingesting an unknown number of "LSD pills." Treated with chlorpromazine (Thorazine), they did respond favorably.

Drug reactions vary. A heroin overdose produces a severe depression, whereas an amphetamine overdose will result in hyperactivity and overstimulation. Violent psychological reactions, varying from hallucinations to severe psychoses (paranoia) may result from LSD use. Immediate medical attention is essential. Nurses should be alert for any unusual behavior not typical of the individual or his age group. Such signs include abnormal dilatation of the pupils, excitability, talkativeness, profuse perspiration, staggering, mental confusion, disturbances in perception, and general personality changes. The nurse can best assist these patients by a calm, supportive manner and a quiet atmosphere. She should make a careful attempt through conversation to make the patient aware of reality.

Sincere concern by the nurse for the addict can, in some cases, help build a communication bridge back to society that will help rehabilitate the individual. Unfortunately, such successes have been less frequent than the failures.

Child abuse (nonaccidental injury)

The term "child abuse" includes many types of physical, mental, and emotional neglect or injury. Hundreds of children are killed annually, and thousands of others are permanently harmed at the hands of adults, usually their parents.

Affected children commonly manifest abrasions, lacerations, skull fractures, intracranial bleeding, and multiple long bone fractures in various stages of healing, as well as personality disturbances and mental impairment. One type of child abuse in which the victim is characterized by severe physical injury and neglect was in the past called the *battered child syndrome*. Neglected, nonaccidentally injured children brought to the hospital are typically under 3 years of age, frequently boys. They are many times born out of wedlock, unwanted, mentally retarded, and/or physically malformed. The children are often too young or too afraid to talk.

Parents of such children are described as emotionally immature and unready to accept the responsibilities of parenthood. Often, they are burdened by adverse social conditions, financial strain, and personal frustration. Some have reversed roles with their children, expecting them to provide love, gratification, and fulfillment to meet their own needs. Many of these parents were rejected and battered in their own childhood. They are repeating familiar parental behavior experienced in their young years.

Recognition. Certain clues may help identify these children. When first admitted to the hospital, neglected and nonaccidentally injured children shut their eyes, turn their heads away, and cry irritably, in contrast to well-nurtured children who characteristically cry loudly and reach out for their parents. The skillful observer may recognize the difficulty when parents offer no reasonable explanation regarding the character, circumstances, or nature of the trauma sustained.

One 2½-year-old boy entered the hospital to have his leg "checked." He weighed 19 pounds, one front tooth was missing, a fingernail was pulled off, his head and face were covered with skin lesions, and his right femur was broken (see Fig. 34-3, p. 527). The only information offered by his mother was, "He was very clumsy and stumbled in the yard." Two weeks passed before he would turn to look at anyone. His parents visited once in a period of 2 months. Suspicion should always be aroused when any of the following are noted: abnormal uncleanliness, malnutrition, multiple soft tissue injuries or burns in various stages of healing, and illness obviously caused by a lack of medical attention. Often, the behavior of the child shows he has no real expectation of being comforted or helped.

Reporting. Because parental neglect and abuse is difficult to understand, it may go unrecognized. Children may recover from their injuries and go home, only to be battered again. The alert nurse is usually the first to suspect that a child has been abused. She should carefully chart what she observes and *report* the situation to the physician at once! Every state requires that the physician report his suspicions to the police department or to the appropriate child protection service in the community. After a written report has been submitted, the case is carefully investigated. The physician participating in good faith in making a report is immune from civil or criminal liability. Willful refusal to report child neglect or abuse constitutes a misdemeanor.

Protection. As part of public comprehensive child welfare services, most communities have established "protective services" for neglected and abused children. The purpose of a protective service is not only to provide care and protection for the child but also to help parents who "want to be good" but for some reason are unable to assume their role. Why else do parents bring their neglected and battered children to the hospital? They always run the risk of punishment. Could an abused or neglected child be their way of actually asking for help?

Management of this serious problem may range from professional counseling and the introduction and explanation of various community services involved in child care to criminal court action. Juvenile courts have power over "neglected children," but according to recent studies, criminal prosecution is a poor means of preventing child abuse. Usually, criminal proceedings divide the family and cause parents to hate their children. Legal action is only advisable when all other means of protection and prevention have failed.

unit eight
Suggested selected readings and references

Boyd, E. M.: The safety and toxicity of aspirin, Am. J. Nurs. 71:964-966, May, 1971.

Condon, A., and Roland, A.: Drug abuse jargon, Am. J. Nurs. 71:1738-1739, Sept., 1971.

Egan, M. C.: Combating malnutrition through maternal and child health programs, Children 16:67-71, March-April, 1969.

Ferro, F.: Our forgotten children need your help: support the bill of rights for foster children, Parents' Magazine and Better Homemaking 49:24, July, 1974.

Fishbein, M.: How "nearly perfect is milk"? Med. World News 15:56, June 14, 1974.

Foote, F. M.: Death from a caustic detergent, Health Serv. Rep. 88:131-132, Feb., 1973.

Freeman, B., Korsch, B. M., Negrete, V. F., and others: How do nurses expand their roles in well child care, Am. J. Nurs. 72:1866-1871, Oct., 1972.

Gelles, R. J.: A psychosocial approach to child abuse, Nurs. Digest 2:52-59, April, 1974; condensed from Am. J. Orthopsychiatry 43:611-621, July, 1973.

Gesell, A., and Ilg, L. B.: The child from five to ten, New York, 1946, Harper & Row, Publishers.

Gil, D. G.: Violence against children: physical abuse in the United States, Cambridge, Harvard University Press, 1970.

Green, M., and Haggarty, R., editors: Ambulatory pediatrics, Philadelphia, 1968, W. B. Saunders Co.

Greenfield, J.: Advances in genetics that can change your life, Today's Health 51:20-24, 58, Dec., 1973.

Hankin, L., Heichel, G. H., and Botsford, R. A.: Lead poisoning from colored printing inks, Clin. Pediatr. 12:654-655, Nov., 1973.

Hecht, M.: Children of alcoholics are children at risk, Am. J. Nurs. 73:1764-1767, Oct., 1973.

Heydman, A. J.: Intestinal bypass for obesity, Am. J. Nurs. 74:1102-1104, June, 1974.

Huenemann, R. L.: A review of teen-age nutrition in the United States, Health Serv. Rep. 87:823-829, Nov., 1972.

Hurd, J. L.: A new perspective on Head Start health care, Health Serv. Rep. 87:575-582, Aug.-Sept., 1972.

Kauff, R. E., and Kimball, J.: Making the annual pediatric evaluation more relevant to the needs of the child, Clin. Pediatr. 13:490-495, June, 1974.

Kempe, C. H., and Helfer, R. E., editors: Helping the battered child and his family, Philadelphia, 1972, J. B. Lippincott Co.

Klein, A., and others: Improved prognosis in congenital hypothyroidism treated before age three months, J. Pediatr. 81:912-915, Nov., 1972.

Lefrancois, G. R.: Of children, 1973, Belmont, Calif., Wadsworth Publishing Co., Inc.

Leonard, C. O., Chase, G. A., and Childes, B.: Genetic counseling: a consumer's view, Nurs. Digest 1:79-89, July, 1973.

Lillbridge, C. B.: A simple system to block toddlers from reaching toxic ingestibles, Clin. Pediatr. 12:441-444, July, 1973.

Lin-Fu, J. S.: Childhood lead-poisoning—an eradicable disease, Children 17:2-9, Jan.-Feb., 1970.

Matheny, A. P.: Assessment of children's behavioral characteristics: a tool in accident prevention, Clin. Pediatr. 11:437-439, Aug., 1972.

Nelson, W. E., Vaughan, V. C. III, and McKay, R. J.: Textbook of pediatrics, ed. 10, Philadelphia, 1975, W. B. Saunders Co.

Pillari, G., and Narus, J.: Physical effects of heroin addiction. Am. J. Nurs. 73:2105-2108. Dec., 1973.

Report of the Committee on Infectious Diseases, part I, ed. 17, Evanston, Ill., 1974, American Academy of Pediatrics, pp. 1-15.

Savino, A. B., and Sanders, R. W.: Working with abusive parents—group therapy and home visits, Am. J. Nurs. 73:482-484, March, 1973.

Schmitt, B. D., Jordan, K., and Hamburg, F. L.: The role of the pediatrician in helping children develop a sense of responsibility, Clin. Pediatr. 11:509-513, Sept., 1972.

Shaw, B. L.: Emergency care for near-drowning victims, RN 33:49-50, July, 1970.

Shirkey, H. D., editor: Pediatric therapy, ed. 5, St. Louis, 1973, The C. V. Mosby Co.

Shumway, C. A.: Iron deficiency anemia, Pediatr. Clin. North Am. **19**:855-864, Nov., 1972.

Sokol, A. B., and Houser, R. G.: Dog bites: prevention and treatment, Clin. Pediatr. **10**:336-338, June, 1971.

Standards of child health care, ed. 2, Evanston, Ill., American Academy of Pediatrics, 1972.

Taif, B.: Foods and nutrition: obesity in childhood, J. Pract. Nurs. **24**:16-19, Jan., 1974.

Warner, R. W., Jr.: Preventing drug abuse: where are we now? Nurs. Digest **1**:21-27, Sept., 1973; condensed from Personnel and Guidance J. **5**, April, 1973.

Wetzel, N. C.: The baby grid, an application of the grid technique to growth and development in infants, J. Pediatr. **29**:439-454, 1946.

Wolman, I. J.: ABC's of artificial infant feeding, Clin. Pediatr. **11**:8A, March, 1972.

unit nine
The child, the family, and the hospital setting

22

Hospitalization of the child

For most of us, regardless of age, hospitalization is a necessary but not particularly welcome interruptive interlude in our daily life style. In many cases a stay in the hospital is not planned, and we suddenly find ourselves in a rather strange world with many of our normal social defenses (such as family and community role, privacy, and clothes) weakened or removed. This turn of events is disruptive enough for the adult, but it is potentially even more so for the impressionable young child.

PREPARATION FOR HOSPITALIZATION

Not too many years ago the preparation of a child and his parents for the experience of hospitalization did not receive much consideration. Emphasis was placed on the child's disease rather than the fact that he was a particular person with certain capabilities and needs who happened to be ill. Typically, the parents brought little Mary Lou to the pediatric ward, signed some papers, and said a rather hasty and usually tearful good-bye. In some cases Mary Lou was placed in a special semi-isolation admission area to be observed for 24 to 48 hours for the possible onset of contagious disease before being transferred to the main pediatric ward. Little was done to prepare her or her parents for this sudden change in their pattern of living.

Today, although we still have a great deal to learn about the child, his needs, and family relationships, we do recognize that

the old approach and many of the old methods were incomplete and unnecessarily traumatic for all concerned. Recently, there have even been attempts to shorten hospitalization or avoid it altogether by more reliance on out-patient departments and Surgi-centers designed for minor operations and recovery requiring less than a day. The modern nurse recognizes that the family may have a great deal to offer the hospitalized child, and when properly prepared and supported, the parents may be able to help the child during a difficult but, we hope, also a potentially constructive period in his heretofore brief experience with life.

The parents

The heart of the problem in preparing the child for hospitalization lies in the preparation of his parents, who are then best able to help their child. It is imperative that parents receive sufficient knowledge of the child's illness so that they readily understand the need for hospitalization. It is also necessary for parents to have some understanding of the tests and treatments to be given and the risk and discomfort involved.

A child's morale will inevitably reflect his parents' outlook. When parents are inadequately prepared, they cannot adequately prepare their child. It is extremely important that the parents have sound information about the child's illness, confidence in their physician's recommendations, and the

The child

According to his level of understanding, the child should be told why it is necessary for him to go to the hospital. Truthful assurance is the best guide. The truth is less frightening to a youngster than the ideas his imagination can invent. Children who are not given the true reason for hospitalization often believe that they have been punished or sent away because they have been naughty. Of course, if the truth is to be supportive, the child must have confidence in his parents and other authority figures based on previous experience of their trustworthiness. Such an attitude cannot be established in a day. Its foundation is laid during the first year and perpetuated through each stage of life.

Telling a child about surgery is a highly individual matter. Information about the impending operation will depend on his age, his level of understanding, and his emotional makeup. Usually a brief, simple explanation of what is wrong and what must be done to change it or make it better will help the child develop a sound and healthy attitude. A detailed and accurate explanation of the operation is not necessary; the child needs the truth, but not always the whole truth. The belief that an event has been explained relieves tension.

Pediatric units in hospitals throughout the United States have developed methods to prepare parents and children for hospitalization. Colorful booklets and pamphlets, telephone calls, hospital tours, preadmission or orientation parties, and the use of television sets all have lessened the trauma of admission to the hospital. Advising parents of procedures and inviting the child and his parents to visit the hospital before admission help the child to know what to expect. Allowing the child to share in the planning for his hospital stay or helping to pack his suitcase is sometimes rewarding.

A child should know in advance what the hospital is like. He should be told simply and in a matter-of-fact manner about such things as the differences between hospital beds and beds at home, the use of the bedpan and urinals, the baths in bed, the spe-

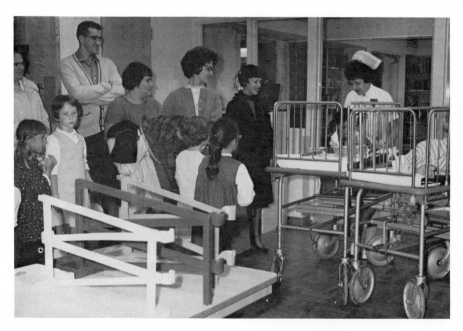

Fig. 22-1. Inviting the child and his parents to visit the hospital before admission helps them to know what to expect. (Courtesy Children's Health Center, San Diego, Calif.)

cial schooling, the playroom, and the food service. If 4-year-old Jimmy knows in advance about the big, wiggly scale that he must stand on to see how heavy he is and some of the other things that will happen at the hospital, he is less likely to be shocked when he faces them directly.

It is not always possible, necessary, or desirable for the child to know everything that will happen. All the child needs to know is enough to assure him that what happens is according to plan and that Mother will be at his side whenever possible. When she cannot be there, kind friends, physicians, and nurses will help care for him until he can go home again.

Printed information sheets to be completed by parents, ideally prior to admission, are helpful. They request brief back-

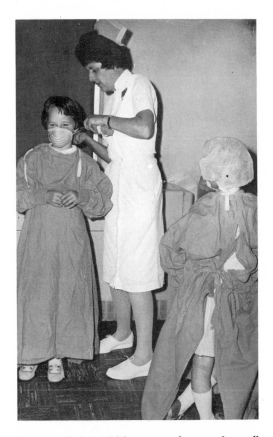

Fig. 22-2. If the child knows in advance what will happen, she is less likely to be shocked when she faces the situation directly. (Courtesy Children's Health Center, San Diego, Calif.)

ground material regarding the health history, habits, skills, likes, dislikes, fears, and family composition of the young patient; this information assists the staff in individualizing his care.

Liberal visiting hours, rooming-in facilities, and appropriate parent participation in care have made it much easier for the mother and father to continue their supportive role and help counteract any sense of isolation or desertion the child may harbor. However, no matter how well a child is prepared for hospitalization, he may still cry at the prospect of treatment, needles, and pain. Explain to the parents that this is a natural reaction and encourage them to stay with their child, since they are best able to comfort him with the thought that he will feel better when it is over. Usually the mother's presence helps the child to weather each interference as it comes and greatly reduces the risk of emotional trauma.

SEPARATION ANXIETY
The young child

Considerable evidence has shown that under certain circumstances the child may view hospitalization as desertion by his parents and thus may be profoundly affected by his hospital experience. When parents of a young child are unable to come to the hospital for prolonged periods, the hospitalized child is exposed to numerous traumatic factors resulting in frustration of those inborn needs that are normally met in a family environment. As a result, the child may fail to thrive physically, socially, and psychologically. In extreme cases, maternal deprivation may be manifested as a general marasmus, or wasting away.*

The effects of separation do not always manifest themselves immediately. The emotional aftermath of hospitalization may appear in such forms as night terrors, fears, negativisms, regressions to earlier, more

---

*Beelicka, I., and Alechnowicz, H.: Treating children traumatized by hospitalization, Children 10:194-195, Sept.-Oct., 1963.

babylike, clinging behavior, and protracted hostilities. In some cases the effects may not appear until later in life.

Studies have pointed out that in children between 1 and 4 years of age the risks involved with parent-child separation are greatest. These risks taper off beyond 5 years of age but never disappear entirely during childhood.

Separation anxiety is characteristic of all young children who have established a healthy parent-child relationship. The phenomenon of "settling in," or adjustment to hospitalization and separation, is deceptive. Robertson* found that children under 4 years of age experience three phases in the

*Robertson, J.: Young children in hospitals, New York, 1958, Basic Books, Inc., Publishers, p. 48.

process of settling into the hospital: protest, despair, and denial. These emotional phases may not be as severe when pediatric policies are more enlightened, but they are probably still there.

At first the young child *protests* the separation. He cries aloud for "Mama," shakes the crib, throws himself around, and is alert for any signs of his mother's return. The nurse may pick up the child and try to quiet him, but this is to no avail. Telling a child to stop crying only conveys to him that he is not understood and adds to his feelings of helplessness. This phase may last for a few days or even up to 1 week.

During the phase of *despair* the child becomes apathetic and withdrawn, which is sometimes confused with acceptance. Instead of crying, he sobs. The hope of the

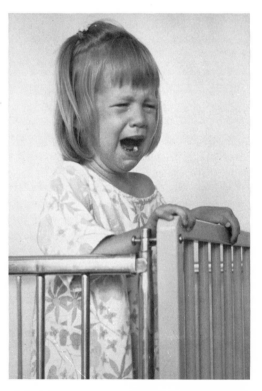

Fig. 22-3. Protest. The day after admission, the child (Marie, 2½ years old) cries aloud for "Mama," shakes the crib, and is alert for any signs of her mother's return. (Courtesy Children's Health Center, San Diego, Calif.)

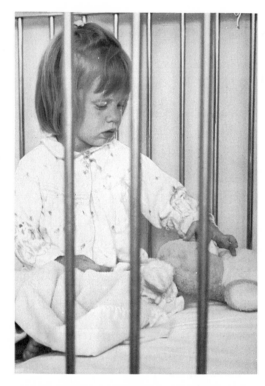

Fig. 22-4. Despair. Four days after admission, the child has become apathetic and withdrawn. She does not understand why her mother has left her or why she is in the hospital. (Courtesy Children's Health Center, San Diego, Calif.)

return of his mother fades, but the wish for her return remains. During this quiet stage, distress seemingly has lessened, and the nurse presumes that he is "settling in." When his parents arrive, he may turn his face away and cry aloud. He does not understand why he is in the hospital. He rejects his parents as they seem to have rejected him. Parents spend most of visiting time trying to get the child to respond to them more normally, and just as the child brightens up, they may leave again. The child's piteous cries on the mother's arrival and departure lead the nurse mistakenly to think that he is better off without his parents. The nurse who understands the reason for the child's behavior can be of great help to the mother who dreads coming back because she anticipates the distress of her

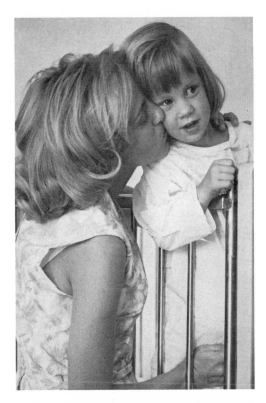

Fig. 22-5. Denial. Eight days after admission, the little child cannot tolerate the intensity of distress, so she represses the need for mother. When her mother comes, she seems hardly to know her, is happy and gay. (Courtesy Children's Health Center, San Diego, Calif.)

child. The mother needs to realize how much her child needs her, and she should be encouraged to come often. When she leaves, she should be sure to tell the child when she will come back. It is unfair for a mother to tell her child that she is going for a cup of coffee. Children have lain awake all night waiting for mothers to return.

Gradually, the stage of *denial* follows despair. The child begins to show more interest in the surroundings, is more responsive to nursing attention, and actually denies the need for his mother. When his mother comes, he seems hardly to know her, is happy and gay throughout the visit, and may even wave good-bye. Psychologists have explained this phenomenon by theorizing that because a young child cannot tolerate the intensity of distress, he represses the need for his mother. However, after he returns home he often demonstrates his disturbed feelings by regressive babylike behavior and is forever clinging to his mother. This only confirms that his complacency in the hospital was a facade.

The school-age child

The school-age child is not so prone to separation anxiety if his illness is short. The child has learned to rely to some extent on adults and other children when away from home. He can understand that hospitalization is a temporary situation and why his parents come only at certain times. School-age children seem more bothered by the disease process and its treatment. Imagination persists strongly throughout these years, and often fantasies and fears of mutilation influence the degree of emotional reaction. Older children worry about the hospital costs. If by chance they feel responsible for causing their illness their worries are intensified.

Long-term hospitalization imposes numerous anxieties on children of all ages. During a serious illness even an older child has a great need for his mother and can tolerate her absence only for short periods. He needs to know that his parents will be there when he needs them most and that he is loved and missed. (See Chapter 24.)

GROWTH AND DEVELOPMENTAL NEEDS

Each child comes to the hospital with his own individual makeup and achieved state of development, a unique past experience, and his own methods of dealing with anxiety. The nurse can encourage emotional growth by accepting the child as he is and by assisting him to continue in his present stage of development. For example, often a child is expected to conform to hospital rules by staying in his crib when, in essence, he has had the run of the whole house prior to hospitalization. Unless acutely ill, a child may refuse to stay in bed. The nurse should not arbitrarily urge the child to "stay there." She should be aware of the dangers of restricting the child to his crib when otherwise he could be ambulatory. For the toddler, sustained restriction of movement may lead to a severe state of anxiety and hostility. Whenever his basic motor urge is thwarted, the child becomes frustrated and angry and may regress. This drive is constructively handled by the wise nurse who is able to devise ways to allow the child freedom to move about safely.

• • •

This discussion has highlighted the psychological risks of hospitalization that are real and well documented. However, it is comforting to note that children usually are able to survive the event of hospitalization without significant emotional scars. It is largely the nurse's function to see that the original trauma is slight and the scars minimal.

23

Rehabilitation of the long-term pediatric patient

For most children the period of hospitalization is brief—a day or two, perhaps a week. Increasingly, the trend is to shorten the treatment period away from home whenever possible; a shorter stay in the hospital has psychological, social, and financial advantages for the child and his family. However, for a few patients, hospitalization is still prolonged. The severely ill child who has a long, complicated convalescence, the child undergoing elaborate orthopedic corrections, and the teen-ager with a damaged spinal cord who is struggling to recapture skills once considered automatic and to adjust to new expectations and goals are all examples of relatively long-term pediatric patients. The following is a brief discussion of the needs of boys and girls who stay in the hospital for extended periods; it emphasizes the nursing perspectives, challenges, and skills of a relatively new specialty within a specialty, that of pediatric rehabilitation.

In a general sense, the definition of rehabilitation is "to restore to a functional state." Those patients and families who have suffered devastating physical disabilities characteristically need a coordinated multidisciplinary team that considers not only the physical but the sociological, emotional, vocational, and spiritual aspects of the patient's total situation. The rehabilitation of children is made more complex by their continuing need for normal growth and development in the face of disability.

Pediatric rehabilitation is based on at least two concepts: first, that each person is unique and has individual basic worth, and second, that the task involves a committed group of people working together as a team with a common goal. The overall goal of pediatric rehabilitation is to foster maximal growth, development, independence, and personal fulfillment within the limitations of the handicap. There are many allied health professionals on the core rehabilitation team: doctors, nurses, physical and occupational therapists, speech and hearing pathologists, medical social service workers, dieticians, financial counselors, teachers, and educational consultants. Representatives of other specialty areas, such as psychology, psychiatry, psychometric testing and vocational counseling, as well as community agencies are available as needed. There are team physicians for each specialty, and the community physician, public health nurse, and teacher are invited to be part of the team for their patient. Each team member evaluates the patient, makes recommendations in writing, and participates in patient planning conferences. The patient and family are, of course, prime members of the team and are included appropriately in conferences where current status and progress are discussed and new goals are set.

The need of the area served by the rehabilitation center should dictate the types of patients seen. Patients with spinal cord injuries and incapacitating birth anomalies, such as myelomeningocele (spina bifida), usually make up a large part of the patient load. Those with Guillain-Barré syndrome (a polyneuritis), cerebral palsy, muscular dystrophy, juvenile rheumatoid arthritis, severe scoliosis, osteogenesis imperfecta, and other complex physical problems are also

341

appropriately treated in a rehabilitation setting.

Generally speaking, any patient with a devastating injury or illness that produces lasting or permanent physical disabilities can and should be handled by the rehabilitation team. Nursing principles of rehabilitation must be initiated at the onset of illness or injury in order to prevent complications and further loss of function. Realistically, many of these children initially require specialized lifesaving care, which can be delivered more effectively in intensive care or medical-surgical units. Hopefully, the principles of both acute and long-term care will be delivered simultaneously. When the patient's condition has stabilized and he is no longer "ill" as such, it is time

---

INITIAL NURSING ASSESSMENT OUTLINE
BASIS OF NURSING CARE PLAN

Introduction	Name, age, chief complaint or problem, circumstances of present injury or illness, referring physician
History	Past injuries, illnesses, hospitalizations
Vital signs	Temperature, pulse, respiration, blood pressure
Allergies	Reactions to drug, food, airborne particles, contact
System check*	
Neurosensory	Level of consciousness, orientation, cranial checks, intellectual level, balance, coordination, sensory abnormalities, emotional stability
Integumentary	Turgor, general condition, complete description of lesions, condition of mouth
Musculoskeletal	Muscle strength, range of motion, motor abnormalities, amputations (Follow-up evaluation by PT)
Respiratory	Pattern and sound of respirations, URI? cough? Pulmonary function studies (Follow-up evaluation by PT and IT)
Urinary	Vocabulary? Normal voiding or ostomy? Continence? Urinary draining devices, catheter size, date of last change
Gastrointestinal	Vocabulary? Schedule: time, frequency, BM consistency, normal movement or ostomy? Effect of diet?
Diet	Type, likes and dislikes, time and amount; method: bottle, PO, gavage, etc.
Health supervision	Dates of last dental, eye, and hearing exams; performed by? Immunizations? Safety problems?
Growth and development (activities of daily living; motor skills)	Independent, with assistance; dependent: feeding, turning, transfer, bathing, dressing, toileting, standing, walking (Follow-up evaluation by OT and PT)
Equipment brought	Cane, crutches, walker, wheelchair, braces, appliances, scooterboards, etc.
Current medications and treatments	Medication: dosage, time, route, effects? Treatments: time, duration, specifics
Family composition	Parents, marital status, age, siblings, extended family, resources (Follow-up evaluation by MSS)
Social and educational interests	Level of education, special friends, hobbies, security items, community contacts
Understanding of injury or illness	By patient, by family
Specialized care needs	

PT, Physical Therapy; OT, Occupational Therapy; IT, Inhalation Therapy; MSS, Medical Social Service.

*In making this assessment, one should ascertain the status of the patient before his injury or illness.

to consider transfer to the rehabilitation unit.

A rehabilitation program ideally involves an inpatient unit, an out-patient clinic, and the community agencies. They all function to help the patient and family progress smoothly from onset of illness or injury back to the home and community as a functioning, worthwhile member of society.

Throughout the patient's progression from the initial care facility back to his home and community there must be no surprises. The transition of the patient to units, wards, agencies, and levels of any program must be done smoothly without interruption or breaks in continuity. The patient, family, and team members must be kept informed of the patient's status, program, and goals. Continuity in care during and after transfer to the rehabilitation unit takes the coordinated effort and skills of all the persons involved. One person must coordinate the process of admission. Frequently, this is the responsibility of the nurse.

Unit staffing of a rehabilitation unit needs to be 30% to 60% above the usual medical-surgical levels. Fastidious nursing care, continual teaching, and reinforcement are required. Independence comes with patience, repetition, and allowing the patient or family member to "do" rather than the traditional "doing for." The program is expensive, and the cost must be passed on to the patient, insurance companies, and government agencies; but the independence gained may in the end reduce the total financial outlay. Needless to say, the patient, family, and rehabilitation team must expend great amounts of physical and emotional energy as well as monetary resources. Perhaps the former is more difficult to supply.

Before contributing to the formation of an individualized nursing care plan, each team member must assess the patient's current status. A logical, systematic approach will assure the inclusion of all important facts in this nursing assessment. (See the chart on p. 342 for a suggested assessment outline.)

Using this evaluation of the patient's current status and pertinent history one can formulate nursing interventions for existing and potential problems. When the patient's progress is sufficient, as shown on the unit and during progressive home passes, discharge plans are finalized. Discharge should also be coordinated by one person. There should be a home visit prior to discharge to help plan for program needs or physical changes within the home. These will be evaluated during progressive pass experiences. Prior to discharge, arrangements for the following must be made: community public health nurse follow-up, admission to a regular or special school, methods of obtaining supplies and medications, return appointments to community physicians, and phone numbers of team members.

After discharge, regular visits to a rehabilitation clinic enable the team to reevaluate each patient with feedback from the school, public health nurse, and other outside agencies.

PSYCHOLOGICAL SUPPORT OF THE LONG-TERM PATIENT AND HIS FAMILY

The very character and severity of an injury or disease may be a source of considerable stress, but the prolonged isolation from normal surroundings, the strange environment of the hospital, and frequent encounters with the many different people involved in patient care make hospitalization particularly difficult. The limited experience and development of the child increases the potential for emotional trauma at this time. Three recommendations seem particularly appropriate for the nursing of children and young people with long-term illnesses: maintain a sense of trust; protect the child from fear, frustration, and pain; and facilitate social interaction and contact with the community.

A sense of trust is best fostered in children when their parents trust the people working in the facility. This trust is gradually developed as the parents and child learn that the staff, demonstrating forethought, accessibility, and reliability as well as technical skills, cares about them. It may be strengthened through the use of the primary nurse concept or the fairly consistent assignment of one or two nurses for each child's care. Trust also increases as the staff helps the family in its grief for the child who is injured or is born with defects. These parents mourn the loss of the well or perfect child as though he had died. Grieving as a result of injury or malformation is similar to that associated with fatality, though the terminology used may vary (see p. 361). The loss is resolved in three stages: (1) shock and denial, (2) developing awareness, and (3) restitution. The immediate response of shock and disbelief is often still present upon arrival at the rehabilitation unit. Statements such as, "When will my child walk again?" and "When he is better, things will be like they were before," demonstrate the denial. Each statement does not require refuting but certainly should not be reinforced. The counseling person should reinforce reality through understanding but factual discussion of the patient's status, problems, and required nursing care. Involving the family in the delivery of care helps in all three stages and permits the family to feel useful, important, and needed.

The second stage of mourning is demonstrated by increasing awareness and feelings of guilt and anger. Laments of "Why me?" "It's all my fault," "If only I'd have looked sooner," and "I shouldn't have let him go," poignantly demonstrate the guilt. Anger is often directed toward the child for being careless or disobedient. One parent may accuse the other of being at fault. Often anger is directed at the hospital staff since this outlet is often "safer" than accusing a family member. Criticism of nursing care, the physician, or staff personalities are the most common manifestations of this anger. Understanding the cause of these feelings enables the staff to support the family. Reassurance that the accident was unpreventable (if, indeed, it was) will help. Giving the parents information about

their child's condition and involving the family in the delivery of care and decision making are necessary. Nonjudgmental listening and prompt attention to problems will help smooth the way toward the third stage of grieving: restitution.

This last stage involves the sharing of grief with others and, hopefully, the undergirding support of relatives and friends. When a loved one dies, the funeral allows the family to accept their loss. In the case of disability, the family frequently substitutes ritualistic behavior such as an exact time for visitation, weekly visits to a special doctor, or daily trips to church. Some families seem to adjust to the changes imposed by disability better than others. Unfortunately, the stresses are great, and family dissolution all too often results. Trust helps ease these stresses. Trust through open communication helps the family work through the problems.

It is impossible and probably undesirable to protect a patient completely from fear, pain, or even frustration. However, these unpleasant feelings may be reduced. Since children need to do little to prepare themselves in advance for most procedures, the knowledge that a certain procedure will be done need not be shared until just before its actual performance. Then the child should be told in simple, truthful terms how the test or nursing activity will affect him and what he can do to help. If children are told about unpleasant procedures too far in advance, unconscious fantasies and fears may be activated. Opportunities to verbalize and to express themselves through drawings, play acting, or music should be made available. Feelings that cannot be put into words need to find an outlet before they in turn become symptoms.

This need for emotional release ties in with the need to facilitate social interaction and contact with the community. The maintenance of social contacts and outside relationships is sometimes difficult for a child with flagging energy and extended illness. Yet the knowledge that one still has such relationships encourages stability and incentive and usually makes return to the neighborhood after hospitalization less traumatic. Short, chaperoned trips into the community to recreational areas, cultural centers, or just visiting friends can also be a method of maintaining one's place in the important world outside. These passes should begin as soon as the family has been given necessary instructions and have demonstrated competence in the child's care. Much support and encouragement are often needed.

The addition of a recreational therapist to the staffs of many hospitals is a welcome event. This specially prepared professional helps patients participate in a wide range of constructive activities either in groups or as individuals. A monthly newspaper planned by the children and young people, hobby fairs, and picnics on nearby lawns have also been successful.

Whether in the rehabilitation unit or regular hospital area, the convalescing long-term patient should be given the opportunity and responsibility of continuing his education. Ideally there will be a classroom for ambulatory patients and provision made for tutors from the public school system. Telephone tutoring is also available in many areas. Education is extremely important to those capable young people whose vocational choices may be somewhat narrowed.

COMMON DIAGNOSES ENCOUNTERED

Three common diagnoses found in rehabilitation units are: spinal cord injuries, congenital anomalies of the central nervous system, and traumatic brain injury. Since students working on the rehabilitation unit will frequently meet patients with these problems, they are discussed briefly below.

Spinal cord injury

Children suffer spinal cord injury less frequently than adults do. Other than spinal defects associated with birth anomalies, such as myelomeningocele, spinal cord problems occur almost exclusively in teen-agers as a result of auto or, less frequently, diving accidents. Although the spinal cord is partially protected by bone, shearing or torsion forces can destroy or severely damage the cord. The affected portion of the body is determined by the level of spinal injury. The higher the cord injury, the greater the resulting disability. The paraplegic patient (paralysis or functional loss involves lower extremities) can be totally independent; the quadriplegic patient (paralysis or functional loss involves all four extremities) may need supervision or assistance. The more hand function available, the more independent the patient will be. A patient with lower spinal cord involvement may be limited to the loss of bowel and bladder function and perineal sensation.

The application of lifesaving measures is, of course, of initial importance in the management of the patient with spinal cord injury. Immobilization and stabilizaton of the spine is paramount. In the hospital this is most frequently accomplished by a turning frame (Fig. 23-1) and skeletal traction. During this time of bony healing the complications of bed rest must be prevented. This involves meticulous skin care, periodic range of motion, adequate fluid intake, venous support stockings, bowel and bladder programs, and special respiratory care. The patient with injury at midtrunk level or above requires more than position changes and coughing. Because the respiratory muscles have been affected, blow bottles and intermittent positive pressure breathing (IPPB) are valuable. An upper respiratory tract infection is a serious threat to this patient.

The higher the level of the cord injury, the less tolerance the patient displays for an upright position. The application of elastic hose from toes to groin or of a snug-fitting corset prior to sitting helps prevent pooling of blood in the lower extremities. Gradually (over a period of days), increasing the angle of the wheelchair back and lowering the legs helps prevent dizziness, vertigo, perspiration, fainting, and other signs of hypotension. When these symptoms occur, tipping the wheelchair back to lower the patient's head relieves the symptoms.

Below the level of injury, temperature regulation is affected in these patients since skin nerve endings that combine with the central nervous system are not functioning to control temperature. The skin does not perspire to aid cooling, nor do the muscles shiver to produce heat. Therefore, the patient's skin may be injured by extremes of heat or cold that he cannot perceive unless he is made aware of this possibility. Also, the patient's response to an inflammatory process may register a higher body temperature than is usual for that type of problem. Control is usually obtained by uncovering the patient or using aspirin suppositories. Tepid sponges will generally lower the most difficult fever.

In the patient with an injury above mid-trunk, or T6, a complication known as autonomic disreflexia may arise. This is a very serious rise in the blood pressure that can conceivably lead to a cerebrovascular accident (CVA). Signs and symptoms include: flushing, headache, sweating, feelings of nasal stuffiness, goose bumps, bradycardia, and a rapid increase in blood pressure. These result from sympathetic system activity and are usually related to physical stimuli, such as bladder and bowel distention, severe pressure sores, or urinary tract infection. Less frequently, external stimuli may trigger autonomic dysreflexia. Treat by elevating the patient's head and removing the stimulus. If the patient does not improve, hexamethonium chloride can be given. Patients who are subject to such episodes should be fully instructed in self-care before discharge.

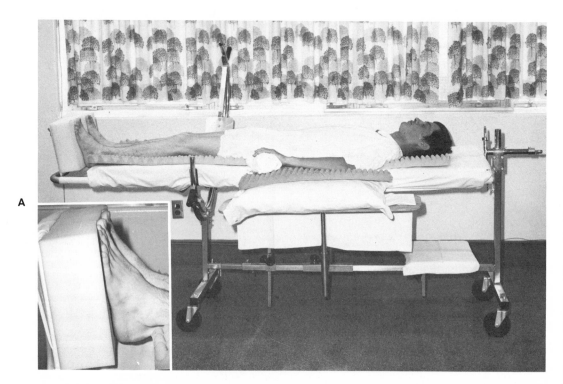

Fig. 23-1. **A,** Supine position on Stryker wedge turning frame, used for spinal injuries or extensively burned patients. **B,** Patient placed in wedge ready for turn. (Only one nurse necessary.) **C,** Prone position on frame. The patient who has control of upper extremities can eat and read. (Courtesy Children's Health Center, San Diego, Calif.)

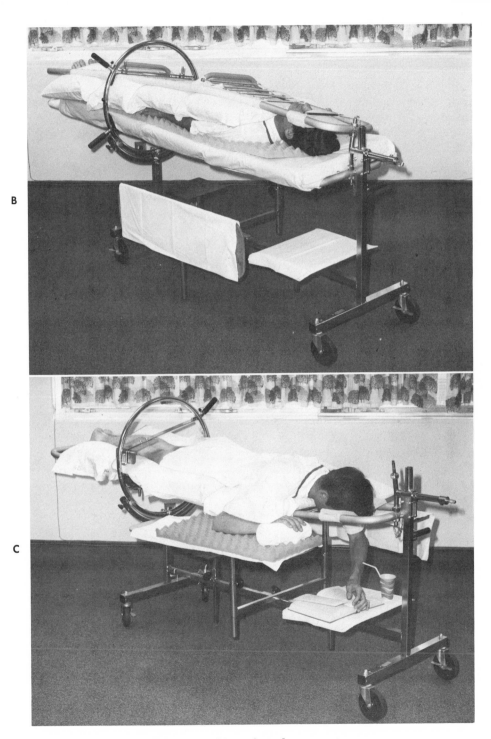

Fig. 23-1, cont'd. For legend see opposite page.

Spina bifida with myelomeningocele

Myelomeningocele, the protrusion of spinal cord fibers through an abnormal vertebral opening into a meningeal sac on the back of the infant, occurs in approximately 2 or 3 of every 1,000 births. These children require initial habilitation rather than rehabilitation in the strict sense of the term. The physical problems of these boys and girls are similar to those experienced by children with low spinal cord injury. Usually the protruding sac is excised shortly after birth. Preventive skin care, range of motion, and bowel and bladder programs are taught to the family. The child learns to care for himself as he grows older. The development of hydrocephalus may be a complication of myelomeningocele. Close observation for signs of abnormal head growth is needed. (For discussion of types of ventricular shunts used to help control head enlargement see pp. 228 to 230.)

In these patients, the effects of gravity, the lack of supportive muscles, and, occasionally, uneven growth makes a straight spine difficult to achieve. Without the use of external support and possible surgery, a patient may literally sit with his rib cage resting on his thighs. The hips may also be affected; many are subluxed or dislocated. Often the feet are clubbed. Urinary tract complications are frequently seen. Urinary tract diversion (Bricker procedure) is often done if there is upper urinary tract destruction due to infection (see Fig. 23-5).

The patient born with a myelomeningocele seems to accept his handicap and body image more easily than the person who has lost normal function. In either case, the emphasis is placed on remaining function. The family must realize that, generally, no mental retardation is present. The child should be treated normally with the realization that he requires a certain amount of preventive physical care. In our society, value is placed on youth and athletics, and the loss of physical abilities does not enhance a child's self-image. The value of the person, as opposed to the body itself, should be taught.

In order for the patient to obtain a satisfying job in adulthood, education is a necessity, and guidance may be helpful. A regular school and college are preferred for their psychosocial value. Psychometric and vocational testing may help in the selection of a school.

By the time a child reaches puberty the problems of sexual awareness will be complicated by questions regarding sexual performance in relation to the disability. The male patient with myelomeningocele is probably unable to have an erection or any sensation in the genital area. The male patient with spinal cord injury has no sensation but may have erections. Although procreation is possible, only a small number have had children. The female patient with spinal cord injury or myelomeningocele may conceive and bear children without sensation. However, patients with spinal cord injuries who are seeking reassurance regarding sexual relationships should appreciate that the most important aspect of a sexual intimacy is a caring relationship and that coitus is only one of many "normal" alternatives to satisfaction. The patient can be an adequate sexual partner through oral and manual stimulation. The patient may physically be unable to attain orgasm but can derive a great deal of pleasure from satisfying the partner.

Brain injury

The symptoms of patients who have received brain injury from auto accidents, tumors, or other causes vary according to the severity of the injury and the areas of the brain affected. The minimally injured child may virtually recover or have only a limp or speech defect; another child may be severely damaged and nonfunctional. Patients who make progress and are likely to regain function are seen in the rehabilitation unit.

Initial lifesaving management seeks to prevent complications. Tracheostomy and ventilation equipment are frequently indicated and careful suctioning techniques and tracheostomy care are required. Positioning may be modified to accommodate the tracheostomy. If placed in a prone position, the patient may need thick padding for chest and head with an open area at the neck to allow adequate space to prevent tracheostomy obstruction. The use of IPPB in addition to turning and positioning helps prevent pneumonia.

Frequently the brain-injured patient will assume characteristic postures. In decerebrate patients, the arms are typically stiff and extended at the patient's sides. The fingers and thumbs of the hand form a C. The legs and ankles are also extended, and in the instance of severe brain damage, the back arches backwards in the opisthotonic position. Another characteristic position assumed is labeled "decorticate." The patient clenches his hands, flexes his elbows, and draws his arms in on his chest. The overall posture resembles the fetal position. The main injury is thought to be in the cerebral cortex.

The physical needs of the patient may be considerable and in many ways not unlike those of the patient with spinal cord injury. However, this patient typically regains awareness and orientation slowly. Sensory stimulation is thought to be valuable. Conversation (even though it may be only one sided at first), a nearby radio or TV, pictures of the family on display, a calendar, and clock help improve orientation. The physical and occupational therapists work with the patient in developing both fine and gross motor coordination. Although strong, the patient may be unable to feed or dress himself. Activities of daily living (ADL's) are introduced early in therapy so that the patient can hopefully begin to achieve some degree of independence. Speech, intellect, and emotional stability are typically affected. Psychomotor testing and educational counseling are helpful. The more severely affected children usually attend special schools for the handicapped.

A child with an impaired intellect and functional body may ultimately be happy and satisfied. A child with a reasonable intellect and severe physical dysfunction, such as aphasia (loss of normal speech) or ataxia (loss of normal gait), understands his condition and frequently has much difficulty adjusting.

At puberty the person with brain injury also has awakened sensual interest. Parents must be cautioned that as a result of their injury, some patients may be overly friendly and invite unwanted sexual encounters. The problems of marriage and possible child rearing are difficult and must be considered on an individual basis.

PHYSICAL ASPECTS OF REHABILITATION

The complications of prolonged bed rest and immobility represent the greatest dangers to the life of the long-term patient (Fig. 23-2). Examples of such complications are:

1. Motor and sensory loss of superficial nerves, skin ulcers, and skeletal deformities due to pressure.
2. Muscle wasting and shortening (contractures), bone calcium loss, ankylosis of joints, edema, venous stasis, and thrombosis from disuse atrophy.
3. Urinary tract infection, stones, constipation, and fecal impaction related to poor fluid intake and positioning.
4. Hypostatic pneumonia from pooling of secretions in the lungs.
5. Depression and psychological disorders resulting from the isolation and interference in normal activities.
6. Disturbance in normal growth and development.

The meticulous application of a few basic nursing principles can prevent many of these complications from occurring. These principles are discussed below.

Routine skin care

An adequate blood supply keeps the skin functioning and in repair. A lack of blood to an area will cause deprived cells to die. The small vessels in the skin form a network that supplies the skin from all directions. Any pressure, such as that from

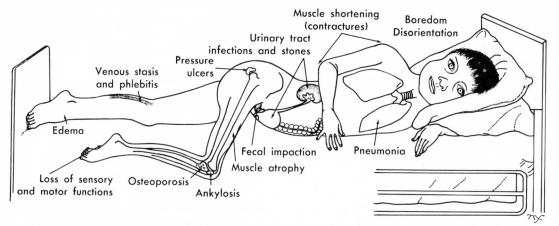

Fig. 23-2. Complications of prolonged bed rest. Of course all of these complications may not be seen in every patient.

Response to pressure: the sequence of events	What you see
Caution signs	
1. Area pinkness, leaving area in a few minutes.*	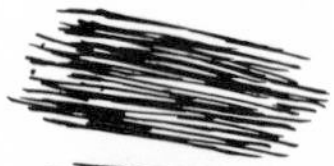
2. Discrete darker reddish spot persisting up to 1 hour.*	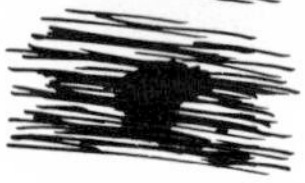
3. Discrete darker reddish spot persisting over 1 hour to several days. The more time needed for the area to regain color after a finger blanching test, the more time needed for return to normal.	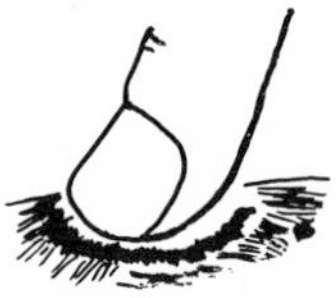
Pressure sores or decubitus ulcers	
4. An unbroken or open blister, sometimes with no color change. May be confused with burn; takes days to heal.	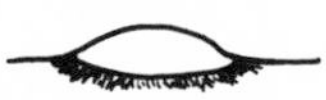
5. A partial-thickness ulcer, damaging part of epidermis; heals from bottom and edges; takes days to heal.	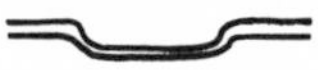
6. A full-thickness ulcer, damaging full depth of epidermis; heals only from edges; takes days to weeks.	
7. A penetrating ulcer, involving bone and connective tissue; takes perhaps months to heal.	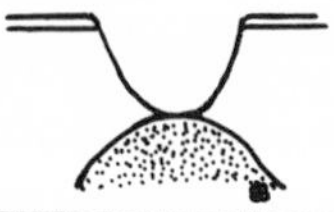
*Best time to treat to prevent sequence. Practice prevention: total body inspections twice daily; pressure point inspections with each position change.	

Fig. 23-3. Skin signals.

sitting, standing, lying, braces, shoes, or appliances, causes compression of these small vessels and does not allow blood to the cells. Where bony prominences (such as the hips, sacrum, and knees) are close to the surface, there is no muscle tissue to pad or distribute the pressure evenly, and considerable pressure, which can cause great damage to the skin, develops. The sequence of events leading to skin breakdown and the sores or lesions that result are described in Fig. 23-3.

When red marks are seen, the child must not bear pressure on that area until the skin has returned to normal. Any surface that comes into contact with the skin must be suspect. Soft, moldable surfaces distribute pressure over a larger area, and any one spot receives less pressure and less damage results. If you recall the difference between sitting on a concrete step and a well-upholstered chair, you will appreciate why items such as foam rubber mattresses, wheelchair cushions, and soft leather shoes are encouraged.

For the patient who is wheelchair bound and who lacks sensation over the buttocks area, it is imperative that he relieve pressure over the bony ischial prominences. The method for relieving pressure is called a chair "lift." For the paraplegic patient it consists of lifting the buttocks by using the arms of the wheelchair to raise oneself or alternately shifting from side to side. Recommended frequency for the paraplegic patient is every 20 or 30 minutes for 30 seconds. This activity should soon become automatic so that the paraplegic does it without having to think about it. The quadraplegic patient must have assistance to relieve this ischial pressure.

The use of new braces, shoes, or different positions or postures must always be instituted gradually and fequently evaluated. (See the following chart for suggested schedule.)

In addition to pressure-caused skin problems, one must be aware of the danger of burns, bumps, scratches, and even pimples. Burns can be caused by hot car upholstery, sunburn, hot sand at the beach, spilled hot drinks, and other accidents. Though they may appear to be minor, these can be very serious and must be seen by the doctor. Any abrasion or scratch that involves a pressure-bearing surface, must be completely healed before pressure bearing is resumed. Diaper rashes and irritations that do not quickly respond to the application of Desitin ointment or zinc oxide should be examined immediately before a severe problem results. Pimples on weight-bearing surfaces should be cleaned gently with mild soap and water and observed closely for

---

SUGGESTED SCHEDULE FOR SKIN TOLERANCE CHECK

Trial periods	*Observations of pressure areas (red marks)*

1. Beginning period—15 min.
   Increase by 15-min. periods according
   to tolerance until 2-hr. level is reached.
	Clearing in 15 min. or no pressure area
	   seen, increase trial period by 15 min.
	Clearing in 30 min., repeat trial period.
	Clearing in 45 min., reduce trial by 15 min.
	Persists 60 min. or more, call doctor for in-
	   structions.

2. After 2-hr. level is reached, trial periods may be increased to 30 min.	Use same clearing time evaluation, but substitute 30-min. trial periods.

NOTE: Any interruption in the use of a brace, appliance, or position may require a reevaluation period. Prolonged intervals between their use may mean starting again at the beginning of the schedule. When any pressure area is detected, check methods of positioning. Cocoa butter applied daily to bony prominences helps keep skin supple.

increasing size and severity. Because of poor blood supply to scar tissue, healed sores may leave scars that are prone to future breakdown and may interfere with the child's ability to hold a job and live a normal life as he grows into a responsible adult. A small amount of time spent daily in prevention will save a great deal of time, trouble, and money later. Remember: (1) never permit any pressure on reddened areas, blisters, or sores; (2) increase positioning times according to the guidelines; and (3) regularly check total body skin, using mirrors as necessary. Teach the child and the family these precautions. By the age of 10 or 11 the child, with supervision, should be assuming responsibility for his own skin care.

If a patient with an existing pressure sore is admitted, some treatment must be undertaken. There are many theories regarding what to put on a pressure sore. The fact is that one can almost say, "Put anything on it but the patient!" No weight bearing should be allowed. It may be possible to avoid the one position that causes pressure; however, if there are ulcers in several different places, you may have no alternative but to carefully position the patient on the affected side. If this must be done, pressure must be relieved from the ulcer by bridging either side of the ulcer with foam rubber pads or pillows, thus freeing the lesion itself from pressure. But circular or doughnut-shaped supports are not recommended.

Pressure sores must be kept clean. Whatever agent is used, cleaning must be done gently to preserve the new delicate epithelium being formed. Half-strength hydrogen peroxide on applicator sticks effectively cleans away drainage. If the ulcer is infected, an antibiotic should be applied topically. A small pressure sore may be left open to the air to dry. If pressure sores are covered, use a nonadherent dressing so that the new epithelium will not be damaged.

Large ulcers are better managed by moist dressings. A fine-mesh gauze pad, such as an eye pad, is cut to the exact size of the

crater and moistened with normal saline solution. The area is covered with a piece of plastic, such as Saran Wrap, and taped down with paper tape to prevent drying. The dressing is changed every 4 to 6 hours, depending on the drainage present and how long it stays moist. If it is allowed to dry, soak the gauze off in order to preserve the new epithelium. As the ulcer heals, the gauze is reduced in size until finally one can leave the shrunken ulcer open to the air.

Positioning

In the discussion of skin care we have underlined the importance of relieving pressure by turning and changing position. Proper anatomical positioning can help prevent skeletal deformities, muscle shortening (contractures), and venous stasis. There are six basic positions from which to choose: back (supine), abdominal (prone), either side, sitting, and standing. These can all be modified to a certain degree. Positioning problems vary according to the diagnosis and individual needs of the patient. The stick-man chart (Fig. 23-4) shows how to prevent pressure areas, contractures, and sensory and motor disturbances through regular protective position changes.

Venous pooling and the danger of thrombosis can be decreased by the careful use of Ace bandages or thigh-high, closed-toe support stockings to help collapse the superficial leg veins. To further prevent venous stasis, as well as muscle shortening and contractures, a full range of motion should be carried out. It is the nursing responsibility to range joints *without* stretching muscles. The bywords are gentleness and patience. The hands and fingers are exceptionally delicate, and specific instructions about appropriate range should be obtained from the doctor or the physical or occupational therapist. Overzealous range of the fingers could make the hand less functional later.

Position changes also lessen stasis of fluid in the lungs. With regular deep breathing, blow bottles, and coughing (if

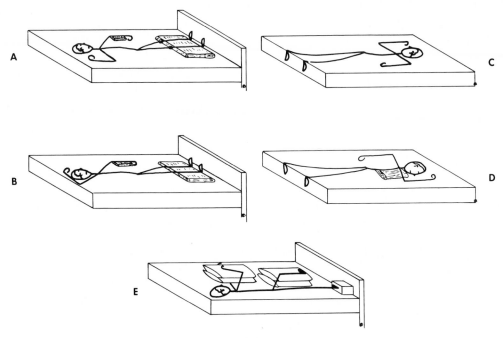

Fig. 23-4. A and B, Supine positions with angle of arms changed. C and D, Two prone positions. A small pad is placed under the shoulder for additional support. E, Side-lying position. Note support for lower foot and two pillows for upper leg and arm.

necessary, stimulated by a suction catheter), pneumonia may be prevented. Changing position and forcing fluids will also help prevent urinary stones and constipation.

Naturally, as soon as the patient is physically able to tolerate a wheelchair, he should be placed in the more normal sitting position, even if he is still comatose. This maneuver adds a position to his repertoire and lets the patient see people and his environment from the more customary vertical perspective, which helps to prevent disorientation.

Depression, disorientation, and hallucinations can result from prolonged horizontal positioning and social isolation of the normal individual. This, added to the physical and emotional trauma of an injury, is a tremendous problem. Anything that will stimulate and orient the mind—people, predictable, pleasing routines, a clock or calendar—is helpful. Frequent visits by the nurse (just to say "hello") help. Conversation with the patient while in the room or delivering care is essential. The presence of parents and siblings and the friendship of another patient who has experienced a similar injury and made progress helps tremendously.

Interference with growth and development, manifested by disrupted bone growth, delay in reaching skill or functional milestones, or inability to play normally, occurs too frequently in the young disabled child. He must have the chance to explore and move about the floor and, if possible, to achieve the vertical position. His environment should be as "homey" as possible and include measured amounts of supervised responsibility and freedom appropriate for his age, abilities, and general condition.

Urinary bladder care

Based on the neurological involvement, neurogenic bladder can be classed as uninhibited neurogenic bladder, reflex or spastic bladder, and autonomous neurogenic bladder.

353

Uninhibited neurogenic bladder. This condition results from an upper motor neuron lesion that may be a residual of traumatic brain injury, brain tumors, or multiple sclerosis. The patient may be aware of a full bladder but, like the small child, unable to prevent voiding. The preferred program consists of bladder retraining—sitting the patient on the toilet on a regular schedule (for example, every 2 hours) and limiting fluids in the evening. Since the patient is not intentionally incontinent, criticism and scolding are inappropriate as well as ineffective. Praise for appropriate voiding and matter-of-fact redressing after incontinence encourage success and desired behavior.

Reflex or spastic bladder. A spinal cord destroyed above the reflex arc results in a reflex bladder that may be a residual of traumatic spinal cord injury, tumors within the canal, or multiple sclerosis. The patient is unaware of a full bladder and has no voluntary control of voiding. In these patients the sphincter is contracted, and the bladder usually incontinently empties, leaving a large amount of residual urine.

Bladder management of this type of patient has characteristically been by continuous internal catheter drainage during the acute phase of the illness. Following this phase the patient then has a "catheter freedom trial." The catheter is removed, and a regular fluid intake is maintained. After approximately 4 hours, the patient sits up in bed and attempts to initiate voiding. This can be stimulated by: (1) pressing or tapping sharply over the fundus of the full bladder, (2) straining, (3) pulling pubic hair, (4) stroking the inner thigh, or (5) lifting the buttocks off the bed, using an overhead frame. If the patient voids, he should be instructed to note the presence of any sensation or aura of a full bladder prior to voiding, such as a feeling of fullness, flushing, pressure, or any unusual sign. This then would become the signal for the patient to trigger the full bladder and void in a urinal, an external urinary collection device, or on the toilet.

Sometimes the patient's bladder will empty when full but will not respond to triggering. In this instance an external collection device would be most helpful unless the times between voiding are consistent or the patient has a predictable aura and time to reach a toilet. If the patient is unsuccessful in voiding after several attempts, the catheter is then replaced.

If the patient successfully voids, a residual urine is obtained after each voiding. When the amount of urine obtained by catheterization directly after voiding is 10% or less than the amount of urine in the full bladder, the patient is termed "balanced." When a patient is balanced, the likelihood of infection is small, and the catheter may be left out. If the voiding trials are unsuccessful, the patient must continue to use a catheter connected to a leg bag or external collection device.

In some rehabilitation centers selected patients with internal catheters have their catheters clamped intermittently during the day for a designated period of time (usually 2 hours). After the 2-hour period the catheters are unclamped and allowed to drain for 10 minutes. They are then reclamped, and the cycle is repeated. This is done to allow the bladder to fill and hopefully maintain capacity and tone.

A recent trend in rehabilitation centers is toward intermittent catheterization. Compared with the use of a long-term indwelling catheter, intermittent catheterization is preferred because it lowers the incidence of infection and increases the chance of a balanced reflex bladder. The passing of a small-gauge, straight catheter on a regular schedule (for example, every 4 hours) can be taught to family members or in some cases to the patient. The aim is to empty the bladder when full without permitting distention. By keeping a regular fluid intake and limiting fluid prior to bedtime, the patient can sleep through the night and establish a regular daytime schedule.

Autonomous bladder. A lack of functional nerve connections between the bladder and the spinal cord creates an autono-

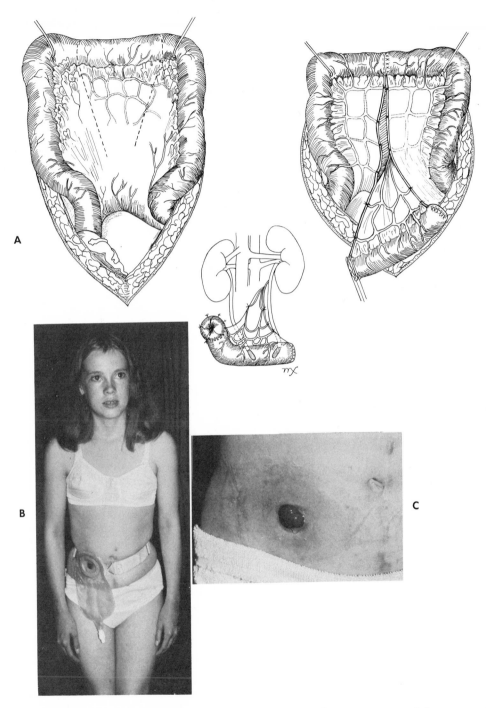

Fig. 23-5. A, Ileoconduit, ileoloop diversion, or Bricker procedure. A segment of ileum is removed maintaining its mesenteric attachment. The ureters are transplanted into an open pouch constructed from the ileum. The ileal pouch is brought to the surface of the abdomen and drains urine continuously. **B,** A type of urinary drainage collection bag for daytime use. **C,** Close-up of uncovered ileoconduit stoma.

mous bladder. It is seen in patients with myelominengocele, cauda equina injuries, or in those who have had radical pelvic surgery. Their bladder and sphincter are flaccid. The patient has no sensation and has continuous overflow incontinence. Some believe management can be obtained by Credé's maneuver (the application of pressure above the fundus of the bladder downward toward the perineum). Others do nothing but let the urine drain. Residual urine, infection, urinary backflow (reflux), and eventual destruction of the upper urinary tracts may follow. The patient often requires a urinary tract diversion to preserve the upper tracts.

Such a diversion is also called an ileal conduit, ileal loop diversion, or a Bricker procedure. A urinary tract conduit is constructed from a separated loop of ileum. The ureters are transplanted into this loop, and a permanent opening into the abdominal wall is constructed (Fig. 23-5). Urine is then collected by means of bag affixed over the draining stoma by adhesive. There are many bags of this type available. They should be fitted individually to each patient. The enterostomal therapist has received special training in the selection, fitting, application, and maintenance of ostomy bags. Since the appliance is a very important personal item and many parts are reusable, the nurse should never discard any part unless directed by the patient or responsible family member. The loss of one part may render the appliance useless until replacement is made.

Catheter care. Indwelling catheter drainage is by suprapubic or Foley catheter. Proper catheter care can prevent infections, abscesses, and periurethral fistulas. The male patient with a Foley catheter usually has more problems. The smallest catheter that will drain without clogging is desired. This will permit exudate to pass around the catheter and out the urethra. The catheter must be taped to the abdomen so that the penis and catheter are directed toward the upper body. This prevents the catheter from being accidentally pulled, causing

damage to the sphincter or urethra. It also eliminates the constant movement of the catheter and penis and irritation and destruction of urethral mucosa. This position prevents excessive pressure against the inside of the urethra by the elimination of the normal S curve from the penis to the bladder. Any dried drainage at the meatal-catheter junction must be removed to allow the exudate to flow out. In one method of crust removal, hydrogen peroxide and applicator sticks are used. The penis should be retracted along the catheter and cleaned well. Any exudate from the urethra should be expressed manually. Many programs follow this cleansing with the application of a water-soluble ointment, such as Betadine. Catheter care should be done at least daily and as often as needed to prevent crusting.

Foley catheters in females should be taped to the thigh. The catheter and periurethral area may be cleaned with mild soap and water or diluted Betadine solution (not Betadine scrub because of the detergent it contains.)

The suprapubic catheter should be cleaned of crusting as described earlier. Some units apply a water-soluble ointment, such as Betadine or polymixin B. A split gauze pad is usually placed at the site of the catheter's entry into the abdomen.

In patients with long-term indwelling catheters, bladder irrigation is indicated to prevent stone formation. One of the most effective irrigants is Suby's solution, which will dissolve crystals in the bladder. The solution is vigorously instilled and drawn back into the syringe for a total of approximately 30 seconds, then discarded. Acid urine inhibits growth of urea splitter organisms, such as *Proteus* and *Klebsiella*. Urinary acidification can be accomplished with large intakes of cranberry juice, prunes, plums, or vitamin C tablets. Citrus juices and carbonated beverages make urine alkaline. Good catheter care, bladder irrigations, urine acidifiers, and forcing fluids will help prevent infections, stone formation, periurethral abscess, and fistulas. Feeling "sand" encrustations when rolling the catheter between the fingers is a signal for catheter change (usually at intervals of 4 to 6 weeks).

External urinary collection devices. For the child who does not require an indwelling Foley catheter, an external device is desired. Unfortunately, there is no successful device for girls, and diapers must be used. As the child grows, custom-fitted plastic pants may be purchased or made from patterns. Since urine may contribute to skin breakdown, a protecting ointment should be applied with each diaper change.

There are many collection devices available for boys. Those that combine a penile sheath and a truss or athletic supporter appliance are generally undesirable. The need for extra elastic straps that may cause chaffing and pressure points seem to be hazards to hyposensitive or anesthetic skin.

For boys from 6 to 9 years old, small, medium, or large finger cots can usually be connected to rubber tubing and a leg bag to make a very satisfactory, inexpensive collection device. The modified finger cot is attached to the penis with nontoxic ostomy cement and a narrow ring of elastoplast that does not touch the skin itself. This can remain on several days without leaking, but it must be removed daily for penile skin inspection. The Heyer-Schulte Company of California now produces a similar ready-made collection device in diameters of 16 mm. through 30 mm. in 2-mm. graduations. This can allow for precise fit, decreased skin problems, and longer wearing time.

Bowel care

Neurogenic bowel may be classified in the same way as neurogenic bladder. Uninhibited neurogenic bowel results in defecation without volitional control when the rectum fills. The reflex, or spastic, bowel exhibits above-normal rectal sphincter tone. When the rectum fills, frequent automatic, partial emptying results. In autonomous neurogenic bowel the rectal sphincter is flaccid and frequent small stools may result.

When the patient has lost normal control, a bowel program should be established early. This helps protect already vulnerable skin from rashes and breakdown. Then, too, the socialization of the older child can be drastically affected by soiling, obnoxious odors, and diapers. Most regular schools will not enroll these children. Furthermore, as an adult, tolerant friends are few and accepting employers are essentially nonexistent.

An adequate program consists of: (1) keeping the stool normal or slightly firmer than normal (as soiling is more likely to occur if it is soft or liquid) and (2) scheduling evacuation time. Each child is an individual and his program must be tailored precisely to his needs. Therefore, one child's program may not be identical to that of another child with a similar problem.

There are many factors that influence bowel patterns. Diet has a very great effect. Disruption of eating patterns—skipping meals, eating extra meals, changing meal times, amounts, or types of food eaten—may disturb the program by causing constipation or diarrhea. By trial and error, one learns exactly what foods constipate or loosen the stool for each patient. Generally, citrus juices, prune juice, and bulk (or roughage) items, such as raw vegetables and nuts, tend to loosen the stool. Inadequate fluid intake and foods such as bananas and cheese will constipate. Gas-forming items, such as beans and cabbage, may cause diarrhea. Most of these foods are not a problem unless eaten in larger than normal quantities. A normal, stable diet with sufficient fluid intake will usually keep the stool as desired. If possible, any changes in factors affecting bowel habits should be added singly so that the effect of each change will be known.

Bowel patterns are also affected by physical activity. Inactivity usually constipates, while great increases of activity may speed the movement of food through the digestive system and cause accidents. Aging, a change of climate or community, altered living patterns, anxiety, and stress may all have their effect.

There are a number of reflexes, techniques, and agents that can assist us in establishing a sound bowel program free of accidents. These include the gastrocolic reflex, digital stimulation, abdominal straining, stool softeners, and bisacodyl (Dulcolax) suppositories.

The gastrocolic reflex is an increase in the peristaltic muscle activity of the large bowel after the stomach has distended from ingestion of food or warm liquids. Therefore, about ½ hour after a meal is a logical time to carry out a bowel program. If the stool is too hard in spite of fluid and dietary measures, stool softeners, such as dioctyl calcium sulfosuccinate (Colace) or dioctyl sodium sulfosuccinate (Surfak), which retain water in the stool, may be used.

Dulcolax is a safe means of chemically inducing peristaltic movement of the large bowel. It is more predictable and safer than irritating laxatives or mineral oils that could decrease vitamin absorption. A Dulcolax suppository is inserted high up in the rectum, against the side of the bowel wall so that it will dissolve and be absorbed easily. Dulcolax usually dissolves in 10 to 15 minutes, reaching peak action in another 10 or 15 minutes.

Digital stimulation does not refer to the digital removal of stool from the rectum. It is a gentle circular motion made by a gloved finger inserted ½ inch against the rectal sphincter muscle. The patient may be positioned on his left side or may sit on a raised toilet seat. This gentle motion will both relax and dilate the rectal sphincter and cause peristaltic muscle contractions of the large bowel. This procedure should be continued for 10 to 15 minutes. It can be used in conjunction with suppositories or by itself. As evacuation occurs, one should gently pull the rectum to one side and allow the stool to be eliminated.

Although any number and combination of these techniques and agents may be used in the child's bowel training, the program should start with the least and the simplest. The time of day for evacuation should be chosen with regard to previous bowel habits, daily schedules, time limitations, and personal preferences. A reasonable time seems to be about ½ hour after the morning or evening meal. Once a time is selected, it must remain consistent within ½ hour.

For a child with a spinal cord injury, one possible routine might be: (1) immediately following breakfast, insert one half of a Dulcolax suppository as high as possible into the rectum (The amount is dependent upon age and size of the child; too much causes abdominal cramping, too little, no action.); (2) wait 10 to 15 minutes, continuing personal care; (3) place the child on a "potty chair" or toilet with his feet touching the floor so that the hips are flexed into the squat position; (4) have the child lean forward against the thighs (to increase intra-abdominal pressure), and massage the abdominal muscles. Encourage him to strain at the same time. (Have children who do not understand blow on a toy balloon.) If diarrhea should occur, it is wise to check for impaction because liquid feces can seep around the impaction, resulting in false diarrhea.

Consistency in the program is essential. Some young children may require the program twice a day. A bowel program takes time, patience, and attention to detail but in most instances is very rewarding.

• • •

The broad goal of pediatric rehabilitation, to foster growth and development, independence, and personal fulfillment, represents a tremendous challenge. It requires all the support of the family, patient, and rehabilitation team. Its rewards may be delayed but are definite, nonetheless.

24

The dying child, his parents, and the nurse

Few nursing assignments are more challenging than helping a mother and father and their sick child who is afflicted with an illness that is invariably fatal. Since the nurse cannot change the reality of the tragic situation, she frequently feels sorrowful. Probably no human experience cuts so deeply into the center of one's heart as the loss of a child.

Understanding a child's concept of death will help the nurse know what to say. Understanding the ways in which his parents may react to the prospective death and one's own feelings about death will relieve some of the nurse's stress. This knowledge should enable the nurse to provide helpful support to the parents and the kind of tender reassuring care the child needs.

A CHILD'S CONCEPT OF DEATH

A child's concept of death is dependent to a considerable extent on his age, since there are different levels of understanding at different ages. Young children do not perceive of death as final or terminal. For children 3 to 5 years of age, death is denied; it is only a change of some kind and is not permanent. Children 5 to 9 years of age recognize death but cannot conceive of it as resulting from chance or a natural happening. Causation is personified. Death to them is like part of a game of cowboys and Indians. Everybody kills each other off, and then they resurrect themselves and play another game. Hence, when someone dies, in the child's mind the event is usually thought of not only as a deprivation but also as a personal abandonment. It may be considered a hostile act on the part of the person who died.

Children 9 years of age and older achieve a realistic concept of death as a permanent biological process. A child over 9 years old is capable of integrating the concept of "not being" if his parents can do so. However, he is comforted by the thought that his death (and theirs) is yet far away.

In view of the preceding information the nurse can readily understand the reasons why children need not be told of their fatal illness. Children generally accept, without obvious panic, the restriction imposed on them as a disease progresses. However, until their energy diminishes, they want to do the same things that other children do. A very bright 3½-year-old boy was nearing the terminal phase of cancer. He seemed so weak that we had his breakfast brought to his cribside instead of serving it in the dining room where most of the little patients ate. For days he hardly ate at all. One morning he asked if his food was cooking. When his tray arrived, he cried aloud and would eat nothing. Knowing that he was hungry, we decided to prop him up and move his crib to the dining room. There he was able to finish every bite without assistance. Even near the end when vomiting occurred after eating, his cries on removal from the dining room could be heard by all. As the child's energy diminishes and death approaches, he has less interest in his surroundings and sleeps most of the time.

Children rarely manifest an overt concern about death, probably because they attempt to repress their anxiety concerning it. Nevertheless, the older child should be allowed to express his fears verbally if he is capable or through play media if he is not. Highly susceptible to the attitudes of his parents, the child will likely sense the gravity of the situation and will need to ventilate his feelings. Often the child should be reassured that his illness is not his fault and is not a punishment for anything he did.

What to tell the child

If by chance the older child does ask about dying, a statement such as, "You have a serious illness, but no illness is without hope and you should remember that,"* is likely to be believed and reassuring. If the child sees or asks about the death of another child, you might say, "Johnny was very sick and died." This implies that the inquirer is not as ill as was his friend. Answer questions simply and always truthfully. Keep in mind the child's level of understanding.

Three stresses of terminal illness

In addition to having illnesses that cause considerable distress, children suffering from terminal illness are subjected to three stresses common to other hospitalized children: separation from mother, traumatic procedures, and isolation. Modification of hospital routine and procedure must be considered.

Separation from mother. Depriving a mother and child of each other when permanent separation will soon take place would be particularly unfortunate. The child wants his mother. Encourage her to touch him. The warmth of physical contact is the most primitive and basic nonverbal comforting technique we possess. It can communicate a solace or comfort to the frightened child that words can never produce.

Traumatic procedures. When parents are helped to understand the reasons why tubes are inserted, intravenous feedings are ordered, blood is withdrawn, or other treatments are initiated, they feel better satisfied. Parents are usually best able to con-

sole and protect their children from fear. Remember, the nurse is best able to help a child allay his fears through his parents. By helping parents to understand, you will have helped the child.

You can also help the older child by transferring his attention and concern from his incurable illness to other *curable* problems or symptoms he may be experiencing. Listen with interest and attention to all his complaints, particularly ones related to intercurrent infections, such as rashes, that can be eliminated. The child can receive enormous reassurance and relief if these complaints are treated intensively. Wahl* calls this method of relieving anxiety "trading up." One month before his death, a 12-year-old leukemic boy stated that he had a cold. Because there was bleeding from all body orifices it was difficult to recognize his symptoms. However, once aware of the preceding information, we treated his cold vigorously. His attention was diverted from his never-ending bloody diarrhea and his many painful intravenous feedings and blood transfusions. Nearing the last stages of life, he succeeded in one last remission; "trading up" illnesses increased this boy's courage as he survived 4 more weeks.

Isolation. Finally, do not isolate the dying child from his friends, relatives, or staff. Usually you cannot conceal a child's death from other children in the ward. They know that "room 101" is the place where children go to die. Furthermore, the most dreaded possibility does not seem to be that of dying but that of dying alone. Children feel secure with other children, and they know nothing too terrible can happen when Mom is there. Encourage parents and relatives to say when they will come back. It implies a promise, "I will see you again, and you will have nothing to fear in the interim." Although relatives and staff are encouraged not to isolate the child, the nurse should not permit constant or unduly

---

*Wahl, C. W.: The dying patient, Consultant, Nov., 1961, Smith, Kline & French.

*Wahl, C. W.: The dying patient, Consultant, Nov., 1961, Smith, Kline & French.

prolonged visits that the child may interpret as a "death watch."

PARENTAL REACTION

One of the nurse's most important roles in the management of the child with a terminal illness is helping the grieving parents.

Integrating the event

Integrating the tragic event of death into their life experience is most difficult. The parents' reactions to the prospective death of the child may be likened to the mechanism of separation anxiety. However, it has much deeper meaning than most separation anxieties that parents and children face.

The mourning process

Anticipation of the forthcoming loss is often accompanied by mourning. The process of resigning oneself to the inevitable outcome usually begins before the child dies, and the parents must be allowed this period of mourning that involves a concentration of interest and energies, self-examination, self-condemnation, and guilt. The parents ask themselves and others, "Would it have made a difference if we had called the physician earlier? Did the child inherit the disease from one of us?" The nurse allows the parents to voice their guilt and reassures them by the gentle and understanding way she answers their questions.

The nurse can help relieve the suffering of parents who are mourning if she has insight into the feelings that they are experiencing. According to Bowlby,* there are three phases in the natural mourning process: protest, despair and disorganization, and hope and rebuilding. Mourning is the process of healing that helps us face and recover from loss. The normal healing process takes a year or more. The clearest evidence of recovery is the ability to remember comfortably and realistically both the

---

*Bowlby, J.: Process of mourning, Int. J. Psychoanal. **42:**331, 1961.

pleasures and disappointments of the lost relationship. The following predictable steps in the mourning process—protest, despair and disorganization, and hope and rebuilding—permit a judgment that healing will occur.

Protest. The first phase is characterized by a general tendency to protest or deny the diagnosis of disease or its fatal outcome. In trying to deny the facts, many strong emotions are brought into play—anxiety, yearning, anger, and guilt. Parents cannot quite believe that this could happen to their child. Often a parent's attitude is one of suspicion, hostility, and constant criticism. Hope for the child is stressed but in a nonspecific way. The parent tells himself, "Something will be discovered." He wants to try anything that might offer hope for a cure no matter how irrational it may seem.

Anxiety is manifested by an intense need to weep, an empty feeling in the abdomen, and loss of appetite. With anxiety there is yearning, longing for a sign that a cure will be found and the child will get well. Guilt feelings are constantly expressed in tears, "If only I had done this or that, if only I had notified the physician sooner." It is natural and necessary to cry, to be angry, and to feel guilty. These are all healthy signs of normal grief. It is a stage in the gradual process of accepting a great loss.

Involvement of parents in the physical care of the child is extremely important in facilitating parental adaptation. But although parental participation in the care of the sick child is desirable, it should not be at the expense of the emotional and physical well-being of the remainder of the family. (Siblings may be disturbed during this period and may require considerable parental support. Parents should be encouraged to divide their time among the various members of the family as the situation warrants.) Mothers and fathers usually want to be with their sick child and need to feel that they personally have done everything possible for the child. Feelings of guilt are somewhat relieved by the expenditure of personal effort in the care of the child. Parents are allowed and encouraged to participate realistically in the physical care of the child by bathing, feeding, or entertaining him and escorting him to the laboratory and x-ray departments. Thus parents become integrated into the ward program, and communication with ward personnel is enhanced.

During the initial period on the ward, mothers physically cling to their children. They are involved solely in their care. After a while parents desire to help as effectively as they can with the care of other children. Assisting them to the playroom and reading to a group rather than just their own child are examples of this desire. Manifestations of this capacity (to help other children) mark a turning point in parental adjustment that reflects acceptance of the child's illness and ultimate death.

Despair and disorganization. Facing and accepting the reality of the fatal illness, parents feel helpless. Life is stripped of meaning. Active, realistic efforts to prolong life typify the early part of this phase.

The mother spends most of her time ministering to the needs of her sick child. During this time the nurse must be aware that the mother's attempts to cope with the situation may fluctuate from gentle, assured bedside care to inappropriate exhausting activity. At one moment she may express exaggerated gratitude to the nurses and medical staff, in the next she is overly critical. Her emotions may range from philosophical resignation to sentimentality. She is emotionally fragile and inconsistent.

The reality of the fatal illness and its meaning begins more and more to penetrate the mother's consciousness. Her denial of the character of the illness may disappear, but hope of a cure persists. Her hope is more specific now, often related to particular scientific efforts.

During this period, mothers cling less to their children and encourage them to participate in ward activities. Parents should be encouraged to express their feelings of depression and defeat during moments away from the child. This helps them move

beyond the initial shock and recognize some of the specific things they still have to offer their child. Every attempt must be made to enable parents to see the continuing value of their function as parents, despite their feelings of despair and helplessness in the face of death.

As the child's physical energy begins to diminish, preoccupation with measures that involve treatment of the disease begins to subside, and parents are interested in relieving the child's discomfort and pain. Although they continue to hope that their efforts will save the child, the intensity of the expectation is gradually reduced. Emotionally they are separating themselves from the child.

Hope and rebuilding. The third phase is characterized by a calm acceptance of the child's impending death. Separation from the child is no longer an adaptive problem for the mother. Mother remains with the child whenever possible but with adequate consideration for the remainder of the family. For the first time, the mother expresses a wish that the child could die so that his suffering would end.

Many parents never reach this third phase of mourning during their child's illness. It may not be until after the child dies that the third phase begins. With the loss acknowledged and the depth of pain plumbed, new people, relationships, and activities become meaningful. Some parents take interest in such organizations as the Cancer Society, Cystic Fibrosis Association, etc. By so doing, the mourner is able to reduce preoccupation with self and the dead child. This allows the mother to reinvest feelings in her other love objects—her husband, her remaining children, or close relatives. The length of the grief reaction and how a person finally adjusts to his new social environment depends, Lindermann* says, on the success of what is called the

*Lindermann, E.: Symptomatology and management of acute grief. In Parad, H., editor: Crisis intervention: selected readings, New York, 1965, Family Service Association of America.

"grief work." By this he means the transition of responsibility for the deceased to other areas of activity and the formation of new relationships and the readjustments this necessitates.

THE NURSE AND THE DYING CHILD
Feelings toward death

Awareness of one's feelings toward death is essential to acquiring the ability to give comprehensive nursing care to the dying child and his parents. Information about the child's concept of death and his parents' fears is not enough. To give sensitive and supportive care to the dying child, the nurse needs help in understanding her own fears about death.

Understanding the concept of death

Fear of death is the most inescapable and realistic of human fears. Fear and anxiety lead to convictions of immortality on a conscious or unconscious level and are universal in all men. We recognize that other people must die but feel an inward assurance that it need never happen to us.

To learn about death, Wahl[*] suggests that we look at the unconscious mind. The mind may be likened to an iceberg. One seventh of it (the conscious) shows above the water and six sevenths (the unconscious) lies below.

The unconscious is continually active. Its thought processsses are illogical. To the unconscious mind, death is never possible in relation to the self. The unconscious is like the mind of the child before he learns to rationalize. Death is never the result of chance or natural happening. When a child has strong feelings of hostility toward a person, he might say, "I hate you, I wish you were dead." If by chance this person dies, the child concludes, "Because I wished this thing, it happened. Therefore I am responsible."

Death of loved ones is viewed as a deliberate abandonment on their part because

of something the child has done. His mother and father died because they hated him. These are the kinds of concepts a child forms. Unconsciously, fear of death involves these same kinds of concepts in adult life.

Each of us feels or reacts differently to the death experience. If this reality (death) is so painful that we handle it by either immersing ourselves in it or utterly denying it, it will be difficult for us to fulfill our role as nurses. We ought to let ourselves recognize, at least to a limited degree, the awe and fear that all of us experience in the face of death. Fear of death is handled in several ways: (1) by a religious belief in immortality, (2) by a denial of the awe felt for death, (3) by withdrawal from the dying child, and (4) by the formation of various phobias or compulsions. As nurses, we are involuntarily influenced by illogical but protective defenses in the presence of impending death. However, if we are to help parents who are experiencing deep grief and distress, we are not to ridicule them or isolate ourselves from them. We are not to punish them in this way. We must become aware of our own feelings. We must try to better understand how we ourselves feel about death.

Courage

Nursing the dying child requires courage. The nurse must remember that courage is not the absence of fear but the willingness and ability to function in its presence. Nurses who care for dying children and counsel their parents must preserve a sympathy and empathy and yet be free enough of emotional involvement to do their work commendably well. We should not become so personally involved with the dying child that we neglect the other children who have an equal need for nursing care.

Group therapy for parents

Recently there has been a trend in university centers to set aside one evening weekly for the staff to meet with the parents of leukemic children. Common prob-

---

[*]Wahl, C. W.: Death, tape recording of lecture, UCLA, November, 1958.

lems are shared in these small mutual support groups. Discussions have centered around the nature of leukemia and its treatment, as well as the emotional problems faced by parents, siblings, friends, and staff. Most of the groups intermittently include physicians, nurses, a social worker, and a psychiatrist. As a result, parents and staff have shared increased understanding of each other's problems. The meetings provide opportunities for parents to meet unit doctors and nurses in a more relaxed setting with ample time for discussion. Specific benefits from these meetings include: mutual support during times of stress and uncertainty; the realization that discipline of the child is still desirable; and the possibility for sharing feelings about death and dying. But perhaps the most important benefit is the opportunity for parents to share and identify with one another on a level common to each. This kind of group interaction can be a meaningful and effective source of emotional support for parents of children with other fatal diseases as well.

Basic concepts of religion

The comfort the nurse can give to the parents of the dying child is important. Knowing their religious belief concerning death may be a great help. Often the nurse will observe that parents with deep faith in God find real comfort in their religious beliefs. For Catholics and Protestants who believe in personal immortality, there is great solace and comfort in the conviction that they will one day rejoin their loved ones.

In the Jewish faith the concept of immortality is not clearly defined. Judaism teaches that perhaps there is a life after death, but the only immortality of which man is certain is the immortality he achieves while he is still alive or through his descendants. Knowing the basic concepts of the vari-

ous religious faiths concerning death may be of great assistance to the nurse. The nurse is not expected to be a theologian nor should she attempt to share her religious beliefs concerning death unless she is asked, but the nurse can help the child and his parents by supplying physical and emotional support and the comfort of spiritual counsel by contacting any clergyman the parents desire. This spiritual advisor, especially one who has added skills in personal counseling to his religious training, can well be the one to whom a parent may turn. He can communicate comfort to parents when friends and relatives are helpless.

Death is inevitable but no less difficult because of its inevitability. Just as it may be the nurse's privilege to help parents and their infant at the event of birth, it may also be her privilege to ease and comfort a mother and father and a small human being who has come to life's last hours. May she do so with gentleness, reverence, and skill.

unit nine
Suggested selected readings and references

Avey, M.: Primary care for handicapped children, Am. J. Nurs. **73**:658-661, April, 1973.
Azarnoff, P.: Mediating the trauma of serious illness and hospitalization in childhood, Children Today **3**:12-17, July-Aug., 1974.
Bell, A.: Day surgery: a concept of care for the pediatric patient, Offic. J. Assoc. Operating Room Nurse **19**:623-631, March, 1974.
Belmont, H. S.: Hospitalization and its effects on the total child, Clin. Pediatr. **9**:483-492, 1970.
Bergmann, T., and Freud, A.: Children in the hospital, New York, 1965, International Universities Press.
Blake, F. G.: The child, his parents and the nurse, Philadelphia, 1954, J. B. Lippincott Co.
Blake, F. G.: Immobilized youth: a rationale for supportive nursing intervention, Am. J. Nurs. **69**:2364-2369, Nov., 1969.
Boone, D. R., and Hartman, B. H.: The benevo-

lent over-reaction—a well-intentioned but malignant influence on the handicapped child, Clin. Pediatr. **11**:268-271, May, 1972.

Bowlby, J.: Processes of mourning, Int. J. Psychoanal. **42**:317-340, 1961.

Connors, M., and others: Ostomy care: a personal approach; cone irrigations; a letter to parents, Am. J. Nurs. **74**:1422-1428, Aug., 1974.

Degroot, J., and Kunin, C. M.: Indwelling catheters, Am. J. Nurs. **75**:448-449, March, 1975.

Delehanty, L., and Stravino, V.: Achieving bladder control, Am. J. Nurs. **70**:312-316, Feb., 1970.

DiLeo, J. H.: Children's drawings as diagnostic aids, New York, 1973, Brunner/Mazel, Inc.

Downey, J. A., and Low, N. L.: The child with disabling illness—principals of rehabilitation, Philadelphia, 1974, W. B. Saunders Co.

Erikson, E. H.: Childhood and society, New York, 1960, W. W. Norton & Co., Inc.

Evans, A. E.: If a child must die, N. Engl. J. Med. **278**:138-142, 1968.

Folck, M. M., and Nie, P. J.: Nursing students learn to face death, Nurs. Outlook **7**:510-513, Sept., 1959.

Guimond, J.: We knew our child was dying, Am. J. Nurs. **74**:248-249, Feb., 1974.

Hardgrove, C., and Warrick, L. H.: How shall we tell the children? Am. J. Nurs. **74**:448-450, March, 1974.

Heffron, W. A.: Group therapy sessions as a part of treatment of children with cancer, Pediatr. Ann. **4**:102-112, Feb., 1975.

Krenzel, J., and Rohrer, L. M.: Paraplegic and quadriplegic individuals, Chicago, 1966, The National Paraplegic Foundation.

Kubler-Ross, E.: Anger before death, Nurs. '71 **1**:12-14, Dec., 1971.

Kubler-Ross, E.: What is it like to be dying, Am. J. Nurs. **71**:54-61, Jan., 1971.

Kubler-Ross, E.: Letter to a nurse about death, Nurs. '73 **3**:11-13, Oct., 1973.

Langford, W.: The child in the pediatric hospital, Am. J. Orthopsychiatry **31**:667-684, Oct., 1961.

Lascari, A. D.: The family and the dying child: a compassionate approach, Med. Times **97**:207-215, May, 1969.

Lindermann, E.: Symptomatology and management of acute grief. In Parad, H., editor: Crisis intervention: selected readings, New York, 1965, Family Service Association of America.

Lore, A.: Adolescents: people, not problems, Am. J. Nurs. **73**:1232-1234, July, 1973.

Loxley, A. K.: The emotional toll of crippling deformity, Am. J. Nurs. **72**:1839-1840, Oct., 1972.

Marlow, D. R.: Textbook of pediatric nursing, ed. 4, Philadelphia, 1973, W. B. Saunders Co.

Mason, E. A.: The hospitalized child: his emotional needs, N. Engl. J. Med. **272**:406-413, Feb., 1965.

McDermott, J. F., Jr., and Akina, E.: Understanding and improving the personality development of children with physical handicaps, Clin. Pediatr. **11**:130-133, March, 1972.

Miller, P. G., and Ozga, J.: How to answer the question "Mommy, what happens when I die?" Nurs. Digest **11**:76-79, May, 1974; reprinted from Ment. Hyg. **57**:21-22, Spring, 1973.

Petrillo, M., and Sanger, S.: The emotional care of the hospitalized child, Philadelphia, 1972, J. B. Lippincott Co.

Plank, E. N.: Emotional care as a priority: approaches to implementation, ACCH J. **3**:11-14, July, 1974.

Prugh, D., and others: Study of emotional reactions of children and families to hospital and illness, Am. J. Orthopsychiatry **23**:79-106, Jan., 1953.

Rehabilitative aspects of nursing; physical therapeutic nursing measures, concepts and goals, New York, 1966, National League for Nursing.

Robertson, J.: Young children in hospitals, New York, 1958, Basic Foods, Inc., Publishers.

Scanlan, M., and others: Quadriplegic adolescent, Nurs. '72 **2**:29-32, June, 1972.

Sculti, K.: Parent discussion group, Am. J. Nurs. **74**:1480-1482, Aug., 1974.

Shore, M. F.: Planning for children in the hospital, Bethesda, 1965, National Institute of Mental Health.

Solnit, A. J., and Green, M.: The pediatric management of the dying child, Part II. The child's reaction to the fear of dying. In Solnit, A., and Provence, S., editors: Modern perspective in child development, New York, 1963, International Universities Press.

Tiedt, E.: The adolescent in the hospital: an identity-resolution approach, Nurs. Digest **1**:20-29, July, 1973.

Wahl, C. W.: The dying patient, Consultant, Nov., 1961, Smith, Kline & French.

Washington guide to promoting development in the young child, Seattle, 1970, University of Washington School of Nursing (mimeographed material available from the University).

Wu, R.: Explaining treatments to young children, Am. J. Nurs. **65**:71-73, July, 1965.

Yancy, W. S.: Approaches to emotional management of the child with a chronic illness, Clin. Pediatr. **11**:64-67, Feb., 1972.

25

Hospital admission and discharge

First impressions are important, especially when a parent and his child are involved. At times hospitalization of a child may be planned, and a previsit to the pediatric department may be possible to reassure parents and patient, but for many families hospitalization comes as an abrupt, unscheduled, and basically frightening experience.

A cordial, smooth introduction to hospital life, extended by a nurse who is sincerely interested in the family involved, will do much to ease the anxiety inherent in the situation. All good nurses minister to more than the hospitalized patient's needs. They are alert to the needs expressed and unvoiced by all family members. However, perhaps nowhere more than in the care of the child is the nurse's response to the entire family so crucial. If the trust of the parent or guardian can be secured initially, the nurse has obtained vital cooperation, a less tense, more rested mother and father, and a more relaxed child. A few more minutes spent at the time of admission may save hours of time later on.

If first impressions are important, so are last contacts. The dismissal may be a most helpful period for the parent, or it may be a confusing "getaway." The following discussion is intended to help the nurse function well in these two eventful situations.

ADMISSION
Identification

The admitting nurse should be introduced or introduce herself to both the new patient and his parents. In many hospitals identification of the patient is accomplished through use of a bracelet, which should be checked for accuracy. Unfortunately, some of the children will be from broken homes. The parent's surname may be different from the child's. This should be clearly and discreetly noted to better understand the situation and avoid embarrassing incidents. To help the staff know their small patients better, many pediatric departments send out questionnaires to the parents of prospective patients requesting helpful information regarding the abilities, habits, likes, and dislikes of the child. Nicknames and special vocabulary used by the child are also investigated. It is good to know that 3-year-old Edmund Atherton Barnstow III responds to "Barney" and loves grape-flavored Popsicles.

Qualifications of a pediatric nurse

The pediatric nurse should feel friendly toward and comfortable with children. She should wish for them the best the future can hold and gain great satisfaction in helping the child become better equipped to meet the demands of life. Her loving concern for children should be expressed through a warm but not "gushy" approach. Children can readily detect people who genuinely care about them. Those nurses who find it difficult to work with children because of inexperience with or isolation from this age group need not feel that they will never function successfully in a pediat-

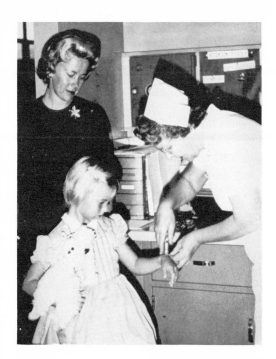

Fig. 25-1. "And here is your bracelet, Mary Lou." (Courtesy Children's Health Center, San Diego, Calif.)

ric area. But they must really want to learn to know children and think of them as persons and not as *problems*. If nurses are willing to be patient and alert, if they are adaptable and imaginative, and if they are knowledgeable, kind, and understanding, then they possess the potential assets for pediatric nursing.

Nurses many times find the pediatric area emotionally taxing. It is sad indeed to see a tender, innocent child suffer or a young boy or girl whose life had been bright with promise suddenly struck down by disease or death. We do not know all the answers to the philosophical questions created by such circumstances, but we do know that these children and young people and their parents need help. There must be those who are willing to try to help them and are especially prepared to do so.

The nature of a pediatric nurse's responsibilities dictates that she possess an ample portion of both fortitude and *discretion*.

She must think at least twice before she speaks. Detailed or crucial information about a patient must come from an authoritative source, such as the *nursing supervisor* or *attending physician,* and should only be given to those directly involved, usually attending personnel or parents. Well-meaning but curious casual inquirers should not be given diagnoses or progress reports. Finally, the nurse must develop the capacity for benevolent self-criticism and evaluation of her own actions so that she may constantly improve her ability to meet her patient's needs.

Nurse-parent role

The newer concepts of pediatric care do not picture the pediatric nurse as an authoritarian dispenser of knowledge and skill, who alone has the ability to meet any need of the small patient. She is not a substitute mother, usurping the biological or legal mother's position. However, she is a practitioner who has the advantage of special practical and theoretical education and training not available to most mothers, and she is a person who cares about children, sick or well. The aims of the pediatric nurse and the child's parents should be basically the same—to help develop each child's potential to the optimum level and produce a creative, contributing member of society who finds high purpose in life and a role worth pursuing. The family learns from the nurse, and the wise nurse learns from the family.

The amount of parental participation in the care of the hospitalized child depends on the condition of the child and the response and abilities of the parents. To say that they should be allowed to do nothing when they have probably had total responsibility for the child until he was admitted to the hospital is often unrealistic and even unkind. On the other hand, if the mother gives the child his bath, feeds him, and completes his routine hygienic care alone, much valuable observation of the child is lost by nursing personnel. At times, instead of obtaining more relaxed, cooperative parents, an exhausted, worried mother and father may result. Perhaps, when the parent and child seem to gain much from parent participation in his hospital care, it is best to carry out such care with the nurse helping the mother and vice versa. Then cooperation is enhanced, observation and reporting is more accurate, and any legal complications of parental care are absent or minimized.

Some parents are unable to share constructively in the care of their hospitalized children. Others do not wish to participate. Occasionally, children may be more relaxed when mother and father do not participate. Parental anxiety caused by possible feelings of guilt, inadequacy, or frustration may be sensed by the child and cause him, in turn, to be anxious. In certain cases the child may be confused about the role of the parent when the mother is at the bedside and the nurse must minister to the small child. In this situation, asking the mother to take a brief rest period until the procedure is completed may benefit both parent and child. For the most part, however, the presence of the parents is a real asset to the child. The mother and father, depending on the condition of the child, can help and be helped by sharing in the admission of the child. They may aid by undressing him, positioning him for temperature readings, helping with feedings, and providing the comfort of their presence. However, no parent should be made to feel that unless he or she is at the bedside the child will not receive complete and loving nursing care. This would cause many anxieties. Nor should parents be made to think that they are neglecting their duty to the child unless they are at the bedside almost constantly. The liberal visiting privileges now extended to parents in most pediatric hospitals are designed to ease tensions, not to create them. To sum up these paragraphs, we would use again the often repeated comment found in many nursing texts: "The modern pediatric nurse is mother's friend and helper—not mother's substitute."

Orientation

If the circumstances of hospital admission and the patient's age and condition permit, the child and his parents should be shown briefly around his unit and be introduced to other children. The parents should be introduced to key personnel and shown where such conveniences as the public telephone, rest rooms, the public dining area, and waiting rooms are located. Many children receive a simple toy such as a hand puppet or coloring book at the time of admission, which helps to entertain and to pass the difficult periods of waiting for examination or surgery. The nurse should be sure the child has something appropriate at the bedside for diversion. A specially beloved toy or blanket may be brought from home. The nurse should make sure that any personal toys or clothing left at the hospital are carefully labeled. In most cases the use of the child's own clothes, with the exception of bathrobes and slippers, is discouraged because of the high incidence of loss in the hospital laundry, despite attempts to avoid such confusion.

When the nurse is speaking to children, it is psychologically good technique to bend or crouch down to their eye level for special introductions, serious talks, or mutual enjoyment. No one likes to talk to knees or stretch his neck to look up all the time!

Nursing procedures

The patient is usually admitted directly to his own unit. During the admission, it is customary to secure the following:

1. Pertinent information regarding his habits, vocabulary, possible allergies, normal diet, preparation for hospitalization, and family structure. This type of information may be obtained on a form filled out by the parent while the admission is in progress if it was not secured before the actual hospitalization.
2. His height, weight, and age.
   a. Babies are routinely weighed without clothes.

b. Be sure that the scale is covered with a diaper or technique paper and is balanced before weighing!

c. This information is used to:
   (1) Determine dosages of medications.
   (2) Determine general condition and progress.
   (3) *Note:* All children with diarrhea and vomiting or intake-output problems are routinely weighed every morning before breakfast.

3. His temperature.
   a. Glass or electronic (rectal, axillary, or oral) thermometers may be employed depending on the policy of the hospital and desire of the physician. The method may be altered depending on child's age, diagnosis, condition, and tolerance of the method.
   b. Never leave a child alone while taking his temperature (oral, rectal, or axillary). When rectal temperatures are secured, always have one hand on the thermometer and another on the child to assure safety and accuracy.
   c. Nonoral temperatures should always be taken when:
      (1) The child has seizures or poor muscular control. (There is danger that the child may bite the thermometer, causing self-injury.)
      (2) The child has difficulty keeping his mouth closed because of oral surgery, general condition, or breathing difficulties.
      (3) The child is receiving oxygen by mask, nasal catheter, or cannulae.
   d. Remember, rectal temperatures on the average are 1° F. higher than oral temperatures, whereas axillary temperatures are one degree lower. All rectal temperatures of 100.0° F. or over and all oral temperatures of 99.0° F. and over should be re-

ported to the head nurse or team leader as soon as determined.
   e. In a few instances, rectal temperatures may be contraindicated (rectal surgery, diarrhea, or ulceration).

4. His pulse.
   a. For infants, an apical pulse rate is secured by placing a stethoscope between the left nipple and the sternum. It is too difficult to secure an accurate radial pulse rate.
   b. Other pulse points may be used in the older child (the temple, the neck) if there is difficulty keeping the wrist still.
   c. Pulse determinations may be made in most cases by timing for 30 seconds and multiplying by 2 on the very young child.
   d. Irregularity and quality as well as rate should be noted.
   e. The activity of the child should be taken into account. (For example, the pulse of a sleeping child should be so labeled.)
   f. For rate ranges, see Table 25-1.

5. His respirations.
   a. The rate and the character of respirations are important. The nurse should be alert to detect sternal retractions and Cheyne-Stokes respirations.
   b. For rate ranges, see Table 25-1.

6. His blood pressure.
   a. The correct-sized cuff is very important. The cuff should cover two thirds of the upper arm measured

Table 25-1. Approximate pulse and respiration rates at rest based on age[*]

Age	Pulse	Respiration
Birth-1 mo.	110–150	30–50
1 mo.-1 yr.	100–140	26–34
1-2 yr.	90–120	20–30
2-6 yr.	90–110	20–30
6-10 yr.	80–100	18–26
Over 10 yr.	76– 90	16–24

[*]Pulse and respiration rates become slower with age.

from the shoulder to the elbow.

b. It is sometimes difficult to determine the blood pressure of an infant. If regular auscultation is not helpful, the systolic pressure may be secured by palpation of the brachial pulse as the cuff is gradually deflated. In some areas a Doppler or arterial pressure transducer apparatus may be used. Still another technique, called the "flush method," may be employed. The distal portion of an upper or lower limb is made pale by the application of wrappings or manual pressure. The blood is prevented from entering the blanched hand or foot by an inflated cuff. The cuff is slowly deflated and the systolic reading recorded when a flush, indicating the passage of blood beyond the cuff into the exposed hand or foot, is noted.

c. Any unusual activity of the child just prior to or during the blood pressure determination must be noted. Try to obtain this reading while the child is quiet.

d. Blood pressures are often taken to determine the onset of shock or increasing intracranial pressure.

e. For some average readings, see Table 25-2.

7. His general appearance and behavior as evaluated through observation.
   a. Overall clinical *appearance*.
      (1) In no acute distress.
      (2) Mildly ill.

Table 25-2. Some average blood pressure readings based on age*

Age	Systolic	Diastolic
Newborn	50	
1 month	80	
4-6 yr.	90	60
7-10 yr.	100	64
11-14 yr.	110	70
15-20 yr.	114	74

*Blood pressure increases with age.

(3) Severely ill.

b. Growth and development.
   (1) Appropriate for age and sex of child.
   (2) Special physical considerations such as orthopedic problems, imperfect vision, deafness, speech or language barriers, malnutrition, obesity, cosmetic defects, prostheses (dentures, glasses, contact lenses, artificial eyes, limbs), history of seizures, and general vigor.
   (3) Cultural, intellectual, and emotional considerations, such as cultural heritage (for example, Mexican-American), mentally retarded or gifted, parent-child-nurse interaction, and initial response to hospitalization.

c. Skin manifestations.
   (1) Unusual color, flushed, pale, cyanotic, or jaundiced.
   (2) Unusual birthmarks.
   (3) Rashes, bruises, possible boils, blisters, possible infestations (body or head lice, scabies).
   (4) State of cleanliness.

d. Nervous system manifestations.
   (1) Level of consciousness.
   (2) Abnormally dilated or unequally dilated pupils.
   (3) Tremor, twitching, or periods of blank staring.
   (4) Limp, flaccid extremities.
   (5) Bulging fontanels.
   (6) One-sided or lower extremtiy weakness or paralysis.

e. Other signs and symptoms important to note on admission.
   (1) Diarrhea, nausea, vomiting, abdominal distention (type of stool or emesis).
   (2) Nasal drainage, coughing. (Signs of respiratory tract infection noted in a child scheduled for surgery should be reported immediately. Surgery may be cancelled.)
   (3) Difficulty in voiding.

All these observations do not make the nurse a diagnostician. She simply observes as accurately as possible and reports.

Collection of specimens

In addition to the preceding measurements and observations, the patient is routinely scheduled for urinalysis and blood examinations.

Urine specimens. The collection of a urine specimen in a child over 2½ years old is not usually difficult. The collection of a specimen from an infant or young toddler poses real problems. Various methods have been recommended. Most pediatric areas use small adhesive-backed plastic bags that adhere to the perineal region or base of the penis (Fig. 25-2). These are usually satisfactory except when the child has a rash or perineal excoriations. The bag must be checked frequently to avoid losing the precious commodity! Occasionally the so-called metabolic bed is used to obtain specimens—particularly if the specimen collection is prolonged (see p. 414).

Blood samples. A blood specimen is usually not secured by the nurse, but she may help restrain the child as the physician or laboratory technician takes the specimen. It may be obtained from a toe, heel, or finger prick, an arterial puncture of the arm, or a venous puncture in the arm or neck. If the child must be restrained and if he is old enough to understand, he should be told that the hands, sheets, or other appliances that may be employed are used to help him hold still so that the physician can help him get well. He should not think of the restraints as a means of punishment. Various types of restraints are used during a child's hospitalization. These are discussed in Chapter 26. Common procedures or diagnostic tests that may be ordered at the time of admission (spinal puncture, Clinitest, sweat test) are also discussed in Chapter 27.

Diet and fluid orders

The diet of a newly admitted child depends, of course, on the reason for the hospitalization, his age, and his general condition. Patients scheduled for pending surgery may be allowed nothing to eat or drink. The diet is ordered by the attend-

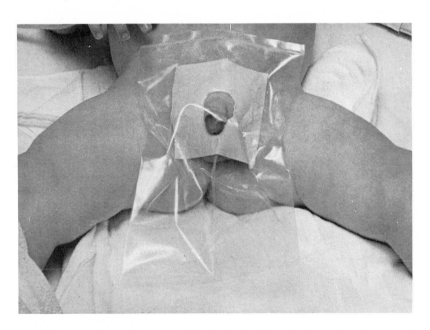

Fig. 25-2. Application of an adhesive-backed plastic bag for collection of a urine specimen. Be sure it isn't upside down!

ing physician. Children may have many allergies often involving not only pollens, animal furs, fibers, and dust but also common foods. Chocolate, milk, wheat products, tomatoes, oranges, and strawberries are among the frequent offenders. Nurses should be alerted to these problems and the allergic manifestations they usually cause. The cultural patterns of some patients may cause feeding problems and poor acceptance of the routine hospital diet.

Admission responsibility

The member of the nursing team who has the responsibility of actually admitting a patient will depend on the condition and needs of the child. In certain situations the admission may be made in its entirety by a registered nurse. At other times it may be a joint or delegated responsibility carried out by both the registered nurse and the licensed vocational nurse.

DISCHARGE
Plans for dismissal

The discharge day is usually extremely busy for the parent. Arrangements must be made for transportation (after all, Mary, in a hip spica cast, won't fit in the family Volkswagen). A baby-sitter for the other children in the family may be necessary while mother takes her home. Maybe father will have to take time from work to provide transportation. Unless special arrangements are made, the child usually must be dismissed in the morning to avoid a hospital charge for an additional day. If mother will have little help after her child comes home, she will be busy trying to shop and run errands not immediately possible when the child first returns home. If possible, the nurse should write out any instructions for home care concerning observations to be made or medications and procedures prescribed, rather than rely on oral instructions to the parents. The arrangements for the next follow-up visit to the physician should be clear.

Preparation for home care
Helps in convalescence

If convalescence at home is expected to be prolonged, more preplanning is necessary. The location of the sleeping quarters of the child may need to be changed to save steps and provide greater opportunity for observation. Special equipment may need to be improvised, rented, or purchased. Provisions for help by a visiting nurse may be desirable. A tentative schedule providing the needed care and rest for the convalescent but still allowing the other members of the household opportunity to pursue a fairly normal range of activity and relaxation is desirable.

Possible behavior changes

Parents should be alerted that hospitalization affects children differently. Occasionally, children will have a period of difficulty readjusting to life at home. They may regress developmentally, and activities that they had already mastered previous to their illness may not be attempted. Irritability and wetting by a previously toilet-trained child are quite common.

Actual leave taking

At the time of discharge, every attempt should be made to send all of the child's belongings home with the parent. (The isolation department may recommend some restrictions.) Return trips to the hospital to pick up articles left behind are annoying. Bedside stands, closets, cupboards, bedclothes, and flooring must be carefully scrutinized.

Before actually leaving the hospital premises, the parent (or responsible adult) must sign a form indicating who is taking the child. Great care must be taken that the person given responsibility for the child at the time of discharge has the legal right to assume that responsibility. At this time a final check is made regarding any medications to be taken home or special instructions to be given.

If at all possible, the child should be taken to the point of actual transfer (usually to a car) in a wheelchair, a rolling bassinette, or on a gurney. He must always be accompanied by a nurse or hosiptal employee.

• • •

Admissions and discharges are part of the everyday pattern of hospital routine. The nurse must remember that they are far from routine for most of the patients and parents who find themselves within the sound of her voice and influence of her actions.

26

Basic patient needs and daily planning

Every patient has individual needs that, because of their unique combination or background, are particularly personal and special. At the same time, these needs may be said to represent the needs of all people because they usually fall into broader, more basic categories of care. For this presentation, the patient's needs have been grouped to form seven areas of discussion.

BASIC PATIENT NEEDS

The nursing staff is responsible for helping to provide the following:
1. Safety
2. Observation
3. Diagnostic tests
4. Supportive procedures
   a. Aiding respiration and oxygenation
   b. Regulating body temperature
   c. Positioning
   d. Adequate nourishment and fluid balance
   e. Cleanliness
   f. Rest
   g. Diversion and self-expression
5. Medications and special treatments
6. Rehabilitation
7. Recording of events

Safety

The problem of safety is constant in any hospital. In a pediatric hospital it seems to be constant and compounded. The environment must be continually evaluated to prevent accidents. The patients are often too small to regulate their own surroundings and lack the judgment to evaluate their environments properly. Unrestrained or unattended children in high beds or cribs should always have the bed or crib sides securely raised. No nurse should turn her back on an unrestrained child in a crib with the side lowered. Children who have climbing urges should have crib nets properly applied to form a tightly fitting net roof (Fig. 26-1) or be placed in a plastic-domed bed unless supervision is constant. Beds of inquisitive boys and girls should be at a "no touch" distance from wall electricity, suction, and oxygen outlets. Toys should be checked for sharp

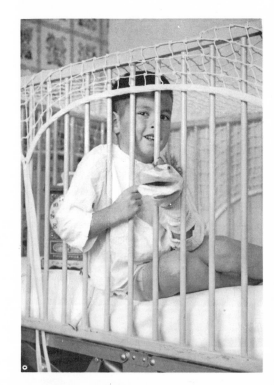

Fig. 26-1. This little boy was a climber at night. A crib net was applied over the top of his bed before lights out. (Courtesy Children's Health Center, San Diego, Calif.)

edges, points, or potential danger. Plastic bags should not be used for storage of toys or playthings. Notices of known allergies should be clearly posted in the child's unit. All equipment should be in good working order and used properly. Special precautions should be observed when administering oxygen. When a child is transported in a wheelchair, in most instances a waist or

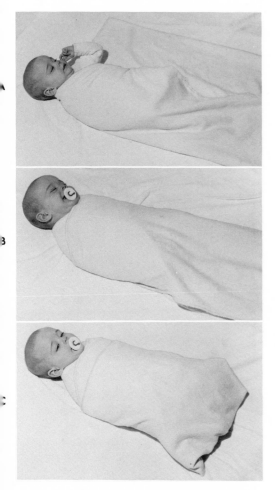

Fig. 26-2. Covered chest mummy wrap. **A,** Center the baby's head at the edge of the "short side" of an open baby blanket or sheet. Place one arm at his side and pull the blanket snugly over his shoulder, arm, and chest and tuck the blanket under the baby. **B,** Position the opposite arm similarly and pull the opposite corner over and around the baby. **C,** Open out the loose end of the blanket and bring it up and around the baby snugly. (We do not generally advocate pacifiers but believe they have a place in certain situations.)

jacket restraint should be used to avoid the possibility of his tipping forward or sliding down. Unnecessary traffic and congestion in the halls should be avoided.

An important component of safety is firm but kindly discipline. Explaining to the child who is old enough to understand the reason for some rules often works wonders. Good discipline also means realistic expectations and prompt follow-through by the nurse responsible for supervising behavior. It means that nurses must not give choices when no alternatives are possible. It also means offering a choice when the ability to choose would bring pleasure, importance, and a sense of self-direction or achievement to the child. Promises kept, a "yes" that means "yes" and a "no" that means "no," and a loving regard for the ultimate welfare of the child are extremely significant in maintaining good discipline.

Sometimes the child must be restrained during a treatment to protect him from himself. Such restraint should never be presented as a punishment but as one way to help the child hold himself still for a little while. An example of such a restraint is the "mummy wrap" (Fig. 26-2). A commercial "mummy restraint" used in many emergency rooms is the Olympic papoose board shown in Fig. 26-3. Another type of control used to prevent a child from touching his face or pulling on a gavage tube is elbow restraints, which are usually fastened to the child's hospital gown. However, elbow restraints are not effective if the child can reach his face with a toy or an implement without bending his arms. To control leg and arm motion, specially constructed ankle and wrist restraints (Fig. 26-4) or the time-proved clove hitch tie (Fig. 26-5) may be used. A pediatric Posey belt may sometimes be employed to allow some movement in bed and yet prevent the patient from getting up. A jacket restraint is pictured in Fig. 26-6.

Restraints must be removed periodically to check circulation and exercise the body part involved. They should be so constructed that they will not become tighter

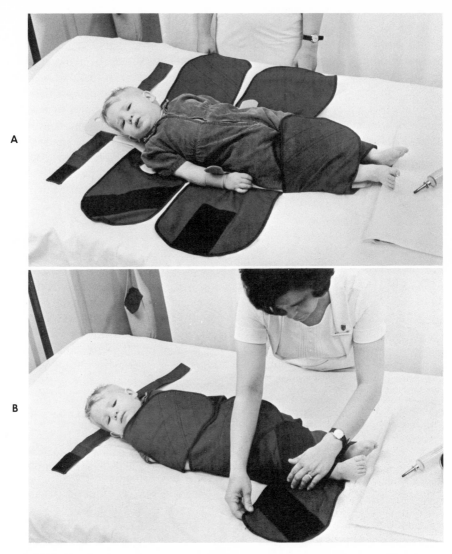

Fig. 26-3. Preparing to restrain a child for gastric lavage using the Olympic papoose board. Various wraps are possible with the velco-lined restraining folds. (Courtesy Olympic Surgical Co., Inc., Seattle, Wash.)

with increased tension and impair circulation or endanger respiration.

Observation

Provision for observation is crucial to the welfare of the patient. To plan and pursue the therapy of a patient intelligently, enlightened observation must become an inseparable part of the patient's care. Observation of the patient should be made especially in the light of his diagnosis. If the diagnosis is pneumonia, for example, the fact that the child is pale and has a frequent, loose cough producing thick, white mucus is significant. Sometimes negative observations are important to make. It is important to record that a child admitted because of convulsions has had no seizures for a certain period. The observation that a child hospitalized for vomiting and diarrhea retained a feeding and had no stools for a specific interval may be significant.

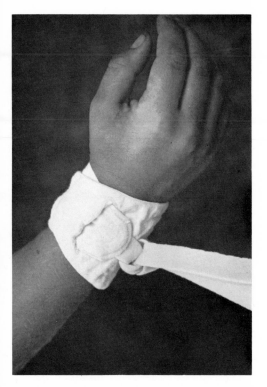

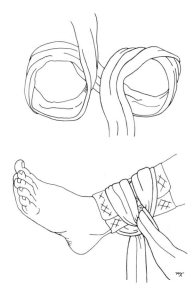

Fig. 26-4. Wrist restraint. The cuff portion encircles the wrist, with one end pulled through a slit in the opposite side. The ties are then knotted around the wrist and fastened to the bedframe with a bow tie. It may also be employed to restrain an ankle.

Fig. 26-5. Application of the clove hitch restraint. The formed loops are placed one on top of the other and the body part put through the opening. The body part should always be previously padded.

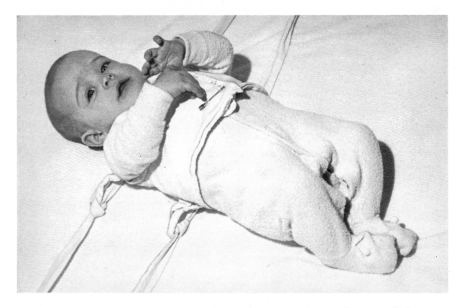

Fig. 26-6. Restraining jacket. The ties are fastened to the bedspring frame, and the pins are placed in front. It may also be used as a wheelchair restraint for small children.

Pediatric procedures

When observing the patient and recording his appearance, activity, and treatment. refer back to his diagnosis. What would be especially important for the physician or supervising nurse to know? A change in a child's bed placement may sometimes be needed to observe him more closely.

Diagnostic procedures

The diagnostic procedures ordered must be understood so that adequate preparation, execution, and follow-up may be provided. It would be impossible to describe within this brief text all the diagnostic procedures encountered by the nurse in a pediatric setting. But for some of the more common tests and a description of specimen collection, consult Chapter 27 and the hospital procedure manual.

In the morning be careful to determine if any of your patients should not receive anything to eat or drink and are posted NPO. After a test for which a patient has been fasting, be sure to inquire *if* the patient may resume his diet. If so, see that the prescribed foods or liquids are secured.

Supportive procedures

Various types of supportive procedures and techniques are used to maintain or improve the physical and emotional resources of the patient. These may include special provisions for aiding respiration or oxygenation, regulating body temperature, positioning, maintaining fluid balance or nutrition, relieving pain, or improving body function. They also include the interest and love expressed by parents, family, friends, and nurses and the physical and spiritual serenity promoted by the development of trust. The use of oxygen and humidification equipment is discussed in a separate chapter as are the methods of regulating body temperature. Positioning of the bed patient, however, is described in the following paragraphs.

Positioning the patient

Even the child who is ambulatory and active needs to be supervised so that he does not develop poor posture habits that will interfere with the optimum function of his body and cause him to look less than his best. The child in bed, particularly if he must remain fairly quiet for long periods, must be especially helped to maintain good alignment, functional positions, range of motion, and good tissue health for all body parts. (Read also section on skin care and positioning in Chapter 23, pp. 349 to

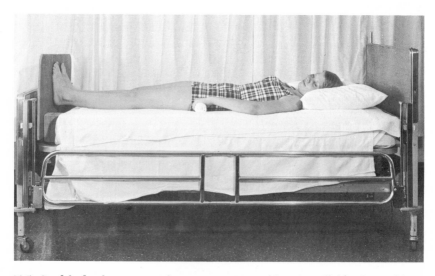

Fig. 26-7. Good body alignment in the supine position. (Courtesy Children's Health Center, San Diego, Calif.)

353.) Barring special treatments involving traction, casting, or specifically ordered body placement, the child in bed should have a posture, when in supine position (on his back) or in prone position (on his abdomen), similar to that which would be considered in good alignment if he were standing. Included in this section are some illustrations showing some of the do's and don't's of positioning.

If a patient remains in bed for an extended period without adequate foot support or with tight covers pressing down on his feet, he will develop a tightening of the Achilles tendon, or heel cord, causing *foot drop,* which makes walking difficult. One leg is often allowed to fall outward toward the side *(external rotation);* and the knee in a common flexed position, if not changed often, can result in fixation and *contracture* in a relatively short period. Positioning the arms across the chest and a partially flexed head position decrease respiratory capacity. Such arm and hand positions (very typical of the arthritic patient), if maintained, cause flexion contractures of the shoulder and elbow and *wristdrop,* with loss of function in the hand.

Fig. 26-7 illustrates how good alignment

may be achieved with the help of a footboard, pillows, and hand rolls. Incapacitated teen-age patients usually need considerable help. It should be noted that a type of foot support is being employed. The knees are straight up, rotated neither to the inside nor outside. Sometimes this correct position is maintained in part by a rectangularly folded blanket that has been partially slipped under the buttocks of the patient. The long protruding end is then rolled under tightly toward the thigh to stabilize the leg in neutral position. A rolled towel or *small* pillow placed under the calves may help relax the knee joints and lift the heels off the bed just enough to relieve pressure. Some patients appreciate a small pillow placed in the small of the back. The arms are alternately rotated for comfort. Soft hand rolls help maintain functional finger-thumb relationships.

When the patient is in the prone, or abdominal, position (Fig. 26-8) his toes should be either over the end of the mattress pointing down between the foot of the bed and the mattress or positioned over the edge of a pillow. A thin pillow support under the abdomen takes pressure off the chest and reduces the lumbar curve. The arms are usually comfortable if abducted

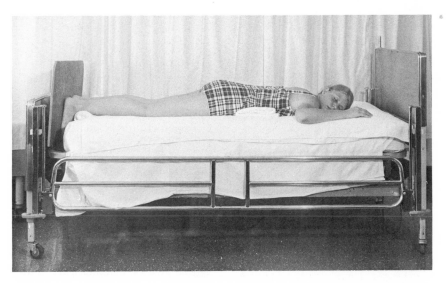

Fig. 26-8. Good body alignment in the prone position. (Courtesy Children's Health Center, San Diego, Calif.)

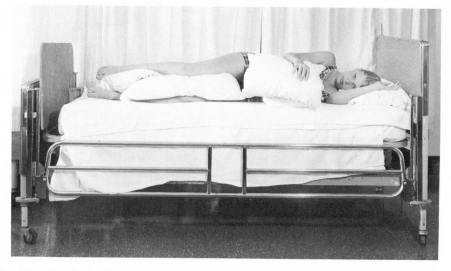

Fig. 26-9. Good body alignment in the side-lying position. (Courtesy Children's Health Center, San Diego, Calif.)

and flexed. No pillow may be required under the head.

The side-lying position is often preferred. The main problem with this position is the strain placed on the hip joint and lower back by the upper leg if it is allowed to fall forward. For a patient who has no back or hip problems and is able to move freely, this is no great difficulty. However, if these problems or conditions exist, this leg position should be avoided by the addition of one or two pillows supporting the upper leg as in Fig. 26-9. Sometimes a pillow tucked lengthwise against the back is comforting. A support for the upper hand relieves the chest.

Good positioning and frequent turning (every 2 hours or less) will do much to comfort the patient; avoid respiratory, circulatory, and urinary complications; reduce deformity; and speed rehabilitation. Infants and toddlers do not require such elaborate supports to maintain alignment and prevent deformity, but they do need to be frequently turned and positioned if they do not move themselves. An older infant or young toddler often sleeps with his head and chest down on the mattress, face turned to the side, while his knees are pulled under his abdomen to make his but-

tocks form the highest point of his sleeping silhouette. This is a perfectly normal and characteristic posture for this age. A young infant should not be left unattended flat on his back because of the danger of aspiration. A rolled blanket should be placed at his back to maintain a side position.

Nourishment and fluid balance

Diet. The diet of a patient does not consist of the type of diet order that the physician writes on the patient's chart. It is not that easy. The diet of a patient consists of what he eats, drinks, and retains of that which has been sent from the kitchen or prepared by the nursing staff in response to the physician's order. Some diets look beautiful on paper but, unfortunately, are not eaten by the person for whom they have been prepared.

Before a tray is served to a patient it should be carefully checked to see that it is compatible with his diet order, food allergies, abilities, and cultural or religious background. Nuts, raw carrots, and celery should not be served to toddlers who do not know how to handle such "chewy" foods. They sometimes suffer from aspiration. Common diets served in the pediatric area are clear liquid, full liquid, soft, high protein, high carbohydrate, low residue, diabetic, and salt or sodium restricted. Students should review these diets in a diet manual.

A child must often be helped at mealtime. A nurse cannot simply put a tray on a bed or crib table and expect even an older child to automatically eat. His utensils should be appropriate. The food must be easily available and attractive. Toddlers often do well if placed in a high chair for feedings. Some young children prefer to try to feed themselves, but very young children enjoy being held during meals. Bibs and nurse's feeding gowns again ease laundry problems.

Infants often drink better if they have a "breathing space" between the time they finish their solids and are offered their formula. Infants and toddlers who need a greater fluid intake may be offered fluids before solid foods when appetites are sharpest to encourage fluid acceptance. Plastic bottles should be used with older infants who enjoy "holding their own." Young children may sometimes be fooled into eating unwelcome vegetables if they are disguised with pureed fruit.

Whether it is necessary to record every bit of food eaten by a child depends on his diagnosis and condition. A diabetic child would require very close observation and recording of food intake. Any food left on his tray must be reported in detail so that a replacement may be calculated and prepared by the diet kitchen. Usually, the dietitian wishes all the trays of diabetic patients to be returned separately to the kitchen for evaluation after meals. The true diet of a patient with any metabolic, growth and development, digestive, or feeding problems should certainly be carefully recorded. Some of the trays of these patients will also be returned to the dietitian for evaluation. This would include most medical patients and some surgical patients. The intakes of children who are long-term patients with fairly stabilized conditions could be adequately described as "ate well," "ate fairly well," or "ate

poorly." *All* pediatric patients are routinely on measured fluid intake, expressed in cubic centimeters (cc.) or milliliters (ml.). Many are on measured fluid output.

Hydration. Fluid intake is really of greater immediate importance than solid feeding. The hydration of a child is extremely important. A young child may become dehydrated more rapidly than an adult. An infant is especially vulnerable, having a greater surface area and higher metabolic rate per unit of weight than an adult. Maintaining an adequate fluid intake is one of the very important responsibilities of the bedside nurse. The amount of fluid that is urged depends on the size and condition of the child. An infant needs about 2¼ ounces per pound (150 ml./kg.) of body weight per day to maintain hydration and more if he must combat preexisting dehydration.

An older child will probably do well on fluid intakes of 1,500 to 2,000 ml. per *day,* depending on his individual needs. Students are reminded that patients who are immobilized in casts or traction apparatus and all those with indwelling urinary catheters must have special attention to assure an abundant fluid intake.

ENCOURAGEMENT. Assuring oral intake often calls on a nurse's ingenuity, patience, and persistence. Small amounts taken frequently are tolerated better by the ill child than copious amounts taken rapidly, no matter how willingly. Fluids taken rapidly are often not retained by children who are ill, upset, or excited.

The kinds of fluids that may be offered a child depend on his diet order and any allergies he may have. Clear fluids include any liquid through which one may see the bottom of its container—water, bouillon, strained fruit juices, Popsicles, gelatin, and soft drinks. A full liquid diet would include unstrained fruit juices and milk products such as ice cream, sherbet, milk shakes, and creamed soups.

Learning which fluids the child has accepted well in the past may save time. Offering a choice is often helpful. Sometimes the manner in which fluids are offered is significant. Some older babies seem insulted by a bottle and drink well from a cup. Others regress and will only take fluids well from a bottle with a certain kind of nipple. Some small children are accustomed to warm milk, others like it cold. Older children often reject milk unless it is ice cold. A nurse who is able to sit down with the child beside her or in her lap and offer fluid as part of good companionship is more likely to be successful than the nurse who expresses her frustration in constant verbal harassment. In some cases the use of straws, doll tea-party dishes, colored ice cubes, or a paper star on Johnnie's fluid intake record may help. Popsicles are usually very acceptable. Just plain water should not be forgotten in the search for fluids. With older children, the factual knowledge that other steps (intravenous feedings) will be necessary to assure hydration if oral fluid intake is too low may encourage drinking. For most children, a carton of milk and a glass of fruit juice at breakfast, a glass of some other fluid or dish of ice cream or gelatin equaling approximately 200 ml. during midmorning, soup and beverage at lunch and a midafternoon liquid snack fulfill the responsibilities of the day nursing shift.

RESTRICTION. Patients scheduled for operative procedures are usually not allowed any oral intake for several hours before their surgeries. After the procedures the amount and type of fluids offered may be restricted. After heart surgery oral liquid intake may be limited to 300 ml. during the morning and offered only in small quantities for an extended period. Some postsurgical patients will be allowed nothing by mouth for a considerable period after their procedures, receiving their fluids parenterally (by other routes than oral, such as by vein) until the physician believes that oral administration could be profitably attempted. The child who has had stomach or intestinal surgery will be offered very small amounts at a time initially to ascertain his tolerance and to decrease stress on the surgical site. Infants with severe cases of diarrhea and vomiting are usually allowed nothing by mouth or placed on a limited oral intake to rest the gastrointestinal tract. Fluids in these cases are also administered *parenterally*.

Fluid and electrolyte balance. It has become increasingly apparent in recent years that the content and volume of the body fluid is a key consideration in the maintenance of cellular health and therefore the health of the total individual. The body organs and systems function to maintain the proper internal and external cellular environments and enable the survival of the person. The following brief simplified discussion of fluid and electrolyte balance is included in the belief that an understanding of this area of biology will become more and more necessary for the general public as well as the bedside nurse.

The body functions in sensitive equilibrium. One of the most delicate balances maintained by the body is demonstrated by the composition of body fluid. Major ingredients of this fluid are water and certain chemicals termed *electrolytes*. Electrolytes are so called because they develop electrical charges when they are dissolved in water. Some electrolytes carry a positive charge and are called *cations*. Negatively charged electrolytes are called *anions*. In either case, the electrolytes may be referred to as *ions*. There are also a small number of chemical compounds found in body fluid that do not ionize or carry electrical charges. Organic compounds such as glucose and urea are the main nonelectrolytes of body fluid.

Body fluid occupies three permeable compartments (Fig. 26-10): blood vessels, tissue spaces (interstitial areas outside of tissue cells), and the areas inside the cells. *Extracellular* fluid (ECF) is located within the blood vessels and between the tissue cells, and *intracellular* fluid (ICF) lies inside the tissue cells.

Every tissue cell is surrounded by a semipermeable membrane that permits selective passage of certain substances and

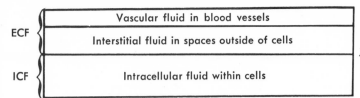

ECF	Vascular fluid in blood vessels
	Interstitial fluid in spaces outside of cells
ICF	Intracellular fluid within cells

Fig. 26-10. Body fluid compartments.

free passage of water molecules in both directions. Water always passes from the more dilute to the more concentrated solution. This transfer of water and ions between the intracellular and extracellular compartments is called *osmosis*. In health a dynamic equilibrium of electrolytes and water is maintained between the two areas. Therefore, although each of the fluid compartments of the body contains electrolytes, the concentration and composition of electrolytes in the water of each compartment varies. The electrolytes found in the fluid inside the cells differ greatly in amount from those found in the fluid outside the cells. Interstitial fluid in the tissue spaces is similar to plasma (the fluid portion of the blood), except that it contains very little protein. In interstitial fluid the principal cation is sodium, and the main anions are chlorides and bicarbonates. Intracellular cations are mostly potassium and magnesium, whereas the anions are chiefly phosphates and bicarbonates. Thus chemical differences exist between the extracellular and the intracellular fluids.

Acid-base balance. The acidity or alkalinity of a solution depends on the concentration of hydrogen, or the H ions present. An acid may be simply defined as a compound that has enough H ions to give some away. A base or alkali is a compound possessing few H ions. An increase in H ions makes a solution more acid, and a decrease makes a solution more alkaline. The concentration of hydrogen ions is expressed by pH. A neutral fluid has a pH of 7.0 (a lower pH means higher hydrogen ion concentration). An acid solution has a pH value below 7; an alkaline solution has a pH value above 7. The acid-base balance of the blood is maintained in an extremely narrow pH range, normally 7.35 to 7.45. Any slight deviation from this range causes pronounced changes in the cellular functions. This in turn may threaten life. Blood is normally slightly alkaline (pH 7.4). The acid-base balance is maintained by the action of the lungs, kidneys, and buffer systems. The lungs assist in maintaining this equilibrium by varying the rate at which CO_2 is blown off, retaining CO_2 in acidic form when blood plasma is getting too alkaline or increasing the respiratory rate when the plasma is becoming too acid. When disturbances in blood pH are primarily due to disease or abnormalities of the respiratory system, the problems resulting are termed either *respiratory alkalosis* or *acidosis.* The kidneys assist in maintaining the normal pH of blood by regulating the rates of excretion of acids and bases in the urine. Excessive retention of base or loss of acids through diseases of body systems other than the respiratory apparatus results in *metabolic alkalosis;* likewise, excessive retention of acids or loss of base produces *metabolic acidosis.*

Chemical buffer systems protect the acid-base balance of a solution by rapidly offsetting changes in its ionized H concentration. Buffer systems defend and maintain the pH of body fluids by protecting against added acid or base.

Fluid volume. The volume of blood plasma, interstitial fluid, and intracellular fluid normally remains relatively constant. Any blood plasma changes that take place during illness usually reflect changes in all the body fluids. Since plasma is relatively easy to obtain from the body and the other fluids are not, it is the chosen fluid for analysis.

Fluid balance. Fluid balance is main-

Table 26-1. Major electrolytes and imbalances

Electrolyte	Deficit	Excess
Sodium (Na⁺)—normal value 136-143 mEq./L.*	*Hyponatremia* Na⁺ below 135 mEq./L. Muscular weakness; abdominal cramps; clammy skin; weak, rapid pulse; hypotension; drowsiness; confusion; coma Predisposing factors—excessive sweating and water intake; gastrointestinal suction and excessive oral water intake; glucose water infusion without sodium; diarrhea	*Hypernatremia* Na⁺ above 150 mEq./L. Thirst; dry skin; loss of skin elasticity ("doughy" tissue turgor); fever; weight loss; scanty urine formation; confusion; stupor; seizures; circulatory embarrassment Predisposing factors—sodium chloride infusion; inadequate water intake; watery diarrhea; renal concentrating disease; anorexia; nausea; vomiting; high fever Additional feeding factors—undiluted cow's milk‡; boiled skim milk; powdered electrolyte mixtures; salt and sugar mixtures; bouillon soup, etc.
Potassium (K⁺)—normal value 4.1-5.6 mEq./L.	*Hypokalemia†* K⁺ below 4.0 mEq./L. Weak pulse; hypotension; muscular weakness; diminished reflexes; cardiac arrest Predisposing factors—diuretics; diarrhea; vomiting; gastric suctioning	*Hyperkalemia* K⁺ above 5.7 mEq./L. Nausea; apprehension; muscular weakness; confusion; hypotension; cardiac arrest Predisposing factors—burns, excessive tissue damage; excessive infusion of potassium; kidney disease; severe dehydration with scanty urine formation
Calcium (Ca⁺⁺)—normal value 10-12 mg./100 ml. (5-6 mEq./L.)	*Hypocalcemia* Ca⁺⁺ below 9 mg./100 ml. Tetany; tingling around mouth and fingers; muscular cramps; convulsions Predisposing factors—hypoactive parathyroid; malabsorption syndromes; chronic renal disease; distressed newborns	*Hypercalcemia (rare)* Ca⁺⁺ above 12 mg./100 ml. Vomiting; constipation; polyuria; abdominal pains Predisposing factors—prolonged bed rest; overactive parathyroid; overdose of vitamin D
Bicarbonate (HCO₃)⁻— normal value 19-26 mEq./L.	*Metabolic acidosis* (HCO₃)⁻ below 12 mEq./L. Apathy, drowsiness or lethargy; deep, rapid breathing (Kussmaul type) disorientation; stupor; weakness; coma Predisposing factors—diabetes mellitus; starvation; kidney insufficiency; excessive parenteral NaCl; severe diarrhea; salicylate intoxication	*Metabolic alkalosis* (HCO₃)⁻ above 30 mEq./L. Depressed, shallow respirations; hypertonic muscles; tetany; disorientation Predisposing factors—vomiting (pyloric stenosis); ingestion of alkalies; gastric suction; diuretics

*Milliequivalents per liter (mEq./L.).
†Potassium may be given intravenously only after urinary output is well established.
‡Hill, L. F.: Infant feeding: historical and current, Pediatr. Clin. North Am. **14**:265, 1967.

Table 26-2. Approximate daily intake and output of water in children whose body surface equals 1 square meter

	Intake	Output
1,500 ml.	liquids food metabolism (oxidation of food)	900 ml. kidney 500 ml. lungs and skin (insensible loss) 100 ml. intestine
1,500 ml.		1,500 ml.

tained chiefly by the kidneys, which are influenced by various hormones. A cardinal principle of fluid balance is that fluid intake must equal fluid output (Table 26-2). The store of water in the body comes from ingested liquids and foods. Water leaves the body via the kidneys, lungs, skin, and intestine. Water loss through the skin and lungs always increases when respirations are increased, fever is present, the environment is very warm, or the skin is injured or burned. Any condition that interferes with an adequate intake of fluid or produces excessive fluid loss threatens the life of the young child.

Fluid imbalance. Fig. 26-11 illustrates that plasma is the only portion of body water in contact with the external environment. It is the first fluid storage supply to be tapped in gastrointestinal disturbances (vomiting, diarrhea, rapid respirations, or deficient fluid intake). Interstitial fluid is the reservoir that responds most easily to the shifting fluid conditions present in disease (for example, overhydration causes edema, and dehydration causes the skin to lose its turgor and become wrinkled). The intracellular compartment represents the largest reservoir and is the least accessible. Here water is lost or gained over a period of days. Without water, a well infant in a temperate environment can live about 3 days, and an adult can survive about 10 days.

Electrolyte disturbances in children. With regard to fluid and electrolyte balance, several differences between the infant and older child must be considered. A newborn infant's weight is approximately 80% water, the older child's is 70% water, and the adult's is 60% water. This percentage varies with the amount of fat. Since fat is essentially water free, a lean individual has

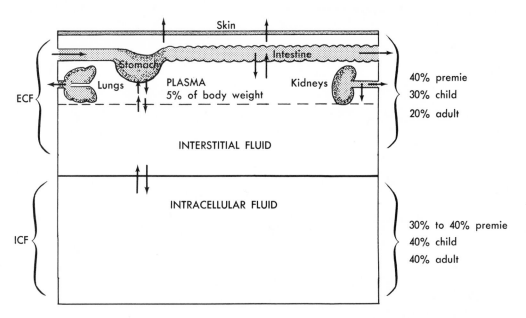

Fig. 26-11. Relative fluid balance in children and adults expressed in percentage of total body weight.

a greater proportion of water to total body weight. The proportion of intracellular fluid to body weight remains comparatively constant at all ages. Extracellular fluid constitutes about 40% of the infant's weight as compared with 20% of the adult's body weight. An infant, then, may approach a fluid loss of 10% of his body weight before a severe fluid deficit occurs. A weight loss of 5% represents a severe fluid volume deficit in the adult. However, remember, 10% of a baby's body weight is not very much!

Although the infant's body has a relatively greater fluid content per pound, he is *more vulnerable* to fluid volume deficit than is the adult. He ingests and excretes a relatively greater daily water volume because of several factors peculiar to his age group. The infant's body surface in relation to his body weight is three times that of the older child. Therefore he loses a relatively greater amount of fluid through the skin and gastrointestinal tract. His high metabolic rate produces more waste products, which must be diluted for excretion. His immature kidneys are less able to concentrate urine, thus adding to the volume of urine. Accumulation of acidic wastes (because of the high metabolic rate and immature kidneys) stimulates respiration,

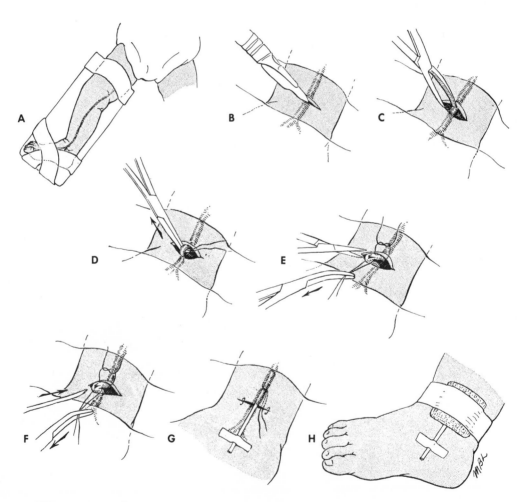

Fig. 26-12. A cutdown procedure. Great care is necessary in immobilizing the leg to prevent impairment of circulation and pressure areas. A cutdown may be used for a number of days to help maintain fluid balance or administer medication.

causing greater evaporation through his lungs. Infants may react to infections with higher temperatures, which also result in a higher water loss from evaporation. As the nurse reviews these facts about the infant's body fluid balance, she can more readily understand why the infant, at one twentieth the adult's weight, requires one third as much water. He requires five times as much water per kilogram of body weight (150 ml./kg./24 hr., as compared with 30 ml./kg./24 hr. in the adult). The infant may exchange half his extracellular fluid volume daily. The adult may exchange only one sixth his extracellular fluid volume. Infants and young children may become severely dehydrated in a short time.

DEHYDRATION. Inadequate fluid intake or excessive fluid loss causes dehydration. It is almost always associated with fever, burns, vomiting, diarrhea, hyperventilation, or hemorrhage. Dehydration seldom denotes water loss alone but rather loss of fluid volume, electrolytes, and water. During periods of dehydration, plasma volume is usually maintained at the expense of interstitial volume.

Early signs of dehydration in a patient are dry lips and mucous membranes, diminished urinary output, reduced weight, and lethargy. Moderate dehydration is further characterized by depressed fontanels, sunken eyeballs, loss of skin turgor, and a 5% to 10% loss of weight. As dehydration increases, the child becomes acutely ill, and his circulation may begin to fail. His skin is grayish, his pulse rapid and weak. Temperature elevation and low blood pressure are characteristic. Recorded output is scant, and weight loss is obvious, 10% or higher. Apathy, restlessness, and even convulsions may occur.

Intravenous therapy. Because many times it is difficult to perform and maintain a conventional intravenous infusion for prolonged periods in the small child, a *cutdown* may be performed (Fig. 26-12). This is a minor but important surgical procedure that is usually completed in the treatment room. The physician "cuts down" to

a vein, directly exposing it. A small plastic tubing is inserted into a minute nick in the vein and sutured in place. This tubing is then joined to the intravenous tubing.

Whether fluids are administered through a cutdown or a needle puncture through the skin into a vein of the scalp or extremity, it is important that the amount of fluid being given the child be gauged very carefully to avoid overloading the circulatory system. The rate of flow ordered should be known, marked on the bottle, and meticulously observed. The use of special pediat-

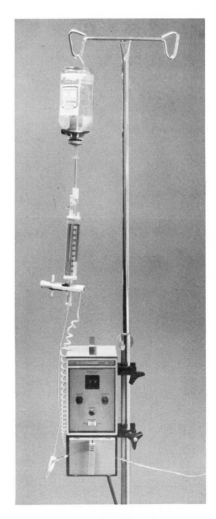

Fig. 26-13. One example of an infusion pump that may be set for a specific amount of fluid delivery. (IVAC Corp., San Diego, Calif. Courtesy Children's Health Center, San Diego, Calif.)

ric intravenous counting chambers or bags that simplify calculation is almost a necessity. Although a number of semiautomatic infusion sets (Fig. 26-13) have added a special margin of safety to administering fluids, the nurse must continue to keep a close watch on the flow rate, the infusion site, and the child's response to the fluid therapy. The infant and small child must be appropriately restrained to avoid dis-

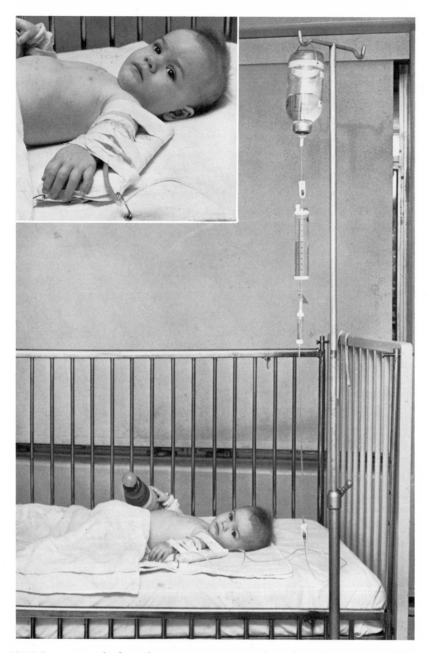

Fig. 26-14. Intravenous feedings for a young patient with prolonged vomiting and diarrhea. Side rail down for illustration only. The arm board is pinned to the bedding. Inset shows arm immobilization. (Courtesy Children's Health Center, San Diego, Calif.)

lodging the infusion. The nurse should be aware that changes in the child's position may slow or speed the infusion, and she should frequently observe the rate of flow in the drip chamber (Fig. 26-14). Extreme care should be exercised in moving the patient. The vocational nurse shares responsibility for observation of the intravenous apparatus with the supervising registered nurse. If a vocational nurse observes an infusion running more rapidly than ordered she may slow it to the known ordered rate, but she must immediately contact the supervising nurse regarding her action, since there may have been a change in orders or some reason for the increased infusion rate. The insertion point of the needle must be checked frequently to detect infiltration or inflammation. Pain and swelling are signs of possible dislocation of the needle.

The responsibility for observation is even greater if the child is receiving blood. There is more danger of circulatory overload, tissue damage, and untoward reactions. Patients receiving blood should be carefully watched and, when necessary and possible, questioned regarding back or chest pain or chills. The temperature, pulse, and respiratory rate should be frequently determined to detect any possible incompatibility. Hives may occur.

Parenteral hyperalimentation. Some children who cannot tolerate oral or nasogastric feeding can now survive by intravenous alimentation. Under strict aseptic conditions a silicone rubber catheter is inserted through the neck, passed into one of the jugular veins, and threaded down to the superior vena cava. By means of a constant infusion pump, a concentrated life-sustaining solution can be given at a uniform rate into the large vein where it will dilute rapidly and thereby prevent thrombosis and phlebitis. Total parenteral hyperalimentation provides glucose, proteins, minerals, vitamins, and fluid necessary for normal growth and weight gain. Hyperalimentation is also possible using peripheral veins, but the risk of tissue damage is considerably greater.

There is a newer modification of intravenous therapy, the so-called Heparin Lock

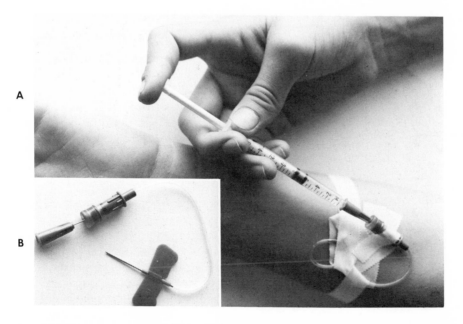

Fig. 26-15. Heparin Lock with needle in diaphragm. Child injecting heparinized saline solution into Heparin Lock on arm.

IV, for patients receiving intermittent intravenous medicines. It allows more mobility without the need for continuous intravenous fluids or frequent venipunctures. The Heparin Lock IV consists of a butterfly scalp vein needle attached to plastic tubing sealed by a rubber insert that is maintained in a certain manner to assure patency and sterility. Because selected patients and parents are being taught this technique, it is given here in some detail, though licensed practical or vocational nurses in the hospital setting would probably not routinely have the responsibility of its maintenance.

TECHNIQUE FOR USE OF HEPARIN LOCK IV

Equipment:
1. Alcohol sponge
2. Tourniquet
3. A special No. 25-gauge butterfly scalp vein needle with associated plastic tubing and rubber cap insert (Heparin Lock)
4. Heparin-saline mixture—prepared with 30 ml. saline solution mixed with 1 ml. of 1,000 units per ml. heparin (The heparinized saline mixture is kept refrigerated and can be used for 72 hours before being discarded.)
5. 22-gauge, 1-inch needle—to insert into lock initially
6. Tuberculin syringe—for heparinized saline
7. 35 ml. syringe or metriset for administration of medication
8. 25-gauge, ⅝-inch needle for subsequent clearing of the tubing with saline solution

Procedure:
1. The 22-gauge, 1-inch needle is inserted through the disinfected rubber diaphragm of the Heparin Lock so that blood will advance into the tubing when the vein is entered.
2. The butterfly needle is then usually inserted into an arm vein and taped into position.
3. Heparinized saline mixture is injected into the tubing with the tuberculin syringe until it replaces the blood.
4. The needle is then withdrawn from the rubber diaphragm.

Note: Before and after the administration of intravenous medications or in the event that any blood is seen in the tubing, the tubing of the Heparin Lock is cleared with 0.5 to 1 ml. heparinized saline mixture. Careful instructions and return demonstrations must accompany the out-patient use of this device.

Cleanliness

Satisfying the need for cleanliness is almost entirely the responsibility of the nursing staff. The way in which it is met depends on the condition of the individual patient and the facilities of the pediatric unit.

Bed bath. A bath is usually administered each day to prevent skin irritation and provide refreshment, stimulation, and comfort. It also serves as an excellent period for patient observation and evaluation. Bed baths are given to patients who are quite ill, are especially susceptible to chilling and respiratory tract infections, have dressings or incisions to be protected, or who are in traction or casting routinely. Most children with elevated temperatures usually have bed baths, although occasionally a tepid tub bath may be ordered to reduce fever, a treatment that may also be a period of cleansing. Bed baths are carried out in essentially the same manner for children as for adults. A bath blanket or towel should be used for a covering, and, except in the case of an infant, the area should be curtained or screened. Unless contraindicated, a good light should be available for the bath area to aid in the detection of any special changes in skin color, rashes, or other abnormalities.

PERINEAL CARE. The child should be helped with the care of his genitalia if he is too young to cleanse the area properly. Any irritation of the penis or labia should be reported. If the little boy is uncircumcised, no extraordinary force should be exerted to retract the foreskin, nor once retracted should it remain so, but observation of the area for cleanliness and possible inflammation should be made. Occasionally, more formal perineal care using an irrigation technique will be desirable to encourage cleanliness, especially in the case of older girls having their menses.

NAILS. The nails of young children often need attention. Cleaning and cutting the nails when necessary should be part of the daily care. Usually, the nails may be cut or filed without an order except when the patient is a diabetic or has peripheral circulatory disorders.

ORAL HYGIENE. Oral hygiene should also be carried out routinely. However, remember that a child with a recent cleft lip, cleft palate, or dental repair usually is not allowed to have a brush or anything hard in his mouth. For those too young to have more than two or three teeth, oral hygiene may be a simple drink of water, but for older children the essentials of good care of the teeth should be taught. A small toothbrush that can easily fit into the mouth is needed. Massage of the gums and correct up-and-down brushing of the teeth are important health habits and often make food and fluid intake more pleasant. Cracked or dry lips may be lubricated with petrolatum.

Bed patients are usually dressed in pajamas or gowns, but sometimes if the child is convalescent, a bright dress or striped tee shirt may be a big lift to the morale of the child and parents.

Unit care. Part of the daily care of the patients is the care of his unit. The bath is not technically complete until the unit is clean and orderly. Whether a complete linen change is necessary depends on its condition. Most children's beds need frequent changes, but do not use linen needlessly!

The patient's bedside stand should be neat (inside and out), and the unit furniture wiped down with a moist paper towel. The aim is not to have each little bed "just so" with a neat and clean but unhappy occupant but to cut down on confusion and reduce safety hazards. A child *needs* to have his toys and a certain amount of freedom in his bed activities. But he is not aided by mounds of equipment taking over his bed or crib. In some hospitals, special bags are available for toy storage. The patient's room should be comfortably warm and well ventilated but free from drafts.

Tub bath. When tub baths are allowed, the amount of supervision required depends on the age and condition of the child. Young children should never be left alone

because of danger of burning from the hot water faucet, drowning, or falling while trying to climb out. Teen-agers usually resent much observation in the tub room and many times need only a minimum of supervision. Unless a prolonged tub bath is ordered for treatment purposes, the bath should not be too extended. There is greater possibility of chilling, and others may be waiting in line. When facilities are available, there is a greater tendency than formerly to give hospitalized children tub baths. Be sure to clean the tub well after each child is finished.

PROLONGED TUB BATH. A prolonged tub bath lasts at least 20 minutes. It may be ordered to relax the muscles before physical therapy, to help remove dressings or crusts, or to apply a certain soothing medication to the skin, such as oatmeal or Alpha-Keri. To help the patient relax in the bath and get his whole body in contact with the water, a pillow may be constructed from a rolled bath blanket to raise the head out of the water while the child lies flat in the tub. If a rubber headrest is available, it may be used for this purpose.

TABLE TUB BATH. The infant who may have a tub bath is placed in a smaller basin for greater security and easier handling. The following procedure could be used for a newborn infant whose umbilicus has healed or, with modification, for an older infant. It may be carried out at the bedside or at a special table or counter. The instructions are written to help the new mother at home bathe her newborn infant, but the principles are the same. Only the organization of equipment may be different. The older child, who enjoys the bath and is able to sit steadily, may have more freedom in the tub and could be soaped while he is in the water.

TABLE TUB BATH

Materials needed:
1. Baby bathtub, large basin, or bathinette
2. Tray with
   a. Mild soap, dish
   b. Jar of cotton balls and twists
   c. Jar of safety pins

391

d. Bottle of baby oil or lotion
e. Capped 4-ounce baby bottle of sterile water
f. Small box of tissues
3. Large heavy towel or mat (possibly placed on several thicknesses of newspaper on the surface used for drying and dressing)
4. Newspaper or hamper for dirty clothes discard
5. Paper bag or handy wastebasket to receive waste
6. Two soft towels
   a. One on which to undress and inspect baby
   b. One for drying baby
7. Two soft washclothes or paper mesh squares
8. Baby clothes (clean)
   a. Diaper
   b. Shirt
   c. Kimono
   d. Receiving blanket
9. Apron

Procedure:
1. Check the temperature of the room (72° to 75° F. and free from drafts).
2. Wash hands thoroughly, put on apron.
3. Assemble equipment (the kitchen table is a good place).
   a. Tray of baby supplies
   b. Tub on newspapers on table
   c. Mat or heavy towel for undressing and drying (next to tub)
   d. Wastebasket slightly under table
   e. Newspaper on seat of chair to receive dirty clothes; clean towel for drying on back of chair
   f. Clean clothes and blanket stacked in order of use
   g. Tub one-third full of water comfortable to your elbow

Note: You may want to put a bottle of formula in warm water to be ready to give to the infant.
4. Place the infant on the mat.
   a. Inspect the eyes, and wash the lids with sterile cotton and water if any discharge is present, proceeding from the inner corner of the eye outward. With older infants, a fresh washcloth or cotton dipped in clear water is sufficient. Inspect the ears.
   b. Wash his face with the washcloth and clear water from the tub. Dry.
   c. Soap the scalp; support the infant, using the football hold, if possible. The infant's head should be over the tub, and his ears should be covered with the nurse's fingers. Rinse the scalp carefully. Dry.
5. Remove his shirt and diaper. If the buttocks are grossly soiled with stool, discard

the washcloth used for the cleanup and use another to continue the bath or use tissues for initial cleanup.
6. Quickly soap the infant's entire body, except the head, paying special attention to body creases and the area under the chin.
7. Lift the child carefully into the tub, feet first, using appropriate holds.
8. Rinse the soap off the infant quickly.
9. Lift the infant back to the clean towel on the mat. Pat him dry. Oil or lotion may be used sparingly on the body creases.
10. Inspect and clean the genitalia with cotton balls. Dress the child quickly in clean clothes and wrap him in a receiving blanket.
11. Offer drinking water and inspect his mouth. Feed the child his formula.

Shampoo. The state of the patient's scalp, his general condition, and the length of his hair will determine the need for a shampoo.

Whether a shampoo for an older child must be ordered by the physician depends on hospital policy, the condition of the child, and the type of shampoo contemplated. Many children can easily have their hair shampooed by lying on a gurney with their head extended over the end next to a sink or tub. A trough to guide the water may be constructed of plastic or rubber sheeting. If a wall spray hose is used, great care should be taken in regulating the water temperature before the water touches the child.

If the child is bedfast, a simple head basin and trough may be constructed from two bath blankets rolled together lengthwise (like a snake) and curved into a horseshoe shape with the open end pointing toward the side of the bed. This form is draped by a plastic or rubber sheeting to make a waterproof basin that leads off the side of the bed into a large bath basin or baby tub. Some hospitals use inflated Kelly pads. A few have bed shampoo basins available, similar to those found in beauty salons. The hair must be rinsed of suds until squeaky clean. Some patients like a vinegar or lemon rinse. Hair should be dried quickly to avoid chilling.

Rest

Personal and environmental cleanliness and order should promote rest, but rest is not automatic. Nap times must be provided and promoted. Most children do best with a rest period after lunch lasting at least an hour. Other nap times should be encouraged, depending on the needs of the child. Shades should be drawn, the television set turned off, the area straightened up, and the child covered comfortably. A reminder of something pleasant that can happen when the child has rested is often helpful in making the nap more acceptable.

Diversion and self-expression

A convalescing child should not be expected to sit or lie quietly all day long without diversion and opportunities for self-expression. Although rest is very important, a child may rest better when allowed moderate activity during the day. To stay perfectly still is impossible and the attempt may be fatiguing in itself. The nurse can

Table 26-3. Play-and-get-well chart

Age	Interest	Toys	Books
Infant (Birth-1 yr.)	Toys that attract the eye, make little sounds, and tempt grasping hands	Bright hanging objects; large plastic rings; string of gaily colored rings; rubber toys that squeak; tinkling bells	None (enjoys a song or lullaby)
Toddler (1-3 yr.)	Toys that enable parallel play, provide security and attention, and help development of muscle coordination	Nest of blocks; mallet and wooden pegs; trucks and cars; cuddly toy animals; large dolls; rocking horse; toy telephone; musical toys; kiddie car	Large linen picture books; nursery rhymes; ABC books; farm and zoo animal stories Likes the same story over and over again
Preschooler (3-5 yr.)	Toys that stimulate child's imagination and develop creative abilities	Nurse and doctor sets; trains and trucks; Tinker Toys; cabin logs; magnets; toy army men; record player; hand puppets; crayons and color books; dolls and clothes; simple puzzles; modeling clay; scrapbooks; cuddly toy animals	Dr. Seuss books; Golden Books; once-upon-a-time stories Enjoys stories about airplanes, trains, and police and fire stations Likes to look at pictures while being read to
Early school age (6-9 yr.)	Application of mental as well as physical skills Interest and enjoyment in playing with children of same sex Realistic toys that bring child into contact with world outside hospital	Craft sets; models; picture painting; stamp collection; string marionettes; spool knitting; beadwork Games such as Monopoly, checkers, and Clue Paper and pencil games; jigsaw puzzles; paper dolls	Comic books; riddle books; crossword puzzles; fairy tales; adventure stories; simple science book; how and why books; who-when-where books; *Highlights*
Middle school age (10-12 yr.)	Adaptable to group activities Combine companionship and challenge and co-ordinate work and play in teams	Card games; photoelectric football; science toys; chess; checkers Skill games such as sculptoring and wood carving Walkie-talkie; telescope; transistor radio; camera; television; picture viewer	Comic books; school textbooks; biographies; adventure stories Junior classics such as *Heidi, Little Women, Treasure Island, Robin Hood, Alice in Wonderland, Andersen's Fairy Tales, Aesop's Tales*

help by supplying appropriate toys, providing suitable television programs, setting up controlled group play for patients in the same room when possible, playing with the child herself, or asking for the help of the "play lady" or auxiliary worker. She may enlist the aid of occupational or recreational therapists if they are available. A hospital library may supply interesting books for pleasure or help with schoolwork.

Play is a learning activity that promotes physical, mental, emotional, and social growth. In play a child develops new abilities, acquires knowledge about himself, and explores the feel, look, and taste of the world around him. He uses play to express what he is thinking and feeling and to relate and interact with others. Dramatic play is recognized as a form of emotional release.

The nurse can help children choose the play materials that will be fun and satisfying. The following principles should be kept in mind when choosing toys: (1) suitability for a particular age, (2) safety, and (3) durability.

Choosing the right play materials at the right time is not an easy task. However, an understanding of the wide variety of play interests can often give helpful clues.

Every child needs a well-balanced toy selection for all-around development. The choice should be planned to stimulate: (1) social play, (2) dramatic play, (3) creative play, (4) manipulation and constructive play, and (5) active physical play.

Play activity is as vital to growth as medicine, food, and sleep. What is the worth of a healed body if the mind is permanently limited from lack of opportunity to grow socially and emotionally?

Medication

The administration of medication to young children entails special skills and knowledge. It is a particularly heavy responsibility because dosages vary so greatly from child to child, as the result of weight, body area, and metabolic differences.

General principles

Pediatric dosages may be calculated in different ways by physicians. Young's rule uses age as a basis for determination.

Young's rule:

Child's dose =

$$\frac{\text{Age of child in years} \times \text{Average adult dose}}{\text{Age of child in years} + 12}$$

More helpful, since the size of children the same age may differ, is Clark's rule, based on weight:

Clark's rule:

Child's dose =

$$\frac{\text{Weight of child in pounds}}{150} \times \text{Average adult dose}$$

A newer concept in computing pediatric dosage is based on the surface area of a child. Some dosages must be individualized for the specific child by his physician.

Giving medication is sometimes difficult because the child often does not recognize the need for the medicine and many, despite the kindliest approach, resist its administration. However, although the licensed vocational nurse is not given major responsibility in the administration of medicines in the pediatric area, she should know the principles involved and receive practice in giving selected medications to children during her pediatric experience.

As with the administration of medication anytime, the following factors must be identified:
1. The right patient
2. The right medication in the right form
3. The right dosage
4. The right method of administration
5. The right time of administration

Before any medication is given, it should be identified on a medicine card and checked against the physician's order. In some hospitals, orders for certain medications must be renewed after a certain time. Common medications that are often automatically stopped unless reordered are broad-spectrum antibiotics and narcotics. Medications that are ordered on an "as necessary," or p.r.n., basis must be checked to see when they were last given to avoid too frequent administrations. It also must be determined whether the need for the medication truly exists. The nurse should look up any unfamiliar medication before assuming the responsibility of its administration. She should know its common usages, contraindications, side effects, common dosages, and peculiarities of administration.

Common measurements

Before giving medications, the nurse should review the common measurements used in the metric and apothecary systems and frequently used conversions. There should be an easily read table available for her reference. Some of the most common conversions follow:

1 dram or ʒ	= 4 ml.
1 teaspoon or tsp.	= 5 ml.
1 tablespoon or tbsp.	= 15 ml.
1 ounce or ʒ	= 30 ml.
15 or 16 minims or ℳxv or ℳxvi	= 1 ml.
gr. xv	= 1 Gm.
gr. i	= 0.06 Gm. or 60 to 65 mg.

Oral medication

Preparation. If possible, medications for children are prepared as solutions for greater ease in administration. Suspensions must always be shaken well before being poured. Most may be diluted, although it is not wise to dilute medicines more than a few milliliters to wash out the measuring container. The child may not take the increased volume easily. Placing a medication in a baby's formula is also precarious. If he refuses to take all the formula, how much has he taken? Was the medication evenly distributed throughout? These are difficult questions to answer.

Administration. Before giving any type of medication, check the patient's identification. Many hospitals now do not rely on bed tags; patients may change beds. Most have a system of banding or identification bracelets. Very young children cannot identify themselves. It is imperative that the nurse be positive of her identification. If the child is old enough he should be asked in addition, "What is your name?"

Always place a bib on a small child before administering oral medications. Such a simple maneuver will save many extra changes and important minutes of the nurse's time, best used in other ways. Remember, if a child is given water or other fluid to wash down a pill, this liquid must be recorded on his intake.

Fluid medications may be given fairly easily to infants when placed in a nipple fitted in a standard ring (used on ring-and-disc–type baby bottles). The baby sucks out the medication while the nurse supports his head to prevent aspiration. Small medication cups are also employed. Syringes may also be used to administer oral fluids, thus increasing the accuracy of the dose. The medicine is poured slowly with the baby in sitting position or with his head elevated. Rubber-tipped medicine droppers may be helpful too. Pills and capsules must be crushed or opened for small children under 5 years of age. The medication may be placed in a cherry syrup, honey, or jelly and given from a spoon. Many of these medications are bitter so that a good disguise must be used.

The child who takes his medicine well should be praised for being such a "big boy or girl." If a child finds it difficult to take medicine, he should be made to feel that his nurse understands some of his distaste and fear and wants to help him during this brief but difficult period. Although a young child may be helped by gentle restraint in the administration of medicines (the nurse may hold the child on her lap with one of his hands wedged behind her and the other controlled by her encircling arm and hand), pouring medication down the throat of a struggling, crying youngster is an invitation to aspiration, early emesis of the medication, and subsequent trying periods when medicine time comes again. At times a child will respond much better if he is allowed to hold the cup and drink at his own rate. Many of the small, disposable

medicine cups are safe play objects for successful medicine takers, who, in turn, med-
icate dolls and stuffed toys. A child must
never be told that he is taking candy when
he is receiving a medication. The two ideas
seem to become easily confused, and many
toddlers have raided medicine chests in
search of something more appetizing but
have settled for orange-flavored aspirin.

Intramuscular injections

When the nurse gives an intramuscular injection to a child she usually needs a second
person to help support, distract, restrain,
or comfort the child receiving such an injection. If the child is old enough to understand, the nurse should explain the procedure just before administering the injection.
The resistant, tearful child might be told

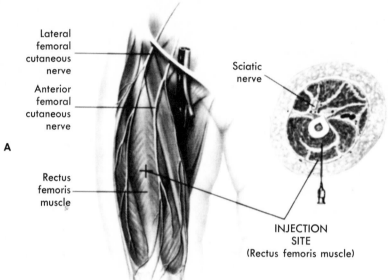

Fig. 26-16. Site of injection chart. The most desirable sites for pediatric intramuscular injections
are: **A,** the rectus femoris muscle; **B,** the vastus
lateralis muscle; **C,** the deltoid muscle. (Courtesy
Ross Laboratories, Columbus, Ohio, 43216.)

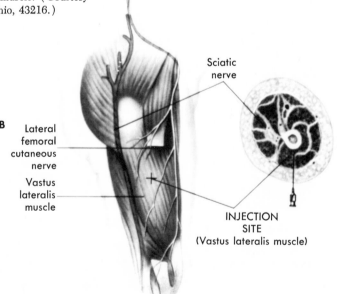

that the medicine will help him get better so that he can go home sooner. The infant or younger child needs to be restrained adequately to assure safe and correct administration of the drug. For most infants and children, an injection means simply "hurt" and may establish a lasting fear. To lessen his fear and to maintain a degree of trust, the nurse should always comfort the child by holding him afterward. When dealing with an older child, she should indicate that she understands why he reacts the way he does.

In final preparation for intramuscular injection, 0.2 to 0.3 ml. of air is drawn into the syringe. When the syringe is inverted, the bubble rises and serves to clear all the solution from the needle into the tissues and prevent backflow.

Equipment
Damp antiseptic sponge
1 or 2 ml. syringe
22-gauge, 1-inch needle for infants and children
23-gauge, ¾-inch needle for tiny infants

Because the gluteal muscle is not well developed in the infant or young child, and permanent sciatic nerve damage is possible, the buttocks are never used for an intramus-

cular injection. The most desirable sites for pediatric injections are the lateral and anterior aspects of the thighs, the deltoid areas, and the soft tissue inferior to the iliac crests. The medicine and syringe should be completely prepared and ready for use before the nurse enters the child's room.

Method. The site is cleansed with the antiseptic damp sponge, using a circular motion. The skin is pulled taut. In young children who have minimal muscle, the needle is inserted at a slightly oblique angle; if the child is large and well developed, it is inserted perpendicularly. The plunger is pulled back to assure that the needle is not in a blood vessel, and the medicine is injected slowly. When the air bubble leaves the syringe, the sponge is placed over the needle, the needle is quickly withdrawn, and the area is gently wiped with the sponge. A bandage is placed over the site. Many older children seem to be helped a great deal if they can grasp the crib sides with their hands and count during an injection. Some gain satisfaction in helping to put on a Band-Aid after the procedure. Afterward, a child should be comforted by the nurse adminstering the injection, if possible. After all, she is not his enemy but a special friend, and everything should be done to help him recognize this.

Suppositories

Aspirin, sedative drugs, and bowel stimulants are often given to children in the form of rectal suppositories. Most of these suppositories may be lubricated with a jellylike material before insertion. Since they are often refrigerated to preserve their shape, warming them, unwrapped, in a clean hand for about a minute may be helpful. The nurse should wear a clean glove or finger cot for the insertion of the suppository. The child should be asked to take a deep breath, if possible, and the medication should be pushed about 2 inches past the rectal sphincter. After insertion, pressure should be exerted on the buttocks, holding them together for more than a minute, or

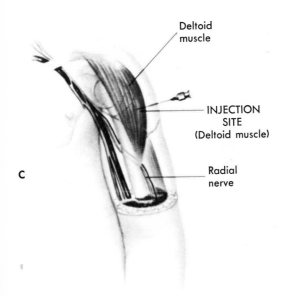

Deltoid muscle

INJECTION SITE (Deltoid muscle)

Radial nerve

C

the suppository may be ejected and its effect lost.

Nose drops

Nose drops are ordered fairly often for infants and children. They are primarily used to combat nasal congestion and make breathing, eating, and drinking easier. In the case of an infant, nose drops may be ordered 20 minutes before meals to improve sucking and formula intake. If the nose is very congested, gentle suctioning of the nasal passageway may be indicated before the drops are administered. It will do no good if the drops only roll in and out again or do not remain in the nose! Young children do not understand the reason for nose drops and may need to be gently restrained by a second person or a modified mummy restraint. The child should be lying down with the head tilted back over a folded towel or small pillow. The dropper should be pointed slightly toward the top of the nasal cavity. The child should remain positioned for several seconds after the instillation. Oily nose drops should be avoided because of the possibility of aspiration and lipoid pneumonia.

Eardrops

Eardrops are still used occasionally in the pediatric area. They should not be cold but close to body temperature or warm. Cold eardrops are painful. The child's head should be resting comfortably on the bed, turned with the ear to be treated exposed. The young child's ear should be pulled down and back to straighten the external auditory canal. After instillation, cotton should not be routinely inserted because it may interfere with drainage of discharge to the exterior or serve to soak up the recently instilled medication.

Eyedrops

Eyedrops, when ordered, should not be dropped on the cornea but instilled in the lower conjunctival sac while the child, lying flat, tries to look at the hair on top of his head! After instillation of the eyedrops, the eyes should be lightly closed, not squeezed shut, since this may force out the medication. It is a good practice with some toxic medications such as atropine to put a little pressure at the inner angle of the eye after the drop has been placed to prevent drainage into the nose through the tear duct.

Topical medication

Ointments or creams may be applied to the skin with a finger cot or buttered on gauze with a sterile tongue blade if the area is to be covered with a sterile compress. Liniments and lotions are often applied with clean hands or cotton balls, depending on their contents and the condition of the area to be treated.

Special treatments

Special treatments related to the particular physical problem that the child may be facing are discussed in separate chapters describing procedures involving the various body functions, systems, or diseases.

Provisions for rehabilitation

As convalescence progresses, provisions for rehabilitation may be necessary to recapture skills lost during illness. This usually begins during hospitalization and continues after discharge. In some cases the problem involved is not so much rehabilitation as *habilitation,* or the formation of skills not previously mastered. This is particularly true of patients suffering from neuromusculoskeletal problems. Emphasis is placed on the development of function with the least cosmetic defect and maximum appearance of normalcy. Priority is placed on skills needed for daily tasks. The hospital may have a special rehabilitation unit (see Chapter 23).

Physical therapy

Those engaged in the specialty of physical therapy concern themselves primarily with the treatment of disease and injury by physical agents such as heat, cold, electricity, and water. The most common techniques used involve therapeutic exercises in and out of water. These specially prescribed exercises are fundamental to the treatment of delayed motor development and respiratory, orthopedic, and neuromuscular disease. They are designed to prevent and correct deformities, increase muscle strength and function, and establish normal postural reflexes. The physical therapist institutes normal patterns of motion and teaches coordination, balance, walking, and stair-climbing (with and without orthopedic appliances), as well as other activities of daily living. Thus, through the careful selection of techniques, he or she prevents deformity, relieves pain, and promotes functional capacity.

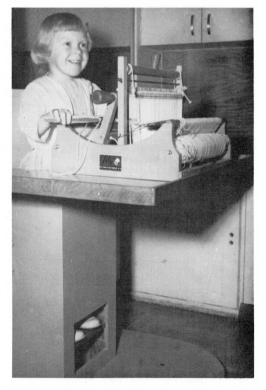

Fig. 26-17. Susan enjoys her weaving in occupational therapy. The stand-up table with a little gate at the back helps her maintain balance. The finger exercise encourages the joint movement that is so necessary for rheumatoid arthritis patients like Susan. (Courtesy Children's Health Center, San Diego, Calif.)

Occupational therapy

Occupational therapy is more often concerned with the maintenance or stimulation of small muscle control necessary for the accomplishment of more refined but equally important skills involving finger and wrist manipulation. Occupational therapy uses many crafts to motivate and involve the patient in activities that strengthen muscles or are psychologically stimulating. Weaving, ceramics, shell jewelry manufacturing, woodworking, and painting are usually just means to an end—a better-functioning patient. Often the occupational therapy department can help by locating or fashioning equipment to aid the patient in carrying out necessary activities of daily living (ADL's): appliances that help malfunctioning hands to hold combs and toothbrushes, special cups, plate guards, angled spoons and forks to help with eating, and elastic shoestrings and long-handled gadget sticks to help with dressing are just a few of many possible examples (p. 550).

Other specialties

Speech therapists and hearing specialists may be part of the efforts to better fit the child or youth for life and meet his needs for communication and participation. A bedside teacher provided by the public school system may help to make the return transition from hospital to regular school less difficult. Greater provision for socialization, according to the developmental needs of the child, may need to be considered to provide for optimum personality development for children undergoing long-term hospitalization. A sense of individual worth, importance, and purposefulness should be fostered.

• • •

An appreciation of the importance of each individual and the contribution he may make to his world should be part of the nursing perspective of the staff. If the child or youth is personally incapable of making a constructive contribution, then society itself may become a source of

399

growth and hope by channeling efforts toward rewarding research and increasing compassion and understanding. A nurse should have a faith that will recognize the tragic realities of life without destroying its sweetness, a philosophy that will allow her to give without becoming empty and brittle, and an outlook that carefully measures minutes in the light of an eternity.

Recording

Although the recording of nursing observations and care may seem to be of minor importance when compared with the proper execution of these responsibilities, clear, concise, and appropriate record keeping is a nursing necessity. It serves as a permanent record of the patient's treatments, medications, and changing condition. It is especially important to have a clear record of the pediatric patient who often, because of his age, lacks communication skills. The nurse's notes may help influence therapy, may be important in research studies, and may become of specific legal importance.

The notes should be hand printed in ink. Errors in charting should never be erased. A line should be drawn neatly through the error in such a way that the entry may still be read and the portion labeled "error." All notes should be signed with the first initial, last name, and title of the person making them. Some comment or an appropriate summary statement should be made concerning the pediatric patient's condition or activity about every hour. In recording, one should always ask oneself, "What is the reason for this child's hospital entry? What signs and symptoms would be significant to record? Is there any change in his condition? Is the intake and output record accurate?" If the child has had any bowel movements, they should be described in terms of amount, consistency, and color. Of course, treatments and medications and patient reactions also form part of the record and are recorded after they are completed or administered. The visits of physicians and parents and relatives should be noted. The nurse should not be too wordy, but she should give an accurate description of the condition of her patient. Good charting for most nurses is not automatic. If it develops, it is the result of concentrated effort and experience. Each hospital will probably have a different form to use, but the principles of charting will remain the same.

DAILY PLANNING FOR PATIENT CARE

After the basic needs of patients have been identified, learning to plan nursing care to meet the needs of patients takes time, ingenuity, and experience. The student requires guidance in executing care so that priorities in need are recognized and work progresses safely and efficiently, benefiting all the patients and staff.

Nursing staff organization and utilization

The planning of the nurse's tasks will depend in part on the organization and work patterns of the ward or nursing area to which she is assigned. The several ways in which care may be rendered are as follows:

1. A nurse may have the responsibility for the total care of a patient under the direction of the supervising head nurse. She would watch for changes in his condition and concern herself with his safety, general hygiene, nutrition, special medications, and treatments. The LVN or LPN usually functions in this way with patients having relatively stabilized conditions or when complex nursing care is not indicated. They may work as private duty or staff nurses. If this type of assignment is made consistently with the same patients, it is similar to the primary nurse concept. This type of assignment is being utilized with increasing frequency.

2. A nurse's responsibility may be for a specific group of patients but involve only certain types of functions. One nurse may observe a patient and render hygienic care and simple treatments. Another may provide supervision, observation, medications, and special treatments. Usually, a nursing

aide, orderly, LVN, or LPN would have the former responsibilities, and a registered nurse would perform the latter, although in hospitals for the chronically ill and in convalescent settings, the LVN or LPN may be given more responsibility for medications and treatments. This has been a common nursing pattern.

3. A nurse may be assigned to a nursing team, which is responsible for all patients in a specific area. The team may consist of registered nurses, LVN's or LPN's, nurse's aides, and orderlies. The team leader, usually a registered nurse working under the head nurse, gives specific detailed patient assignments to each of her team members. In addition, she acquaints all team members with the general condition and primary needs of all the patients in their total area of responsibility. Some functions are literally performed at the same time, for example, taking temperature, pulse, and respiration and passing trays. Others are performed by the assigned team nurse or the supervising registered nurse as the need of the patient involved dictates. The LVN or LPN may be assigned observation responsibility, general hygiene, treatments, and medications, depending on her patients and the medications involved. Periodic conferences involving the entire team are held to report and discuss patient needs and ways in which they can best be met.

In pediatrics, nursing patterns involving LVN's or LPN's most often have included numbers 2 or 3 above. Pediatrics is a specialty that deals with many variables. Because of the young ages and immature development of many of the patients, some procedures that would not be considered complex in certain settings become more difficult when their performance involves a pediatric patient. Medication dosages must be calculated often and closely scrutinized. When making nursing assignments, a supervisor must consider not only the level of nursing preparation represented by the personnel but also the experience and individual capabilities of the nurses involved.

Individual planning and organization

When given her morning assignment and report, a nurse must plan her individual care in order to accomplish her goals in the best way possible. The head nurse, team leader, or student instructor may assist in this planning.

Usually, the best beginning is a *quick* tour of all the patients assigned to check on any immediate needs. The following things could be done during the tour:
1. Introduce the nurse to the child and/or parent, when appropriate.
2. Check the general safety of the patient's environment.
   a. Restraints and side rails, crib nets.
   b. When necessary, intravenous apparatus for rate of flow and possible infiltration.
   c. Humidification devices for function.
   d. Oxygen equipment.
   e. Inappropriate toys.
3. Help set up and supervise breakfast, when appropriate, checking diet for accuracy.
4. Evaluate the need for supplies.
   a. Linen.
   b. Sizes of underwear, dresses, trousers, shirts, hospital gowns, or pajamas.
   c. Procedural supplies.
      (1) Dressing supplies.
      (2) Solutions—irrigating sets, etc.

After this brief "grand tour" the patient's needs must be evaluated again. In deciding which patient should receive basic care first, one must consider the following:
1. Any prior appointments that have been scheduled for the patients.
   a. X-ray examination or therapy.
   b. Physical therapy.
   c. Speech therapy.
   d. Bedside tutoring.
   e. Scheduled dressing changes.
2. General condition of the patient.
   a. As a general rule, the patient who is least comfortable has the priority.

401

b. Presurgical patients who have had their preoperative medications are usually not disturbed.

c. Patients who are sleeping and need the rest may, at the discretion of the supervising nurse, be left temporarily undisturbed. Sleep may be their most pressing need.

3. Types of treatment that are ordered and when they are to be given.

a. Enemas would ordinarily be given before the bath and bed change.

b. Shampoos would ordinarily be given after the bath but before the bed change.

c. A patient's care would preferably be completed before a blood transfusion or other infusions are started.

d. Ideally, sterile dressings are best changed when local movement, bed making, mopping, etc. is at a minimum.

4. Hospital routine.

a. Taking the temperature, pulse, and respiration is routine on most patients. The time at which it is done depends on the hospital policy and the type of nursing organization pattern followed. Many team patterns say that all TPR's should be taken before or immediately after the breakfast period and the results recorded on a special sheet handy for quick perusal by nurses and physicians.

b. Meal schedules. Children usually need more supervision and aid than adults. Babies are usually fed their ordered solids, bathed, and then given their formula.

A good rule to follow that saves steps and time during the morning is, if possible, never go anywhere empty-handed. There is usually something that needs to be carried to or from a patient's unit.

May an active brain, gentle skill, and good humor accompany your many steps.

27

Common diagnostic tests

A day does not pass in a busy hospital without many diagnostic tests being performed. The tests may entail the services of the clinical laboratory, the x-ray department, the operating room suite, or other specialized areas. They may be performed in the nursing unit. Although the nurse does not need to know the details of all these procedures, she should know the purpose of the test, whether patient preparation is necessary, the general procedure followed during the test, its effect on the patient, and the follow-up care needed.

For convenience the tests described in this chapter are arranged in table form and grouped as follows: tests of blood specimens, tests of urine specimens, tests of stool specimens, miscellaneous specialized tests, and x-ray tests. Only those tests commonly performed and of special interest in obstetrical or pediatric areas are described. The details of each test frequently differ from hospital to hospital. The nurse is advised to consult the procedure manual of the institution where she is employed before participating in any test.

TESTS OF BLOOD SPECIMENS
General considerations

1. Blood specimens are secured by the physician, the laboratory technician, or, occasionally, the nurse.
2. Blood specimens for chemical analysis must be collected after a period of fasting, unless otherwise specified. Water, however, may be allowed in *small amounts.*
3. Blood specimens are obtained by the following methods:
   a. Prick of the great toe, heel, earlobe, or finger. The blood is col-

lected by pipette or capillary tube; equipment is supplied by the laboratory.

   b. Venipuncture.
   (1) Various sites may be used in children (Fig. 27-1):
      (a) Infants—jugular, femoral, or scalp vein; occasionally veins of the arm
      (b) Children 2 or 3 years old or more—usually veins of the arm
   (2) Necessary equipment includes the following:
      (a) Tourniquet or blood pressure cuff
      (b) Antiseptic and sponges
      (c) Needles, Nos. 20 to 22 (depends on vessel size), 1 to 1½ inches
      (d) Syringes, sterile and dry (size depends on amount of specimen)
      (e) Collecting containers or tubes, with or without anticoagulants, other special tubes as needed, and rack
      (f) Glass slides
      (g) Band-Aids
4. Nursing care during the collection of blood specimens usually consists of explaining the procedure to the young child and helping support or restrain him.
5. Blood specimens must be collected, labeled, transported, and checked into the laboratory properly. Immediately after collection, invert tubes containing anticoagulant eight times to assure mixture—do not shake. If an ad-

Text continued on p. 410.

Table 27-1. Tests of blood specimens

Test	Purpose and rationale	Preparation of patient and/or specimen	Special considerations	Normal value
Albumin, globulin, total protein, and A/G ratio (usually performed together)	To aid in diagnosis or in evaluating treatments of many diseases, including those of liver and kidney Blood may produce excessive globulin when albumin is abnormally displaced or lost, causing change in blood plasma ratio	Fasting patient Specimen—6 ml. clotted venous blood		A/G ratio—1.5:1-2.5:1 Total protein—6-8 gm./100 ml. serum (lower level for newborn infant)
Antistreptolysin O titer	To aid in diagnosis of suspected rheumatic fever (not specific for this disease) Indicates presence of antibodies formed to combat recent streptococcal infection	Nonfasting patient Specimen—5 ml. clotted venous blood		Up to 200 units/ml. serum
Arterial blood gas (children and adults)	To evaluate respiratory exchange and acid-base balance	Specimen—1 ml. from arterial puncture collected in heparinized syringe	Specimen in syringe placed in ice for transport and immediate exam	Pco_2 35-45 mm Hg Po_2 75-100 mm Hg pH 7.35-7.45
X Bleeding time	To determine time needed for small cut to stop bleeding (involves constriction of small blood vessels) Prolonged bleeding time in thrombocytopenic purpura and other blood disorders	Nonfasting patient Basic procedure—standardized puncture wound made in fingertip, earlobe, or forearm, drops of blood produced removed with filter paper every 30 sec. Time needed for bleeding to end noted		1-6 min., depending on details of procedure
X Blood counts Platelet count (thrombocytes)	To aid in diagnosis of bleeding tendencies, thrombocytopenic purpura, aplastic anemia, etc. Platelets necessary for coagulation	Nonfasting patient Specimen—drops of capillary or unclotted venous blood (if automated procedures used, larger sample may be necessary)		200,000-500,000/mm.³
X Red blood count (erythrocytes)	To aid in determination of primary blood disease or effects of secondary disease on blood Red blood cells carry	Nonfasting patient Specimen—drops of capillary or unclotted venous blood (if automated procedures used, larger sample may be necessary)	Newborn infant has higher red blood count than adult	Adult; 4.5-5 million/mm.³

Table 27-1. Tests of blood specimens—cont'd

Test	Purpose and rationale	Preparation of patient and/or specimen	Special considerations	Normal value
Red blood count—cont'd	oxygen and carbon dioxide Elevated counts may indicate dehydration or polycythemia; low counts hemorrhage, red blood cell destruction, or failure in red blood cell formation			
White cell count (leukocytes)	White blood cells help combat infectious organisms Blood levels usually elevated in infections, may be elevated in blood diseases (leukemia) Depressed levels may result from blood disease and toxic drugs or chemicals	Nonfasting patient Specimen—drops of capillary or unclotted venous blood (if automated procedures used, larger sample may be necessary)	White blood count averages 20,000/ $mm.^3$ at birth; however, counts as high as 38,000/$mm.^3$ may be considered normal White blood count gradually falls with age; approaches that of adult by 3 yr. of age	Adult: 5,000-10,000/ $mm.^3$
White blood cell differential	To aid in diagnosis of certain diseases by study of white blood cell percentages Five main types of white blood cells; certain diseases cause alterations in proportions of different cells found in circulating blood	Nonfasting patient Specimen—drop of fresh or unclotted blood spread on glass slide, strained, and examined under microscope	Usual percentage pattern of type of white blood cells for adults: Neutrophils—50%-65%, increased during infections; eosinophils—0%-6%, increased in allergic conditions and parasitic infections; basophils—0%-1%, increased in some blood disorders; lymphocytes—25%-40%, increased in some viral and bacterial infections and leukemia; monocytes—0%-10%, increased during some infections	
Blood culture	To identify microorganisms that may be circulating in bloodstream Drug sensitivity test usually performed subsequently if organisms found	Nonfasting patient Special venous blood container with culture media Often ordered when high temperature spikes present	Operators should not speak during collection of specimen to avoid contamination Inside of container lid or stopper should not become contaminated; specimen to laboratory immediately Preliminary reports may be available in 36 hr.	Normal blood is sterile

Continued.

Table 27-1. Tests of blood specimens—cont'd

Test	Purpose and rationale	Preparation of patient and/or specimen	Special considerations	Normal value
Blood sugar	To aid in determination of abnormal glucose metabolism Disorders of blood sugar include hyperglycemia, caused by diabetes mellitus, liver diseases, or other endocrine overactivity; hypoglycemia, caused by tumor of islets of Langer**hans** (in pancreas) or other endocrine disturbances; insulin-glucose imbalance, caused by diabetic treatment	Fasting patients unless otherwise ordered Specimen—3-5 ml. venous blood in tube with sodium fluoride		80-120 mg./100 ml. (Folin-Wu method) 65-110 mg./100 ml. (Ortho-toluidine method)
Blood types Major groups	To determine blood type for possible transfusion or maternal-newborn blood studies	Nonfasting patient Both unclotted and clotted blood desired for transfusion cross matching		Four main blood types found in general population: A—38% B—12% AB—5% O—45%
Rh factor	To determine blood type for possible transfusion or maternal-newborn blood studies	Nonfasting patient Both unclotted and clotted blood desired for transfusion cross matching		85% of Americans, Rh+ (positive); 15% of Americans, Rh— (negative)
Blood urea nitrogen (BUN)	To determine kidney disease or urinary obstruction Urea, a waste product of protein metabolism, normally excreted by kidney; if urinary system fails, blood urea levels will be elevated	Fasting patient Specimen—5 ml. clotted venous blood		7-20 mg./100 ml. blood
Carbon dioxide–combining power (carbon dioxide capacity)	To aid in determination of acidity or alkalinity of blood High carbon dioxide–combining power may be result of persistent vomiting, hypoventilation, or excessive administration of ACTH or cortisone	Nonfasting patient, unless otherwise ordered Specimen—8 ml. venous blood, completely fill test tube to avoid air contact		Adult: 55 vol. %, 24-32 mEq./L. Child (under 2 yr.): 40-60 vol. %; 18-28 mEq./L.

Table 27-1. Tests of blood specimens—cont'd

Test	Purpose and rationale	Preparation of patient and/or specimen	Special considerations	Normal value
Carbon dioxide—cont'd	Low carbon dioxide–combining power may be found in diabetic acidosis, severe diarrhea, certain kidney diseases, and hyperventilation			
Clotting (coagulation time)	To determine time needed for blood to clot outside body Many factors necessary for normal clotting; clotting may be slow in hemophilia, anticoagulant therapy, etc.	Nonfasting patient Several methods, using fresh venous or capillary blood		Wide range, depending on method used
Coombs'	To detect weak or incomplete type of antibody reactions Used especially to diagnose erythroblastosis fetalis, caused by Rh incompatibility	Nonfasting patient Specimen—2-5 ml. clotted or unclotted blood, depending on laboratory methods and type of test ordered	Direct or indirect Coombs' tests may be ordered	Direct Coombs' test negative
C-reactive protein (CRP)	To aid detection of inflammation and tissue breakdown Nonspecific test, often used to aid diagnosis of rheumatic fever and infarctions	Clotted capillary blood or clotted venous blood may be used, depending on technique employed		Normally, no C-reactive protein present
Glucose tolerance	To aid in determination of abnormal glucose metabolism More sensitive than single fasting blood sugar determination	Fasting patient, except for glucose; oral or intravenous glucose tolerance tests may be ordered Fasting blood and urine specimen secured; calculated oral or intravenous dose of glucose given fasting patient Concurrent periodic blood and urine specimens may be ordered during 2-5 hr. period	Patient's current weight determined to calculate amount of glucose to be given; unsweetened lemonade or carbonated drinks, commercially prepared for this purpose, may be used to dilute glucose Testing procedures differ according to basic reason for test (possible hypoglycemia or hyperglycemia); procedure man-	Normal range: Oral—peak of not more than 150 mg./100 ml. blood, return to fasting level within 2 hr. Intravenous—return to fasting level within 1 hr.

Continued.

Table 27-1. Tests of blood specimens—cont'd

Test	Purpose and rationale	Preparation of patient and/or specimen	Special considerations	Normal value
Glucose tolerance—cont'd			ual of individual hospital should be consulted	
Hematocrit (Hct.)	To determine relative proportion of cells and plasma in blood Most reliable screen test for anemia—low in anemia, high in polycythemia and dehydration	Nonfasting patient Specimen—4 ml. or less of unclotted venous blood Specimen measured into a special hematocrit tube and spun; height of resulting column of packed red blood cells checked	Newborn infants have higher normal values than older children or adults; a low of 35 may be seen at about 2-6 mo. of age	Adult: Male—40-50 mm. red blood cells/100 mm. of column height Female—35-45 mm. red blood cells/100 mm. column of height
Hemoglobin (Hgb.)	To determine amount of hemoglobin in blood available for transport of oxygen Hemoglobin levels help determine color of blood; amount of red blood cells and level of hemoglobin in blood are not always parallel	Nonfasting patient Specimen—capillary or venous blood in oxalated tube	Newborn infants have higher normal levels than older children or adults (14-19 gm.); low of 11 gm. may be seen at 3-6 mo. of age	Adults—12-16 gm./100 ml. of blood
Protein-bound iodine (PBI)	To aid in determination of thyroid function Increased concentration of protein-bound iodine in blood may indicate hyperthyroidism; a decrease, hypothyroidism	Fasting patient Specimen—8 ml. clotted venous blood	Patient must not have had any previous iodine-containing substances (for example, intravenous pyelogram or gallbladder visualization) during preceding 6 mo.; administration of thyroid hormone may be discontinued for preceding 14 days	Adults: 3-8 μg./100 ml. serum
Sedimentation rate	To aid in detection of inflammation and tissue breakdown Nonspecific test, which, when elevated, may point to rheumatic fever activity, arthritic infections, and infarctions	Nonfasting patient Specimen—4 ml. unclotted venous blood Blood measured into a calibrated thin tube, and level of the formed elements settled in a certain time noted	If patient anemic, "corrected sedimentation rates" may be reported	Depends on equipment—0-20 mm./hr. (Wintrobe), 10-13 mm./hr. (Westergren)

Table 27-1. Tests of blood specimens—cont'd

Test	Purpose and rationale	Preparation of patient and/or specimen	Special considerations	Normal value
Serology test for syphilis RPR, VDRL	To aid in detection of syphilis Legally required before marriage in some states; routine at prenatal examination; some hospitals require on all admissions	Nonfasting patient Specimen—5 ml. clotted venous blood	Nonspecific tests— false positive and false negative results may be obtained Handle report of positive results discreetly	Negative

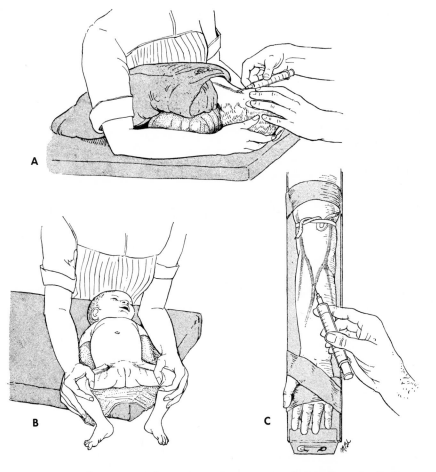

Fig. 27-1. **A,** Suggested restraint and positioning for puncture of a jugular vein. **B,** Suggested positioning for a femoral puncture. **C,** Suggested arm restraint in preparation for venipuncture for blood samples, intravenous medication, or infusion. The arm board should be well padded.

dressing machine is available, stamping the paper tape with the patient's charge-a-plate will easily assure the inclusion of the patient's name, unit, physician's name, and date on the label. A laboratory requisition form should accompany each specimen. The fact that the specimen has been sent should be recorded.

TESTS OF URINE SPECIMENS
General considerations

1. Urine specimens, except for bladder taps, are secured by the nurse.
2. Urine specimens may be obtained in various ways, depending on the physician's orders. Specimens may be ordered regulating the preparation of the patient or the timing of the specimen collection.
   a. Routine voided specimen. No special preparation usually needed. The patient is asked to void into a clean container (*Note:* Children and some adults do not understand the word "void"; select terminology in accord with the age and education of the patient. Little children may say "peepee," "tinkle," "number 1," "pass water," or "urinate.") The patient should be told not to put toilet paper in with the specimen. If the patient is menstruating, a routine voided specimen will be of no diagnostic value. A "clean catch" or catheterized specimen may be ordered, or the test deferred until later.
   b. Voided "clean catch specimen." Special preparations are made before the specimen is collected.
      (1) Necessary equipment includes the following:
         (a) Five or six sterile cotton balls
         (b) Betadine solution in squeeze bottle or bowl
         (c) Paper bag or other waste receptacle
         (d) Sterile or clean collecting

bottle, depending on situation; specimens for culture always collected in a sterile container
         (e) Clean gloves
      (2) For female patients the perineum is carefully cleansed with cotton balls saturated with Betadine solution. The labia are retracted, and each cotton ball is used only once, moving from front to back. After the urinary stream begins, the collecting bottle is positioned to collect an adequate specimen. Older patients may be able to carry out the procedure alone if properly instructed. Younger patients may find it difficult to void when directed. Little girls may be washed off and placed directly on a sterile bedpan if unable to void with the labia retracted. If the patient is well hydrated, the request for a specimen is more easily fulfilled. A midstream collection kit includes everything necessary for the collection of sterile specimens.
      (3) For male patients the glans penis is carefully washed with Betadine solution, and the foreskin, if present, is retracted to assure proper cleansing. When the patient begins to void, the container is positioned to collect an adequate specimen. Older boys and young men often carry out this procedure alone or with the assistance of an orderly.
   c. Three-glass specimen (for male patients). The glans penis is cleansed. Three sterile urine specimen bottles are labeled No. 1, No. 2, and No. 3. The patient begins the urine stream, voiding approximately 20 ml. in bottle No. 1. Without interrupting the urine stream he voids

Table 27-2. Tests of urine specimens

Test	Purpose and rationale	Preparation of patient and/or specimen	Special considerations	Normal value
Addis count	To aid in diagnosis of type of kidney disease present (acute, latent, or chronic nephritis, etc.) Cells and casts in urine sediment secured from 12-hr. specimen counted, and amount of each compared	Patient usually dehydrated—no fluids after breakfast until next morning and dry lunch and dinner At 8 P.M. patient begins 12-hr. urine collection After genitalia cleansed, saved specimens are voided directly into special container At 8 A.M. specimen closed and pretest diet resumed	Not performed on patients with severe kidney disease Special preservative must be placed in container	Results variable, depending on disease present
Phenolsulfon- phthalein (PSP)	To determine ability of kidney tubules to excrete dye Dye excretion decreased in chronic nephritis and urinary tract obstructions, increased in certain liver diseases	Procedure differs in various hospitals; consult laboratory manual for details Equipment—venipuncture equipment, 1 ml. dye solution, and urine specimen bottles Principles—patient empties bladder, and specimen discarded; patient is hydrated (no coffee or tea); physician injects 1 ml. of dye solution; specimens collected in separate bottles at various intervals, usually 15, 30, 60, and 120 min. after injection	Warn patient that urine may be pink or red after injection of dye because of pH of urine	Elimination of 63%-84% of injected dye in 2 hr.
Routine urinalysis				
Acetone	To determine presence of ketones in urine, a possible sign of developing acidosis	Usually done by nurse for diabetic patients; 1 drop of urine placed on Acetest tablet, and after 30 sec. color change compared with scale	Diabetic patients may have urine specimen free from sugar but containing acetone, although this is not common	No acetone present normally
Albumin	To detect loss of plasma albumin through kidney	Amount needed depends on method used		Usually no albumin present; however, orthostatic or postural albuminuria

Continued.

Table 27-2. Tests of urine specimens—cont'd

Test	Purpose and rationale	Preparation of patient and/or specimen	Special considerations	Normal value
Albumin—cont'd	May indicate kidney disease, heart failure, drug poisoning, or toxemia of pregnancy			sometimes occurs in absence of disease Albuminuria is common finding in newborn infant
Glucose	To detect presence and amount of glucose in urine, possibly caused by diabetes mellitus	Less than 1 ml. urine needed Clinitest—follow directions issued with Clinitest tablets; The "5 drop" and/or "2 drop" method may be ordered Clinistix—simple to use but most expensive; follow directions	When performing the Clinitest, observe reaction—rapid passage through green, tan, orange, and finally to dark shade of greenish brown indicates amount of glucose is over 2% in "5 drop" method; continue testing with "2 drop" method, which indicates up to 5% glucose Be sure to follow timing instructions explicitly Do not touch tablets; store away from heat and sun; watch for deterioration	No glucose usually present
Gross appearance (color, clarity)	To aid in estimation of degree of hydration and ability of kidneys to concentrate urine			Color depends on amount of hydration—may change markedly from one time to next Smoky urine may indicate hematuria; cloudy urine, abnormal sediment
Microscopic studies Cells	Red blood cells and white blood cells found in urine in kidney disease	Specimen of urine placed in centrifuge and sediment examined microscopically	Presence of red blood cells or white blood cells in voided specimen of mature female has little significance, since these results may be caused by contamination Recheck of catheterized specimen indicated	No red blood cells May be a few white blood cells May be a few epithelial cells

Table 27-2. Tests of urine specimens—cont'd

Test	Purpose and rationale	Preparation of patient and/or specimen	Special considerations	Normal value
Casts	Casts, representing abnormal sediment in urine, may be formed of many substances passing relatively slowly through tubules; presence usually indicates kidney disease	Specimen of urine placed in centrifuge and sediment examined microscopically		Rarely found normally
Specific gravity	To measure density of urine Detects presence of many abnormal substances, but does not identify them High specific gravity may occur in albuminuria, glycosuria, and dehydration Test also indicates patient's ability to concentrate urine	Tested with a urinometer (calibrated float) or T.S. meter		1.003-1.030 (adults) 1.002-1.006 (newborns after ingestion of milk)
pH	To determine acidity or alkalinity of urine	Strip of Nitrazine paper is dipped into urine or placed in a baby's diaper; color change compared to scale	pH should be measured quickly because urine becomes alkaline on standing Sometimes alkaline urine is needed to keep excreted substances soluble during sulfadiazine therapy or blood or tissue destruction), and therapy is directed to this end	4.5-7.5 (urine is usually acid, but pH may vary to maintain pH of blood)

about 100 ml. into bottle No. 2. Without interrupting the urine stream he continues to collect the specimen in No. 3 until his bladder is empty. The assistance of the orderly or a male nurse may be needed.

d. Catheterized specimen. Male catheterizations are performed by a male nurse or orderly; female catheterization technique has been described in Chapter 13. The urethra of the female infant curves downward; therefore, the catheter should be inserted in a slightly downward direction. Urine specimens for culture are always collected in a sterile container.

e. Percutaneous bladder aspiration (bladder tap). This specimen is obtained by a physician. The patient is placed in a supine position on a firm surface. The abdominal area is cleansed with antiseptic. The puncture is made above the pubis with a No. 22 (1-inch) or No. 21 (1½-inch) needle. A 5- or 10-ml. syringe is attached to aspirate a specimen in a sterile manner. This procedure should be delayed if the infant voids just before it is scheduled. Afterwards, the tap site is covered by a Band-Aid.

f. Timed specimen. This specimen usually consists of voided urine, although it may involve drainage from a urinary catheter. To begin the specimen collection, have the patient empty his bladder. Note the time. Discard this first urine specimen. Label a large collection bottle with the patient's name, his physician's name, and the time the discarded urine specimen was voided. This is the start of the test. Collect all voided specimens for the ordered period in this single large collection bottle. If a special preservative is not used, keep the bottle in the refrigerator. At the end of the period have the patient empty his bladder again and add this specimen to the total collection. Send the total specimen to the laboratory. Since this represents the total urine output of a patient within a known period, the collection *must* begin with an empty bladder. Twenty-four-hour urine specimens are notoriously difficult to obtain in pediatrics, especially from little girls. One of the newer methods employs a modified incubator, crib, or bed in which a nylon screening device is placed above a drainage unit. (This is sometimes called a "metabolic bed.") The child is positioned on the screen. As she voids, the urine is "filtered" through the screen.

Table 27-3. Tests of stool specimens

Test	Purpose and rationale	Preparation of patient and/or specimen	Special considerations	Normal value
Fat determination	To confirm diagnosis of steatorrhea (excess fat in stools), signs of celiac syndrome	Patient on normal diet 2 or 3 days before test Timed specimen usually ordered		Between 15% and 25% of weight of fecal sample
Occult blood	To detect presence of fecal blood, which is changed by process of digestion	Usually random specimen used If positive, patient is on meat-free diet for 3 days and another specimen obtained	Diet containing meat may sometimes cause positive result	No occult blood
Timed stool specimen	To determine amount of certain substances excreted in feces in given time	Patient should not void or place tissues in bedpan with stool Determine date and approximate time of previous defecations; this will be start of test collection; refrigerate total specimen until complete and then take to laboratory		

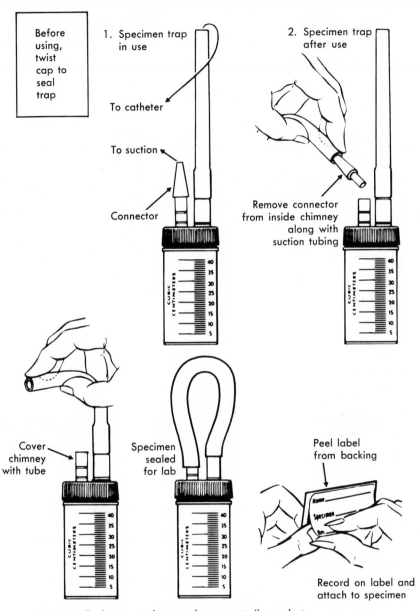

Sterile
Unless package is damaged or opened

Before using, twist cap to seal trap

1. Specimen trap in use

To catheter

To suction
Connector

2. Specimen trap after use

Remove connector from inside chimney along with suction tubing

Cover chimney with tube

Specimen sealed for lab

Peel label from backing

Name
Specimen
Date

Record on label and attach to specimen

Directions: Peel open package and expose sterile product.

To create suction inside bottle: Attach suction tubing to firm connector. When procedure is completed, remove firm connector from cap with suction tubing attached. Do not touch bottle cap with suction tubing if suction tubing is not sterile.

To direct specimen into bottle: Insert distal end of catheter connection inside latex tube.

Fig. 27-2. A sterile specimen trap, helpful in securing sputum specimens. (Courtesy Clinical Products, Sterile Specimen Trap, Chesebrough-Pond's, Inc., Hospital Products Division, Greenwich, Conn. 06830.)

3. Urine specimens should be properly collected, labeled, transported, and checked into the laboratory with proper requisitions. Urine specimens should be sent promptly to the laboratory unless protected from deterioration by a preservative or refrigeration.

TESTS OF STOOL SPECIMENS
General considerations

1. Stool specimens are obtained by the nurse.
2. Stool specimens are obtained by collection from a bedpan or diaper or, occasionally, by rectal swab. They are placed, with tongue blades, into a clean cardboard receptacle. The entire specimen need not be sent to the laboratory unless a timed specimen is

ordered or the reason for the stool collection is the detection of a tapeworm head. Specimens for ova and parasites or culture should be sent to the laboratory immediately.
3. Stool specimens should be collected, labeled, transported, and checked into the laboratory immediately and properly.

TESTS OF SPUTUM
General considerations

1. Occasionally sputum specimens are requested for culture and sensitivity studies. Sputum specimens are quite difficult to obtain from young children. Even older children and adults may find it difficult to produce material originating in the bronchial tree.
2. Specimens are best secured from co-

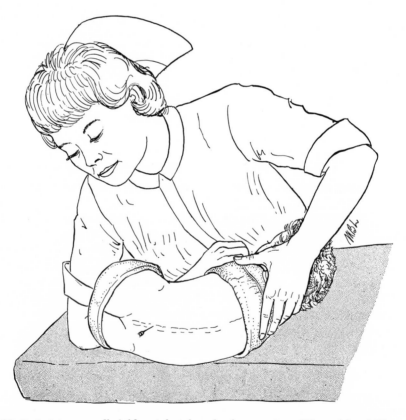

Fig. 27-3. Restraining a small child or infant for a lumbar puncture. When older children (2 to 3 years old) are positioned, the child's head may be tucked under an elbow, and the nurse may have to lean over her charge in a gentle but firm fashion to maintain positioning.

Table 27-4. Miscellaneous specialized tests

Test	Purpose and rationale	Preparation of patient and/or specimen	Special considerations
Electrocardiogram (ECG or EKG)	To aid in determination of irregularities in electrical impulses controlling heart action and to help diagnose heart damage	Usually no special preparation except simple explanation; no pain involved Leads positioned on various parts of trunk by technician	
Electroencephalogram (EEG)	To aid in determination of abnormalities in brain waves Useful in diagnosing convulsive disorders, brain tumors; estimating cerebral activity	Simple explanation Young children need to be sedated before test Testing takes approximately 1 hr.; no pain involved Electrodes placed on scalp with adhesive substance by special technician in quiet atmosphere	
Fetal lung maturity Foam stability test (Shake test); positive result usually indicative of fetal lung maturity L/S (lecithin/ sphingomyelin) ratio; 2:1, or 2, usually indicative of fetal lung maturity	To detect the presence of surfactants denoting fetal lung maturity and possibility of respiratory distress syndrome	Amniocentesis necessary to secure sample of amniotic fluid for analysis	Used to best advantage to determine time of elective cesarean procedures
Lumbar puncture	To obtain cerebrospinal fluid specimens for cell count, chemical analysis, culture, or gram stain Spinal fluid glucose lowered in cases of meningitis Spinal fluid protein elevated in meningitis or subarachnoid hemorrhage White blood cell count moderately increased in encephalitis; greatly elevated in most cases of meningitis	Inform child just before procedure Positioning: place child on side with knees drawn up sufficiently to arch back, or in sitting position with his spine curled forward to increase the spaces between vertebrae for needle insertion Child must be supported and maintained in position throughout procedure	Three specimens properly labeled, transported, and checked into the laboratory immediately Normal value in children: Pressure 70-200 mm of H_2O Cell count 0-8 WBC (under 5 yrs) and 0-5 WBC (over 5 yrs), 0 RBC Protein total 15-40 mg./100 ml. Glucose 50-90 mg./ 100 ml.
Sweat test	To help detect presence cystic fibrosis Abnormal amount of sodium chloride present in perspiration of affected persons Positive sweat chloride 60 mEq per liter or higher Positive sweat sodium usually 10 mEq per liter higher than sweat chloride	Plastic bag technique—extremity to be used is washed, dried, and enclosed in clean plastic bag (heating pad may be applied); when adequate perspiration evident, bag is carefully removed without touching the inside, and perspiration allowed to collect in bottom of bag; bag closed and transported in upright position to laboratory Pilocarpine iontophoresis: an electric current via attached electrodes drives pilocarpine into skin of forearm, stimulating local sweat production in about 5 min.; a specimen of perspiration is then absorbed into gauze or filter paper; usual time for sweat collection is 30 min.; sample is weighed and analyzed	

Table 27-5. X-ray tests*

Test	Purpose and rationale	Preparation of patient and/or specimen	Special considerations
Barium enema	To aid in diagnosis of lower bowel pathology by outlining colon with radiopaque material May be part of treatment for intussusception	Cathartics or cleansing enemas may be ordered on previous day or morning of test Clear liquid diet may be given 1 day before test until test completion Barium enema given in x-ray department when patient is under fluoroscope; examination takes 1 to 2 hr. Enema or cathartic may be ordered after roentgenograms completed	Carefully note and record patient's bowel movements after procedure
Brain scanning	To provide a visual display of abnormal tissue within skull; useful in diagnosing brain tumors	Injection of radioactive isotope (Radionuclide pertechnetate [^{99m}Tc]) Before scanning, minimum wait of 15 to 60 min. after IV injection	
Cystogram	To aid in diagnosis of urinary obstruction or other abnormality by visualization of bladder, ureter, and urethra with radiopaque material during filling and emptying of bladder	Urethral catheter inserted prior to procedure Bladder emptied Radiopaque material injected into bladder and x-ray film taken Catheter removed	
Voiding cystourethrogram		Roentgenograms taken during voiding process	
Ciné cystourethrogram	To determine whether reflux appears or increases at voiding pressure	Continuous fluoroscopic pictures taken during voiding process	
Gastrointestinal series (G. I. series)	To aid in diagnosis of stomach and small bowel pathology by outlining areas with radiopaque material	Night before test, patient may have light supper No food, fluids, or medications after midnight until 6-hr. x-ray studies completed X-ray department gives barium under fluoroscope Patient remains NPO until x-ray department gives release after 6-hr. studies If 24-hr. studies ordered, no enema or cathartic given until studies completed Check for enema or cathartic orders when test completed	

*If the nurse is holding or positioning the child during the x-ray procedure, she should wear a lead apron.

Table 27-5. X-ray tests—cont'd

Test	Purpose and rationale	Preparation of patient and/or specimen	Special considerations
Intravenous pyelogram (IVP)	To detect kidney or urinary disease by intravenous dye injection followed by abdominal roentgenograms	Cathartic or enema ordered to clear bowel on day before test Patient may eat light dinner with little fluid Fluids, food, and medications withheld after midnight Roentgenograms of abdomen taken before and after intravenous injection of dye by physician Fluids usually forced after completion of test	Allergy to iodine is contraindication to routine technique
Pneumoencephalogram	To detect abnormalities of brain by injection of air or oxygen into spinal canal Lumbar puncture done, and and some spinal fluid withdrawn and replaced by air, which rises to ventricles of brain, forming characteristic outlines	Patient NPO 6 hr. before test; given preoperative sedative and analgesic; may be done under local or general anesthetic in x-ray department After procedure, patient kept flat and observed carefully; headache, nausea, and vomiting fairly common; signs of increasing intracranial pressure should be reported; treated as postoperative patient	
Ventriculogram			Similar to pneumoencephalogram, except air introduced directly into ventricles through burr holes in skull Performed in operating room

operating patients after IPPB treatment or chest therapy (cupping, vibration, and postural drainage).

3. For those who cannot cooperate, the use of a sterile specimen trap connected to a suction apparatus has been helpful (Fig. 27-2).

28

The child surgical patient

Not too many years ago the child was considered, in many ways, to be a miniature adult. Old photographs reveal that he was dressed like an adult, and at times he received similar treatment. However, age does make a difference. Anatomical relationships, physiological activity, and psychological responses are greatly influenced by the phenomena of normal growth.

This chapter discusses some of the differences that set the child apart from the adult and reviews a few routines and procedures encountered fairly commonly when nursing the pediatric surgical patient.

CHILD-ADULT DISTINCTIONS

The following list of child-adult distinctions is not complete, but it may prove helpful in the evaluation of the needs of children.

1. The metabolic rate of infants and young children is much greater proportionately than that of adults. Children are growing and need to be fed more frequently.

2. Abnormal fluid loss is more serious in the infant and young child than in the adult. Fluid intake and output must be calculated very carefully, including fluid loss from diaphoresis or wound drainage. A 7-pound infant who sustains a blood loss of 1 ounce (30 ml.) has been compared with a 150-pound man who has lost 600 ml. of blood.

3. The child lacks the reserve physical resources that are available to the adult. His general condition may change very rapidly, almost without warning.

4. The body tissues of the child heal quickly because of his rapid rate of metabolism and growth.

5. The child usually needs proportionately less analgesic than an adult patient to obtain relative comfort after surgical procedures.

6. The young child lives more in the present than an adult does. This may be both to his advantage and disadvantage. "Now" is understood and very important, but he has difficulty understanding "later." On the other hand, he usually does not become upset by anticipating unpleasant future problems or prospects or worrying about finances or loss of a job!

PREPARATION FOR SURGERY

When relatively simple surgery is contemplated, there is a growing trend toward 1-day hospitalization or the performance of operative procedures at out-patient Surgi-Centers. However, many youngsters are still formally admitted to a hospital even for minor surgery.

The child entering the hospital for surgery may have had considerable preparation for the event, or he may have had none. The condition for which he is admitted may be relatively simple to correct, or it may entail an operation of considerable complexity and risk. He may have had numerous previous admissions and know many of the staff by name, or he may never have seen a blood pressure cuff, call light, or bedpan.

Psychological preparation

The nurse should remember that in all contacts with patients, regardless of age, there should be explanation and emotional support adapted to the individual's ability to understand and his personal needs. She should also remember that as parents are reassured, the confidence they gain in turn helps support the child.

Physical preparation

Patients being admitted for surgery should be especially evaluated for the presence of respiratory infection and signs of malnutrition. Occasionally, surgery may be delayed until the general condition of the child improves.

Physical preparation for surgery usually (except in emergency situations) begins the night before the procedure. Although some children may be admitted to the hospital early in the morning of the day of minor surgery, most come into the hospital the previous afternoon.

If orthopedic surgery is planned, the child is usually given a Betadine bath as ordered in the evening. The body part to be involved in the surgery is carefully washed and inspected. The fingernails or toenails of any extremity involved are cleansed and trimmed. In many cases the ordered shave of the operative area is delayed until the morning of surgery, unless the surgery is scheduled very early. For some types of surgery, preparatory enemas may be ordered.

Food, fluids, and oral medications are withheld as ordered, depending on the type of surgery planned, the age of the child, and the time of the procedure. The fact that the child must not receive anything by mouth should be conspicuously posted. The child should be told of the fact so that he does not think that he has been forgotten when the breakfast trays are passed. Any loose or missing teeth should be noted and recorded on the chart.

Sedative and analgesic drugs are given, usually in two stages. Preliminary sedation is usually ordered approximately 2 hours before surgery. Analgesic and atropine compounds, which prepare the patient for general anesthesia, are routinely given "on call." Every effort should be made to see that the child is allowed to rest after receiving his preoperative medications. The room should be dimmed and quiet and the side rails in place.

After the child is taken to surgery in his crib or on a cart, his unit is prepared for his return. His bed, if present, is made up according to his postoperative needs, and any special equipment desired is placed conveniently. An orthopedic patient may need bed boards under the mattress, an overbed frame and trapeze, and extra plastic-covered pillows. Other equipment that may be required, depending on the individual, includes a suction machine, intravenous standard, oxygen mask, mist tent, bed lift, and properly sized restraints.

POSTOPERATIVE CARE
Immediate observation

When the patient returns to the nursing unit from the recovery room, his general condition must be noted. Periodically, his pulse, respirations, and, possibly, his blood pressure are determined and recorded. Until the patient is responsive and alert, he should be kept on his abdomen or side unless the surgery performed contraindicates these positions. The nurse should note the condition and placement of any dressing and describe any apparent drainage. The presence of a plaster cast or mold should be noted. Casted extremities should be elevated, and frequent checks for circulatory disturbances should be made. Intravenous infusions should be checked for possible infiltration and correct rate of flow. The child should be protected from harming himself (pulling out needles or tubes or tampering with suture lines) by the use of an appropriate restraint, as necessary. Urinary catheters should be connected to dependent drainage and stabilized properly to the bed with a safety pin and rubber band to prevent the formation of a dependent loop of tubing, which obstructs drainage. The type and amount of urinary drainage should be observed. The patient's skin color and temperature are checked. The nurse must always watch for and quickly report signs of shock—low blood pressure; cold, moist, pale, or cyanotic skin; rapid pulse; dilated pupils; and restlessness.

Diet

Whether the child will be allowed oral fluids after he is responsive will depend on the physicians orders and the child's general condition. Sometimes surgical patients are not allowed oral fluids for a considerable period; instead, they are fed intravenously. When oral feedings are introduced, they are begun gradually, and the patient's tolerance is observed. The routine post-surgical diet follows this sequence with modifications for different ages—clear liquid, full liquid, soft, and regular. Rich, spicy, highly seasoned, or gas-forming foods should be avoided.

Ambulation

Early progressive ambulation for the general surgery patient is the rule in the modern care of patients. In only a few cases and situations will the physician delay ambulation beyond the first postoperative day. The general surgery patient usually has orders to stand at the bedside and take a few steps the day after surgery. The nurse should be sure to follow these orders because judicious ambulation strengthens the patient, aids in the restoration of gastrointestinal function, and helps prevent such complications as pneumonia and the formation of blood clots and pressure areas.

When the patient's condition or young age makes it impossible or inadvisable for him to get out of bed, the nurse must be sure that he is turned frequently, receives good skin care, and breathes deeply at intervals. The physician may order the use of "blow bottles" or intermittent positive pressure treatments to aid lung expansion.

After surgery, toddlers and preschool-aged youngsters usually move about quite spontaneously in their cribs or beds; ambulation presents few problems for them. However, older children may express the same timidity and fear of pain that most adult patients exhibit when asked to move or get up and may need a great deal of initial support and encouragement from their parents and the nursing staff.

Fortunately, in most cases it is not long before these same youngsters are enjoying the freedom of the playroom. Most will recover quickly and gather together their little hoard of treasures and say their "good-byes" in a few days. At times some possessions are overlooked; one nursing staff fondly remembers Bobby, who left his turtle in the linen closet!

COMMON PROCEDURES

A few of the common procedures encountered when nursing pediatric surgical patients are described in the following pages. Some of these treatments may also frequently involve medical patients. They will include skin preparation for surgery, cleansing enema, dressing change, gavage feeding, gastrostomy feeding, urinary catheter irrigation, and irrigation of nasogastric or intestinal tubes.

SKIN PREPARATION FOR SURGERY

Purposes: To cleanse the area of prospective surgery to help prevent infection, provide a clearly visible operative field, and carefully inspect the skin for possible pustules, lesions, or signs of poor circulation.

Materials:
1. Sharp, sterile razor
2. Clean bowl for warm water
3. Prescribed soap or antibacterial solution
4. Waterproof pad or sheeting
5. Towels (2)
6. Washcloth or gauze sponge
7. Clean cotton applicators, if the areas to be "prepared" involve the umbilicus or toes
8. Nail clippers, if extremities are involved
9. Bath blanket or drawsheet
10. Gooseneck lamp

Procedure:
1. Check the order, the operative permit, and the time preoperative medications will be given. The preparation should be finished before the medications must be given.
2. Identify the patient.
3. Explain the procedure to the patient according to his level of understanding. Small children usually respond to the explanation, "We're going to wash your tummy to make

it very clean." When you are ready, begin by doing just that. Explain as you work. As the child gains confidence, you may show him the tiny hairs on his arm and talk about how adults shave. Run your finger along his skin to show him how the razor feels. Suggest that it may tickle a little but that he will help by being very still.

4. Position the lamp and raise the bed to a convenient working level.
5. Wash your hands.
6. Place the waterproof pad and towel under the patient to protect the bed.
7. Prepare and place the warm water and ordered antibacterial agent conveniently. (Some physicians may order a dry shave.)
8. Apply tension to the skin with the washcloth or a gauze sponge as you shave. (If the feet or fingernails are very dirty, they may be soaking in a basin of warm water while the adjacent areas are being shaved.)
9. Crouch down frequently to look *across* the surface of the skin to check for remaining hairs.
10. Retain your "prep setup" until the skin preparation has been checked by the team leader, head nurse, or instructor.
11. Record the procedure. Any skin lesions (for example, pustules) must be reported. Pustules are *not* to be opened. Razor nicks should be treated with direct pressure with a sterile sponge and reported. Great care must be used in shaving, especially in areas

of old scars, insect bites, or bony prominences, where nicking may easily occur.
12. In some cases a povidone-iodine (Betadine) scrub of 10 minutes may be ordered after the shave is complete. The physician may order the prepared area wrapped in sterile towels until surgery.

CLEANSING ENEMA (Fig. 28-1)

Purposes: To cleanse the lower bowel prior to surgery, relieve constipation or flatulence, and aid in the expulsion of parasites.

Materials:
1. Rectal catheter or tubing and clamps, appropriately sized
   a. For infants, size 12 to 16 French
   b. For young child, size 12 to 20 French
   c. For older child, size 16 to 22 French
2. Container of ordered solution
3. Lubricant and wipes
4. Asepto syringe barrel or enema can or bag, depending on the amount of fluid to be given and the size of the child
5. Ordered solution (kind and amount) at 105° F. when given

Note: Disposable enema setups may be easily used for some patients depending on amount of solution needed.

Procedure:
1. Identify the patient.
2. Explain to the child what will be done as you do it according to his level of under-

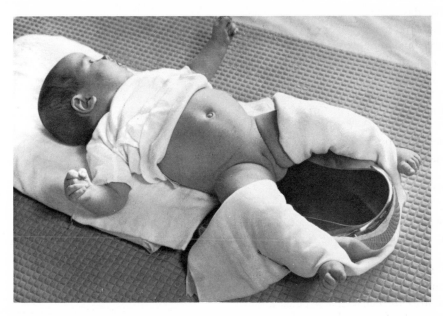

Fig. 28-1. One way of positioning an infant for an enema. The restraining diaper is centered under the tip of the pan and then brought up and over the infant's legs and pinned to itself.

standing. In the case of the very young child, understanding will not be complete, of course, but the tone of voice and the socialization such explanation offers can be helpful. Telling a small child that you are "going to put a little water in where we take your temperature to help you go to the bathroom," sometimes helps.

3. Screen the unit and position the child. A number of positions are advocated when giving an infant or toddler an enema.

a. For most children the side position with the upper leg flexed seems to be the most comfortable. The left side is preferred because this placement puts the descending colon lowest. However, a left-sided position is not absolutely mandatory. In fact, some investigators question the supposed advantages of left-sided placement. Infants and small toddlers often do well if placed on a firm pillow, which has been draped with a lightweight plastic sheet and covered with an absorbent towel, with their hips pulled to the edge. The plastic extends over the side of the pillow into or beside a curved basin or small bedpan, which is placed snugly against the buttocks just below the rectum. For warmth, the child is covered by a bath blanket or towel.

b. If the infant is very active and a nurse has no one to help maintain him in a side position, the infant may be gently restrained in supine position over a small bedpan. His back and head are supported by a small pillow or folded bath blanket. His buttocks are placed over the bedpan and his legs gently drawn to either side and secured by a diaper placed under the bedpan and drawn up and over the lower extremities and pinned to itself as illustrated in Fig. 28-1.

c. Older children with sphincter control are usually positioned on their sides and given enemas in basically the same way as any adult.

4. Place the ordered amount and type of solution in a can or Asepto barrel attached to a rectal tube. Expel the air from the tube and lubricate the tip. Do not occlude the eyes of the catheter.

5. Gently insert the tubing approximately 2 to 3 inches into the rectum and observe the flow. Hold the container of solution no higher than 12 to 18 inches above the patient's hips.

6. Observe the patient closely during the procedure for an increase in respiratory and pulse rates and exhaustion.

7. As needed, put the child on a bedpan or potty chair, or allow him to go to the bathroom.

8. Remove equipment and tidy up the area.

9. Record the procedure and the results obtained.

STERILE DRESSING CHANGE

Purposes: To protect the incision or wound from contamination by replacing wet dressings, allow direct observation of the incision or wound to evaluate the healing process, increase the cleanliness and comfort of the patient, and, in some instances, apply local medications or carry out irrigations that assist in treatment.

Materials: Materials vary according to the area to be dressed, whether sutures are to be removed or local debridement attempted, and the wishes of the physician. Generally, the following supplies are needed, although not all the supplies listed are needed every time. Simple dressings may require only sterile compresses, handling forceps, adhesive tape, and a discard bag.

1. Dressing tray containing the following
   a. Basic instrument kit with sterile
      (1) Suture-remover scissors
      (2) Clip removers
      (3) Sharp-pointed suture scissors
      (4) Tissue forceps
      (5) Smooth forceps
      (6) Small hemostat
      (7) Probe
   b. Wrapped, sterile cotton applicators
   c. Wrapped, sterile dressings of various thicknesses and sizes
      (1) Thick, absorbent pads (ABD pads)
      (2) 4 × 4-inch and 2 × 2-inch gauze squares (flats)
      (3) Nonadherent dressings (Telfa)
      (4) Soft gauze dressings that have been fluffed out (fluffs)
   d. Various sizes of gauze roller bandage and Ace tensor bandage
   e. Various sizes and kinds of adhesive tape

2. Sterile gloves (used when the area to be dressed is large or difficult to manage)

3. Large paper bag to receive old dressings

4. Clean kidney basin for antiseptic pour-off overflow

5. Bandage scissors

6. Appropriate antiseptic, irrigating solution, or medication

7. Clean paper towels

Procedure:

1. Select a time when there is little bedmaking or mopping activity in the area. These activities increase the bacteria count in the air.

2. Identify and screen the patient and explain the purpose of the dressing change according to his level of understanding. At times positioning assistance may be needed.
3. Drape the patient appropriately.
4. Adjust the lamp, if needed; position and open discard bag and kidney basin, if needed.
5. Wash your hands.
6. Open only those supplies needed.
7. Place sterile handling forceps on the edge of a sterile wrapper—points on the sterile surface, handles over the edge.
8. Remove bandages or adhesive tape (Always pull tape toward the incision or wound to prevent undue strain or pain.)
9. Lift off the top dressing, your hand protected by a clean, folded paper towel or clean plastic gloves. Contact only the side of the dressing that was exposed to the exterior. Drop dressing and towel or glove into open paper bag.
10. Lift off any remaining inner dressing with the sterile handling forceps. Be careful not to pull drains, if present. Dressings that stick to the skin may usually be moistened with a small amount of sterile saline solution to facilitate their removal.
11. Cleanse the area gently of any old drainage present with mild antiseptic or ordered solution and sterile gauze sponges mounted on handling forceps. Pour the solution onto the sponge over the discard kidney basin. Dry the area with a sterile compress.
12. Place a dressing, appropriate for size of the incision and amount of drainage present, using handling forceps.
13. Secure with adhesive tape, Elastoplast, or Montgomery tapes.
14. Discard used dressings, wash your hands, and tidy up the area.
15. Record the procedure and the condition of the wound or incision. Describe the type and amount of any drainage present and report any unusual odor. Note any skin irritation caused by adhesive.

GAVAGE FEEDING USING AN INDWELLING NASOGASTRIC TUBE

Purposes: To avoid mouth and lip motion when it may endanger surgical repair, nourish a child who is too weak to be fed orally in the normal fashion, and supplement oral feedings when nutritional buildup is imperative and sufficient intake by normal means is impossible.

Materials:
1. Sterile Asepto or piston-type syringe (If the child is receiving sterilized formula, a sterile syringe will be secured for each feeding. If he is not receiving sterilized formula, the nurse may wash and store the syringe in a clean manner for use next time.)
2. Container of formula (infants who receive sterilized formula will have the tube feeding sterilized)
3. Glass of water (bottle of sterile water for infants)
4. Towel or napkin
5. Perhaps bib and infant seat

Procedure:
1. Identify the patient and explain the procedure according to his needs and level of understanding.
2. Briefly warm the formula, if necessary, so that it will be tepid at the time of the feeding. (Feeding cold formula, if not given by Barron pump or slow drip, can be upsetting to the patient and may initiate vomiting.) Evaluate the consistency of the feeding: Is it too thick? Will it clog the tube? Volume must also be considered. Many times you cannot dilute a feeding and administer the entire amount to maintain the caloric count ordered. Such a feeding would overload the stomach.
3. Unless contraindicated, raise the backrest of the bed of a child or place a baby on his side, head elevated. This position lets gravity aid the flow of the formula.
4. Protect the area next to the tube opening with a towel. Put a bib on an infant.
5. Test the position of the end of the tube by each of the following methods:
   a. Observe the length of the tube exposed.
   b. Place the open end of the tube under water and watch for a flow of bubbles on expiration. Some gas in the stomach may cause an occasional bubble, but it will not cause a flow of bubbles synchronized with expiration.
   c. Inject approximately 1 to 5 ml. of air (depending on patient) into the tube. Listen with a stethoscope just below the sternum for sound of air passage. Withdraw the air and suction further for evidence of stomach contents, or, if ordered, measure entire aspirate to help determine digestion of previous feedings and current stomach capacity.
   d. Ask the patient to hum, if possible. If the tube is in the trachea, the patient cannot hum.
6. Continue with the administration of the formula. In most instances allow the formula to flow by gravity. Exerting additional pressure may be dangerous. If the flow is sluggish, raise the barrel. If it is too fast, lower the barrel or pinch the tube. If

425

the flow has stopped, change position of the patient slightly. If the flow still does not continue, *gentle* pressure with a syringe bulb or piston may *start* the flow. If no response is forthcoming, the tube must be removed and another inserted. If the infant is crying, flow will be slower than when he is quiet.

7. Add more formula before the barrel is empty to avoid introducing additional air into the stomach. If the tube is to be left in place, when the formula is finished (just before the last few drops leave the barrel), add approximately 15 ml. of water to rinse the tube. (Failure to include this step will cause a clogged tube.) If the tube is to be removed, pinch it tightly before and during its quick removal to prevent drops of formula from entering the airway.

8. Any infant must be bubbled after gavage just as he would be bubbled after routine oral feeding.

9. Record the amount and type of feeding and the tolerance of the patient.

GASTROSTOMY FEEDING

Purpose: To provide nourishment via a tube that has been surgically inserted through the abdominal wall into the stomach because of obstruction or surgical repair of the child's oroesophageal tract.

Materials:

1. Tray containing the following:
   a. Syringe barrel (sterile for small infants receiving sterilized formula)
   b. Container of formula (sterile for small infants)
   c. Container of water (sterile for small infants)
2. Towel or napkin

Procedure:

1. Identify patient and explain the procedure according to his needs and level of understanding.

2. Warm the formula if necessary so that it will be tepid at the time of the feeding. (Feeding cold formula, if not given by Barron pump or slow drip, can be very upsetting to the patient and initiate vomiting.) Evaluate the consistency of the feeding: Is it too thick? Will it clog the tube? Volume must also be considered. Many times you cannot dilute a feeding and administer the entire amount to maintain the ca-

loric count ordered. Such a feeding would overload the stomach.

3. Keep the patient flat, if possible, during the gastrostomy feeding.

4. Attach the syringe barrel to the tube and fill with formula before unclamping the tube. (*Note:* There may be orders to aspirate the contents of the stomach into the barrel. The amount aspirated is noted, and it is allowed to return to the stomach. The feeding to be given is decreased accordingly to prevent overloading.)

5. Unclamp the tube and allow the fluid to flow slowly by gravity. Never use pressure of any kind to start the flow of formula into the gastrostomy tube. This may cause unwanted backflow into the esophagus.

6. Continue to add formula to the barrel before it completely empties to avoid introducing air into the stomach.

7. Finish the feeding by adding 15 to 30 ml. of water to rinse the tube. Clamp off the tube before all the water leaves the barrel to avoid introducing air into the stomach. (*Note:* In some cases involving infants, the physician may order that the tube not be clamped but be left opened with the barrel attached and elevated above the baby's body. The formula is allowed to return to the barrel as the child cries or changes position.)

8. Record the amount and type of feeding and the tolerance of the patient.

URETHRAL CATHETER IRRIGATION

Purposes: To prevent the clogging of the catheter by blood clots, salts, or cellular debris and instill medication into the bladder.

Materials:

1. Tray containing the following:
   a. Sterile syringe
   b. Sterile solution basin
   c. Sterile drainage basin
   d. Sterile 4 × 4-inch gauze squares, towel, or catheter cap
2. Ordered solution (e.g., physiological saline)
3. Basin of warm water to heat solution to tepid temperature.

Procedure:

1. Check the order and identify the patient.

2. Explain the procedure to the patient according to his needs and level of understanding.

3. Place the solution bottle into warm water.

4. Disconnect the catheter drainage tubing from the catheter proper. Let the catheter drain into the drainage basin. After allowing the contents of the drainage tubing to flow into the collecting bottle, place the sterile end in a sterile 4 × 4-inch gauze square, towel, or cap.

5. Pour the ordered solution into the basin and draw the ordered amount into the syringe.

6. Inject the ordered amount of solution slowly into the catheter. Momentarily pinch off the catheter and disconnect the syringe. Allow the flow to return by gravity. (*Note:* Some neurological patients, by special orders, have more vigorous catheter irrigations in which the irrigating fluid is injected "with conviction" and is aspirated three or four times before being removed from the bladder and catheter.)

7. Evaluate the amount and the character of the returned drainage.

8. Reconnect the catheter and drainage tubing.

9. Report to the team leader or supervising nurse any difficulty experienced with the irrigation.

10. Record the procedure, the kind and amount of injected solution, and the character and amount of the return flow. Note the reaction of the patient.

IRRIGATION OF A NASOGASTRIC OR INTESTINAL TUBE

Purposes: To prevent the clogging and assure the patency of an indwelling nasogastric or intestinal tube. The tube may have been inserted for the following reasons:

1. To prevent vomiting

2. To relieve postoperative abdominal distention, discomfort, and pressure on surgical repairs

When the tube has been inserted for the reasons cited, it is attached to some type of suction or drainage device. Usually the suction ordered is intermittent, occasionally it may be continuous. High or low negative pressure may be prescribed. Sometimes only gravity drainage is ordered. Most children are placed on low intermittent suction. Irrigation is only carried out when the wishes of the physician concerning the individual case are known.

Materials: Unless the type of surgery would make it necessary to employ sterile technique, the materials used to irrigate a tube must be kept meticulously clean but need not be sterile. The type and amount of irrigating fluid to be used is ordered by the physician. Physiological saline solution is frequently requested. The amount to be used will depend on the size of the child and the type of surgery performed.

A setup would usually include the following:

1. Syringe (10 to 30 ml., depending on amount to be used)

2. Basin or solution reservoir

3. Clamp

4. Towel and emesis basin

5. Ordered solution

Procedure:

1. Identify the patient.

2. Explain to the child according to his level of understanding. For young children it is usually sufficient to say that you are putting a little "water" in the tube.

3. Draw up the amount and kind of solution ordered in the syringe.

4. Place a folded towel and emesis basin under the junction of the tube leading to the suction apparatus or gravity drainage.

5. Turn off any mechanical suction device.

6. Clamp the tubing that leads to the suction or drainage bag and disconnect the two parts of the tubing; wrap the end of the tubing that leads to the suction machine in a towel, cover it with a cap, or hang it from a support on the machine.

7. Fit the syringe of irrigating fluid into the patient's tube and gently instill the ordered amount. Whether the nurse will be allowed to withdraw any of the irrigating solution with the attached syringe will depend on the preferences of the physician.

8. Detach the syringe, and reconnect the tube either to the suction machine (removing the clamp and restarting the suction) or to the gravity drainage. (Recheck any suction setting.)

9. Remember, this patient is usually not allowed oral fluids except perhaps *small* amounts of ice chips. However, lubrication of the nares, renewal of the tape maintaining the tube's position, and oral hygiene are fairly frequent patient needs.

10. Record in the patient's output record the amount of irrigating fluid used. (*Note:* If a tube is not draining and resistance is encountered during an attempted ordered irrigation, the nurse should notify her supervisor immediately.)

29

Aiding respiration and oxygenation

The process of respiration brings oxygen into the body for circulation to the individual cells via the bloodstream and removes waste products, carbon dioxide, and water from the body. In some diseases the transfer of oxygen to the tissue cells is made very difficult by a breakdown in the anatomy or physiology concerned. To aid the handicapped processes, various procedures, apparatuses, and medications have been developed to help clear the airway, enrich the oxygen content of inspired air, stimulate or maintain adequate respiratory effort, or achieve the proper circulation of blood.

Within the last few years inhalation therapy, a technical speciality devoted to the maintenance of optimal respiratory exchange and prevention of respiratory disease, has developed. In many hospitals an inhalation therapist will supervise gaseous therapy (such as intermittent positive pressure or special tents) and aid in resuscitation measures.

HINDRANCES TO OXYGENATION OF THE BLOOD

To understand the rationale of many of the treatments ordered the student should review the structure and function of the respiratory system. The passageways from the exterior of the body to the microscopic air sacs, or alveoli, which make up the functional tissue of the lungs, must remain open to assure proper oxygenation. Any obstruction, whether caused by the position of the tongue, aspiration of a foreign body, edema, a tumor, the presence of tenacious secretions in the laryngotracheobronchial "tree," or spasm of the bronchioles, will lead to respiratory difficulty. Any condition such

as pneumonia, emphysema, tuberculosis, or a malignancy that causes a depletion in the ability of the lung tissue to receive air and transfer oxygen and carbon dioxide may cause respiratory distress. Any interruption in the mechanisms of breathing that creates an intermittent suction (negative pressure) in the thoracic cavity through contraction of the diaphragm and intercostal muscles (because of nervous system stimulation caused by carbon dioxide buildup in the bloodstream) will also affect respiration and therefore oxygenation. Of course, in the final analysis the circulatory system must also be adequate to deliver the oxygen to the final destination, the individual microscopic body cells.

The most accurate way to determine the extent of oxygenation in a patient's blood is by chemical analysis of the oxygen and carbon dioxide level in a blood sample.

SECURING AND MAINTAINING AN AIRWAY
Position

The first concern in aiding breathing always involves the airway. Occasionally it may be obstructed because of the position of the tongue. This may be true in the case of the unconscious patient; the tongue is not actually swallowed, but it may fall backward and obstruct the pharynx. An open airway may be obtained by placing the patient on his back with his head in "sniffing" position and his lower jaw held up. This returns the tongue to normal position. At times the insertion of a plastic oropharyngeal airway will be helpful.

If the airway is obstructed by a foreign body or secretions, the emergency relief usually attempted *first* involves gravity

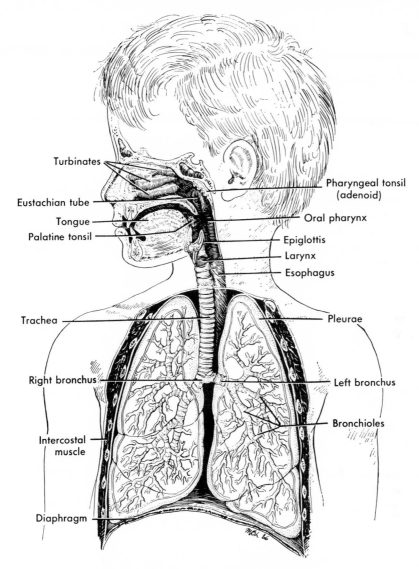

Fig. 29-1. Normal respiratory tract.

drainage. Occasionally the bronchi may need to be visualized with a special instrument called a bronchoscope for removal of the foreign body.

To prevent aspiration, a child in danger of vomiting or regurgitating should be maintained on his side or abdomen. If this is impossible because of other more important considerations (such as type of surgery, or administration of an anesthetic), the head should be lowered and turned to the side during episodes of nausea and vomiting.

Suction

Suction of the naso-oropharyngeal passages or even deeper suction may be necessary to clear the airway. Suction may be accomplished by using a bulb syringe, a simple manual suction catheter (DeLee trap), or a catheter setup attached to wall or portable suction. The following points about procedure should be remembered when a catheter is used:

1. The suction apparatus should be personal for each patient and kept free from contamination. Some hospitals

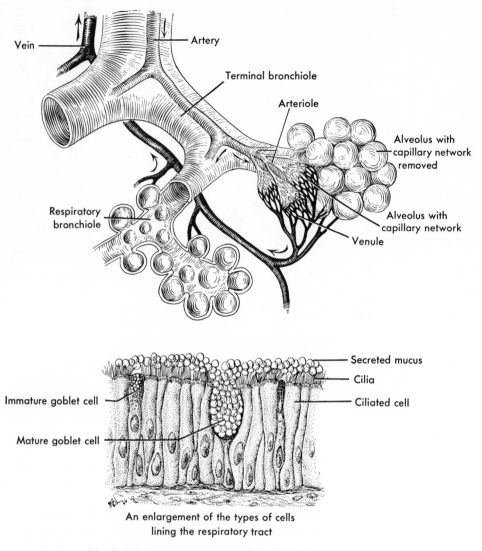

An enlargement of the types of cells
lining the respiratory tract

Fig. 29-2. Microscopic anatomy of the lower respiratory tract.

now employ a "use-once-only-and-throw-away" catheter technique.

2. The drainage bottle should contain about 1 inch of disinfectant solution at the outset to thin out the secretions, ease its cleaning, and reduce the number of bacteria in the bottle. It should be opaque or covered with a small pillowcase.

3. Catheters should be lubricated with water before use to assure greater ease of insertion.

4. During catheter insertion, the suction should be temporarily discontinued by pinching the catheter or uncovering the Y-tube control to avoid depleting the patient's supply of oxygen or injuring the mucous membranes.

5. The lowest amount of suction necessary should be applied. Suction should not be prolonged; suction administered too frequently may aggravate congestion instead of relieve it.

6. The catheter and tubing should be immediately rinsed after use to prevent clogging and stored conveniently

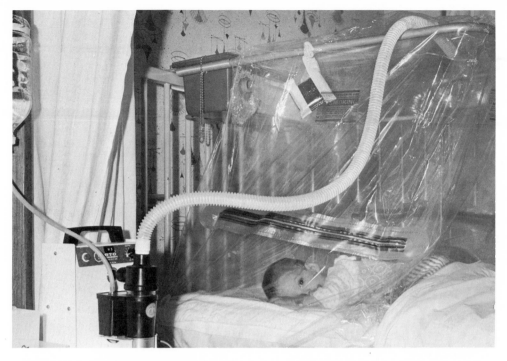

Fig. 29-3. Ultrasonic mist has gained favor because the small mist particles penetrate the respiratory passages better than former misting techniques. The equipment is compact and relatively easy to handle. In real therapeutic situations the mist may be so dense that the child is obscured. Side rail down for picture only. (Courtesy Children's Health Center, San Diego, Calif.)

in an aseptic manner, unless the catheters are not reused.

7. The child usually will need to be restrained during the procedure.

Humidification

Sometimes secretions are so thick that they are difficult to drain by gravity or suction, and various procedures and agents may be used to thin out the secretions. These may take the form of simple moist inhalations provided by a convenient cool mist humidifier at the bedside or under a canopy or tent. (Warm mist or steam tents have been almost entirely replaced because of the danger of burns.)

A form of aerosol therapy that has been found to be effective in liquefying thick respiratory secretions is that provided by the *ultrasonic nebulizer* (Fig. 29-3). This unit, although generally used with a tent, is not dependent on a gas source for mist formation, produces fine penetrating water particles, is quiet, and occupies little space. It employs sterile distilled water. It has been used particularly by cystic fibrosis patients. However, the small infant in such a dense water-aerosol environment must be observed carefully for overhydration, since relatively large amounts of water can be absorbed from the lung into the circulation. Infants may be weighed frequently to assess the amount of such absorption, and fluid intake modifications may be necessary in certain cases. Patients should be removed from the mist tent at intervals.

Medications

Medications are frequently ordered to aid in clearing the airway.

Nose drops. Nose drops, such as phenylephrine hydrochloride (Neo-Synephrine), may be ordered to shrink mucous membranes and ease nasal congestion.

431

Expectorants. Oral expectorants, which increase the bronchial secretions and may help thin mucus, are occasionally ordered. Common medications of this type are potassium iodide and glyceryl guaiacolate.

Aerosols. Acetylcysteine (Mucomyst) reduces the thickness and tenacity of mucus. If a vial of acetylcysteine is opened and not completely used, it should be stored in the refrigerator and used within 48 hours. In tents a 20% volume solution is usually ordered.

Isoproterenol hydrochloride (Isuprel), commonly administered in aerosol form, helps dilate or relax the bronchioles to relieve spasms, shrinks swollen mucous membranes, and reduces the secretion of thick mucus. When isoproterenol hydrochloride is used, the heart rate must be carefully watched, since this medication may cause an abnormally rapid pulse (tachycardia).

• • •

If the airway is impaired because of spasm of the bronchi or bronchioles, as is often the case in asthmatic attacks, the addition of other medications to relax the bronchioles may be needed to relieve wheezing and respiratory distress. Chief among such medications used is the very powerful epinephrine (Adrenalin).

Some anatomical alterations of the respiratory system are difficult to treat and may be of long duration. However, some of the swelling and/or distortion of lung tissue and bronchioles may respond to the use of antibacterial drugs or medications used for specific chest diseases such as tuberculosis. Abnormal dilatation of the air sacs, or emphysema, may be particularly persistent and troublesome in the asthmatic child. Air is typically breathed in and depleted of its oxygen content. The air sacs have lost their normal elasticity, and cannot force the "old air" out of the lungs properly. Another full breath of well-oxygenated air cannot be taken, since the "old air" still occupies some space in the air sacs. Real distress may develop, especially on expiration. Medication such as epinephrine and a calm, reassuring

manner on the part of the nurse help, but structural changes may be enduring.

Postural drainage and percussion techniques

Some respiratory diseases (for example, cystic fibrosis and emphysema) produce such exaggerated amounts of tenacious secretions deep in the lungs that it may be difficult for the patient to expel them even with the aid of medications, humidification, and suction techniques. These secretions interfere with proper pulmonary ventilation and set the stage for frequent respiratory tract infections that further endanger the patient. Another way of promoting drainage of a clogged or potentially obstructed respiratory tree is through the use of breathing exercises and selective postural drainage consisting of positioning, cupping, and vibration, followed by purposeful coughing.

When physical therapists are available, they usually perform these maneuvers and instruct the family if continued treatment is necessary at home. In the event that physical therapists are not available, nurses may be asked to learn the techniques. Anyone responsible for performing them should be specially instructed and initially supervised in their use. The following brief explanation is not intended to take the place of such instruction.

The treatment is most effective when preceded by aerosol therapy and is enhanced by diaphragmatic breathing. It may be prescribed as a prophylactic as well as a therapeutic measure.

Various postures assumed by the patient help drain different parts of the lungs. Therefore the position or positions in which the patient is placed depend on the site of his congestion and the general aims of his therapeutic program. In general, the placement of the patient enlists the forces of gravity and the sweeping action of the respiratory cilia in clearing the lungs. Any constrictive clothing should be removed. The patient's knees and hips should be flexed in the various positions necessary, so

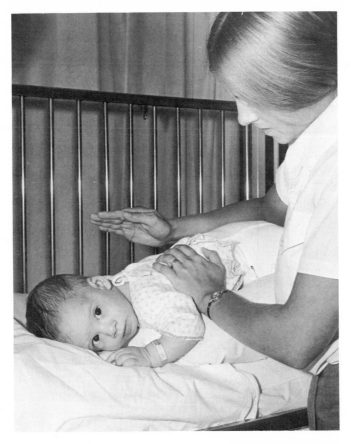

Fig. 29-4. The physical therapist is performing the early morning, before breakfast ritual on a small patient with congenital structural weakness of the bronchi. Scheduled cupping and vibrating have proved particularly helpful. (Courtesy Children's Health Center, San Diego, Calif.)

that relaxation will be promoted, and there will be less strain on the abdominal muscles when coughing is encouraged. When the patient's head must be lowered, usually all that is needed for an infant or young child is a well-positioned, firm pillow (Fig. 29-4). An older child may have to assume a modified jackknife position, lying over an elevated knee-gatch. A teen-ager may be able to hold his head and chest down crosswise over the side of the bed, while helping to support himself by grasping a low stool. However, he should not be left alone in this predicament! A baby or toddler may respond best when positioned on the nurse's or therapist's lap. This therapy should be done before meals or at least an hour after eating. It is never initiated if the patient is

hemorrhaging or in pain. Percussion is usually begun in the upright position and terminates with the head lower than the rest of the body.

Two basic maneuvers are used: (1) cupping, also known as clapping or tapping, and (2) vibrating. The first is performed with the palm of the hand raised, the fingers and thumb forming the sides of a firm cup. When the cupped hands are gently but abruptly applied to the patient's chest wall, the wrist is alternately flexed and extended. A characteristic hollow sound is produced. The technique is continued about 30 seconds over the affected area while the patient both inhales and exhales. It is then followed by the vibrating motion done only while the patient is exhaling slowly. This second maneuver is accomplished by tensing the hands, arms, and shoulders and producing gentle and fine vibratory movements on the chest wall. It is continued only during slow expirations. The two maneuvers are then repeated several times, depending on the tolerance of the patient.

Percussion techniques should not be used over the spine, kidney area, abdomen, sternum, or developed breast tissue. Coughing should be encouraged as needed.

Laryngoscope

If a patent airway cannot be maintained through positioning, simple suction, insertion of an oropharyngeal airway, humidification, percussion, or administration of appropriate mucus-thinning or bronchodilatory medications, the larynx may be visualized with a laryngoscope and an endotracheal tube inserted for suction and ventilation The laryngoscope blades and endotracheal tubes must be of an appropriate size, or they are useless.

Tracheostomy

If continued airway obstruction is observed or contemplated, a surgical opening of the trachea (tracheostomy) may be created to provide an artificial airway and allow easier access to the trachea for suction. Care of a patient with a tracheostomy is a very serious responsibility.

The adult or child who has had a tracheostomy usually cannot speak or make any vocal noise unless the opening of the tracheostomy tube, which retracts the surgical incision, is temporarily covered. For any person who has previously been able to communicate well orally and for the young child who lets his wants be known by crying, failure of oral communication, accompanied by respiratory problems, is extremely frightening.

Children with tracheostomies should be placed in areas where they will be under constant observation. When appropriate, signal cords or handbells should always be available. For those able to write, a magic

slate or paper and pencil should be near at hand. The method of temporarily closing off the tracheostomy opening with the fingers to speak should be taught to the older child during his convalescence. Temporarily obstructing the tube in this way will also aid defecation. A calm, efficient nurse does wonders in alleviating the anxiety of tracheostomy patients.

A double-walled tube is generally used in the tracheal opening. A second tube, or inner cannula, fits directly inside the outer tube, providing a means of quickly clearing the larger, outer tube if the inner tube becomes blocked. Periodically, the frequency depending on the needs of the patient, the inner cannula is suctioned or removed and cleaned. When the inner cannula has been removed, the outer cannula is also suctioned. The nurse may suction as deeply as necessary to remove secretions. Occasionally, orders are left that small amounts (3 to 5 drops) of sterile physiological saline solution be dropped into the tracheostomy tube to help thin out any secretions before suctioning. If oxygen is being administered, a smal humidification unit may be fitted directly over the tube, or a humidifier may be placed in the patient's room to instill the necessary moisture.

To provide the equipment necessary for the care of a patient with a tracheostomy, a special tray is available at the bedside. Materials necessary for cleaning the inner cannula and maintaining the suction equipment should be on the tray (Fig. 29-5). When caring for a patient with a new tracheostomy, the nurse uses a new sterile catheter and glove each time the patient is suctioned. Complete equipment should include the following items:

1. Sterile gloves
2. Sterile basin of detergent or hydrogen peroxide for soaking the tube and removing mucus and crusts
3. Sterile pipe cleaners to thread through the tube and ensure patency
4. Sterile basin of sterile water for rinsing the tube
5. Antiseptic solution for storage of the

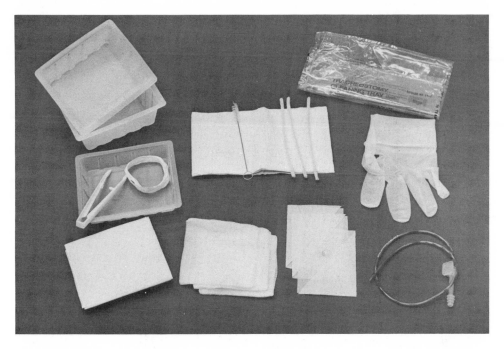

Fig. 29-5. These sterile materials are found in a disposable tracheostomy cleaning tray that is now available. Note the thumb control on the suction catheter. (Courtesy Grossmont Hospital, La Mesa, Calif.)

catheter in use (if catheter is re-used)

6. Extra tracheostomy tube of the same size as the one being used
7. Tracheal dilator or curved hemostat for emergency use to hold a temporary tracheostomy open in the event that the outer tube is accidentally expelled
8. Supply of *lint-free* tissues for wiping away expelled mucus
9. Bottle of physiological saline solution
10. Supply of sterile, lint-free precut gauze tracheostomy dressings
11. Medicine dropper, if instillations are ordered
12. Paper bag taped conveniently to the supporting table to receive waste

Tracheostomy tubes may be made of silver, plastic, or rubber. Parts are usually manufactured to be used together and cannot be interchanged. There are actually three parts to most tracheostomy tubes: the inner cannula, the outer cannula, and the obturator, a small, curved rod ending in an olive-shaped tip. The obturator is placed within the outer cannula at the time of insertion to help keep the tube clear, protect the mucous lining from injury, and help direct the cannula placement. As soon as placement is secured, the obturator is removed. It is then stored in an obvious spot (on the tracheostomy tray or in a clear bag taped to the head of the bed) for use during reinsertion of the outer cannula in case of an emergency. The inner cannula is inserted and locked into place after the withdrawal of the obturator. There are three main types of locks available: a metal flap that turns down over the inner cannula, a knob-turn lock, and an interlocking lateral plastic flange. Tracheostomy tubes are now available with a single cannula (no inner tube). They are manufactured with or without cuffs. A cuffed tracheostomy tube is used principally with ventilators. The inflatable cuff (or cuffs) around the inserted tube blocks the escape of air around the tube and increases the efficiency of the

435

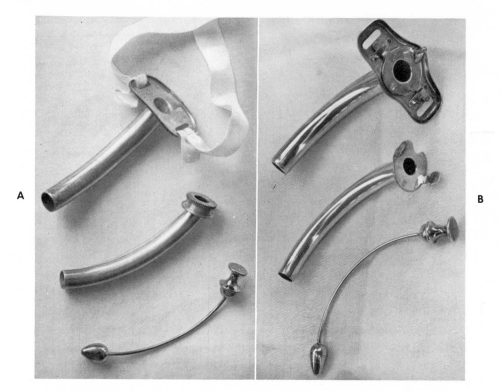

Fig. 29-6. Four types of tracheostomy tubes (shown in descending order, the outer tube, inner tube, and obturator). **A,** On the Hollinger, the head, or knob, on the inner tube rotates to fit under the small lip at the back of the outer tube. **B,** On the Jackson, the small metal flap on the back of the outer tube rotates to hold the inner tube securely. **C,** The plastic Portex, with a pop-in-and-out inner cannula that fits under two opposing flanges. This set comes with two inner cannulae. **D,** A single cannula, double-cuffed tracheostomy tube. The smaller attached tubes are alternately used to inflate two "balloons" around the lower end of the large tube. This device is used when ventilation is assisted by mechanical means.

machine. The cuff must be periodically deflated to prevent pressure injury to the mucous membrane. Fig. 29-6 shows a double-cuffed tracheostomy tube. First one cuff and then the other are inflated and deflated, easing pressure on the tracheal lining.

All the equipment used in the maintenance of a new tracheostomy should be handled in a sterile manner. However, when the tracheotsomy is "old," clean technique is usually followed. All equipment is presterilized before being used on a patient, and the suction catheters, tray, bowls, and solutions are frequently renewed or changed. The suction catheter in use is often stored in an antiseptic solution to reduce the possibility of contamination.

Therefore tracheostomy care of a long-term convalescent patient becomes, in the final analysis, a clean procedure; to insist on throw-away catheter technique would appear to be financially and practically unfeasible. Nevertheless, the nurse must be careful in her technique and wash her hands conscientiously.

A Y-tube connection is recommended on the suction catheter to facilitate its use. Suction is obtained by covering the open end of the Y-tube with the thumb. It is more gentle to the mucous membranes than a catheter, which has been pinched to stop suction during insertion. Insertion of the catheter is made with no suction applied. Suction is applied periodically as the tube is rotated on withdrawal. It has been sug-

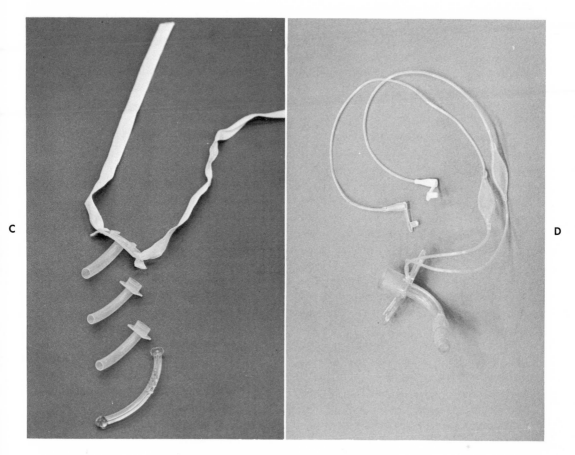

Fig. 29-6, cont'd. For legend see opposite page.

gested that the nurse hold her breath during suctioning so that she will not suction for too long an interval and inadvertently interfere with respiration. (The catheter may partially block the passage of air or remove necessary air.) If bronchial suction is desired, the patient's head should be turned first to one side and then the other during the suctioning process, if possible. This assists the catheter to enter both bronchi instead of following the easiest pathway to the less angled entrance of the right bronchus. Too frequent aspiration should be avoided. Very young children usually resist suctioning. Often better results are obtained if they are positioned on their backs with the shoulders raised on a folded bath blanket and the head dropped back.

Assistance or a modified mummy restraint may be needed.

ENRICHED OXYGEN ENVIRONMENTS
Safety factors

Various methods and devices are used to make inspired air richer in oxygen. The oxygen content of air in a well-ventilated room is about 21%. Therefore any device used to elevate the oxygen content must be capable of administering oxygen of a higher percentage. However, because of the danger of eye damage and loss of sight due to retrolental fibroplasia caused by oxygen excesses in the blood, many devices are set to deliver no more than 40% oxygen to a specific area without a special maneuver. A small premature infant is es-

437

pecially vulnerable to retrolental fibroplasia; nevertheless, there are times when his environmental (ambiant) air must contain more than 40% oxygen in order to meet his needs, which have increased because of respiratory or cardiac problems. The most accurate way of assessing the actual oxygen needs of these infants is by periodic blood gas determinations. The results of these tests are compared with the oxygen concentrations delivered in the hood or incubator, which are monitored at least every 2 hours.

When oxygen is being used, other safety factors involved must be clearly understood to avoid fire. Oxygen readily supports combustion, and all sources of possible ignition of flammable materials should be removed from the environment. Also, safe storage and maintenance of oxygen cylinders, if used, must be carried out to avoid fire and explosion hazards.

Rules for oxygen administration. The following rules should be observed during oxygen administration:

1. No open flames, cigarettes, cigars, matches, cigarette lighters, or candles should be allowed in a room in which oxygen is being used. Signs that read "Oxygen In Use—No Smoking" should be clearly posted.
2. No device that is capable of producing a spark should be operated in the oxygen-enriched environment. Any electrical equipment used must be especially grounded to be safe. Therefore most electrical equipment is prohibited; no standard television sets, radios, vaporizers, heat lamps, electrical beds, or call bells should be used. Occasionally TV sets and hospital equipment are elevated high on special shelves. In this position they can be used in a room where oxygen is being administered since the room is not air tight and the oxygen (which is heavier than air) seeks lower levels.
3. No oil or alcohol rubs should be given in oxygen tents or other closed units.

4. No wool blankets should be used on the bed of a patient receiving oxygen.
5. At no time should an oxygen outlet, tank, regulator, or administering apparatus be oiled, greased, or handled with greasy hands or gloves.
6. All enclosed oxygen units (such as incubators or tents) should be "flushed" with oxygen before the patient is enclosed within them.
7. Because of the potential danger of excess carbon dioxide accumulation, all tents or enclosures should provide some method of ventilation or chemical control that will prevent this problem.

*Rules for use of oxygen tanks.** The following rules are related to the use of oxygen tanks or any cylinder containing gas under pressure:

1. All cylinders contain gas under pressure unless truly empty. If a cylinder falls and the valves are damaged, oxygen may escape with tremendous force. All cylinders must be stabilized with proper supports to guard against falling (for example, strapped to the bed or positioned in an oxygen tank carrier or a heavy metal baseplate).
2. An oxygen regulator must always be used when administering oxygen from a cylinder to reduce the pressure of the oxygen to safe levels before it reaches the patient. The regulator includes a dial, which measures the amount of oxygen remaining in the cylinder, and a flowmeter, which measures in liters per minute the amount of oxygen being administered (Fig. 29-7). The particular type of regulator employed must be thoroughly understood before it is put into use. There are several types, and the details of their operation differ. However, the following principles hold

---

*Many hospitals now have piped-in wall oxygen, but the nurse should also be acquainted with the use of oxygen stored in cylinders.

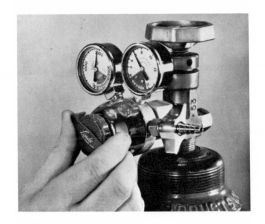

Fig. 29-7. A characteristic oxygen tank with regulator attachment.

3. When discontinuing cylinder oxygen for periods of half an hour or less, simply close the flowmeter. When longer periods without therapy are desired or when one wishes to replace the tank or regulator, proceed in the following manner:

    a. Close the cylinder valve. When the pressure registered on the dial is 0, continue to wait until all the oxygen is exhausted in the flowmeter and the flowmeter indicator also rests at 0. Then close the flowmeter, and detach the regulator if a cylinder change is desired.

Methods of oxygen enrichment

Oxygen tent. A large oxygen tent may be ordered for an older child. Such a tent is usually a plastic canopy suspended from an overhead rod and attached to a cabinet containing a machine, which, when properly adjusted, regulates the tent's ventilation and temperature and may also provide a control for increased humidity along with an orifice for the appropriate oxygen flow (Fig. 29-8). An oxygen tent may be set up in the following manner:

1. If time and the patient's condition permit, place a bath blanket between the bed mattress and the bedspring to prevent snagging the plastic canopy, which can be easily torn. A plastic or rubberized sheet under the sheet covering the mattress will cut down on oxygen loss if the mattress is permeable.

2. Bring the tent canopy and control cabinet to the bedside. Extent the overhead bar, designed to support the tent during use, and expand the tent folds slightly along the bar.

3. Plug in the electrical cord leading to the control cabinet, and turn on the motor.

4. Set the air circulation or ventilation control on the cabinet, if available, halfway between low and high.

5. The temperature control on the cabinet is usually placed at 70° F. How-

true for all types, although the way in which they are fulfilled will depend on the individual apparatus.

a. All cylinders should be momentarily opened by loosening the cylinder valve (out of earshot of the patient) before the regulator is attached. This is called "cracking the cylinder," which produces a sharp, noisy blast. It is done to dislodge any particles of dust from the cylinder valve and prevent injury to the equipment and leakage. The nurse should stand to the side of the cylinder, out of the way of the brief steam, when it is "cracked."

b. Regulators should be attached with a hand wrench to assure a tight connection.

c. Before the oxygen flow is started:

    (1) The flowmeter must be closed.

    (2) The operator must step out of the way, to the side of the regulator-tank connection, in case the regulator should be dislodged as the result of some defect when the flow is begun.

d. The cylinder valve is opened slowly. When the cylinder valve is opened and the needle registering the contents of the tank comes to rest, the flowmeter may be adjusted to the approved amount.

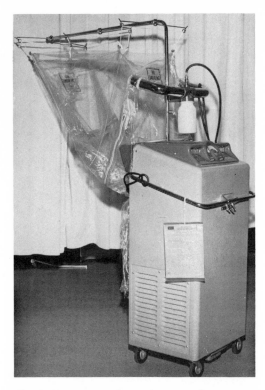

Fig. 29-8. One type of oxygen tent with a temperature control and ventilating humidification units. (Courtesy Children's Health Center, San Diego, Calif.)

ever, even in extremely hot weather the temperature setting should not be more than 10° to 15° F. below the room temperature to prevent shocking the patient when the canopy is lifted and decreasing the working efficiency of the tent.

6. If ventilation deflectors are present in the tent, arrange them so that the cool air entering the tent does not blow directly on the patient.

7. Connect the oxygen inlet tube to the wall flowmeter or oxygen cylinder regultaor and start the flow at 15 liters per minute. Maintain this rate for 30 minutes and then analyze the oxygen concentration. If the ordered contration is attained, the flow is usually reduced to 10 to 12 liters per minute —the minimum flow required to wash out and dilute exhaled carbon diox-

ide. Instead of increasing the oxygen flow to 15 liters per minute for 30 minutes, many times the same concentration can be achieved by holding a flush valve open for at least 2 minutes after the tent has been placed around the patient. Warn the patient that such a valve opening causes a rushing noise as the tent floods with oxygen.

8. Gently place the canopy over the patient in such a way that its sides (skirts) do not touch his face.

9. Many tents of this type seem drafty to the patients. How much protection from cold is necessary depends on the patient's own body temperature. Little girls may wear scarfs and bed jackets, if desired. Boys like hoods and cotton jackets.

10. Mold the tent canopy around the child's body to prevent unnecessary oxygen loss (Fig. 29-9). A folded sheet may be placed at the end of the tent, molded around the child's body, and tucked under the mattress with the tent. If the tent is not tucked in properly, much leakage will occur.

11. When lowering or raising the head of the bed, take care not to catch the tent canopy in the mechanism or put the canopy under undue tension. Many times the patient in an oxygen tent will feel better with the head of the bed moderately raised, if orders permit.

12. Plan nursing care so that the tent is opened as little as possible and many of the patient's needs are met during one interval. The motor blower may be shut off before opening the tent to reduce oxygen waste. Be sure to restart the motor after the nursing care has been completed.

13. High humidity concentrations may be achieved with the addition of jet humidifiers on many of the units. Sterile distilled water alone or additional ordered medications may be used.

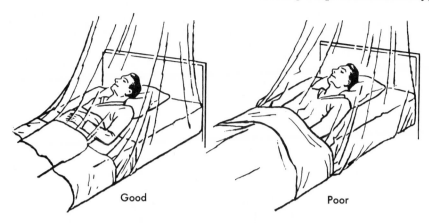

Fig. 29-9. Good and poor methods of draping the tent canopy. To assure proper oxygen concentrations, waste should be minimal. (From Oxygen therapy handbook, ed. 5, New York, 1962, Linde Co., Division of Union Carbide Corp.)

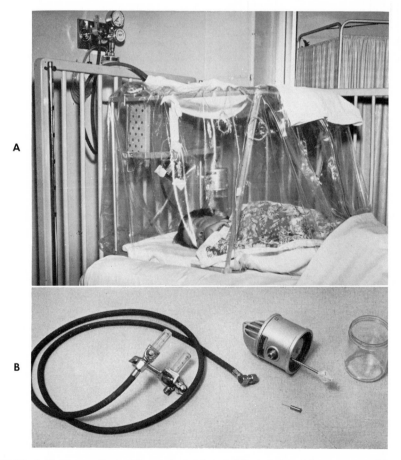

Fig. 29-10. A, Tony, a patient with congenital heart defect, is in a Mistogen tent. The side rail was lowered for the photograph only. **B,** Parts of the humidifier and hose attachment. From left to right: double flowmeter (used if two tents must operate from one wall oxygen outlet), oxygen hose, needle valve, humidifier head with nylon filter attached, and fluid reservoir.(Courtesy Children's Health Center, San Diego, Calif.)

441

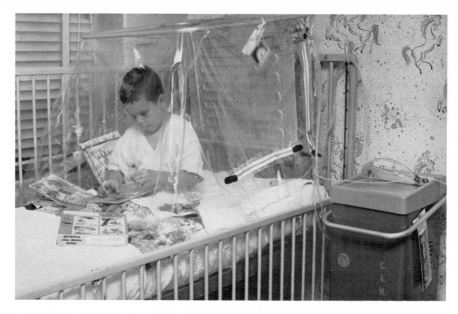

Fig. 29-11. The C.A.M. tent, a newer version of the Mistogen tent, is cooled and ventilated electrically. The working apparatus is not near the patient, and more room is available for activity. This boy has asthma; the side rail was lowered for photograph only. (Courtesy Children's Health Center, San Diego, Calif.)

High-humidity oxygen units. A tent that provides both high humidification and oxygen and rests on top of the bed is often used for younger children. Various models are available. The one shown in Fig. 29-10 is the Mistogen tent to which ice must be added. Fig. 29-11 is a photograph of the Child-Adult Mistogen tent, a newer model that is electrically refrigerated.

Many tents do not include an electric ventilator to circulate the air as do the larger oxygen tents and have a real tendency to overheat. The temperature of a tent that is not electrically cooled and ventilated must be regulated by the addition of ice and frequently checked because temperature may quickly rise. However, the factor that actually determines whether more ice should be added to the reservoir to help cool the tent is the body temperature of the patient. If, for instance, the child has a subnormal temperature, a minimal amount of ice may be used. If the child has an abnormally elevated temperature, a cooler tent temperature will usually be sought and more ice added. Usually tent

temperatures ranging between 68° to 72° F. are satisfactory for covered children with normal body temperatures.

The humidifier used in such tents also differs with the manufacturer. Fig. 29-10, *B*, shows the different parts of the Mistogen humidifier. If this particular humidifier does not produce mist, the following factors should be checked:

1. Is the filter dirty?
2. Is the needle valve clogged?
3. Is the oxygen flow sufficient?
4. Is the fluid level sufficient?
5. Has lint collected inside the metal humidifier head?
6. Is the oxygen hose connection correct?

Sterile water is now being used in most hospitals to try to reduce bacterial growth.

The oxygen liter flow necessary for such tents depends primarily on the size of the tent and the oxygen concentration desired. Flow rates of 4 to 10 liters per minute may be ordered. If the tent has an open top like the Mistogen model, a small blanket may be secured over most of the opening to help increase the humidity and oxygen concentration.

Patients placed in the cool, high-humidity environments produced by such tents must be checked *frequently* to see if their hair and clothing are damp. If the child does not have an excessively elevated temperature, he should have an undershirt under his cotton gown. Infants seem to do best when dressed in long-sleeved, foot-in sleepers.

Nasal cannula. Oxygen may also be administered by nasal catheter or nasal cannula. However, the catheter is rarely used because it is unnecessarily irritating and confining for children. The cannulae used are usually short, paired, open tubes made of plastic or metal that are attached to a larger tube leading to the oxygen supply. These tubes are placed just inside the nostrils. A nasal cannula should be used when only low concentrations of oxygen, less than 35%, are desired. Oxygen administered by cannula should be passed through a humidifier to prevent uncomfortable drying of the mucous membranes. The cannula should not obstruct the nostrils, and the patient should not breathe through his mouth.

Oxygen mask. Oxygen by mask is usually administered through a tube leading from the oxygen supply to a light plastic face mask. Some of the units available are disposable. Masks are capable of administering high oxygen concentrations quickly and are ideal for emergency use. A rather wide variety of oxygen masks is available; some masks allow rebreathing of the first one third of the air expelled with each expiration (the fraction of an expiration richest in oxygen content) along with oxygen from the tank or wall supply. A well-known partial rebreathing face mask is the BLB, named for the initials of its inventors, Boothby, Lovelace, and Bulbulian. A partial rebreathing mask must fit tightly to the face, but a simple face mask that does not provide for rebreathing and is used for emergency or short-term use should not be applied tightly unless an escape valve or opening for carbon dioxide release is present. Nurses should be well acquainted with the particular oxygen equipment used in their setting and should study the manufacturer's instructions.

Incubators with increased oxygen. Incubators are often used in the treatment of newborn infants and small infants. Basically, they are glass or plastic boxes that provide warmth, oxygen, humidity, and easy observation of the infant. They are sometimes used only to provide additional heat, controlled electrically by presetting the temperature control and watching the thermometer inside. In some cases the temperature of the incubator is regulated by the body heat of the baby as determined by a temperature probe taped to the baby's trunk (see p. 198). The desired interior temperature of the incubator is usually about 85° to 89° F., depending on the infant's temperature response. Often, oxygen is added to the environment to ease respiration and relieve cyanosis.

Incubators are available in two basic styles—those that have lift-up lids, which open at the top for nursing care, and those that also provide special side entries for nursing care, such as the Isolette Infant Incubator (Model C-86) shown in Fig. 29-12. The entire plastic hood rocks back for placement of the child inside. A front panel may also be lowered if necessary to provide easier access for procedures; however, if oxygen is being used or incubator temperature is especially important, as much infant care as possible should be accomplished through the side portholes without lifting the hood or opening the side panel. Incubator temperatures and oxygen concentrations (whenever supplementary oxygen is being used) should be recorded at least every 2 hours. The incubator is made up with a pillowcase folded over the mattress; diapers are placed under the infant's head and buttocks to catch drainage. Many times, to aid observations, the infant wears no clothes or only a diaper. The mattress platform may be slanted to aid oral drainage or help prevent regurgitation.

443

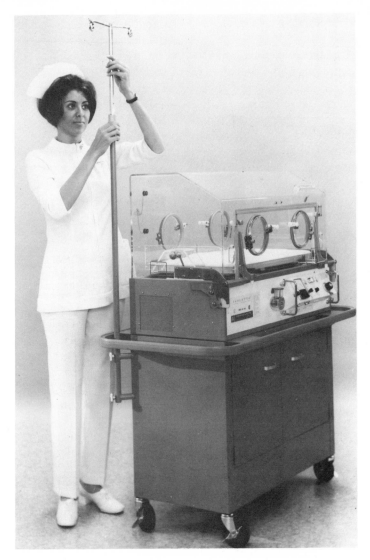

Fig. 29-12. Isolette infant incubator, Model C-86. (Courtesy Isolette-a Narco Medical Co., Warminster, Pa. 18974.)

The humidity of the incubator may be regulated by setting a special control that allows the air to flow over a water reservoir under the incubator deck. However, the warm water in the reservoir may easily become a site of bacterial growth. To combat this tendency, some nurseries have added antiseptics to the water used; others have abandoned the use of the subdeck reservoir entirely. If additional humidity is desired, a jet humidifier may be positioned on the side of the incubator. The amount of

relative humidity desired by different physicians may be quite variable. High humidity supplied by jet humidifiers may be ordered with appropriate aerosol medications.

The nurse may weigh a small infant while he is in an Isolette by suspending him in a muslin hammock attached to a hook, that protrudes through a hole in the incubator roof and is secured to a small scale.

Open, radiantly heated infant warmers

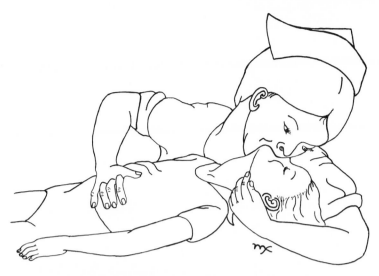

Fig. 29-13. Positioning for mouth-to-mouth resuscitation.

equipped with oxygen hoods, body temperature sensors, and other emergency equipment are now frequently used in addition to enclosed incubators.

STIMULATION AND MAINTENANCE OF RESPIRATORY EFFORT

If respiratory effort is absent or precarious, various methods may be employed to stimulate or maintain respiration. They all presuppose an *adequate airway.*

In the delivery room or nursery if a newborn is not breathing regularly, the nurse often stimulates more effective respirations by rubbing the infant's back, snapping the soles of his feet, or jarring his bed or incubator.

Mouth-to-mouth resuscitation

If respiration has actually ceased, mouth-to-mouth resuscitation is a very practical prompt source of aid, no matter what the setting, since it requires no additional equipment and can be instituted while other methods are being prepared for use. The following is a description of mouth-to-mouth resuscitation:

1. The airway is cleared of any foreign material.
2. The child is positioned on his back with the head in "sniffing" position and the jaw elevated to jut out, clearing the airway of the tongue (Fig. 29-13).
3. The operator places her mouth tightly over the child's mouth and obstructs the child's nose with her cheek. (In the case of infants, both the mouth and nose may be covered by the operator's mouth.)
4. One hand is placed on the child's abdomen to check for distention.
5. Controlled, small puffs of air from the operator's cheeks are blown into the mouth of the infant or young child so that the chest is seen to rise at the rate of 20 times per minute or more.
6. Resuscitation of some kind is continued until the child responds spontaneously or is pronounced dead.
7. *Note:* In the absence of a detectable pulse, the American Heart Association recommends cardiopulmonary resuscitation (CPR) instituted by external cardiac compression (ECC) and artificial ventilation (AV). Patient is placed on firm surface and four quick inflations are given. If one rescuer is present, ECC is performed on infants by depressing midsternum ½ to ¾ inch with two fingers at rate of 80 to 100 per minute. ECC and AV should be

445

alternated in a 15-to-2 ratio. If two rescuers are present, the ratio of ECC to AV is 5 to 1. In case of older child, the heel of one hand is abruptly pushed against the midsternum by the overlying heel of second hand, and force is exerted straight down ¾ to 1 inch toward spine. ECC rate is 60 per minute with same ratio as above. Such emergency resuscitation usually requires two operators. External heart massage is not without danger. However, the danger of injury (broken ribs, traumatized liver) is probably less than the danger of circulatory collapse. It is usually not attempted in cases in which such dramatic efforts would only delay a death that will take place minutes or hours after the treatment is terminated (for example, in a child dying of a malignancy or advanced leukemia).

A nurse should make use of every opportunity to secure practice and instruction regarding resuscitation measures during nonemergency situations. She should know where emergency resuscitation and oxygen-

ation equipment is stored in the area in which she works. This would include knowledge of the location of the following items:

1. Resuscitation apparatus
2. Suction setup
3. Oxygen mask and cylinder
4. Emergency stimulant tray

Ambu resuscitator

A common type of resuscitation apparatus available is the Ambu resuscitator (Fig. 29-14). Use of this resuscitator is much less fatiguing for the operator than mouth-to-mouth resuscitation. The operator may stand or sit behind the supine patient's head with the top of the patient's head stabilized against her body. One hand of the operator holds the mask firmly against the patient's mouth and nose, while tilting the head back and maintaining the forward position of the jaw to clear the airway. With her other hand the operator lightly compresses the air bag in a rhythm of *1, 2, 3, 4, 1, 2, 3, 4*, compressing during the count of 1 and taking her hand completely off the bag for 2, 3, 4. Too rapid, excited compression of the bag will cause greater respiratory dis-

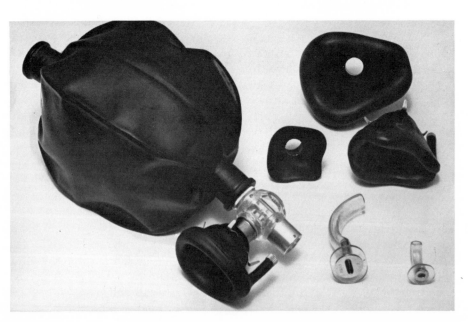

Fig. 29-14. The Ambu resuscitator. Various-sized masks and plastic airways. (Courtesy Children's Health Center, San Diego, Calif.)

tress. The operator should observe the chest rise and allow the patient time to exhale adequately. When the patient makes an effort to breathe spontaneously, the treatment may be discontinued while the patient's respiratory attempts are evaluated.

Positive pressure apparatus

Several positive pressure appliances are available that may, when appropriately "set," sustain respiration artificially for prolonged periods while administering oxygen at predetermined percentages. These various types of intermittent positive pressure machines force air into the lungs through masks and endotracheal or tracheostomy tubes. They may be regulated to automatically cycle at a certain rate and depth of respiration.

Intermittent positive pressure breathing devices are also used periodically on patients to prevent or reduce respiratory complications by expanding the lungs, administering aerosol medication, and helping to thin respiratory secretions. They are especially helpful in the postoperative period. Orders directing their use should include the number of treatments to be given per day, the length of the treatment, the pressure to be used, the oxygen concentration to be employed, and the type and strength of solution to be used in the nebulizer. A face mask or mouthpiece is utilized for this type of therapy.

Although an inhalation therapist usually has the responsibility for these treatments, the nurse should familarize herself with the equipment used in the hospital where she works.

Other devices or techniques used to improve respiratory exchange postoperatively are blow bottles, supervised balloon inflation, or child-powered toy windmills.

Gases other than oxygen

At times gases other than oxygen or compressed air are employed to aid respiration. A patient may breathe briefly in and out with a paper bag over his face, which supplies about a 4% concentration of carbon di-

oxide, or he may be given intermittent breaths of carbogen (an oxygen–carbon dioxide mixture), which helps increase the rate and depth of respiration. Carbon dioxide is a potentially dangerous gas and may elevate respirations and blood pressure seriously. It should be administered only by people who are thoroughly familiar with the equipment and the possible dangers to the patient.

Helium is sometimes used at the bedside in combination with oxygen instead of the normal mixture of nitrogen and oxygen found in air. Such a combination of helium and oxygen is only one third as heavy as air. Use of this combination of gases sometimes eases the respiratory effort necessary for selected patients.

EVALUATION OF RESPIRATORY DIFFICULTIES

If the signals of respiratory distress are unknown, unobserved, or ignored so that proper methods of instituting aid are not begun promptly, the patient will not benefit. A child may be suffering from lack of ventilation, and proper equipment for his aid may be nearby. But unless this aid is given properly, no improvement will result. A nurse should be thoroughly familiar with signs of respiratory difficulty or potential difficulty. Such signs and symptoms of respiratory difficulty may include the following (Fig. 29-15):

1. Depressed or elevated respiratory rate at rest for the age of the child considered (see p. 369 for a pulse and respiration table)
2. Any retractions present
3. Noisy, labored breathing *on inspiration/expiration*
4. Flaring nostrils and the use of facial and neck muscles in attempts to aid respirations
5. Pallor or cyanosis (gray to purple skin coloring) may be localized or generalized and associated with circulatory problems
6. Restlessness, apprehension, and disorientation
7. Inflamed respiratory tree with thick

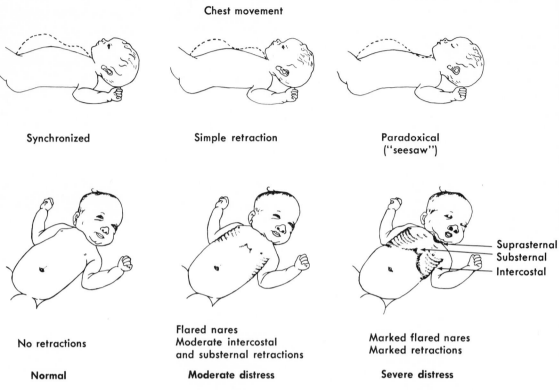

Chest movement

Synchronized

Simple retraction

Paradoxical
("seesaw")

No retractions

Flared nares
Moderate intercostal
and substernal retractions

Marked flared nares
Marked retractions

Suprasternal
Substernal
Intercostal

Normal

Moderate distress

Severe distress

Fig. 29-15. Types of respiration—visible signs of respiratory distress.

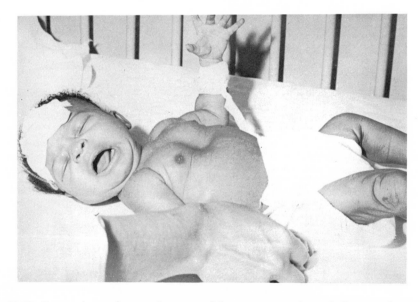

Fig. 29-16. Deep substernal retractions caused by pneumonia (note hollow in chest area). (Courtesy Naval Regional Medical Center, San Diego, Calif.)

nasal discharge and intermittent blockage of the nasal passageways

8. Frequent productive or nonproductive coughing

Note: The absence of coughing is not in itself necessarily a sign of respiratory improvement.

The observation of any of the preceding signs and symptoms deserves prompt report and evaluation. If a child becomes cyanotic and a bedside oxygen unit is available, first make sure that the child's airway is open, then start the oxygen and signal the supervising nurse for assistance and further evaluation of the patient. The pulse rate and respirations should be counted. Many children with circulatory and respiratory problems in which fluid tends to collect in the chest or the abdomen breathe more easily when propped in a semi-Fowler's position or supported in an infant seat (Fig. 29-16).

A breath is such a small thing, but so necessary. One who watches and records respirations is a guardian of life.

30

Traction, casting, and braces

This chapter presents, for initial consideration or review, basic nursing procedures and responsibilities involved in the care of patients receiving therapy in traction, casts, or braces. These patients may be hospitalized for various reasons; fractures, musculoskeletal diseases, and neurological disorders account for most of their diagnoses. For more information regarding specific illnesses in this grouping, the student is referred to Chapter 34, which discusses in greater detail some of these problems and the nursing care they require. However, to avoid needless repetition, the orthopedic nursing entailed in the care of such patients is discussed separately in this section.

TRACTION

Traction, or methods of exerting pull, is discussed first because, at times, it must precede casting. Traction is used for the following reasons:

1. To bring a broken bone back into alignment (reduce a fracture) and provide immobilization for correct union
2. To secure a corrected position to treat a congenital or acquired deformity not involving a fracture (reduce a dislocated hip, scoliosis)
3. To prevent or treat contracture deformities
4. To relieve muscle spasm and pain (back injury)

Basic types

Traction may be exerted manually or by the use of certain appliances. There are two main types of traction—skin and skeletal.

Skin traction

Skin traction helps position the bone indirectly by pulling on the skin and muscles. It is relatively simply to apply and involves no surgical operation. However, only a limited amount of weight may be added with this type of traction, and occasionally the amount of pull possible is not sufficient to produce the desired results. Also, the skin may show signs of irritation—allergic reactions, circulation difficulties, or friction—caused by the supportive wrapping. The attachment of the weight to the skin is usually secured by running strips of adhesive-type material, cotton or perforated plastic-backed adhesive tape, or foam rubber up both sides of the extremity and securing the strips with an Ace bandage. The ends of the strips are then attached to a foot spreader, which, in turn, is connected to the desired weight.

Skeletal traction

Skeletal traction is secured by inserting some mechanical device directly into or through the bone and attaching the prescribed weight. Wires, pins, or tongs may be used to obtain the bone contact. Considerable weight may be attached to such an arrangement, and no bulky or irritating skin wrappings are necessary. Nevertheless, skeletal traction, too, has its drawbacks. Since the bone is actually pierced, there is always danger of infection, and a surgical procedure is involved in both the insertion and the removal of the mechanical attachment. The areas where the holding devices are inserted through the skin must be frequently inspected for signs of inflammation, infection, and drainage.

Nursing considerations

The beginning student often expresses a feeling of perplexity after viewing her first traction patient. Often there seems to be a surplus of weights, ropes, pulleys, and bars, and she wonders how they all fit in to produce a desired result. The mechanical apparatus used may seem quite complex at times, but the basic principles of traction that guide their use are neither numerous nor obscure.

Maintenance of proper traction

The maintenance of proper traction depends on the direction and amount of pull exerted through the use of ropes, pulleys, and weights and the positioning or alignment of the patient. Therefore it is very important that the nurse understand the orders concerning the care of each individual patient in traction and maintain the correct relationship of the various parts of the traction apparatus to the patient. The following points should be noted:

1. Pulleys increase the amount and change the direction of pull on a body part by a weight. A rope should ride properly on a pulley to exert the ordered weight.
2. Weights should not be added or subtracted by the nurse. Too much weight may cause the nonunion of a break; too little weight may cause unwanted overriding and an extremity of unequal length. Weights should always hang freely. They should be frequently observed so that they do not "come to rest" on a rung of the bed, a poorly placed chair, or the floor.
3. The amount of time that traction is to be applied should be clearly understood. Skin traction may occasionally be removed (but such removal is always dependent on the physician's order). Skeletal traction is usually continuous at all times.
4. Ropes should be in good condition and frequently inspected for signs of wear. Knots should be taped for additional safety. Multiple weights attached to the same rope should be taped together so that they cannot easily fall or be removed. Some pediatric-orthopedic areas place the foot of the beds over which weights hang next to the wall to discourage tampering by the small fingers of ambulatory patients.

Countertraction

Pull in one direction must be balanced by pull in the opposite direction for traction to remain effective. This opposing pull is called *countertraction.*

Countertraction may be exerted in various ways. If the weights used to create the initial pull are not extremely heavy, it may only be necessary to keep the patient in a certain placement in bed, checking periodically to see that he has not slipped past the desired place. The patient's body provides the countertraction. The friction of the patient's body against the bedding may also help prevent him from slipping out of position.

If the pull is stronger, the end of the bed where the initial traction is applied may need to be elevated to allow gravity to increase the countertraction created by the patient's body weight. Elevation may be achieved through the use of grooved blocks under two legs of the bed or a mechanical bed lift.

If it is very difficult to maintain the child in proper position in bed, sometimes some types of restraint may be used (a restraining jacket or waist restraint). However, the use of such devices may cause other problems—pressure areas, hypostatic pneumonia, and constipation. The use of restraints must be carefully evaluated.

Sometimes the body part being treated is placed in a type of frame or splint that is lifted off the surface of the bed. When this arrangement is used, a counterweight may often be connected to this frame, exerting force in the opposing direction.

In review, countertraction may be created in four basic ways:

1. Maintenance of body placement in

bed by constant observation and correction, if needed

2. Elevation of the part of the bed next to the weights
3. Use of restraints
4. Application of a counterweight

The method employed depends on the desires of the physician and the responses of the patient. Failure to maintain correct placement in bed while the patient is in traction may (1) cause the weights, which are supposed to create initial pull, to rest on the floor or some other surface and temporarily stop traction altogether, in some cases allowing possible displacement or (2) change the angle of pull and distort the result desired.

Both situations are potentially harmful. When a nurse is told "Keep Susie's hips at the level of the tape markers on the bed," or "Be sure that Roger is kept pulled up in bed," the staff is trying to avoid the situations just described.

Activity and body position

The amount of movement and activity allowed the patient in traction should be understood and promoted, and good body alignment and support should be maintained. Bed boards may be placed under the mattress to prevent sagging.

Some patients are allowed relatively little movement or position change because of their individual musculoskeletal problems or traction arrangements. If the nurse allows these patients to sit up or turn on their sides, the traction may be lost or altered so that no treatment or, perhaps, even real damage may result. A patient who has a leg in a Thomas splint support raised off the surface of the mattress is allowed considerable movement because such a traction maintains proper alignment when the patient's trunk is raised. Even a slight amount of turning toward the splinted leg is usually possible. Such an arrangement is termed "balanced traction." When balanced traction is used in conjunction with an overhead bar and trapeze, the patient enjoys considerably more activity, and

nursing care is greatly simplified (see Fig. 30-9).

Although it is important that the patient not be moved in a way that will disrupt his traction, it is also important that he be moved to the extent permitted to encourage proper body function, elimination, respiration, and circulation and to avoid pressure areas. Exercise and correct positioning of the uninvolved extremities are very necessary to prevent other problems (stiffness or deformity) from occurring in some patients. As in all cases of prolonged immobilization, a high fluid intake should be encouraged. A diet well supplied with roughage and natural laxatives, such as prunes, helps avoid constipation. Special attention should be given to the prevention of foot drop or undesired internal or external rotation of the lower extremities.

Circulation and skin condition

The circulation and skin condition of a patient in traction or other immobilization devices such as casts should be frequently evaluated.

The skin of any patient who is bedfast for long periods with only limited movement permitted must be meticulously observed and protected. Pressure areas are most likely to develop over bony prominences such as the hips, sacrum, ankles, elbows, scapulae, and shoulders. Areas exposed to continuous friction are also likely spots for skin breakdown. If a Thomas splint is being utilized, the skin area under the padded ring must be frequently inspected. The heels of both the affected and nonaffected leg should be carefully observed. Often the foot that is not being treated may develop a sore heel because the patient helps himself move up in bed by digging his good heel into the mattress to obtain leverage. To prevent unnecessary pressures, the bed linen must be kept smooth and tight, and crumbs and other irritating small objects must be eliminated from the bed. Skin traction wrappings may cause circulation and nerve interference similar to that occasionally encountered with the casted patient. Inability to dorsi-flex the exposed big toe of a wrapped af-fected lower extremity should be reported to the physician promptly.

Pressure areas are much easier to prevent than to treat. Frequent inspection, cleans-ing, and massage of susceptible areas and encouragement of as much movement as is allowed and consistent with the patient's well-being will greatly reduce, if not en-tirely eliminate, pressure areas. Every com-plaint of skin tenderness, a burning sensa-tion, or aching should be investigated. It does not take long for a small red area to become an enlarged open sore, particularly in areas where circulation may be already impaired. Any devices that lift a pressure area off a surface must be used with cau-tion and frequently evaluated, since they may sometimes cause circulatory distur-bances themselves. Patients who are para-lyzed or suffer from sensory loss must re-ceive special care and observation. A child in traction should routinely receive back and skin care during his bath and at least twice more during the day shift. The use of an overhead bar and trapeze can greatly facilitate back and skin care when such aids are feasible. If no such arrangement is pos-sible, a nurse may press down on the mat-tress with one hand to allow her other hand to massage, or two nurses may work together to lift the child *slightly* to facili-tate skin care, depending on the type of traction used.

Sometimes the use of imitation or genu-ine lamb's-wool mats under the patient is helpful. Tincture of benzoin applications on closed areas of pressure or potential pressure are sometimes prescribed. The benzoin serves to toughen the areas but may stain the sheets.

Bedmaking

Some hospitals are supplied with special traction linen designed to fit under or around different traction appliances such as the Thomas splint. A special "split" top sheet may be available to use on either side of the splint. More commonly, a large sheet

is simply pulled to one side over the good leg and a light baby blanket draped over the splinted leg at night. Another satisfac-tory and modest arrangement uses two blankets, each contained within a separate folded sheet. One such blanket-sheet com-bination is placed over the chest and ab-domen of the patient, with open edges under the chin; the other is placed on top of the good leg and below the suspended leg, with open edges toward the foot of the bed where they are tucked in. The upper and lower blanket-sheet combinations are then pinned together around the thigh of the leg in traction. This makes a very neat bed. Traction patients may have special snap-on pajamas (tops and bottoms) to fa-cilitate dressing, or perineal drapes or G-strings may be used.

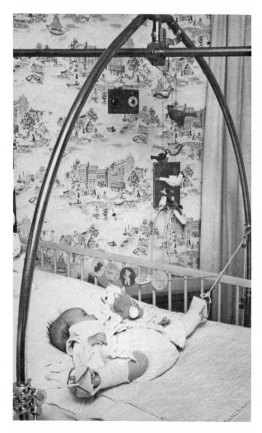

Fig. 30-1. This baby is almost ready for a hip spica cast. Frequent back care is essential. (Cour-tesy Children's Health Center, San Diego, Calif.)

Types of traction equipment

Traction equipment may be quite varied, depending on the individual needs of the patient.

Progressive abduction traction

Figs. 30-1 and 30-2 show types of traction used to achieve progressive reduction of congenital dislocation of the hips. Fig. 30-1 shows an infant who is almost ready for casting. When this child was first placed in skin traction, her legs were suspended at right angles to the bed. Gradually her legs have been abducted until they are almost flat on the bed. When her legs are properly abducted, she will be placed in a plaster cast for further treatment. Such a patient must be carefully observed for developing circulation problems because the leg wrappings may interfere with blood flow. Swollen, cool, or "blotchy" looking toes, slow blanching on pressure, or delayed return of skin color after pressure is released from a toenail bed are all signs that should be promptly reported. The pulse at the ankle may also be checked to detect circulatory problems. This type of patient should be raised slightly during feedings to prevent aspiration. The jacket restraint may be loosened or removed if a responsible party is *at* the bedside, but it should be in place when the child is alone. To make the bed, one nurse may lift the baby's body just enough to allow another nurse to slide the bed sheets under his hips and back. The weights should not be removed. Frequent back care and diaper changes are a necessity.

Fig. 30-2 shows another traction device

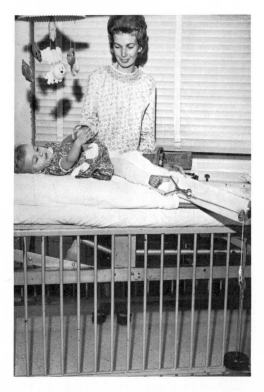

Fig. 30-2. A-frame traction, or a Putti board. Mother stays as much as she can to cheer her toddler. (Courtesy Children's Health Center, San Diego, Calif.)

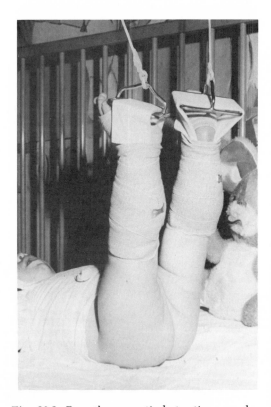

Fig. 30-3. Bryant's, or vertical, traction may be used for infants or young children weighing less than 25 pounds. The pelvis is no longer lifted above the mattress by the traction, since this has been found to be associated with circulatory problems in the legs. (Courtesy Children's Health Center, San Diego, Calif.)

used to treat dislocation of the hip by progressive abduction. It is known as an A-frame, or Putti board. The angle of a padded wedge is progressively widened to produce increased abduction. This type of traction is advantageous because the child may be placed in either prone or supine position and, depending on his physician's orders and the setup, may be carefully turned. Turning helps prevent respiratory problems and pressure areas and encourages appetite.

Bryant's traction

Bryant's traction is often used for the treatment of fractured legs in young children (Fig. 30-3). Nursing care of the child in Bryant's traction is similar to that described for children in the traction pictured in Fig. 30-1.

Russell's traction

Russell's traction, a skin traction using a sling and single rope arrangement attached to one weight supported by multiple pulleys, is used to treat fractures in older children (Fig. 30-4). Because the extremity is suspended, more patient movement is allowed, and nursing care is considerably easier.

Buck's extension

A rather simple, frequently used skin traction for treatment of the lower extremities or lower back is called Buck's extension (Fig. 30-5). Note the adhesive strips on the sides, the elastic bandage wrapping, the foot spreader (to prevent pressure of the adhesive strips against the ankle), the pulley, and rope leading to the freely hanging weight. Some physicians order a small

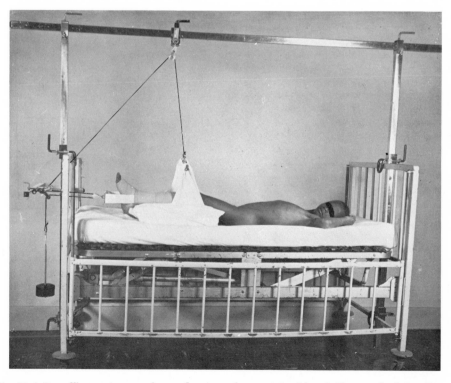

Fig. 30-4. Russell's traction may be used to treat fractures in older children and adults. (From Shands, A. R., and Raney, R. B.: Handbook of orthopaedic surgery, ed. 7, St. Louis, 1967, The C. V. Mosby Co.)

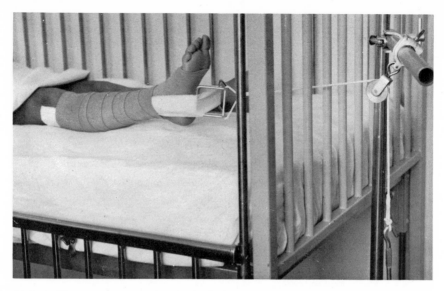

Fig. 30-5. Buck's extension. Note that the heel clears the mattress. Some physicians use a small flat pillow under the leg to provide clearance. (Courtesy Children's Health Center, San Diego, Calif.)

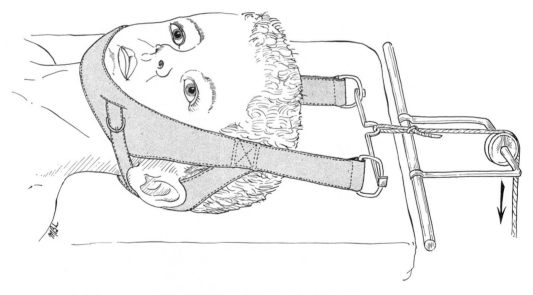

Fig. 30-6. Cervical skin traction with halter.

flattened pillow under the leg just above the Achilles tendon to protect the heel from pressure. In this picture the angle of pull elevates the heel slightly off the bed.

Cervical traction

The patient in cervical traction may have a sling or halter arrangement around the chin and occiput (Fig. 30-6), or he may be placed in skeletal traction, which involves the placement of some type of tongs into (but not through!) the cranium (Fig. 30-7). Orders regarding the placement of the patient, the movement allowed, and whether any elevation of the backrest is permitted should be clearly understood. Patients in skeletal-cervical traction are often positioned in slight hyperextension,

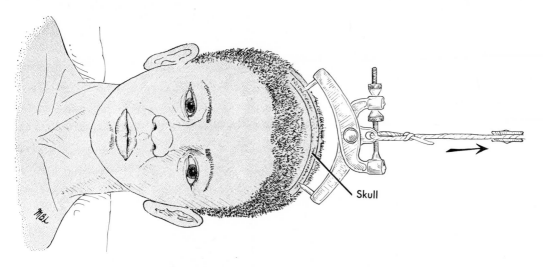

Fig. 30-7. Crutchfield tongs, cervical-skeletal traction.

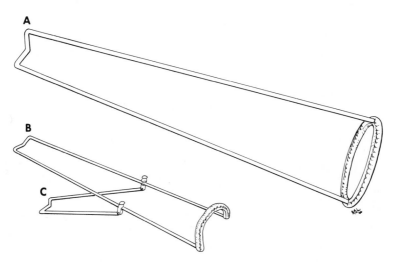

Fig. 30-8. A, Thomas splint with complete ring; *B*, half-ring Thomas splint; *C*, Pearson attachment.

and flexion of the cervical spine is not permitted. If cervical skin traction is used, foam rubber padding may be necessary in the chin area to prevent skin irritation. Gum-chewing may help relieve aching jaw joints.

Pelvic traction

Occasionally pelvic traction may be ordered to relieve lower back pain. Pelvic traction is exerted by use of a pelvic band or girdle attached to a weight or weights. Sometimes a thoracic belt may be used for countertraction. Such an arrangement is designed to relieve muscle spasm and lessen pressure on nerve roots. Pelvic traction may be ordered continuously or intermittently. Many patients are given bathroom privileges.

Balanced traction

As previously mentioned, *balanced traction,* involving the suspension of the affected limb above the surface of the bed, provides the opportunity for more movement or activity on the part of the patient. The patient may raise his hips, have his backrest elevated, or turn slightly toward the side of his splinted lower extremity. An overhead bar and trapeze greatly facilitates lifting. The suspension device takes up the slack created and maintains the line of traction. It is well to remember that, no matter how much these patients want to stay up, they should intermittently rest flat, without the elevation of the backrest, to prevent hip contractures.

Although suspended traction gives

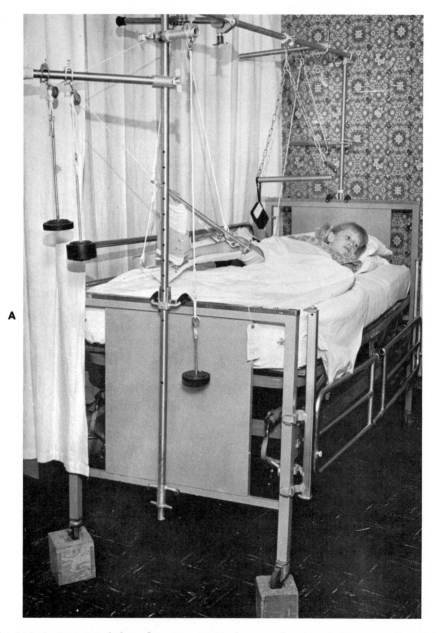

Fig. 30-9. **A,** Patient in balanced traction. **B,** Explanatory drawing. **C,** Close-up view of leg. (Courtesy Children's Health Center, San Diego, Calif.)

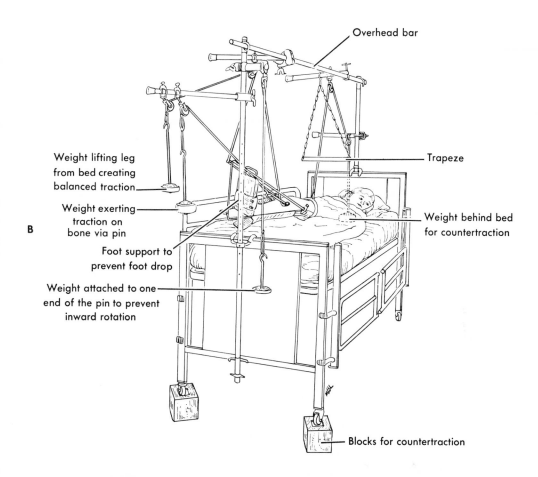

Overhead bar

Weight lifting leg from bed creating balanced traction

Weight exerting traction on bone via pin

B

Foot support to prevent foot drop

Weight attached to one end of the pin to prevent inward rotation

Trapeze

Weight behind bed for countertraction

Blocks for countertraction

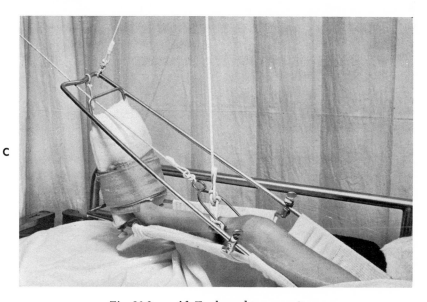

C

Fig. 30-9, cont'd. For legend see opposite page.

greater liberty of movement and effectively relieves heel pressure, the area where the ring of the Thomas splint rests must be frequently inspected for the development of skin problems. Each day the skin may be gently pulled up or down from under the ring and washed, dried, and massaged. The ring itself may be polished with saddle soap. Fig. 30-8 shows a Thomas splint with a complete ring and a Thomas half-ring splint with a Pearson attachment, which is used to actually support the extremity. Fig. 30-9 shows a young girl with a balanced skeletal traction, including an extra support to prevent foot drop and an additional weight to correct a tendency toward pronounced internal rotation of the leg. Not long after this photograph was taken the girl was sent home in a long leg plaster cast.

CASTS

Casts are often applied subsequent to treatment by traction, supplying a form of external immobilization of a body part. Occasionally, a cast may be applied over a skeletal pin, thus helping to continue traction as well as contributing to immobilization. Such a procedure may be called plaster traction. The ends of the protruding pins should be covered with plaster or some sort of protective device to avoid the snagging of clothing or bed coverings or injury to others. Plaster traction allows greater mobility for the patient (when feasible). In addition to immobilization and possible traction, casts may also be a means of aiding proper positioning or resting a body part.

The most common kind of cast consists of plaster-of-Paris–impregnated crinoline bandages that have been applied and molded while moist over some type of soft, protective layer and allowed to dry to a hard, resistant shell. Dry plaster of Paris is a form of calcium sulfate; when mixed with water, it forms the substance known as gypsum. Plastic materials have also occasionally been used to form casts. These are dur-

able, lightweight, and waterproof, but more expensive.

Application of the cast

Because of the "orderly disorder" that invariably accompanies plaster applications, it is preferable to schedule cast work in a room especially designed for such procedures—a room that is easily cleaned and contains all the equipment and supplies usually needed.

Commonly needed supplies are as follows:

1. Materials that protect the skin, to be wrapped around the body part before application of the harsh plaster
   a. Sheet wadding (Webril)
   b. Tubular stockinette
2. Various widths of plaster-of-Paris bandages and strips (splints)
3. Materials to reinforce or protect areas of the cast or body that are under special pressure or strain
   a. Felt
   b. Yucca board
   c. Wire netting
   d. Rubber heels (for leg casts of ambulatory patients)
4. Special tools
   a. Various types of cast knives
   b. Plaster shears
   c. Cast spreaders and cast benders
   d. Manual and electrical cast cutters
   e. A bucket for tepid water to moisten the plaster
5. Other possible needs
   a. Sterile and nonsterile cover gowns
   b. Gloves, caps, and masks

The furnishings of a cast room need not be elaborate. Usually, an examining table, some benches, good lighting, an x-ray view box, and a sink are sufficient. A sink with a plaster trap is convenient because water used to soak the plaster-of-Paris rolls may be discarded into the drain without too much danger of plugging the plumbing. If large body casts or scoliosis jackets are applied, additional supportive frames, tables, or slings will be needed. Newspapers placed on the floor under the working area will aid cleanup.

Preparation of the patient

Some patients undergoing casting procedures are anesthetized to aid muscle relaxation, relieve pain, and facilitate the entire procedure. Patients who have open reductions of fractures or other operative procedures just prior to casting are, of course, always anesthetized. Small children are many times anesthetized for closed reduction procedures. Such patients are given nothing by mouth for several hours before the procedure and usually receive preoperative sedation. If a flammable general anesthetic is used, all precautions against explosions should be taken. The staff must be dressed appropriately and all equipment properly grounded. Even if the use of anesthetics is not contemplated and a closed manipulation prior to casting is the only maneuver scheduled, a preoperative analgesic drug may be ordered and oral feedings temporarily withheld.

Duties of the nurse

The nurse helping the physician in the cast room is responsible for making available all the necessary equipment and supplies. She may also help by preparing the plaster rolls for use. The desired width of plaster-of-Paris bandage is removed from its waxed paper wrapper and immersed on end in water (approximately 105° F.). When air bubbles no longer rise from the roll, the bandage should be lifted from the water. The sides of the closed bandage may be gently squeezed to help remove water and retain plaster. The loose end of the bandage is unrolled slightly, and the roll and its end are handed to the physician for application. The bandage should not be dripping at the time of the transfer. The nurse may also assist by helping to hold the extremity being casted. She may be asked to support part of the newly formed cast. If she does, she should remember to use only the palms of her hands in rendering such support to prevent the formation of pressure areas.

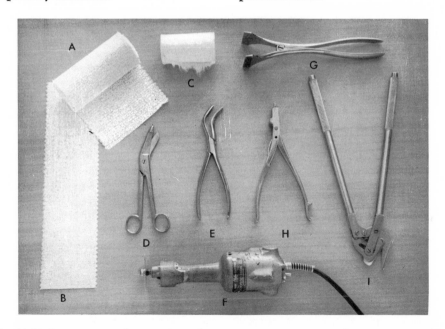

Fig. 30-10. Instruments and materials used in preparing or removing plaster casts. *A*, Plaster roll; *B*, plaster splint; *C*, Webril (sheet wadding); *D*, plaster shears (large bandage scissors); *E*, cast bender; *F*, cast cutter or saw (electrical); *G* and *H*, cast spreaders; *I*, cast cutter (manual). (Courtesy Children's Health Center, San Diego, Calif.)

Cast changes and removal
(Fig. 30-10)

Sometimes a patient must have one cast removed and another applied. The frequency with which a child must have his cast changed depends on his rate of growth, the condition of the cast, and the progress of the desired correction. The cast may be cut manually with a cast knife, which may be shaped like a short kitchen paring knife, and a hand cast cutter. The cut is made along a predetermined line, which may have been dampened by a vinegar solution, hydrogen peroxide, or water from a syringe. A metal strip may be inserted just below the cutting line to protect the body part. An electrical vibrating-blade cast cutter may be used instead. The electrical saw makes a great deal of noise, which sometimes frightens the patient. When the cast has been carefully cut, the sections are separated by a cast spreader, and the padding underneath is released with large bandage scissors. The body part that has had the support of the cast must be gently supported and handled and not forced into new, unfamiliar positions. Sudden lack of support or movement will often cause considerable pain and distress.

Professional opinion differs regarding the care of the skin of a patient who has been in a cast for a considerable time and will almost immediately be enclosed in a cast again. Some physicians want their patients to have baths; others believe that the least amount of handling possible is the best choice. All wish to avoid trauma to the skin, which would lead to trouble during the subsequent period of casting. If the use of a cast will be discontinued permanently or for a considerable time, the physician may order a combination of gentle baths and the application of baby oil to help loosen the crust of old skin and sebaceous material that has collected on the surface of the body part that was under the cast. With patience and time this crust may be removed with no injury to the underlying epidermis.

Care of the newly casted patient and his cast

A newly casted patient may complain of the heat generated by the plaster as it undergoes its physical reaction with the water. This heat of crystallization is transitory; however, in the case of body casts it may cause considerable annoyance. Newly applied casts are soft, damp, and grayish white and have a slightly musty smell. They must be handled carefully.

Transfer of the patient

When transferring a newly casted patient, lift the cast with the palms of the hands, do not grasp it by the fingers. Finger pressure may cause indentations, tissue injury, and disturbances in circulation. If the patient is in a body cast covering the trunk or hips and legs (hip spica), many hands may be necessary to make an efficient, smooth transfer from cart to bed.

Preparation of the unit

The unit of a patient who is having a new body cast applied requires special preparation. Bed boards should be placed under the mattress to prevent sagging. Numerous plastic-covered firm pillows should be available to support the contours of the soft cast.

If the child is old enough and able to benefit, an overhead bar and trapeze should be attached to the bed. The room should be well ventilated to assist in the drying of the cast. Occasionally special cast driers may be available or an undraped heat cradle may be utilized to help speed drying. A new cast should be exposed to the air. However, for modesty's sake a G-string or diaper may be positioned over the perineal area. A fracture pan should be available in the bedside stand. In many hospitals infants and small children in body casts are measured for so-called "cast boards," which hold the child at a slight incline, elevated from the bed mattress (Fig. 30-11). A bedpan is kept positioned under the child at all times, and plastic strips, which are tucked into the perineal

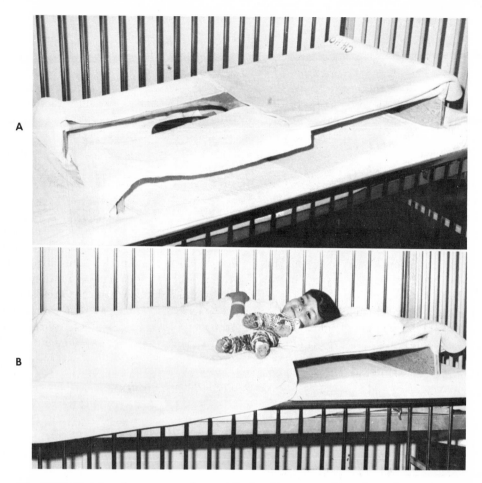

Fig. 30-11. Cast board, premeasured especially for this patient. Note the incline and the positioned bedpan. (Courtesy Children's Health Center, San Diego, Calif.)

area of the cast, guide waste material into the pan below. Very young children who are incontinent may be "taped" with some type of waterproof material as for a urine specimen until the cast is dry enough to be protected against accidental soiling.

In cases of newly casted extremities often all that is necessary for the nurse to have ready in the patient's unit is a supply of firm, waterproof pillows to aid in the elevation of the body part to help prevent swelling. Sometimes elevation is best maintained through the use of a Gatch bed or the placement of pillows under the end of the mattress. The cast, again, should be left exposed to the air to facilitate drying. Most casts dry in approximately 24 hours.

Care of the cast

When the cast is dry, as indicated by a chalky white finish and a hard, nonmoist surface, it should be protected against accidental wetting in the perineal region. This may be done in several ways. Various types of plastic material may be cut to fit under the perineal edge of the cast and to protect the curved band of the cast just adjacent. It may be held in place by pieces of water-repellent adhesive tape. Some pediatric departments use a plastic adhesive tape, which may be cut into wedge-shaped pieces and positioned around and under the perineal rim and on the outer surface (Fig. 30-12). Regardless of the method selected to protect the cast, the waterproof

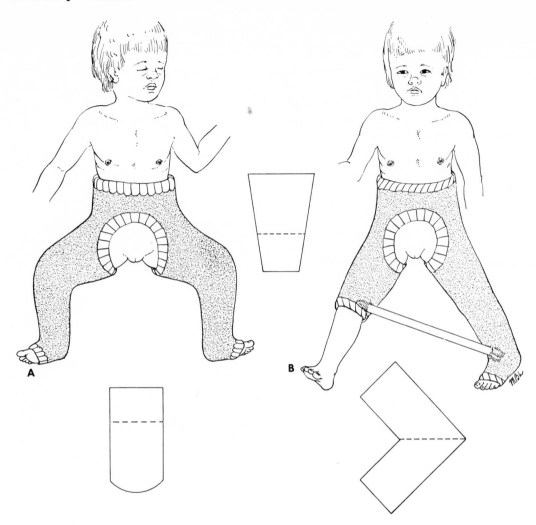

Fig. 30-12. Different types of petalling. **A,** Bilateral hip spica cast. **B,** Unilateral hip spica cast with an abductor bar.

material should not be applied until the cast is dry because the cast may become moldy. In many such cases the strips do not adhere anyway, and all the time spent in applying the plastic is time lost! When the cast is dry, all rough or potentially rough edges of the cast should be covered. This process is called "petalling" because the pieces of adhesive tape first used for this purpose were cut in the shape of flower petals. However, nurses today may use adhesive tape cut like chevrons, circles, or wedges as well as the traditional "petal" to protect cast edges (Fig. 30-12). Petalling keeps small bits of plaster from the cast

edges from falling into the cast, helps prevent skin irritation around the cast, and usually improves the overall appearance of the cast. If tubular stockinette is applied before the plaster bandage during the construction of the cast, it may be neatly trimmed and brought up over the cast edge and secured with adhesive or plaster splints to make a smooth, attractive edging when the cast is dry.

Various methods have been employed to enhance the appearance of a cast and help protect it from damage and soil. Some physicians finish a cast by dusting on plaster powder and rubbing it in. Some apply shellac, varnish, or plastic spray to a dry cast to increase its longevity and help keep it clean. It is best not to get a cast dirty or stained in the first place, but if it does become soiled, the nurse may clean the area with a damp, not wet, cloth and a small amount of white cleanser (such as Bon Ami) or fast-drying white shoe polish. Some dry, dirty areas may be covered by adhesive tape or additional plaster-of-Paris strips. Children should be cautioned against getting their casts damp. Swimming is definitely out!

The preceding paragraphs have been concerned primarily with the cast itself; however, the most important consideration in orthopedic care is not the cast but the patient it encloses. Casts are a great help in correcting various musculoskeletal problems, but they may also cause or accentuate problems. The casted patient must be carefully observed to detect the development of any of these difficulties.

Observation for circulatory complications

A newly casted extremity may suffer impaired circulation. Sometimes circulatory problems compound themselves. Because of injury, operative procedure, or a tight cast application, there may be swelling under the cast. The increasingly tight cast impedes circulation further, and tissue damage may take place. There are certain signs and symptoms of abnormal pressure and swelling that should be reported long before significant tissue damage occurs. They should be sought frequently after casting and periodically thereafter. They include the following:

1. Swelling of the toes or fingers
2. Cold toes or fingers (they should be pink and warm)
3. Pale, cyanotic, or mottled toes or fingers or an absent or delayed blanching sign (Pressure is made on the nail beds to blanch the area. When the pressure is removed, the normal nail color should return immediately. If the area does not blanch, this is also significant because it indicates local congestion and lack of good circulation.)
4. Inability to find a pulse in an extremity (when the area to be palpated is accessible)
5. Inability to move exposed toes or fingers
6. Complaints of the following:
   a. Tingling
   b. Numbness
   c. Burning sensation
   d. Pain
   (Of course, very small children are unable to verbalize these subjective symptoms. They are watched for "fussiness.")
7. Excessive bleeding after surgery, as estimated by bloody drainage seeping through the cast layers (This is rather difficult to evaluate. One should consider the type of surgical procedure involved. Physicians seem to differ in opinion concerning the advisability of circling with pencil the drainage stains on a cast and marking them with the time noted. One orthopedist was heard to say that he thought that such a practice alarmed patients unduly. Perhaps the nurse could make a few guide dots instead of the more obvious circle and mark the time in her written notes if she thought the amount of seepage needed closer observation.)

When possible, the corresponding unaffected extremity should be compared with the casted arm or leg. Some people have cold hands most of the time, with or without casts! Any complaint of a burning sensation or pain should be promptly reported and investigated. Considerable damage may occur in a relatively short period. If such complaints are neglected, the body part may become numb and no additional complaints may be heard for some time, until tissue damage is significant.

A casted extremity that is swelling must be relieved soon. In a hospital situation it would be rare not to be able to call a physician who could take appropriate measures to relieve the pressure. A nurse should not hesitate to call a physician if circulation is impaired even though the hour may be inconvenient. In the unusual situation in which no physician can be contacted, the nurse should be prepared to cut the cast herself. Certainly such a situation would be extraordinary, but if no help will be available for a considerable period, it is better to have a damaged cast than a gangrenous extremity. The usual emergency procedure involves cutting the cast in half and forming an upper and lower or anterior and posterior shell. The inner wrappings should also be cut, since they may cause considerable pressure. The extremity may be maintained in the shell with the halves held opposite one another by elastic bandage. Such a cast is said to be *bivalved*. Occasionally physicians intentionally plan to bivalve casts; such casts provide support but also allow some movement and exposure and facilitate the skin care of an area. Bivalved casts are occasionally used as splints in conjunction with elastic bandage.

Even when the cast is dry and relatively old, the daily care of the patient in a body cast or a hip spica cast should continue to include observation for disturbance in circulation and possible areas of pressure and skin breakdown. The skin next to the cast edges must be carefully inspected and massaged. Alcohol or lotion may be used. The heel and heel cord and the perineum should be especially watched for signs of irritation.

Turning the patient

The patient in a dry body cast is routinely turned at least every 2 to 3 hours in an attempt to prevent pressure sores and promote respiration and elimination. The number of people needed to turn a patient in a body cast depends on the size and general condition of the patient and the age of his cast. Remember the following when turning a patient in a large body cast:

1. If there is a choice, plan to turn the patient toward the nonoperative side.
2. Before turning the patient, pull or lift him to the side of the bed, placing his "turning side" toward the center of the bed. Have the patient lift his hands above his head or, if this is not feasible, have them held against his sides with a towel or diaper placed between the hands and the cast just before turning to prevent injury. Do *not* use the abductor bar to turn the patient. It is held in place with only a few turns of plaster bandage. It helps support the cast, but it is not a handle.
3. If possible, place the protective pillows needed under the cast in the new position before the patient is turned.
   a. If the patient is placed *on his abdomen,* a flat pillow just below the chest area sometimes helps chest expansion and respiration. A small pillow for the head increases comfort. Legs need to be supported to prevent the toes from digging into the bedding and the problem of foot drop. Curved up-and-down contours of the cast also should be protected from strain. The abdominal position is preferred for older children at mealtime to aid in swallowing and self-help.
   b. If the patient is placed *on his back,* a small pillow is needed under his head. Curved up-and-down contours of the cast should be protected from strain and the heels lifted from the pressure of the mattress.
   c. When positioning the patient, be sure that the edges of the cast do not press against the skin. The patient should be made as comfortable as possible.
   d. A young child who is not continent and does not have a cast board may be placed on a sort of horseshoe-shaped pillow arrangement, and a small bedpan or large kid-

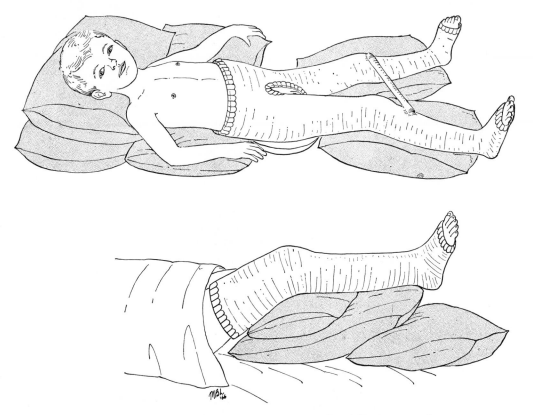

Fig. 30-13. Methods of using pillows to support a cast. The child shown at the top is on a bedpan.

ney-shaped basin may be positioned under the patient with a plastic strip tucked under the cast leading to the pan or basin (Fig. 30-13). Such a pillow support should elevate the child on a slight incline, the head higher than the feet, to prevent urine backflow into the cast.

Safety factors

Children in casts of any type must be carefully observed and taught not to put *anything* down into the cast. Small objects, such as crayons and bobby pins, can cause pressure areas, pain, infection, and a delay in recuperation. The nurse must also be vigilant regarding the use of so-called scratchers, employed to relieve itching. If scratchers are allowed at all, they must be relatively soft, such as a strip of gauze that has

been strategically placed before the cast application is begun. Bent coat hangers and even pipe cleaners may cause excoriation, and we do not recommend them for such purposes. Gently blowing air from a syringe under the rim of the cast may be soothing at times. One must be sure that the child is not scratching a healing surgical incision.

General nursing considerations

Bathing. Parts of the body that might be overlooked during the daily bath are the fingers and the areas between the toes. Plaster crumbs may collect between the digits and cause pressure areas. Cotton-tipped applicators dipped in baby oil help clean these areas satisfactorily. Fingernails and toenails should be kept trimmed and neat.

Diet and fluids. The child who is immo-

467

bilized not only needs meticulous skin care but also special attention to his diet and fluid intake to promote healing and avoid constipation and urinary stasis. A liberal fluid intake should be maintained, and a high-protein diet is often encouraged. At times prune juice or some mild laxative may be indicated to avoid a less agreeable enema.

Support of a casted extremity. When a child with a casted extremity is allowed to be up in a chair, the cast should be elevated and not allowed to become dependent. The physician may order that a casted arm be supported in a sling. There are several types of slings available. The classic sling is formed from a triangular bandage. The fingers are exposed but the wrist is supported and the hand is higher than the elbow. The knot should not rest over the cervical spine; this is uncomfortable and may cause a pressure area. Fig. 30-14 shows a commercially prepared hammock-type sling. It is available in several sizes.

When local swelling of an extremity is present, some physicians order that the arm be elevated with pillows. If such elevation is to be effective, the child's wrist must be higher than his elbow and his elbow must be higher than his shoulder. Occasionally, an extremity may be suspended from a sling attached to an overhead bar or an intravenous standard.

Diversion and intellectual stimulation. A person may be clean, free from pain, on the mend physically, but not particularly happy. The nurse who is interested in the total patient, not just the body in the cast, should help provide proper diversion, intellectual stimulation, and interpersonal contacts for her patients. This is a time when older children can develop constructive hobbies and lasting interests.

Discharge. Of course, many of the casted patients do not remain in the hospital very long. Often, the cast is applied, dried, protected, and petalled, and the patient's discharge is written within 48 hours or less. The family must be instructed in detail

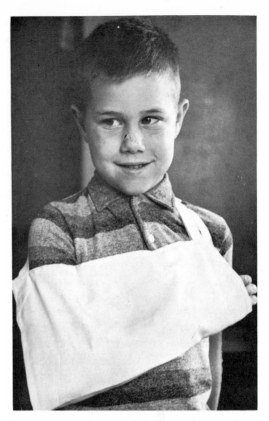

Fig. 30-14. A commercial hammock-type sling. Note that the arm enters the sling from the top, not from the side.

concerning skin care, observation for circulatory problems, cast protection, and cleansing if they are not already familiar with cast care. Appropriate transportation must be arranged. Patients in long leg casts or hip spica casts cannot be comfortably placed in all automobiles!

BRACES

A removable, external support used to maintain position or provide strength to a body part is called a brace. A brace may be made of numerous kinds of material but characteristically is constructed of metal, leather, felt, and lacings. Braces are expensive pieces of equipment. They are individually fitted and produced, and they demand the respect of both patient and nurse. Braces furnish support by exerting pressure on at least three points of the body. There are many different types of braces. The Milwaukee brace for the treatment of scoliosis is one example of a body brace. There are short, below-the-knee braces for ankle or foot support or full-length leg braces for both knee and ankle stabilization. Some patients (cerebral palsy victims) must have combined body and long leg braces because of extensive residual muscle paralysis. Many braces include movable joints, which may be locked with various mechanisms to provide greater stability for weight bearing.

Maintenance of the brace

The routine care of a brace includes protecting it from rust, carefully cleaning and oiling any hinges with a fine-grade oil, and removing any excess oil to prevent staining of leather supports or clothing. It also includes the care of any leather parts by the periodic application of saddle soap, followed by polishing or cleaning with fluids such as benzene. Cleaning fluids may also be used on felt pads. Laces should be maintained intact and free from pressure-causing knots. Shoes incorporated in any leg brace should be frequently inspected for abnormal wear. Any missing part (such as felt kneepads or screws) should be promptly reported because the loss may seriously jeopardize the ability of the brace to fulfill its purpose.

Nursing responsibilities

The nurse and patient should be familiar with the purpose of each brace, the way in which it should be applied and positioned, when it should be worn, the length of time it should be worn, and its mechanism and maintenance. Patients wearing braces should be frequently inspected for bruises and pressure areas. Trial periods should be gradually lengthened (see p. 351). Those wearing leg braces should have well-fitted, "no-hole" stockings. A body brace is usually worn over a cotton shirt. It should be applied with the patient lying flat in bed. Back braces are buckled or laced from the bottom up. They are then adjusted as necessary with the patient in standing position.

The use of braces enables many patients who would otherwise be confined to bed or wheelchair to maintain locomotion and varied activity. Sometimes braces may be ungainly, heavy, and uncomfortable, but they are often a blessing in disguise.

CRUTCHES

Often, a patient is required to use crutches, with or without braces, to be ambulatory. The physical therapist is usually responsible for teaching crutch walking and the particular gait best suited to the individual patient. However, the nurse may be asked to measure the patient for crutches and assist him in developing good habits involving their use.

One method of measuring patients in supine positions for standard-type crutches is to measure the distance from the patient's axilla to a point 4 to 8 inches out from the patient's heel as he extends and adducts his legs. Ideally, he will be wearing the shoes that he will be using while walking. Another method advocated involves subtracting 16 inches from the patient's height. Crutch length will depend also on the condition of the patient and the gait selected.

The nurse should be sure that the rubber guards on the crutch ends are not worn smooth. The patient should not lean on the "armpit rests." The weight of the body should be borne by the hands. It is easier for a patient using crutches to rise from a firm, rather than an overstuffed, chair. When walking with a patient who is learning to use crutches, the nurse should walk behind her patient. In case of difficulty she may grasp the patient by his belt, trousers, or waist.

• • •

Orthopedic nursing can be extremely satisfying. It may take much skill, patience, determination, and time to achieve a straightened back and a corrected foot, but they are well worth all the effort involved.

31

Methods of temperature control and therapeutic uses of heat and cold

The regulation of body heat and the effects of localized temperature change on body parts are significant considerations in the medical and nursing care of many patients. The regulation of body temperature through the use of therapy may not only bring greater comfort to the patient but may also avoid complications that occur in the presence of high fever or abnormal loss of body heat.

Occasionally extremes of body temperature have been induced for therapeutic reasons. Local hot and cold applications are commonly used for treatment. Both the regulation of general body temperature and local reactions to temperature extremes will be discussed in the following paragraphs.

BODY TEMPERATURE
Regulation (Fig. 31-1)

Although the normal oral temperature is usually cited as 37° C., or 98.6° F., these figures indicate only the average normal temperature. Oral temperatures ranging from 36.4° to 37.2° C. (97.6° to 99° F.) are not considered abnormal. Rectal temperatures *average* 1° F. higher than oral readings, whereas axillary temperatures register 1° F. lower, *on the average*. Normal body temperature in a human being represents a balance between heat production and heat loss in the body. The main source of body heat is inadvertently created in the process of carrying out normal body functions. Production of body heat is the result of the activity of all cells, made possible by the oxidation, or burning, of foodstuffs within those cells. Blood, flowing through the various parts of the body, helps distribute heat;

and although measured body temperature differs depending on the method by which it is determined (oral, rectal, axillary, or skin probe), the remarkable fact is that these various measurements record temperatures so similar. Body heat is conserved by the involuntary constriction of the blood vessels of the skin, forcing more blood into the warm interior of the body and cutting it off from cooler areas near the skin's surface; it is also conserved by the automatic reduction of perspiration. Of course, the maintenance of body heat is also aided by the voluntary activity of the person. Adding a sweater or coat to provide better insulation or exercising to increase metabolism and circulation increases the tolerance of cold environmental conditions. Much heat is produced through the activity of the skeletal muscles. When additional warmth is necessary, these muscles will even contract involuntarily to produce heat, a process we call shivering. Conversely, removing insulation, increasing surface evaporation, and reducing muscular activity decrease body heat.

Body heat is lost primarily through the dilatation of the capillaries in the skin, the evaporation of increased perspiration on the skin's surface, and the process of warming inspired air, which is subsequently exhaled.

The part of the body that ultimately controls the unconscious processes necessary for the regulation of heat production, heat maintenance, and heat loss is thought to be located deep in the brain. The part of the brain considered most responsible for heat regulation is the hypothalamus, often

470

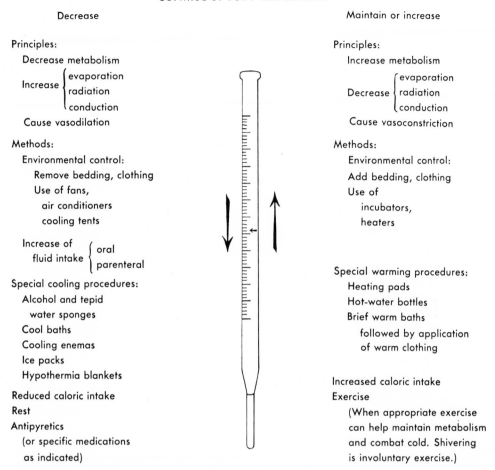

CONTROL OF BODY TEMPERATURE

Decrease | Maintain or increase

Principles:
 Decrease metabolism
 Increase { evaporation, radiation, conduction }
 Cause vasodilation

Methods:
 Environmental control:
  Remove bedding, clothing
  Use of fans,
   air conditioners
   cooling tents
 Increase of fluid intake { oral, parenteral }
 Special cooling procedures:
  Alcohol and tepid
   water sponges
  Cool baths
  Cooling enemas
  Ice packs
  Hypothermia blankets
 Reduced caloric intake
 Rest
 Antipyretics
  (or specific medications
  as indicated)

Principles:
 Increase metabolism
 Decrease { evaporation, radiation, conduction }
 Cause vasoconstriction

Methods:
 Environmental control:
  Add bedding, clothing
  Use of
   incubators,
   heaters

 Special warming procedures:
  Heating pads
  Hot-water bottles
  Brief warm baths
   followed by application
   of warm clothing

 Increased caloric intake
 Exercise
  (When appropriate exercise
  can help maintain metabolism
  and combat cold. Shivering
  is involuntary exercise.)

Fig. 31-1. In health, the body keeps its temperature within safe ranges. However, during unusual conditions or illness, normal temperature controls may be disturbed, and special regulating measures may be needed.

dubbed the "thermostat" of the body. It probably controls the processes of vasoconstriction and vasodilation, the associated activity of the sweat glands, and the involuntary skeletal muscle motion. Perhaps indirectly it influences the appetite and digestive and metabolic regulation through glandular stimulation or control.

In infants and young children temperature regulation is not perfected, and rather wide swings in body temperature occur readily. During the first days of life an infant is more likely to be influenced by the temperature of his environment, hence the frequent use of incubators. Toddlers and young school-age children often react to the common infectious diseases of childhood by running temperatures of 104° F. or more. A child may initiate a temperature elevation during a hard crying spell.

Causes and effects of elevated body temperature

At times a temperature elevation may produce a beneficial effect. In fact, fever is often looked on as a protective mechanism, since it helps kill certain heat-susceptible microorganisms and warns the individual of the possible presence of a pathological process. In the past, fever was even artificially induced in the treatment of certain infectious diseases.

Fever is described as a resetting of the body's thermostat in response to the presence of toxins produced by infection. This resetting of the thermostat interrupts normal heat-dissipating mechanisms. The capillaries at the skin's surface contract, causing the patient to feel cold, and he shivers, sometimes violently, to reduce the feeling of cold. The muscular activity of shivering further elevates the body temperature.

The skin of chilling patients should be kept sufficiently warm to halt shivering while other means of combating excessive internal temperatures or eliminating the initial cause are instituted. An exaggerated elevated systemic temperature—whether initiated by infectious processes, certain chemicals, or elevated environmental temperatures (heat exhaustion, sunstroke)—can cause serious injury, especially if it is prolonged. It can cause dehydration if adequate fluid intake is not maintained. On the other hand, an abnormal rise in body temperature may result from dehydration due to any cause (vomiting, diarrhea, or poor fluid intake). A frequent companion to high fever in children is a convulsion. A common phrase in a pediatric setting is "febrile convulsions." The word "febrile" refers to the state of being feverish. A person who has no abnormal temperature elevation may be called "afebrile."

Causes and effects of depressed body temperature

A depressed body temperature may simply reflect inactivity. The early morning temperature reading may be quite low, only because body processes are at a naturally low ebb. However, an abnormally low systemic temperature may also indicate circulatory collapse or the tiring of basic body processes prior to death.

In cases of cardiac and thoracic surgery it may be particularly desirable to slow down metabolism during surgery and postoperative care by cooling the body to extremely low temperatures to rest the heart and respiratory system. The narrowing of the blood vessels in the skin that results from surface cooling forces the blood into the interior of the body, thickens the blood (increases viscosity), slows the blood flow, and necessitates less oxygen intake. Uncompensated by muscle activity, the drop in temperature is of therapeutic importance. At times during chest surgery the surgeon may elect to actually stop the heart and lungs through the combined use of a heart-lung machine and profound hypothermia, which is cooling the bloodstream through the use of a special temperature-regulating attachment. The use of such techniques has been extremely helpful to the surgeon.

Raising body temperature

At times it becomes the duty of the nurse to carry out techniques to maintain or raise body temperature. This may be done to provide comfort, regulate metabolism, or combat exposure. It may be accomplished most simply by increasing room temperatures, applying more blankets, adding clothing, and offering warm but not hot drinks. In the home situation, placing a child who has been chilled in a *brief* warm bath, dressing him warmly, and tucking him in bed is a time-honored technique.

An infant is most easily warmed by the use of an incubator, a cozy box supplied with a built-in heating unit, or one of the radiant heat infant warmers. In an emergency situation in which no incubator is available the warmest place for a newborn infant would be directly next to his mother, who could share her own body heat.

The application of local heat is helpful in raising total body temperature. The use of hot-water bottles, various heating pads, and hypothermia blankets, which may be regulated to function like giant heating blankets, are discussed in detail on p. 474.

Reducing body temperature

A sponge bath is only one method of reducing temperature, and it is usually not the first or only method employed. There are approximately six basic ways in which one may try to reduce fever or lower body temperature.

Fluid intake. The first method of body temperature reduction involves encouraging fluid intake. It has already been noted that fever may result from dehydration. If oral fluids are impractical because of the state of the gastrointestinal tract or exaggerated body need, many times fluids must be administered intravenously.

Environmental control. Body temperature may be lowered and the patient made more comfortable by attention to the immediate environment. The removal of extra blankets and heavy clothing (unless the patient is complaining of chills and shivering) is often helpful. A well-ventilated, draft-free room may also be an aid. In warm weather well-placed fans, which circulate the air without blowing on the patient directly, may be used.

Medication. Medication may be ordered to help reduce fever; such medications are called *antipyretics.* The most frequently prescribed medications are acetylsalicylic acid, commonly known as aspirin, and acetaminophen (Tylenol or Tempra), the nonsalicylate analgesic and antipyretic. They seem to reduce temperature chiefly by producing greater amounts of perspiration and, therefore, greater cooling by evaporation. For dosages of aspirin see p. 319.

Sponge bath and tepid bath. Tepid water sponge baths are also administered to reduce fever; these have already been described. Sometimes the child will be placed in a tepid tub bath, especially if the child is not sufficiently responsive to other therapy. The child should never be left alone while undergoing such treatment.

Cooling enema. Another method that has been used to reduce fever is the cooling enema. This procedure usually consists of the intermittent administration of cool tap water per rectum. The infant and toddler have little or no sphincter control, and the solution usually returns fairly quickly even before the entire amount to be given is administered. When treating children of this age group, it is usually unrealistic to speak of clamping the tube for several minutes and then siphoning out the remainder of the fluid before repeating the process. However, even the brief introduction of cool fluid into the lower gastrointestinal tract may prove helpful if the child does not become too upset. Infants under 6 months of age usually do not tolerate more than 100 ml. of fluid administered at one time. Infants 6 months and older or toddlers usually are not given more than 250 ml. at one time. The efficiency of the enema should be checked by taking the child's temperature 30 minutes after termination of the treatment.

Hypothermia blankets. Patients with temperature elevations that are exaggerated or fail to respond to other methods of treatment may be placed on so-called hypothermia blankets (sort of K-pads in reverse).

There are several hypothermia blankets manufactured. Although the operating instructions on each may differ, the principles involved are similar. Cold, distilled water or alcohol and distilled water (depending on the model) are circulated through tubes embedded in a plastic mat or mats. The water is cooled and circulated by a refrigeration pump unit to which the pads are attached. With some units, adjustment of the pad temperature is accomplished manually by the nurse, depending on the temperature of the patient. With others, a rectal probe is inserted, which enables the patient's temperature to be continually monitored. The temperature of the patient registered by the probe may regulate the temperature of the pads automatically, according to predetermined temperature settings. Several pads of various sizes may be used, both under and over the patient according to his needs. There is always a light bath blanket or sheet between the patient and the plastic pad. The pad should not be folded or creased, and no pins should be used to secure them. The temperature desired and the time it should be maintained should be ordered by the attending physician.

473

LOCAL APPLICATION OF HEAT
OR COLD
Local application of heat

Local application of heat and cold for the treatment of disease may be ancient therapy, but it is also very contemporary. Local heat is frequently ordered to prevent chilling, relieve pain, hasten superficial abscess formation or the drainage of an infected wound, and relieve congestion in one body part by increasing the blood supply to another.

Effects

The primary effect of locally applied heat is vasodilation of the treated area (the skin becomes warm and pink). Locally applied heat also speeds up metabolism; enhances associated muscle relaxation; increases the temperature of the underlying skin, subcutaneous tissue, and muscle; and even raises the skin temperature of remote body areas. Studies have shown that immersion of an arm in a hot soak will raise the temperature of the big toe. There is controversy regarding the degree of reflex vasodilation achieved in *deep* tissues through the application of surface heat. When the effects of heat are desired in the deep-lying organs of the body, diathermy treatments, using high-frequency currents or ultrasound, are often ordered. These treatments are administered using special equipment and are not usually part of the nurse's responsibility. They more properly lie within the sphere of the physical therapist.

Dangers

The surface application of heat is not without danger. The nurse should never apply heat (other than in the form of extra blankets) without a physician's order.

When an internal abscess or localized infection is suspected (such as appendicitis), local heat should never be applied because of the danger of rupture, subsequent spread of infection, and peritonitis.

Skin temperatures surpassing 110° F. cause tissue damage. However, compresses or soaks that are prepared with solution above 110° F. do not necessarily raise skin temperatures to 110° F. Skin temperatures depend on the extent of the exposure to heat, considering body area, time, method employed, and temperature of the solution.

Water temperatures have been placed by several authors in the following descriptive classifications:

Neutral (warm)	93° to 98° F.
Hot	98° to 105° F.
Very hot	105° to 115° F.

The area receiving heat treatments should be frequently observed for signs of congestion and tissue damage. Nerve endings that detect the presence of hot and cold have the capacity to adjust when temperatures are not extreme and become less sensitive to variations. Temperatures may be increased to an injurious level unless this loss of sensitivity is recognized. Fair-skinned individuals are more likely to be burned than darkly pigmented individuals and should be observed especially closely. Special precautions should be observed when the area to be treated reveals poor circulation or sensory loss. Patients may sustain tissue damage from burning and not realize that they are being burned because of the lack of feeling in the area.

The time interval ordered for heat application should be carefully observed because if significant warmth is applied to a local area longer than approximately an hour (some say 30 to 45 minutes), a reflex vasoconstriction may reduce the blood supply to the area, and a reverse effect may occur.

Methods

Dry heat. Dry heat may be administered by an electric heating pad, a hot-water bottle, or a unit that circulates warm water through a plastic pad. An electric heating pad is rarely used in a hospital setting because of the danger of electrical malfunction and the problems of maintenance and disinfection. Hot-water bottles are not recommended because of the many instances of accidental burning that have resulted from their use. If hot-water bottles are employed for infants and young children, they

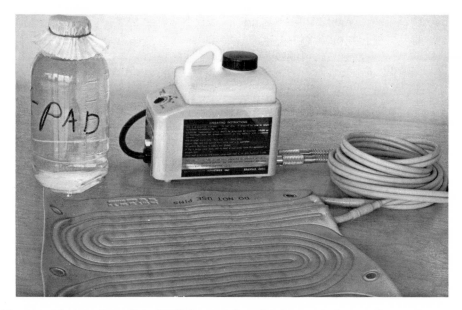

Fig. 31-2. The K-pad circulates distilled water through tubing in a plastic pad at a preset temperature. (Courtesy Grossmont Hospital, La Mesa, Calif.)

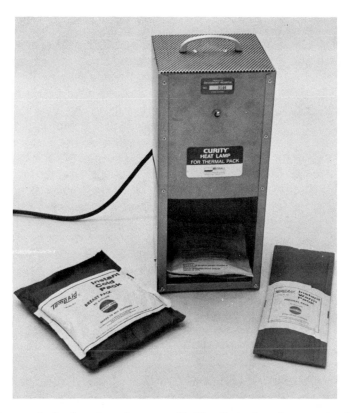

Fig. 31-3. New methods of applying heat or cold. The Curity heat lamp warms foil-wrapped sterile compresses. The instant cold and warm packs are activated by striking the dark circles. (Courtesy Grossmont Hospital, La Mesa, Calif.)

should never contain water hotter than 115° F., although temperatures up to 120° F. are permitted for older children and adults. They should be emptied of excess air, tightly stoppered, and turned upside down to check for leaks. A dry, warm cloth cover should be placed on the bottle to provide proper insulation. Hot-water bottles should not be placed between skin surfaces or under the back.

The plastic pad containing tubing, through which warm water may be circulated at a preset temperature from a bedside heating unit, has become popular. A well-known appliance of this type is the K-pad (Fig. 31-2). Such an apparatus uses distilled water, which is periodically added to a reservoir at the top of the heating and circulating unit. Warm water is pushed out of the unit, flows through the continuous pattern of tubes embedded in the plastic pad, and returns to the heating unit. No pins should be used in stabilizing the position of the various sized pads available. Pads may be tied or taped in place; however, if they are bent, the warm water may not circulate properly. Ideally, a pad should be neatly wrapped in a pillowcase or towel and the tubing covered with stockinette. Detailed operating instructions accompany the unit.

Another method of applying heat to a small area is shown in Fig. 31-3. A chemical mixture contained within a waterproof envelope is activated by abruptly striking a premarked spot. These units are convenient, disposable, efficient, but somewhat expensive.

Moist heat. Moist heat therapy is more penetrating and faster acting than dry heat therapy. Moist heat may be applied locally in the form of hot soaks, packs, or compresses.

HOT SOAKS. If the condition of the young child permits such treatment, soaks of body parts when no open skin areas are involved may be carried out as part of a general bath, depending on the reason for the order. If this is not feasible, basins of water or other ordered solution may be provided at the bedside. If the area to be soaked involves an open lesion or wound that is not too extensive, a sterile container is provided for sterile water, tap water, or other solution. (Tap water from an approved water system is generally accepted as free from disease-producing microorganisms.) However, normal saline solution (properly called physiological saline solution or sodium chloride, 0.9%) is often preferred because it contains approximately the same salt concentration as normal tissue fluid and therefore will not cause abnormal drying or bogginess in the body tissues. Because sterile physiological saline solution is usually readily available in the hospital setting, it is often used for soaks involving small body areas. (Physiological saline solution may be prepared in the home by adding 2 teaspoons of salt to 1 quart of water.) The temperature of hot soaks for children, unless ordered otherwise, is 105° F. (41° C.). The duration of the soak may vary according to orders, but the treatment is usually prescribed for 20 minutes. When the soak is terminated, any open skin area is dried and dressed as ordered.

Soaks involving large body areas are usually carried out in a bathtub. The tub is disinfected before and after use, but the procedure is not really sterile, just clean. Tepid (about 98° F.) body soaks are often ordered for severely burned patients. The soak, in these cases, is not administered as a heat treatment but for the cleansing and debriding action that occurs when the patient's inner dressings are removed in the water and the tub solution is agitated. Frequently such soaks, followed by the application of sterile dressings, are performed in a physical therapy department using a whirlpool bath.

HOT PACKS. Heat applied to the body in the form of packs involves the use of relatively heavy, moist pieces of flannel, which, when properly insulated, hold heat for considerable periods. Since the dramatic decrease in poliomyelitis, hot packs are seldom ordered. In the past they were quite commonly used to relieve muscle spasm.

HOT COMPRESSES. Application of hot or warm compresses, however, is commonly part of a nurse's responsibilities. They may be applied to speed superficial abscess formation, promote wound drainage, or improve circulation. If the skin in the area to be compressed is broken, sterile gauze is used. The following are general suggestions for warm compress application (usually several alternatives in procedure are available):

1. The procedure should be explained to the patient according to his ability to understand and cooperate.
2. The area under the body part to be compressed should be protected by a clean, waterproof material overlaid by an absorbent towel or bath blanket.
3. The sterile gauze pads may be placed in a hot (110° to 115° F.) sterile solution as ordered (usually physiological saline) and wrung with two sterile forceps until dripping stops. The pads may be placed on the designated area and replaced with new compresses about every 2 minutes.
4. In areas where the additional weight will not cause pain or injury, two or three warm compresses may be quickly covered by sterile, lightweight waterproof plastic, and the body part may be wrapped or covered by an insulating towel warmed by an overlying K-pad, a hot-water bottle, or a low-set electric pad.
5. In another method of preparing hot, moist compresses, the dry compresses are placed over the area and irrigated with warm solution using a sterile syringe. The compresses are either changed periodically or wrapped as previously described.

Clean warm compresses are applied in much the same manner, except that sterile precautions need not be observed. Wriggly toddlers usually need to have the compresses gently tied in place and fairly constant nursing attendance to prevent the dismantling of the nurse's handiwork. Great care should be taken not to burn the child.

The child should not be left in a position in which he may come into direct contact with the hot water used for heating the compresses.

Local application of cold
Effects

The local application of cold may also be therapeutic. Cold applied to the skin surface for brief periods (30 to 45 minutes) produces vasoconstriction of the area treated, which helps in the prevention (but not treatment) of swelling, the control of hemorrhage, and the retardation of any inflammatory process. Cold applied for a sufficient period will significantly cool muscles and other underlying organs, either directly or by reflex action. Cold also has an anesthetic quality that may sometimes become of primary importance. The use of ice cubes in the treatment of minor burns illustrates both the anesthetic and vasoconstrictive effects of cold. If applied to the skin for longer periods, cold may trigger a reverse reflex mechanism that results in vasodilation. A corresponding reverse reflex mechanism was noted in the discussion of the effects of the local application of heat.

Dangers

The local use of cold applications, like that of heat, is not without hazard. The skin surface must be frequently observed for mottling and tissue damage. Cold applied to areas in which circulation is inadequate may produce injury (frostbite) and lead to gangrene. The anesthetic quality of cold may make the patient unaware of injury inadvertently produced by other factors.

Methods

Like heat, cold may be used therapeutically in dry or moist form. Moist cold is more penetrating than dry cold.

Dry cold. An example of the application of dry cold would be the typical ice bag or ice collar. Some of these, like the Freez-A-Bag, are prefilled and sealed. Others must be filled. Small cubes and a small amount of cold water are used to fill two-thirds of the bag; all air is pressed out (it delays the transfer of cold), and the bag is capped. The bag should be wrapped in a cover to prevent condensation from wetting the patient or bedding. For effective local reaction, an ice cap or ice bag should be removed approximately every 30 to 45 minutes to observe and allow the skin to return to normal and enable the cold to continue its process of vasoconstriction when reapplied.

Moist cold. Moist cold may be applied in the form of cold, damp compresses, cold soaks, or sponge baths.

COLD COMPRESSES. One may remember the Sunday comic strips, picturing moist cold in the form of raw steak being applied to black eyes to prevent swelling. Steak is an expensive compress, however!

If the body part compressed can tolerate weight, clean cold compresses are best made from washcloths or towels. If a delicate organ like an eye or an extremely tender body part is to be treated, gauze compresses may be used. The adjoining area is protected by a waterproof plastic or rubber sheet lined with an absorbent layer. A basin of water and ice, large enough to accommodate the compresses, should be at hand. The compresses should be wrung out well to avoid dripping, and once applied, they should be left exposed. Covering it would soon make it only tepid as a result of the heating capability of the body. The compresses have to be changed frequently, depending on their size and density and the temperature of the body part to which they are applied.

It is difficult to apply sterile cold compresses because ice is not sterile. However, if sterile technique is necessary, sterile cold solutions may be maintained in a refrigerator and the sterile container packed in ice at the bedside during the treatment. Sterile compresses may be handled in an aseptic manner with forceps or gloves. We do not recommend the use of forceps around the eyes and faces of young children in the usual bedside setting. Their movements are too unpredictable. Wearing gloves is much less cumbersome and is safer.

Light gauze compresses must usually be changed about every minute to maintain their temperature. If any drainage or open skin area is present, the compress should not be reused but discarded.

COLD SOAKS. Cold soaks, often recommended to prevent the swelling of a twisted or sprained ankle, usually consist of cold water in a basin into which an extremity is placed for about 20-minute intervals. Occasionally alternating cold and hot soaks are ordered to stimulate circulation.

SPONGE BATHS. Tepid water sponge baths are fairly frequent procedures in a pediatric setting. Solutions of 25% to 50% alcohol are rarely ordered since there is danger of toxic inhalation and coma if the area is not well ventilated. Four basic techniques are used to reduce systemic body heat:

1. Friction before or during the cool sponging produces greater vasodilation that, when combined with the heat loss caused by evaporation, increases cooling.
2. Strategic positioning of cool cloths over areas where large blood vessels approach the surface of the body (e.g., in the axilla and groin) hastens cooling of the blood.
3. Placement of an ice cap to the head reduces cerebral temperature and lessens the danger of convulsion.
4. Light covering of the part of the body not being sponged and the use of solutions that are not excessively cold protect the patient from chilling. If the patient shivers for a prolonged period as the result of his abrupt exposure to cold, the shivering may actually maintain or raise his temperature. Some texts recommend the application of a warm-water bottle or other dry heat source to the feet of the patient to prevent excessive chilling.

A sponge bath is ordered in response to an elevated temperature; therefore checks of temperature, pulse, and respiration would normally precede it.

TEPID WATER SPONGE BATH

Purposes: To reduce body temperature and relieve discomfort.

Materials:

1. Waterproof sheet
2. Absorbent bath blanket or towels, depending on the size of the child
3. Light bath blanket to place over the patient
4. Basin of tepid or cool water at approximately 70° to 80° F.
5. Small supply of ice to add to the sponging solution, if necessary
6. Four washcloths
7. Wrapped Freez-A-Bag or ice cap for the head (Some hospitals do not include this as part of the procedure.)

Procedure:

1. Explain the procedure to the patient as much as possible.
2. Place the child on top of a waterproof sheeting and absorbent blanket (unless this is already part of the base of his bed) fairly close to the side of the bed so that he may be easily reached. Remove any pillows.
3. Undress the child except for diaper or loincloth and cover him with the light bath blanket.
4. Place the ice cap or Freez-A-Bag under the child's head.
5. Rub the skin of the anterior trunk and extremities briefly with a dry washcloth to bring the blood to the surface, decreasing the sensation of chilling and aiding in heat reduction when the cool moist washcloths are applied.
6. Place cool, moist, but not dripping, folded washcloths on the axilla and groin on the side of the child that you will sponge last.
7. Wash the patient's face and neck with the solution.
8. Expose only the area being sponged. Use firm, long strokes in sponging the upper extremity, thorax, abdomen, and lower extremity on the side farthest from you. Place the washcloths on the groin and axilla of the opposite side. Continue sponging the patient, first the upper extremity, then the thorax, abdomen, and lower extremity.
9. During the sponge bath, periodically evaluate the patient's reaction. How are his color, pulse, and respiration? If he seems to be chilling or shivering excessively, protests and becomes agitated, or if other untoward reactions occur, stop the treatment and lightly cover the patient. Report reactions to the supervising nurse.
10. Turn the patient on his side. Rub and sponge his back firmly.
11. Gently pat the skin dry at the end of the sponge bath with a towel and dress the child in a light gown. The sponge bath should take about 20 to 25 minutes.
12. Cover the child with a light sheet or blanket. Remove the bed protectors and encourage rest.
13. Take the patient's temperature, pulse, and respiration 30 minutes after the sponge bath and report them to the supervising nurse or physician.
14. Record the procedure, the patient's reaction, and the results.

The local use of heat or cold applications can be of strategic importance in patient care. It may involve old principles, but they have proved worthy of our study and application.

unit ten
Suggested selected readings and references

Bahruth, A.: Keeping track of injection sites, Nurs. '73 3:51, June, 1973.

Blake, F. G., Wright, F. H., and Waechter, E. H.: Nursing care of children, ed. 8, Philadelphia, 1970, J. B. Lippincott Co.

Brant, P. A., Smith, M. E., and Ashburn, S. S.: Intramuscular injections in children, Am. J. Nurs. 72:1402-1406, Aug., 1972.

Brown, S.: Easing the burden of traction and casts, RN 38:36-41, Feb., 1975.

Brunner, L. S., and others: The Lippincott manual of nursing practice, Philadelphia, 1974, J. B. Lippincott Co.

Dos and dont's of traction care, Nurs. '74 4:35-41, Nov., 1974.

Egan, D. F.: Fundamentals of respiratory therapy, ed. 2, St. Louis, 1973, The C. V. Mosby Co.

Erikson, R., and Storlie, F. J.: Taking temperatures: oral or rectal and when, Nurs. '73 3:51-53, April, 1973.

Filler, R. M.: Intravenous alimentation. In Smith, C. A., editor: The critically ill child, Philadelphia, 1972, W. B. Saunders Co., pp. 220-238.

French, R. M.: Nurse's guide to diagnostic procedures, ed. 3, New York, 1971, McGraw-Hill Book Co.

Fuerst, E. V., and Wolff, L.: Fundamentals of nursing, ed. 5, Philadelphia, 1974, J. B. Lippincott Co.

Garb, S.: Laboratory tests in common use, ed. 5, New York, 1971, Springer Publishing Co., Inc.

Gormican, A., and Liddy, E.: Nasogastric tube feedings, Nurs. Digest 2:59-63, Jan., 1974. Condensed from Postgrad. Med. 53:71-76, June, 1973.

Gross, R. E.: An atlas of children's surgery, Philadelphia, 1970, W. B. Saunders Co.

Hays, D.: Do it yourself—the Z-track way, Am. J. Nurs. **74**:1070-1071, June, 1974.

Humphery, N. M., Wright, P. S., and Swanson, A. B.: Parenteral hyperalimentation for children, Am. J. Nurs. **72**:286-288, Feb., 1972.

Indyk, L.: Monitoring in children. II. Temperature and blood pressure, Clin. Pediatr. **11**:157-160, March, 1972.

Kaler, J., and Kaler, H.: Michael had a tracheostomy, Am. J. Nurs. **74**:852-855, May, 1974.

Kee, J. L., and Gregory, A. P.: The ABC's and mEq's of fluid imbalance in children, Nurs. '74 **4**:28-36, June, 1974.

Kerr, A. H.: Orthopedic nursing procedures, ed. 2, New York, 1969, Springer Publishing Co., Inc.

Landwirth, J.: Continuous nasogastric infusion feedings of infants of low birth weight, Clin. Pediatr. **13**:603, July, 1974.

Larson, C. B., and Gould, M.: Orthopedic nursing, ed. 8, St. Louis, 1973, The C. V. Mosby Co.

Leifer, G.: Principles and techniques in pediatric nursing, Philadelphia, ed. 2, 1972, W. B. Saunders Co.

McFarlane, J., and Nickerson, D.: Two-drop and one-drop test for glycosuria, Am. J. Nurs. **72**:939, May, 1972.

Odom, J. V.: Going metric, Am. J. Nurs. **74**:1078-1081, June, 1974.

Petrillo, M.: Respiratory tract aspiration: programmed instruction, Am. J. Nurs. **66**:2483+, Nov., 1966.

Sacharin, R. M., and Hunter, M. H. S.: Pediatric nursing procedures, Baltimore, 1969, The Williams & Wilkins Co.

Sato, F.: New devices for continuous urine collection in pediatrics, Am. J. Nurs. **69**:805+, April, 1969.

Scipien, G. M., and others: Comprehensive pediatric nursing, New York, 1975, McGraw-Hill Book Co.

Secor, J.: Patient care in respiratory problems, Philadelphia, 1969, W. B. Saunders Co.

Stein, A. M., Mandell, D., and Ferguson, J.: Multiple fractures: look out for those pulmonary complications, Nurs. '74 **4**:26-32, Nov., 1974.

Tate, G., Gohrke, C., and Mansfield, L. W.: Correct use of electric thermometers, Am. J. Nurs. **70**:1898+, Sept., 1970.

Tepe, P.: A physiological approach to pediatric medicines, Nurs. Clin. North Am. **1**:111+, March, 1966.

Warren, F. M.: Blood pressure readings, getting them quickly on an infant, Nurs. '75 **5**:13, April, 1975.

Wu, R.: Explaining treatments to young children, Am. J. Nurs. **65**:71+, July, 1965.

unit eleven
Common pediatric problems and their nursing care

32
Conditions involving the integumentary system

The integumentary system consists of the skin as well as the hair, nails, sweat and oil glands, and superficial sensory nerve endings. These organs form the first line of defense against body injury. The integumentary system prevents both excessive loss of fluid from the body and the entry of certain poisons and microbes into the body. It is of special importance in the regulation of body temperature, principally through capillary dilatation and constriction and the formation of cooling perspiration. It is of considerable aid in the evaluation of environmental conditions and therefore in the determination of individual safety. Embedded within the tissues of the integumentary system are nerve endings, which relay to the brain sensations of pressure, touch, hot, cold, and pain. The skin can be an important avenue of fluid loss. However, it has only limited powers of absorption.

The health of the skin is often a reflection of the health of the individual. Skin color, hydration, and the presence of detectable surface irregularities and disturbances in sensation may reveal significant information about an individual's health habits and status. The skin may also give clues to a patient's emotional reactions. Involuntarily, we may blush with embarrassment or pale with fright.

LAYERS OF THE SKIN
(Fig. 32-1)

The epidermis is paper thin, and it consists of several microscopic layers. The uppermost layer consists of dead cells ready to be shed from the body's surface. They are constantly being replaced by new cells, which are formed in the lower layers. The lower layers of the epidermis secure their nourishment from the dermis, or true skin, over which they lie.

The dermis, also called the *corium,* is a dense layer of connective tissue well supplied with blood vessels and nerves. It also contains sweat and oil glands and hair follicles, some of which may extend into the deeper subcutaneous tissue. Small muscle fibers may be attached to the hair follicles.

The subcutaneous layer is chiefly fatty tissue in a framework of elastic and fibrous tissue. It serves multiple functions including that of lipid storage and insulation.

The observation of the skin and the description of its condition is often the responsibility of the nurse. Her patients may not be hospitalized primarily because of skin problems. Skin difficulties may be, at times, of secondary importance in the diagnostic picture. However, the condition of the skin is always of significance as the nurse views her patient's total needs.

KEY VOCABULARY

Physicians commonly use certain terms to describe the condition of the skin. Some of the words the nurse may wish to use in her own recording. Others she may not employ, but she should be able to interpret their meanings. These terms are simply defined as follows:

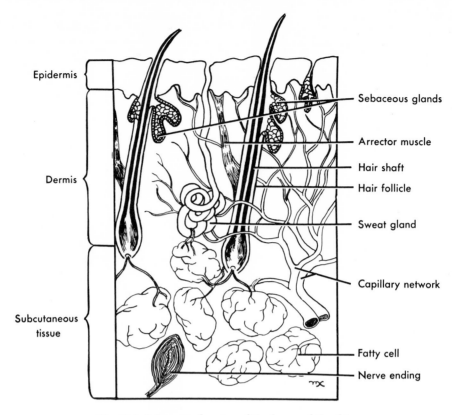

Epidermis

Dermis

Subcutaneous tissue

Sebaceous glands

Arrector muscle

Hair shaft

Hair follicle

Sweat gland

Capillary network

Fatty cell

Nerve ending

Fig. 32-1. Schematic drawing of the layers of the skin.

abrasion (adj., abraded) loss of superficial tissue by friction (chafing).

contusion (adj., contused) a bruise; a black-and-blue mark.

crust (adj., crusted) the temporary covering of a lesion formed primarily by dried blood or serum (scab).

ecchymosis (adj., ecchymotic) a black-and-blue mark.

erythema (adj., erythematous) a reddened area of the skin.

excoriation (adj., excoriated) a superficial laceration; a scratch.

jaundice or *icterus* (adj., jaundiced or icteric) a yellow tinge to the skin or sclerae.

laceration (adj., lacerated) a jagged cut or tear.

lesion any change or irregularity in tissue caused by disease or injury.

macule (adj., macular) a flat spot or stain; the typical measles rash is macular.

papule (adj., papular) a small, solid elevation on the skin; the typical early stage of a pimple is papular.

petechia (adj., petechial) a small bluish purple dot caused by capillary hemorrhage.

pruritus (adj., pruritic) itching.

pustule (adj., pustular) a pus-filled vesicle; a superficial cutaneous abscess.

ulcer (adj., ulcerated) a raw area often depressed or forming a cavity, caused by loss of normal covering tissue.

urticaria (wheals and hives) (adj., urticarial) large, slightly raised, reddened or blanched areas, usually accompanied by intense itching.

vesicle (adj., vesicular) a small elevation of the skin obviously containing fluid such as a blister.

A skin lesion should be described in such a way that the following information is included:

1. Size (described in metric measurements, such as 1 cm. in diameter)
2. Elevation (raised, flat, depressed)
3. Quality (smooth, rough, scaly, moist)
4. Color
5. Distribution (localized, scattered, etc.)
6. Associated sensory disturbances (numbness, itching, pain, burning, etc.)
7. Type of any drainage or exudate noted

COMMON SKIN PROBLEMS

The infant and toddler

Miliaria rubra (prickly heat, or heat rash)

Miliaria rubra is a common problem caused by blockage of the sweat pores. The exits of the sweat ducts are plugged, causing sweat to seep into the dermis or epidermis. This produces a red, pinhead-sized vesicular-papular rash associated with underlying erythema, especially in areas where perspiration is common or friction is frequent. It may be accompanied by considerable itching. Occasionally the rash may include pustular lesions. Prevention is easier than treatment; avoid overdressing children. Any procedure that will reduce the need for perspiration will help improve the condition. Light dusting of the skin with a fine cornstarch or baby powder may be beneficial. Some dermatologists may recommend the use of a skin lotion containing hydrocortisone. In the event of secondary infection an antibiotic drug may be prescribed.

Intertrigo

Intertrigo is often simply called *chafing.* It is commonly found in the folds of the skin where friction is frequent and hygiene may be lacking; examples of problem areas include the creases in the neck and in the folds of the groin and gluteus muscles, where the skin may become quite inflamed. As in miliaria rubra, prevention is more simple than cure. Meticulous hygiene and keeping the area dry and lightly powdered is of great importance.

Seborrheic dermatitis (Fig. 32-2)

Seborrheic dermatitis is a very common dermatitis of infancy. It is a disorder of unknown origin, usually benign and self-limited, but it can be chronic and is often confused with atopic dermatitis. Seborrheic dermatitis is characterized by a scaly eruption (scales may be dry or greasy) on an inflammatory base; it chiefly affects the scalp, eyebrows, eyelids, and pubic regions. In infants seborrheic derma-

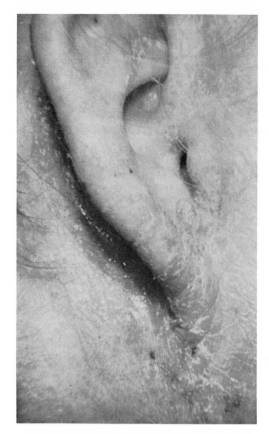

Fig. 32-2. Seborrheic dermatitis. (Courtesy W. W. Duemling, M.D., San Diego, Calif.)

titis is seen most commonly as "milk crust" or "cradle cap," yellowish, slightly adherent large scales found principally on the top of the head. It sometimes is related to a reluctance on the part of the mother to wash the soft spot on the baby's scalp for fear of causing injury. It also develops fairly often in the groin and may become secondarily infected with yeast (*Candida* or *Monilia*) or bacteria. Frequent shampooing and the use of mild medications containing sulfur, salicylic acid, or hydrocortisone are often prescribed for seborrheic dermatitis. In adolescents it is often associated with acne. When the condition involves the scalp, the common name is dandruff.

Some children are affected by another form called intertriginous seborrhea, which is usually moist and involves areas behind the ear and the axillary and inguinal regions.

483

Diaper rash

Infants who have diaper rash are quite often victims of seborrhea. The rash may take multiple forms from simple erythema to blisters and ulceration, depending on the causes. As a group, children with irritation of the diaper area usually have sensitive skins—a predisposition said to be inherited. Unfavorable conditions quickly trigger an unfavorable response. Situations that often set the scene for skin problems are poorly washed and rinsed diapers, infrequent diaper changes aggravated by prolonged use of plastic diaper covers, and incomplete or infrequent washing and drying of the diaper area. Careful attention to cleanliness is necessary. However, overzealous ministrations can cause problems, too!

To reduce the formation of irritating ammonia produced by the action of bacteria on urine, every effort is made to cut down the bacterial population on the diaper area. The use of a gentle antiseptic final rinse, such as methylbenzethonium chloride (Diaparene), is often recommended. The use of antiseptic rinses by diaper laundries is standard practice.

The cautious application of dry heat to diaper rash often improves the skin condition. A gooseneck lamp with a 25-watt bulb may be positioned over the prone infant. Precautions against burning should be observed. The lamp should be out of the child's reach and away from the bed linens. The bulb should be at least 12 inches from the child's buttocks. During heat treatments the diaper area should be free of medications. If the application of heat is difficult, simply exposing the area to the air is frequently helpful. Sunshine, if present, can be used for brief periods, but an infant should be carefully watched for overexposure.

A fine baby powder to decrease area moisture is usually an aid. Desitin, hydrocortisone, and certain antibacterial agents, such as Polysporin and nystatin cream, may be ordered depending on the needs of the particular patient. In general, occlusive medications should be avoided (for example, nystatin cream is preferred to nystatin ointment).

Infantile eczema (atopic dermatitis)
(Fig. 32-3)

Infantile eczema most often appears between the first and sixth month. In most cases it subsides considerably by 2 years of age. It is characterized by skin lesions, which first appear as localized, scaling, red areas usually on the head, neck, wrists, elbows, and knees, although involvement may become progressively more extensive. Fairly rapidly, small vesicles, which break and weep a yellow, sticky fluid, develop in these reddened areas. The fluid dries, forming crusts or scales on the skin. The skin may become thickened and fissured. Since itching is intense, the child invariably scratches the lesions, and thus secondary infection is usually present. Lesions on various parts of the body may be in different stages of development—some quite moist, others dried and scaling. For this reason different types of topical medications may

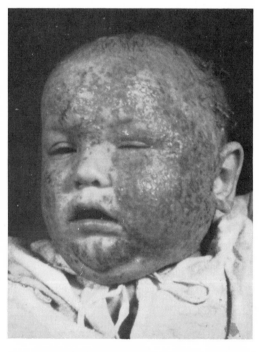

Fig. 32-3. Infant with severe eczema. (Courtesy R. B. Pappenfort, M.D., San Diego, Calif.)

be applied to the parts of the body, depending on the aims of the treatment. Seborrheic dermatitis and fungal infections may be associated with atopic dermatitis. Permanent scarring does not usually occur unless the lesions become secondarily infected or deeply excoriated.

Infantile eczema is considered to be an essentially allergic response. It is, more properly, a symptom of a disorder rather than the disorder itself. Infantile eczema has been called the most frequent manifestation of the allergic state in infancy. It is not always clear, however, just what agents, or *allergens,* cause the dermatitis. Exposure to allergens may occur in any of the follownig ways:

1. By ingestion (common foods causing difficulties in infancy are cow's milk, egg whites, wheat products, and citrus juices)
2. By inhalation (dust, pollen, animal dander)
3. By skin contact with some medications and materials such as rubber, plastic, and wool

Many investigators believe that child-parent relationships and emotional stress play a significant role in the initiation and course of the disease. There is often a family history of allergy manifested by eczema, asthma, or hay fever. Eczema usually improves during the summer months and worsens during the winter. The infants affected usually appear well nourished, and some tend to be overweight.

Many factors must be considered in the treatment of eczema. If possible, the offending allergens should be identified and eliminated from the infant's environment. Secondary infection, if present, should be treated, and itching, scratching and exposure to known infections should be avoided. Treatment of the lesions to clear scaling, minimize discomfort, and improve appearance is continued. Psychologically, supportive care for the child and his family is of great importance.

To identify those substances that help to initiate the dermatitis, a careful history is taken by the physician. For the infant or toddler, an elimination diet is often prescribed in which the foods that are allowed are listed in detail. If the baby is not breast-fed, evaporated milk, goat's milk, or soybean milk may be prescribed. The importance of rigidly following the diet must be impressed on the parents. As time goes on, more foods are added, one by one, to the diet. The child is carefully observed for changes in his skin condition and general health after each addition.

The home environment of the infant must be carefully controlled also. Since many children with allergic symptoms of the respiratory tract show sensitivity to dust, their nurseries are stripped of all drapes, rugs, and fuzzy toys. The crib mattress is encased in a nonallergenic cover, and wool blankets or clothing are eliminated. Although infants do not usually have pets, the presence of a dog or cat in the household may cause significant problems, and so, sad to relate, pets must sometimes find new homes. However, fish and turtles generally do not cause allergies. The house should be frequently vacuumed with special attention to the child's sleeping quarters. Skin testing, with special patches and scratch techniques, in an effort to determine allergens is usually reserved for older children.

A child with eczema should *not* be vaccinated against smallpox because of the great danger of the virus spreading to the open lesions and causing a serious complication called *generalized vaccinia.* For the same reason he should not be allowed to be with other children who have been recently vaccinated. Other immunizations are recommended, however. The eczema patient should also be protected against deliberate contact with people who have staphylococcal, streptococcal, or viral infections such as herpes simplex (the cause of the common fever blister). In many hospitals the child with eczema is placed on isolation precautions; however, routine isolation creates problems of its own—psychological stress and financial strain!

To help reduce scratching, which increases the possibility of secondary infection, various methods are used. Efforts are made to decrease the itching by the use of a minimum of clothing, all softly textured. Diapers are changed frequently. Fingernails and toenails are trimmed short. Formerly, the baby's arms were restrained in some way. Restraints are no longer recommended unless all other methods of control fail.

Different types of medications are used. Systemic antihistaminic drugs may be tried to ease itching. Sedation may be ordered to allow the infant to sleep. Erythromycin may be useful in combating secondary infection. Bacitracin and neomycin are recommended for local application for the same reason. Various topical ointments containing hydrocortisone may be used to reduce inflammatory response if infection is not present.

If coal tar preparations are used, care should be taken not to expose the areas to sunshine because a chemical reaction, which in itself is irritating to the skin, may take place. Jars containing coal tar ointments should be tightly closed to prevent deterioration. Coal tar ointment should be removed in special baths or with liquid petrolatum before a new application is made.

Medications are applied with clean hands or a finger cot or glove. They are generally used on a small area on a trial basis to test skin reaction. Many of these medications are expensive and should not be wasted.

Sometimes special baths or soaks are prescribed for the infant to help remove crusts and reduce pruritus and weeping. Common ingredients added to the bath water are cornstarch, oatmeal preparations (such as Aveeno), or bicarbonate of soda solutions. The water should be tepid, about 95° F. If possible, a small baby bathtub should be used. Sometimes the skin of the infant is so dry that the physician restricts bathing. In routine bathing a soap substitute is regularly used.

Continuous, tepid, wet, medicated compresses are sometimes employed to dry weeping crusted lesions. Therapeutic compresses must be *kept wet* to accomplish the aim of the treatment. This type of compress or gauze bandage is not covered by waterproof material but is left exposed to cool the area by evaporation.

Older children may undergo so-called desensitization procedures. Through the injection of small but gradually increasing amounts of allergen, the body is sometimes able to eventually tolerate the substance without untoward reaction.

The course of infantile eczema is usually not one of steady improvement. The child will improve, have a relapse, and improve again. The parents should be told to prepare themselves for a rather long seige of skin difficulty. However, after 2 years of age a respite can usually be expected. Unfortunately, as eczema disappears other allergy-type manifestations such as asthma or hay fever may develop. The child with eczema is infrequently hospitalized because of the increased exposure to infection (despite precautions), the emotional upset that may occur in the child as a result of the change of environment, and the need for the "maternal figure." However, exhaustion and tension on the part of the mother or father may be considered a factor in obtaining an admission to the pediatric unit of a hospital.

THE PRESCHOOL-AGE AND YOUNG
SCHOOL-AGE CHILD
Impetigo (Fig. 32-4)

Impetigo is a skin infection caused by either coagulase-positive staphylococci or beta-hemolytic streptococci. It is very contagious and serious in newborn infants and fairly contagious but less serious among children and adults. It is often associated with poor hygiene. Inflammation begins with the appearance of reddish spots on the skin, which develop into small blisters. These blisters become pus filled and break, causing thick yellow-red crusts on older children but few crusts on infants. When the crusts are removed, small superficial ulcers are seen. The face and hands are the

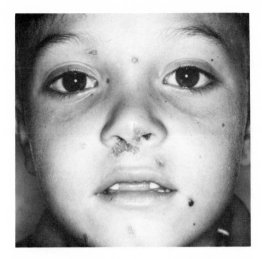

Fig. 32-4. Impetigo. (Courtesy David Allen, M.D., San Diego, Calif.)

areas most frequently affected, but other body areas may become involved. In the hospital, isolation is indicated.

Treatment includes careful cleansing and removal of the crusts, with compresses if necessary, and the use of neomycin-bacitracin ointment. A course of penicillin or erythromycin administered systemically is recommended because of the demonstrated association between certain strains of beta-hemolytic streptococci and nephritis. Also, a more rapid improvement of the lesions is seen when systemic therapy is used. The nurse should be especially cautious in the care of the lesions and disposal of infected material because the infection spreads easily. The child's fingernails should be clipped short. The dermatitis usually responds well to treatment.

Erythema multiforme and the Stevens-Johnson syndrome

Erythema multiforme is a skin condition characterized by the sudden appearance of a macular erythematous rash on the skin and mucous membranes, which may progress to papules and vesicles of exaggerated size in the next stage. It usually is associated with the appearance of respiratory symptoms, fever, and chills. It is more common in boys of school age. Erythema mul-

tiforme has been linked with a type of hypersensitivity reaction to infection or drugs, but the exact cause remains unknown. A rare explosive form of this condition involving the conjunctivae of the eyes is called *Stevens-Johnson syndrome.* This type may be fatal. Treatment consists of symptomatic supportive measures and, in severe cases, short-term, high-dosage steroid therapy and intravenous fluids. Although the child may be seriously ill, he may respond quite rapidly to medication (Fig. 32-5).

Furuncles and carbuncles

Furuncles and carbuncles are deep infections of the hair follicles. They may occur singly or in groups. If the furuncles run together, forming one sore with several draining points, the resulting lesion is called a carbuncle. Carbuncles are not common in small children but are seen with greater frequency among adolescent boys. A furuncle begins as a single papule associated with a hair. The papule becomes a pustule, which enlarges and forms a head. At this time the physician incises and drains the "boil." Warm compresses or soaks may be ordered to prepare the lesion for lancing. If multiple furuncles are present, systemic antibiotic therapy may be prescribed.

Sty, or hordeolum

A sty, an infection involving an eyelash follicle, will usually clear spontaneously or may be incised.

Ringworm of the scalp, skin, and feet (Fig. 32-6)

Ringworm of the scalp, or *tinea capitis,* used to be fairly common among school-aged children and is still seen from time to time, particularly in urban areas. It can be caused by several kinds of fungi. Some types of fungi are contracted from human beings, whereas others are contracted from animals. The fungus attacks hairs at their bases, causing them to break off close to the skin and leave circular balding areas. The scalp in the area of the hair loss may become red and scaly. Mild itching may

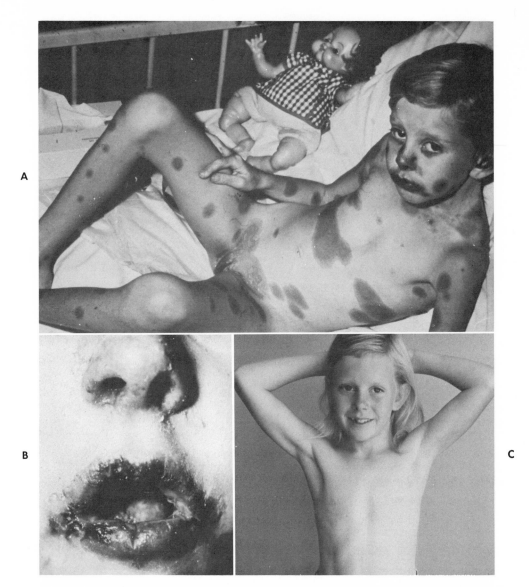

Fig. 32-5. **A,** Six-year-old girl with Stevens-Johnson syndrome. **B,** Involvement of lips and mucous membranes. **C,** Two months later—skin clear. (Courtesy Naval Regional Medical Center, San Diego, Calif.)

be present. Diagnosis is usually made on the basis of the clinical history, an ultraviolet light called *Wood's lamp,* or a microscopic examination of the affected hairs. Some fungi that commonly cause ringworm of the scalp fluoresce brightly when exposed to the rays of Wood's lamp. In the past, treatment of ringworm was quite difficult, and the disease had a tendency to become chronic, usually healing spontaneously at

puberty. Treatment included shaving the head. Boys and girls wore little stocking caps in an effort to cover the hair loss and prevent the spread of the disease. X-ray treatment was sometimes prescribed. The oral administration of the antibiotic griseofulvin has been quite successful. The drug does not kill the fungus but prevents its spread into uninfected cells. As the infected cells are shed or removed, they are

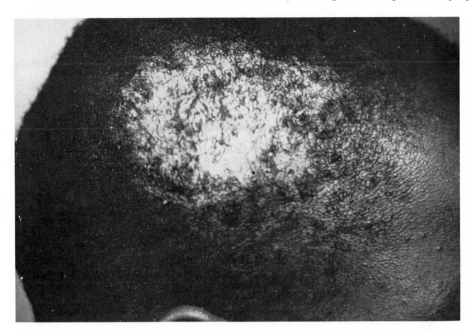

Fig. 32-6. Tinea capitis (ringworm of the scalp). (Courtesy W. W. Duemling, M.D., San Diego, Calif.)

replaced by healthy cells. Clipping of the affected hair after a few weeks of treatment is also desirable. In addition, a local antifungal ointment may be ordered.

Ringworm of the skin is of two main types. One type, *tinea cruris,* involves the groin, and the other, *tinea corporis,* characteristically involves the face, neck, arms, and hands. Although there are exceptions, the classic lesion of ringworm of the skin is rounded or circular with a gradually extending, small, raised vesicular border with central healing. The lesion may vary considerably in size, but it is usually about the size of a quarter. Treatment consists of prevention of scratching and application of one of several topical remedies—ointments containing sulfur and salicylic acid, solutions of gentian violet, or Tinactin (tolnaftate 1%). Local treatment is combined with systemic use of griseofulvin in some cases.

Ringworm of the feet, *tinea pedis,* or so-called athlete's foot, is essentially limited to postpubescent children. Younger children with scaling of the feet usually have some form of eczema. However, it is discussed here with the other types of ringworm. Ringworm of the feet is most often characterized by itching or burning of the feet, blisters, and painful cracks between the toes. At times it may extend to involve other areas and become quite serious. It is caused by several kinds of fungi. Treatment consists of the use of griseofulvin. Better ventilation of the feet and the reduction of sweating in the area are helpful. Frequent changing of socks is a necessity. If the infection has been intense and tends to recur, the advisability of discarding shoes worn during the infection should be considered. Antifungal preparations such as Desenex or Whitfield's ointment are often used locally but are ineffective unless combined with griseofulvin. The feet should be carefully dried. A prophylactic antifungal dusting powder is often advised for susceptible persons. For the protection of other people, victims should not use public showers or swimming pools.

Pediculosis, or louse infestations

Although there are three types of lice—head lice, body lice, and pubic lice—only one type is of significant importance to children, *pediculosis capitis*, or infestation of the hair of the head by lice. This condition is often seen in neglected children of lower socioeconomic levels. However, children who are well cared for may inadvertently become exposed and contract the infestation, much to their parents' shock!

The parasitic head louse causes itching as it travels on the scalp. Small, grayish, oval eggs called *nits* are laid and attached to the base of the hair shafts with a type of mucilage produced by the louse (Fig. 32-

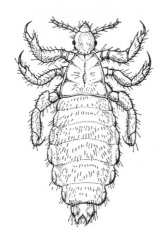

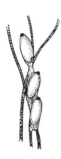

Fig. 32-7. Top, the female head louse; center, an enlargement of nits on hair shafts; bottom, life-sized louse.

7). As the hair grows, the nits become more visible; they resemble tiny flakes of dandruff except that they do not brush out. New lice hatch in 3 or 4 days, and the cycle repeats. Pediculosis is often accompanied by excoriation and secondary infection caused by scratching.

Old-style treatment involved the local use of crude oil or kerosene. More acceptable and very effective are shampoos with gamma benzene hexachloride (Kwell or Gexane). DDT (chlorophenothane) preparations may be ordered. After the end of the treatment, the hair should be combed with a fine-tooth comb to remove the devitalized nits. Warm vinegar solution also aids in the mechanical detachment of nits. The entire family of an affected person should be treated, if possible.

Scabies

Scabies is a superficial infestation by the itch mite *(Acarus scabiei,* or *Sarcoptes scabiei).* The female mite burrows under the skin, making a tunnel about half an inch long, which is visible as an elevated line from the skin's surface. The insect is so small that it is rarely visible to the naked eye. Scabies usually involves those body areas where the skin is moist and thin—between the fingers and toes, in the axillae, and on the groin and abdominal areas. The itch mite causes itching, as the name indicates. Various treatments are now available. Gamma benzene hexachloride (Kwell) may be applied in cream form, or applications of benzyl benzoate emulsion or sulfur may be ordered. Prolonged soap and water baths are usually prescribed before and after the therapy. Again, the entire family of an affected person should receive therapy, if possible.

THE ADOLESCENT
Acne vulgaris

Vulgar means "common," and acne vulgaris is a skin inflammation that is exceedingly common among teen-age boys and girls. It may exist in a very mild form, or it may be extremely severe. There are probably several causes that, appearing together, produce the problem. When acne is present, it first appears, almost without exception, at the time of puberty. Hormone levels in the body are believed to play a role. Many times the parents of the affected child also experienced similar difficulty; therefore, hereditary factors are not discounted.

The sebum, or fatty secretion of the oil glands, is altered by hormones, and several types of skin microorganisms utilize sebum as a food source and change it into irritating fatty acids that cause acne. The pores clog, and blackheads (plugs of keratin, sebum, and microorganisms, also called *comedones,* the primary lesions of acne) form. The pores may also be clogged with dirt, but blackheads are not commonly caused by dirt particles but by oxidation of the top of the plug, a process that may occur no matter how carefully the adolescent washes. Plugging of the oil ducts may lead to papules, pustules, and, at times, cyst formation and permanent scarring.

Since acne most often occurs on the face, shoulders, and back, it is of great cosmetic and psychological concern. The teen-ager should be given professional help during this distressing period so that it is as short and free from complications as possible. Acne fosters a sense of inferiority and social insecurity at a difficult period in life.

Treatment includes a review of general health habits. Little emphasis is now placed on avoidance of carbohydrates and fatty foods such as chocolate, nuts, and peanut butter, and a well-balanced diet is stressed. Lack of sleep, nervous tension, and menstrual problems may lead to a flare-up. Mild cases are treated wtih topical measures such as antibacterial detergent soaps or skin cleansers (Fostex or Acne-Aid) and lotions containing *keratolytic* compounds (salicylic acid, resorcin) and sulfur (Komed, Kummerfeld's) lotion. Girls are advised to avoid oily makeup and moisturizers, but there are numerous tinted antibacterial creams or lotions available that help heal and mask the lesions, a very important psychological

consideration. Frequent shampooing is often very helpful. Patients should be instructed not to press or scratch the lesions because this may break down tissue walls and spread infection. However, despite this advice, most patients find it extremely difficult not to tamper with the lesions they see in the mirror. The physician may remove comedones in his office with a special extractor, or he may give careful instructions to the patient's family regarding the removal of comedones. The drug treatment of choice in advanced cases is either tetracycline or erythromycin to kill the bacteria or hormones to alter the sebum-producing activity of the sebaceous glands.

Usually, acne is self-limiting and subsides in 3 or 4 years. However, severe cases may persist into middle age. The partial removal of scarred tissue may be accomplished, in selected cases, by superficial abrasion, a technique called *dermabrasion.* X-ray treatment is no longer recommended by many dermatologists because of the possibility of causing skin changes later in life and the availability of other therapeutic alternatives.

Herpes simplex

Herpes simplex is a viral infection that often causes an irregular vesicular lesion on the margin of the lip (fever blister) or gums. The blister breaks, and a crust develops and eventually clears. These lesions have a tendency to recur in the same area, causing considerable annoyance, discomfort, and cosmetic concern. Occasionally herpes simplex will take on a more important aspect. It is serious when a newborn infant or very young child is involved because the lesions have a tendency to multiply, and it is serious when the eye is involved because an impairment of vision may result. Local treatment may involve the application of alcohol or ether.

Dermatitis venenata

Dermatitis venenata may be seen at any age; it is an inflammatory skin response resulting from external contact with some irritating substance, such as fibers, plants, synthetics, or adhesive tape. However, it is most often observed in those groups who go hiking in the midst of some poison oak or poison ivy. Signs of skin irritation usually occur several hours after exposure and consist of redness, swelling, and small blisters at the point of contact. Itching is intense. If the patient knows that he has been exposed, the best immediate treatment before the appearance of symptoms is washing the area with a laundry soap and rinsing and drying the area well. Of course, the best course of action is proper identification of the offending plants in the first place and a prudent detour. After the blisters have developed, the urge to scratch must be resisted to prevent spreading. Calamine lotion and cortisone preparations applied locally may help relieve itching.

BURNS

Another problem, which primarily involves the skin but may finally affect many organs and processes of the body, is burns. Burns may be caused by exposure to hot liquids, strong chemicals, direct flame, radiation, sunlight, or electrical current. Toddlers and young children are most often scalded by hot coffee, grease from frying pans, or hot water from unguarded bathroom faucets. Older children are frequently burned when their clothes catch fire while they are playing with matches, using kerosene, or standing too close to household heaters. In the United States approximately 5,000 children are hospitalized because of burns on a given day.

Classification

Burns are classified into four categories, depending on the depth of penetration of the body's surface.

A *first-degree* burn (partial thickness) involves only the epidermis. It is very superficial; a tender, slightly swollen redness results. A common illustration of a first degree burn is the typical summer sunburn. A *second-degree* burn (partial thickness) involves the epidermis and dermis. This cat-

egory is further divided into superficial and deep dermal burns. Some epidermal appendages must be intact in order for these burns to heal spontaneously. Deep dermal burns may change from partial-thickness to full-thickness wounds by infection, trauma, or obliteration of the blood supply to the affected part. A second-degree burn is characterized by blister formation or a reddened, discolored region with a moist, weeping surface. A *third-degree* burn (full thickness) involves the entire dermis and portions of the subcutaneous tissue. The region affected has a brown, leathery appearance with little surface moisture. A *fourth-degree* burn (full thickness) involves subcutaneous tissue, fascia, muscle, and perhaps bone. The tissue appears blackened and contracted. Partial-thickness burns have the ability to heal without grafting. Full-thickness burns need to be grafted in order to heal. It is not always easy to evaluate the depth of a burn immediately after the injury.

It is not only the degree of burn that is significant but also the amount of body surface affected. A person can usually survive a rather extensive superficial burn, but he may tolerate a deep burn only if a small area is involved. In evaluating the extent of a burn on an adult, the so-called rule of nines may be applied; it gives a certain percentage value to each part of the body—a percentage that is almost always nine or a multiple of nine. This method of calculation, unless modified, is not helpful when working with children because of the relatively large size of a baby's or young child's head and the reduced length of his legs. (One example of modification based on size differences is illustrated in Fig. 32-8.)

The area, extent, and depth of a burn determines its severity, and treatment is planned according to severity. *Minor burns* are described as partial-thickness first- or second-degree burns covering less than 15% of the body surface and not involving strategic areas such as the face, hands, feet, or genitalia. Minor burns are treated on an

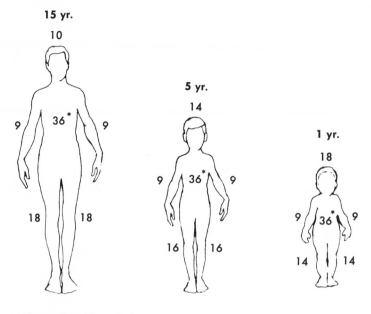

15 yr.

5 yr.

1 yr.

*18 anterior, 18 posterior

Fig. 32-8. Modification of the "rule of nines." (Courtesy Burns Institute, Galveston Unit, Shriners Hospital for Crippled Children.)

outpatient basis. *Moderate burns* are described as partial-thickness second-degree burns covering over 15% but less than 30% of body surface or as full-thickness burns involving less than 10% of body surface. Moderate burns usually require hospitalization. *Major burns* are described as partial-thickness second-degree burns covering at least 30% of the body surface or as full-thickness third-degree burns involving the face, hands, feet, or genitalia or more than 10% of the body surface. Children with major burns always require hospitalization.

Therapeutic management and nursing responsibility
Initial considerations

Any person who is at the scene when someone is burned should first extinguish the fire if the victim's clothes are aflame. If an abundant source of water from a hose or bucket is readily available, it should be used; if not, handy blankets or throw rugs may be employed to smother the flames, since fire cannot continue in the absence of oxygen. If neither water nor blankets are available, the victim should be rolled on the ground or floor to help smother the flames. When the fire has been extinguished, the burned area should be rinsed with cold water. The victim should be taken immediately to a physician's office or, preferably, a hospital for evaluation and care. He should be transported wrapped in a clean sheet and blanket. Time should not be lost in trying to remove the child's clothes. No medication of any type should be administered.

When a burned child is admitted to an emergency room or other hospital receiving area, his clothes should be removed gently, cutting along the seams of the garments if necessary. He should be placed on and covered by sterile sheets in a room with good lighting. All those in attendance should wear face masks. Those in contact with the patient should be provided with sterile gowns and gloves. The severity of his burns will be estimated by the attending physician, and the need for hospitalization will be determined.

Minor burns. Care of minor burns usually consists of cleansing the area with mild soap and water. The technique of immediately immersing the area briefly in cold water or holding an ice cube on the injured surface to reduce pain and edema has become quite popular. The area may be covered with a fine mesh gauze lightly lubricated with an antiseptic or antimicrobial cream. It should be secured with a lightly compressing stretch gauze bandage. The child's tetanus immunization should be validated and given if not documented up-to-date. Acetaminophen (Tylenol) may be prescribed for pain, and the patient should be seen by the physician in 48 hours.

Moderate or major burns. The first phase of therapy when moderate or major burns are present is the maintenance of an *airway* and the prevention of *shock*. The airway is not a problem in all cases, but occasionally, because of the location of the external burn, the inhalation of fumes, or internal burning of the respiratory tract, it is of great importance. An endotracheal tube may be needed. The administration of oxygen may be required. A Levin tube may be inserted to prevent the onset of gastric dilation and paralytic ileus, two complications often resulting from major burns.

Intravenous fluid therapy is usually initiated. In young children cutdowns are performed. With second- and third-degree burns there is danger of great fluid loss and an upset in electrolyte balance. A urinary catheter is usually inserted because the amount and type of urine formation per hour is important in determining the rate of intravenous therapy and providing an index of the patient's general condition. A dwindling urinary output may serve as a warning of developing hypovolemia. A urinary output of 0.5 to 0.1 ml./kg. per hour for a child is desirable. An adult's output would approximate 50 to 60 ml. per hour. Signs of overhydration revealed by excessive output require a reduction in fluids given intravenously. The urinary catheter output should be observed frequently and recorded hourly. Specific gravity determi-

nations are frequently ordered. It is extremely important to report irregularities in the urinary output, the loss of a urine specimen, or an error in the measurement of a urine specimen because of the danger of miscalculating the need for and amount of intravenous therapy. Many blood tests also help determine the kind of fluids that are needed. Frequent hemoglobin and hematocrit studies are carried out. Blood gas studies may be ordered. Overloading the circulatory system is a real possibility unless great care is exercised. Blood typing and cross matching are performed in the event that transfusions may be necessary. The patient is weighed to provide a base line for subsequent weight loss or gain. Vital signs are checked frequently, although meaningful blood pressure readings may be difficult to secure because of the age of the child and the location of the burn area. Some children need central venous pressure determinations.

Hospitalized children with serious burns are treated with low doses of parenteral penicillin to prevent infection by the beta-hemolytic streptococcus. Penicillin is given immediately and during the first 2 or 3 days of treatment to the nonsensitive patient. Thereafter, antibiotics are given as indicated by the patient's clinical course and specific cultures of the wound. Pain medication is administered intravenously to help control shock. There is more pain accompanying a partial-thickness burn than a full-thickness burn because in the partial-thickness burn some nerve endings are still intact. The shock phase of the body's response to extensive burns is usually considered to last from 48 to 72 hours. Most hospitals routinely isolate their burn patients in an effort to prevent or reduce infection.

The vocational nurse should not be assigned the total bedside responsibility of a severely burned child during this critical period, although she may skillfully assist the registered nurse in important aspects of the care. The vocational nurse must understand the principles of the patient's treatment, and as the patient's condition becomes more stable, she will participate more fully in his care.

Types of treatment

Partial-thickness, second-degree burns and full-thickness burns may be treated in several ways—the closed method, the open or exposure method, the modified exposure method, or the silver nitrate regimen. More than one technique may be used with one patient, depending on his needs.

Closed method. If the burned area is relatively small and hospitalization is not indicated, the closed method is usually preferred. When the closed method is chosen for more extensive burns, the treatment involves covering the burned area with various dressings and bandages: first, a sterile gauze impregnated with ointment; next, sterile compresses or fluffs; followed by sterile gauze bandage, Kerlix, or Kling and cotton padding and a snug covering of stockinette. Depending on the condition of the dressing, the condition of the patient, and the physician's preference, this dressing may be left on without disturbance for more than a week, or orders may be written for the inner dressing to be soaked and removed at specific intervals to help in the cleaning of the wound and separation of dead tissue from the burned area. This may be done in the form of Betadine tub baths, whirlpool treatments, or local soaks. All dressing materials should be ready to reapply in a sterile manner after the soak. Through soaks and redressing and/or intermittent surgical debridements, the burned areas are cleaned and the developing granulation tissue is prepared for grafting. Granulation tissue is a deep pink, fragile tissue that bleeds easily. When the tissue is sufficiently prepared, the child will undergo grafting. Donor sites are selected on the patient himself. (Donations from other individuals [other than an identical twin] may "take" temporarily but are later rejected. Such grafts are used to cover the wound and prevent infection in the preparation for skin autographs.) The donor site is usually covered with fine gauze and a pres-

sure dressing. Later, when bleeding has been controlled, the outer pressure dressing may be removed. Donor sites heal in about 2 weeks. The newly grafted area is kept covered. The dressing should be observed for amount and type of drainage and odor. Exposed adjacent areas should be observed for edema and circulatory problems. Grafts are usually firmly attached by the twelfth day after the grafting procedure.

Open method. The open method is particularly helpful in treating children with extensive burns. This method of burn therapy necessitates rigid isolation technique because no dressings are used in the initial period of burn care. A significant advance in the care of these children is the bacteria-controlled nursing unit (BCNU). It consists of a 6- by 10-foot transparent plastic enclosure around the patient's bed. The bed is made with sterile sheets and mattress pad; the air is filtered, humidified, and warmed to keep the child from shivering. The nurse stands outside the unit and puts on shoulder-length gauntlets before inserting her arms through the portals to care for the child. If it is necessary to go inside the unit, personnel must put on a cap, mask, waterproof disposable gown, and sterile gloves; and the door to the unit is opened by another person. These units in combination with new surgical methods of treating burns have resulted in a sharp drop in septic complications. The open method of treatment allows greater motion, reduces the incidence of contractures (thereby speeding rehabilitation), allows direct observation of the involved areas for complications, and reduces odor.

When the open method is used for the immediate care of moderate and major burns, it usually includes washing the involved areas with a physiological saline solution or distilled water, depending on the type of treatment to follow. At the time of admission, the loose skin and blisters of partial-thickness burns are surgically removed by the physician in a procedure called debridement. Full-thickness major burns are now being treated soon after admission by primary (tangential) excision. In the operating room under hypotensive anesthesia, which minimizes bleeding, devitalized burned tissue is cut down to the fascia, and skin grafts are immediately applied. The *immediate coverage* of the burn wound with grafts, medication, or pigskin following debridement or primary excision is very important to the child's recovery. Such treatment should forestall pain, fluid loss, and infection and provide the best environment for reepithelization. Pigskin (a porcine heterograft) serves as an excellent temporary resurfacing material when applied early to debrided partial-thickness, deep

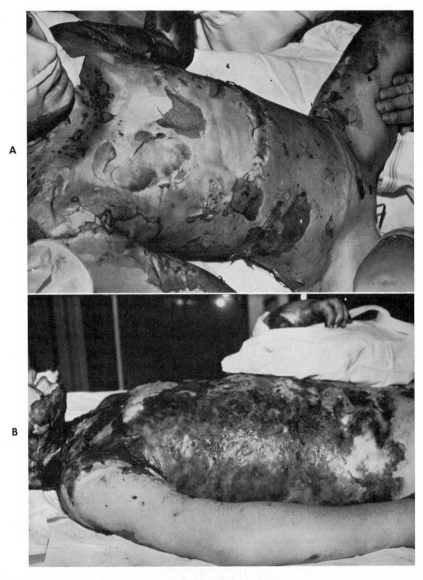

Fig. 32-9. **A,** This 6-year-old child has just been admitted into an emergency room because of second- and third-degree burns. She is receiving oxygen by nasal cannula. **B,** Open therapy was the treatment used. A heavy eschar formed over the trunk. **C,** Escharatomy incisions performed to permit deeper respirations. (Courtesy Matthew Gleason, M.D., San Diego, Calif.)

dermal burns. The pigskin adheres tightly to the debrided burns, and pain subsides. The pigskin survives by diffusion exchange with the host dermis for 1 to 3 weeks. The child feels better and can ambulate early. Changes are rarely needed because exudate and crusting are absent. Epithelial regeneration takes place beneath the pigskin as early as the fourth or fifth day. Gradually the edges of the graft dry, and as healing takes place, the graft peels off. Many people believe that the use of pigskin for partial-thickness, deep dermal burns is a preferable alternative to topical antibiotic treatment. A superior surface without hypertrophic scarring is found 1 to 3 years later. When pigskin is not used to cover partial-thickness burns, the open method causes the gradual natural formation of eschar, a thick black crust composed of the drying wound secretions. This crust serves as a temporary, partial protection against infection. In the case of the little girl in Fig. 32-9, an incision through the eschar was required to release pressure and permit adequate respirations. During this period the nurse may be ordered to gently wash the burned areas with an antibacterial solution and rinse with physiological saline solution. Days later the eschar will begin to separate, and the physician will cut away portions of the dried crust, revealing new granulation tissue. When the granulation tissue is exposed by removal of the eschar, antibiotic-impregnated gauze is usually laid over the open granulation areas. Debridements may continue daily in the nursing unit, or less often, in the operating room.

Full-thickness major burns are preferably covered with autografts, grafts from another part of the patient's body. When a very large area is burned, porcine heterografts or homografts from a cadaver or living donor are used to cover the excised area. These biological dressings seal the raw surface in the preparation for skin autografts.

After surgery, the child is placed in protective isolation or in the BCNU. Twenty-four hour personalized nursing care is essential with particular attention to respiratory therapy, nutrition, the newly grafted area, and the prevention of complications. The use of biological dressings and the BCNU in the treatment of deep dermal and full-thickness burns has revolutionized the treatment and rehabilitation of burn patients.

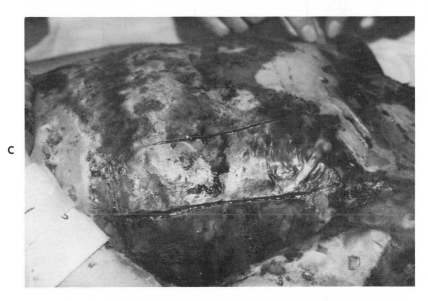

Fig. 32-9, cont'd. For legend see opposite page.

Modified exposure method. With the advent of various ointments and creams that have proved useful in combating common wound contaminants, a kind of modified open therapy has evolved. The patient is usually placed on sterile precautions as well as routine isolation. No occlusive dressings are used. A thin layer of the medication may be applied directly to the injured area with a sterile glove or tongue blade, or the medication may be embedded in sterile gauze strips that are positioned as needed. A spray form may also be available. Some drugs currently employed are as follows:

1. Mafenide acetate (Sulfamylon acetate cream), 10%: This water-soluble medication is particularly helpful in preventing pseudomonal infections.

Each day it should be completely removed for wound inspection by irrigations or baths. It is reapplied every 12 hours or more frequently as necessary. It causes an intense burning sensation when first applied, which is diminished if the cream can be applied directly after the irrigation or bath while the wound is still damp. Allergic reactions (itching and hives) may occur. Acid-base imbalance (acidosis) associated with its use has caused it to lose favor.

2. Povidone-iodine kills both gram-negative and gram-positive bacteria (including antibiotic-resistant strains), viruses, fungi, protozoa, and yeasts. Betadine solution and Betadine ointment contain 10% povidone-iodine; Betadine aerosol spray contains 5% povidone-iodine. It is a film-forming, water-soluble iodine complex that does not sting or stain. It is not associated with electrolyte loss or disturbances in acid-base balance.

The burn wound and surrounding area is initially cleansed with Betadine solution and debrided. In the open method, Betadine solution is applied every 2 hours until healing starts; it may be dabbed with a sterile swab or used as a wet soak or spray. After healing begins, the application varies from every 8 hours to once daily throughout the patient's hospital stay. In addition to specific antiseptic treatment of the burn wound, a total bath (which may include shampooing the hair), using lower concentrations of Betadine solution, is administered at least once a day.

When Betadine ointment is used, three applications to the burn wound are recommended daily, and Betadine aerosol spray may be used periodically throughout the day on areas where it is difficult to maintain the application of the ointment. In the closed technique, impregnated gauze is placed on the burn site and additional ointment is applied to the gauze 4 times a day. The dressing is preceded by a daily whirlpool bath containing Betadine Whirlpool Concentrate.

3. Silver sulfadiazine ointment: This drug is designed to combine the best features of mafenide acetate and silver nitrate therapy. It is active against *Pseudomonas*, painless on application, stainless, and not associated with acid-base imbalance.

Silver nitrate therapy. The old method of treating burns with silver nitrate solution has undergone modification and a dramatic revival. After an initial wash with distilled water, the burned area is flooded with 0.5% silver nitrate solution. The use of this antiseptic is continued by the application of thick saturated compresses directly against the burned surfaces. The dressings must not be allowed to dry out. Saturation may often be maintained with greatest ease by the incorporation of multieyed catheters within the gauze layers. A syringe is used to inject tepid silver nitrate into the exposed end of the catheters to moisten the dressing. To reduce the heat loss that may occur with this treatment, the area compressed should be covered with a dry, but *not* water-tight, sheet or blanket. A clean rather than a rigid sterile technique is sufficient during these treatments. The constant compressing is interrupted only for special salt solution baths (to help maintain the body's fluid balance) and intermittent debridements. Careful, frequent blood studies must be carried out to be certain that electrolyte imbalance does not occur because of the possibility of excessive sodium and chloride loss through the burn site. The use of the silver nitrate therapy has greatly reduced the incidence of infection. It reduces or prevents odor, decreases the need for skin grafting, and usually allows earlier placement of grafts. It also permits greater mobility and therefore seems less likely to be associated with lasting functional loss.

However, this treatment also presents certain peculiar problems. Silver nitrate, although colorless when poured from the opaque storage container, rapidly forms a black stain on almost everything it touches. Unfortunately, it seems to touch almost everything, even when care is used. Bed linen, floors, shoes, uniforms, and woodwork are not exempt! In an effort to be more protected against the black stains, nurses and physicians participating in silver nitrate treatment usually adopt rather unprofessional-appearing dress. Plastic sacks may be cut to allow the head and arms to protrude in a workable manner, and plastic aprons, if available, may be used. Footwear is protected with smaller plastic sacks, or old shoes are worn. Cotton cover gowns that have already been worn during silver nitrate treatment are also worn over the plastic gowns. They may be stained, but they are clean. One burn service reports that they have dyed the linen used on their area a deep chocolate brown. The theory must be, "If one can't beat it, join it!" Rubber gloves are included to protect the hands, particularly the nails. Many stains on fabric can be removed with a solution of iodophor (Wescodyne), 1 ounce to 1 gallon of water, followed by a bleach or exposure to sunshine. Wescodyne is also used to help clean the room. The floor should be covered with plastic. Only old and necessary furnishings should be used.

With this treatment, the patient's skin will become dark and scaly. The film can be gradually washed or peeled off, depending on the areas involved and the physician's wishes. Participating in silver nitrate therapy is a fascinating and unforgettable experience.

Continuing concerns

No matter what methods of burn therapy are selected, all treatment is done to accomplish the following aims:
1. Preserve life
2. Promote healing
3. Prevent infection
4. Prevent deformity
5. Provide emotional and physical rehabilitation

An important part of the nurse's responsibility is the provision of a good nutritional intake. Initially the child with extensive burns will probably be maintained on intravenous hyperalimentation, but fairly soon he may be fed orally with or without a nasogastric tube, depending on his progress. It is very important for the nurse to keep an accurate record of all nourishment and fluids taken. Many physicians will demand a detailed daily intake record kept to be analyzed by the dietitian for caloric and foodstuff (protein, fat, carbohydrate, and mineral) content. Protein consumption is particularly important. Usually supplemental vitamins and iron will be ordered. Vitamin C and zinc are substances believed to be particularly helpful in aiding tissue healing.

A stress lesion called *Curling's ulcer* sometimes develops in burn patients. Nurses should be alert for signs of blood in the stool or nasogastric tube. The child's appetite should not be discouraged with servings that are too large. Feedings should be judiciously planned. The patient should not be expected to eat directly after an exhausting dressing change. A different schedule for the kitchen on some days or better planning of ward procedures on other days may be necessary, but the patient should receive his meals when he can best *eat*. Likes and dislikes should be noted. Sometimes permission to bring food in from home brings forth happy cooperation on the part of both parents and child. The child must be weighed periodically to help determine his nutritional status.

The immediate and long-term positioning of a seriously burned patient is critical in preventing extensive deformity. Although the position of flexion may be the position of greatest comfort to the patient, it will also become the cause of crippling contractures. The posture of extension (Fig. 32-10, A) may at first appear "heartless" but, in the final analysis, such placement of the head and extremities may save the patient weeks, if not months, of needless hospital-

ization and additional pain. The hand brace in Fig 32-10, B, is designed to prevent the development of a claw-type deformity. Note the forced extension of the fingers. This splint and the neck splint pictured in Fig. 32-10, C, are made of a type of plastic, "Orthoplast" Isoprene, that, when molded and fitted to the individual patient, has been quite successful in preventing de-

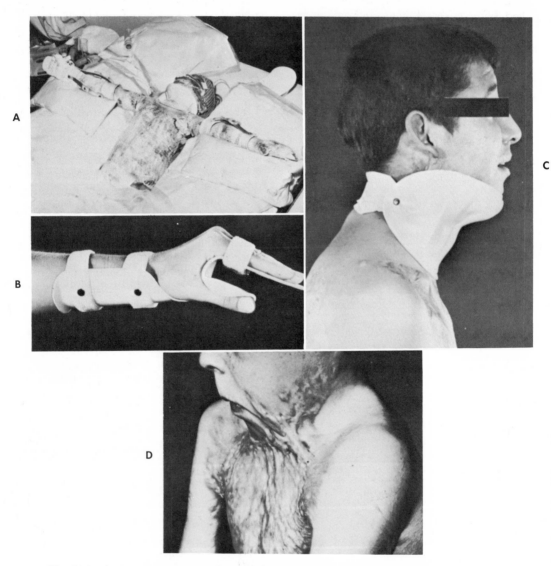

Fig. 32-10. A, Routine positioning for severely burned pateint with lesions involving the trunk, arms, neck, and face. Neck, arm, and hand splints have been applied. Oxygen and mist are being administered. **B,** An "Orthoplast" Isoprene hand splint. Note the extended fingers. **C,** An "Orthoplast" Isoprene neck splint. **D,** An example of the condition the neck splint is designed to help prevent—severe contractures of the chin and neck. (From Willis, Barbara: Am. J. Occup. Ther. **24:**187-191, 1970 [**A, C,** and **D**]; **23:**57-61, 1969 [**B**].)

formities (Fig. 32-10, *D*) that had previously been difficult to avoid. They are applied over a mafenide acetate gauze dressing almost immediately after the patient is admitted. These helpful devices were developed at the Shriners Burns Institute, Galveston Unit, under the direction of the charge occupational therapist, Barbara Willis.*

Active and passive exercises of the affected body parts, if neglected when ordered, may retard convalescence significantly. It is the responsibility of the nurse (and the physical therapy staff) to see that these important movements, which the patient often resists, are carried out. Appropriate exercises plus good positioning to avoid flexion contractures can make a big contribution to the early rehabilitation of the patient (Fig. 32-10).

During the entire period of treatment and observation of the extensively burned patient, the morale of the parents and their child is of tremendous importance. Often the parents feel guilty concerning their child's accident. They may be appalled at the condition of the child and his appearance. Some will be overly protective; others may hardly be able to make themselves approach the child. All will be extremely upset whether they appear so or not. The child may have serious guilt feelings if he considers himself responsible for his injury.

---

*Willis, B.: The use of Orthoplast Isoprene splints in the treatment of the acutely burned child: preliminary report, Am. J. Occup. Ther. **23**:57-61, 1969. Willis, B.: The use of Orthoplast Isoprene splints in the treatment of the acutely burned child: a follow-up, Am. J. Occup. Ther. **24**:187-191, 1970.

Some of these children have had a history of emotional disturbance before their accident. Good communication between the physician, the nursing staff, the parents, and the burned patient is essential. A feeling of acceptance and freedom to talk and not feel criticized for talking are important for both the child and his parents. Simple explanations of treatments take time at the beginning, but they save much time and anguish later on. Nursing personnel, as well as the patient and his parents, may need psychiatric support in carrying out their roles.

Rehabilitation

The rehabilitation of a burned child may be long and exhausting, but despite the pain and fatigue, the end result is well worth the continuing effort. Fortunately, with the use of new surgical techniques the time needed for rehabilitation promises to become much shorter. Splinting, traction, and frequent visits to the physical therapy department's pool or exercise room may be necessary. Plastic surgery may be needed in some cases to relieve contractures or remove keloid formation (exaggerated scar tissue). Special tutoring or educational provisions may be required to prevent educational loss, and social contacts must be maintained, particularly in the case of older children. A positive, constructive attitude toward therapy should be encouraged.

Patients who have been seriously burned will probably be among the nurse's most challenging and difficult responsibilities. They will also be among her most rewarding.

33

Isolation technique and communicable childhood diseases

The student nurse often contemplates her experience with patients suffering from contagious disease with a fascinating mixture of eager anticipation and fear. Both these emotions, when under control, work to her advantage. There is much to learn about the needs of the patients and about safe methods of meeting these needs in this nursing area. There are new words, new techniques, and a new awareness of the unseen. The student must be impressed with the importance of carrying out the isolation, or barrier, techniques recognized in the area where she is working. Any lapse in technique by *anyone* jeopardizes other patients, the entire staff, and, indeed, perhaps the entire hospital.

However, the student nurse should also appreciate that in a number of ways she is probably working in the safest part of the hospital. In the isolation area, precautions are taken that are not observed elsewhere. Nurses in other hospital areas may inadvertently be exposed to contagious conditions without precautions because the conditions, although present, may be undetectable.

KEY VOCABULARY

The following list includes some of the new words the nurse may encounter when working in an isolation area:

communicable or *contagious diseases* disorders caused by small living forms (organisms) or their toxins, which may be passed directly (from person to person) or indirectly (from person to inanimate object, airborne particles, or other living creatures that continue the spread of disease to other persons).

infectious diseases disorders caused by small living forms (organisms) that invade tissue and cause symptoms of illness. (Most infectious diseases are also communicable, but there are exceptions. A person who is suffering from tetanus but has no draining wound would not have to be on isolation precautions; neither would a person with a disease caused by an organism that is present everywhere but causes disease only when introduced unnaturally into the body, such as, an *Escherichia coli* urinary tract infection.)

contaminated in isolation technique, or medical asepsis, this adjective is applied to any person or thing that has touched a patient with a contagious disaese, has touched anything the patient has touched, or has undergone prolonged exposure to such a patient before proper disinfection has occurred. (The student may remember that the word "contaminated" used in a surgical setting means "touched by anything not sterile." In isolation technique it means "touched directly or indirectly by the patient or his excretions or discharges.")

portal of entry the way that infections gain entrance into a person's body, for example, respiratory tract, digestive tract, skin, and mucous membranes, with or without the aid of living creatures (such as insects or mites).

incubation period time that must elapse between the infection of an individual at a time of exposure until the appearance of signs or symptoms of the disease.

carrier person or animal capable of transmitting a contagious disease while showing no outward sign of the disease.

isolation the observance of certain barrier techniques designed to stop the spread of illness by preventing direct or indirect contact with a person with a contagious disease during its period of communicability.

quarantine confinement of a person or group of persons who have been exposed to a contagious disease to a specific place without outside contacts for the duration of the longest usual incubation period of the disease in question.

immunity ability to protect oneself against the development of an infectious disease. Immunity may be natural or acquired. *Natural immunity* may be hereditary—related to racial strengths and the individual capacity for protective antibody formation. It may involve transfer of maternal antibodies to the fetus. *Acquired immunity* may be *active,* with formation of protective antibodies as a result of having actually contracted the disease or of having been exposed to milder or related forms of the organism that causes the disease. Acquired immunity may also be *passive,* with protection gained through the introduction of antibodies already manufactured by some other living creature against a certain disease-producing organism (immune serum globulin [ISG]). Active immunity is relatively long lasting and more desirable than passive immunity. Passive protection is immediate but relatively brief, and there can be unfavorable reactions experienced because of the use of sera from animals.

vaccine preparation containing killed or weakened living microorganisms, which, when introduced into the body, cause the formation of antibodies against that type of organism and thereby protect the individual from the disease.

toxoid preparation containing a toxin or poison produced by pathogenic organisms; it is capable of producing active immunity against a disease but too weak to produce the disease itself.

antitoxin preparation, often *horse serum* rich in specific antibodies, designed to produce passive immunization. (The antitoxins are produced by injecting a horse with a toxoid; after a period of time, antibodies are manufactured and identified in the horse's blood serum; this serum is modified for injection. Some people are allergic to the serum containing the antibodies. Extreme caution must be taken in administering antitoxin.)

ADMISSION TO AN ISOLATION UNIT
Parental needs and fears

Almost without exception, admission to the hospital is a period of strain for the parents and child. The anxiety and feeling of helplessness often experienced by parents is increased considerably when the admission necessitates the use of certain barrier techniques or entry into a special nursing unit labeled "Isolation." The sight of the medical and nursing staff wearing gowns and perhaps masks and the sound of such potentially alarming terms as "contaminated" and "contagious" does not tend to reassure parents. Everything seem so strange. Disquieting and not always accurate deductions often disturb their peace of mind. "If Johnny has to be here, he must be terribly ill. I wonder what the other children here have. Couldn't Johnny catch something else from them?" Parents need a lot of support and instruction at such a time, and both physicians and nurses must contribute the necessary time and effort to provide it.

Unit preparation

Usually the admission of a new patient is anticipated, and an individual isolation unit is set up before his arrival. Patients are not placed in the same room unless it is confirmed that their diagnoses are the same and the attending physicians involved grant permission. The room should be comfortably warm and well ventilated. In addition to a correctly sized bed or crib, bedside stand, and overbed table found in all standard patient units, an isolation unit should include the following items:

1. Laundry hamper and two plastic laundry bags
2. Clothes tree or rack where gowns (if they must be reused) may be hung in a special way
3. Plastic bags for wrapping or collecting objects for home transport and for collecting and preparing trash for discard
4. Disinfectant used to wipe down the furniture after the patient's basic care
5. Antibacterial detergent (such as Betadine) for hand and arm care of the attendants
6. Access to a sink, running water, and a toilet
7. Paper towels in a dispenser
8. Knife, fork, spoon, as needed
9. Clean masks, gowns, and gloves readily available

The following articles, usually necessary for an admission, should also be at hand:

1. Appropriately sized gown or pajamas; diapers and pins, if appropriate
2. Bath towel set
3. Washbasin and emesis basin
4. Bedpan and/or urinal, toilet paper or wipes

5. Coloplast bag or other means to help obtain a urine specimen from an infant or young child, if appropriate

6. Correctly sized blood pressure cuff (plastic coated if possible) and sphygmomanometer

7. Thermometer, petrolatum, and cellulose wipes

8. Scales, properly draped and balanced

9. Soap, lotion or powder, toothbrush and toothpaste, and comb (To cut down on waste, dispensable supplies in small sample sizes are often used.)

10. Emergency equipment, oxygen, and suction machines, as indicated.

It is important that all equipment be in readiness because much time is lost if the nurse must leave the patient to obtain equipment. However, unnecessary equipment should not be brought into the unit, since it would be needlessly exposed to contamination and could not be used for other patients without the completion of certain procedures to render it noninfectious. The safety of an individual patient's unit also depends on adequate, well-planned utility and laundry rooms.

Admission modifications in isolation

Unless a special order is written, usually only parents or legal guardians are allowed to visit a patient in isolation.

In our opinion, the mother should be allowed to put on a gown and be with and assist the child during the admission in most instances. After all, she has already been exposed to the infection, and the reassurance the child gains by her presence is usually significant.

The child's clothes are usually placed in a clean bag and returned to the parents.

Questions are often asked. "What do we do with Johnny's clothes when we get them home?" "What about all the things that Johnny used at home while he was sick?" In most cases it is sufficient to tell the parents to wash his clothes separately, using a hot setting on an automatic washer, regu-

lar laundry detergent, and 1 cup of household bleach if the clothes are colorfast.

If the patient has been placed in strict isolation and no machine is available, colorfast fabrics may be washed by hand after soaking at least 10 minutes in hot water with laundry detergent and 1 ounce of household bleach per gallon of water. It is recommended that any white cotton be boiled 10 minutes in water before using the washing methods described above. Silk, wool, and nonfast colors may be washed by hand or machine in warm water and detergent with the addition of a phenolic household disinfectant such as Lysol (1 cup per machine load or 1 ounce per gallon of water for hand washing). Clothes should be rinsed at least three times if hand washed or washed a second time, without the addition of phenols, if a machine is used. The utensils or machine used may also be disinfected with the use of a chlorine solution rinse.

The former sickroom or sickrooms should be carefully cleaned (preferably vacuumed), damp dusted, and well aired. Objects that the child had handled should, whenever possible, be washed and exposed to sunshine for at least a day. Objects difficult to clean and relatively unimportant probably are best discarded. If the disease is of a serious nature, the discard of some types of objects, for example, stuffed animals, would be preferable. After all, stuffed animals, or their reasonable facsimilies, are usually replaceable. People are not!

The parents should be shown where they may store their coats and purses outside the patient's room when visiting and where the supply of clean gowns are kept and how to put them on. They should be taught simply to take the gowns off, place them in the laundry hamper, and wash their hands just before leaving, and open the door with a paper towel. They should be told to always check at the nurses' desk before taking anything in to the child, since all objects cannot be adequately disinfected, and if an article is brought to a child with a serious disease, it may have to be destroyed when the child goes home. This might cause unnecessary distress! Expendable toys are therefore encouraged. (Television sets may be available for entertainment; check on this for older children.)

When weighing an isolated patient, the nurse must drape and balance the scale before bringing it into the patient's room. The child is weighed and the drape discarded in the laundry hamper. The scale is then cleaned and sprayed with disinfectant.

A urine specimen is collected in the usual way, except that when the specimen has been obtained in the Coloplast bag, bedpan, or urinal, the specimen container to be sent to the laboratory is held by a "clean nurse" while the "contaminated nurse" pours the specimen. The clean nurse is responsible for capping and labeling the specimen. Stool specimens may be collected in a similar manner, using tongue blades to lift the specimen to the cardboard container. If only one nurse is available, the open specimen container may be set on a clean technique paper (a clean paper towel). The stool is then transferred, and the nurse ungowns, washes her hands, covers the specimen, and labels it outside the patient's room. The outside of any specimen container to be sent to the laboratory must always be clean.

ISOLATION TECHNIQUE
Types of isolation

Isolation techniques are designed to accomplish two main objectives: to prevent the spread of any communicable disease that the isolated patient may have and to protect the isolated patient from any outside source of infection.

The first objective is accomplished by erecting barriers between the patient, his environment, and his bodily excretions or discharges and the rest of the hospital and hospital staff. Special protective coverings may be worn by the nursing staff, and special hand-washing instructions are observed. Articles *coming out* of the unit, that is, articles that have been exposed to the

patient for a prolonged period or that have directly contacted his person or his unit, must generally undergo some type of disinfection. This technique also helps to reduce the introduction of secondary infection from outside the unit because the attendants usually wear gowns that are worn nowhere else in the hospital over their uniforms while directly caring for patients.

When the second objective is paramount, as in the care of a noninfectious newborn infant, a type of reverse isolation is practiced. Sterilized linens, clothing, and sterile attendants' gowns and masks may be required, or a clean technique may be judged sufficient. Good hand washing before and after patient care is stressed. No special precautions are taken to remove objects and materials from the room, but there are restrictions regarding the kind of things *going into* the room for use. This same type of technique may be employed with certain burn cases. In fact, burn cases may require the observance of both kinds of isolation techniques concurrently. (This makes nursing doubling interesting and the laundry problem tremendous!) Reverse isolation may also be employed with leukemic children receiving immunosuppressive therapy in the hospital. However, patients on reverse isolation are not routinely treated in a nursing area that serves patients with contagious diseases. Students working in the regular isolation wing usually will not have both types of isolation to deal with, unless a burn patient is ordered on double isolation technique or a child with leukemia develops a contagious complication.

For a long time many hospitals routinely practiced only three categories of formal isolation: strict, regular (or routine), and protective. All forms employed careful hand washing procedures and observance of medical asepsis, but they differed in the details of implementation. Strict isolation usually implied that a gown, mask, and perhaps gloves were used and that the gown could be worn only once. It was employed in those cases in which the infection was airborne and/or of a particularly

505

serious nature. Regular, or routine, isolation implied the use of a gown, with the possibility of its reuse, but not masks or gloves. Protective isolation generally included clean or sterile gowns and masks, depending on the special needs of the patient in jeopardy of infection. However, these three types did not always emphasize the source of infection and mode of transmission of a specific disease and at times imposed greater or less restriction on the patient and his nurse than is now considered necessary.

In 1970, staff members of the Center for Disease Control of the Department of Health, Education, and Welfare in Atlanta, Georgia, prepared for government publication a booklet entitled "Isolation Techniques for Use in Hospitals." This publication describes five different types of isolation, or precautionary techniques, based on the characteristics of the disease and the patient being treated. These different types of isolation may be modified as necessary to fit the individual needs of patients and different patient care areas. All techniques involve *good hand washing* on entering and leaving the room as well as limitation of visitors. In modified summary they are as follows.

1. *Strict isolation* includes a private room with the door kept closed; gowns, masks, and gloves on entering room; and special discard or disinfection of articles. Examples of diseases requiring strict isolation are: staphylococcal and streptococcal pneumonias and congenital rubella syndrome.

2. *Respiratory isolation* includes a private room with the door kept closed, masks for those who must enter the room and who are susceptible to the disease, and special discard or disinfection of articles contaminated with secretions. Gowns and gloves are not considered necessary. Examples of diseases requiring respiratory isolation are: chicken pox, rubeola (2-week measles), pertussis, and pulmonary tuberculosis.

Note: Pediatric nurses routinely wear overgowns with young children on respiratory isolation because of their developmental level. Barrier gowns are used when caring for all infants and toddlers, whether isolated or not. To help prevent spread of the airborne organisms, patients needing respiratory isolation are best placed in a specially ventilated double-doored room that exerts a slight negative pressure when entered, thereby retaining contaminated air.

3. *Protective isolation* includes a private room with the door kept closed, gowns and masks on entering room, and gloves worn by all persons having direct contact with the patient. Articles brought into room should be clean. In some hospitals and situations, all linen in direct contact with the patient is sterilized prior to use. Mattresses and pillows should be covered with impervious, clean plastic. Use of only fresh cleaning equipment is necessary for such units. Persons requiring protective isolation include certain patients receiving immunosuppressive therapy and those with extensive skin lesions vulnerable to infection.

4. *Enteric precautions* include a private room for children, gowns and gloves for persons in direct contact with either the patient or articles contaminated with fecal material, and special discard or disinfection of articles contaminated with urine or feces. Examples of diseases requiring enteric precautions are: infectious or serum hepatitis, salmonellosis (including typhoid fever), shigellosis, and pathogenic *Escherichia coli* gastroenteritis.

5. *Wound and skin precautions* include gowns for all persons having direct patient contact, gloves if contact with infected area or its drainage is anticipated, masks only during dressing changes, and special discard (or disinfection) procedures used during dressing changes and bed making. The mattress and pillows should be covered with clean, impervious plastic. Examples of conditions requiring wound and skin precautions are: staphylococcal and streptococcal skin infections not associated with extensive burns.

Note: Details of care using this classification may be obtained from the 1970 government publication. In addition to the five categories of isolation, precautions in dealing with secretion, excretion, and blood (body discharges) of patients with specific diseases and safe barriers against possible spread of infectious material, are discussed in the booklet.

Personal precautions

The nurse working with patients in isolation must take certain personal precautions for her own safety and for the safety of her co-workers and other patients. Some of these are essential for every nurse to follow, regardless of the area in which she finds herself; others are particularly important when dealing with known infectious conditions. The following precautions should be noted:

1. Fingernails should be short and clean.
2. The nurse should be free from symptoms of contagious illness (upper respiratory tract infections, skin infections, diarrhea).
3. Any open lesion on the hands or face should be reported and evaluated before going on duty. Perhaps a change of assignment would be prudent to protect the nurse.
4. No rings should be worn. A watch, although used, should not be kept on the wrist.
5. A nurse's cap should not be worn while performing bedside care in this area.
6. Eyeglasses, if worn, should be periodically disinfected.
7. Shoes should be kept off chairs and other clean areas. Think where they have been!
8. The nurse's hands should not touch her face.

There are certain areas in a hospital that are always considered contaminated. All floors are contaminated regardless of the location. In most hospitals the entire room of a patient with a communicable disease is considered contaminated *with the exception* of the supply of paper towels inside a dispenser near the sink. This supply is located as far from the patient as possible. At times there is an adjoining anteroom where such supplies are kept and washing and laundry discard facilities are available.

The isolation gown
Occasions for use

An isolation gown should be worn in a unit whenever there is a possibility of contact with the patient or any contaminated equipment in the room. When strict isolation is ordered, anyone going into the room, whether or not she will be touching anything, should wear a gown, mask, and perhaps gloves (depending on what will be done). However, in the case of other types of isolation the attendant may enter several times to bring in supplies and equipment without touching anything already in the room and not be required to gown or wash her hands—if she is *careful*. If the nurse touches something contaminated with her hands, she should, of course, follow the hand-washing technique before leaving the room. A gown should not be worn outside a patient's room once it has been worn inside the room, with the following exceptions only:

1. When transporting a patient for an ordered procedure in a separate tub room.
2. When transporting a patient to some other department for x-rays, therapy, or a change in room or unit.

When a contaminated gown must be used outside the patient's room, the nurse should be very discreet about what she touches and where she goes. When it is necessary to transport a child with a communicable disease through the hospital corridors his wheelchair or gurney should be draped with clean linen. The nurse pushing the whelchair or gurney should have a clean supply of paper towels or tissues, which she can use to open doors or push buttons when her hands are contaminated. She should also have a bag in which to discard these tissues after use. The child should wear a mask if his disease is spread through droplet contamination. He should be properly restrained to prevent falling and covered to prevent chilling. If the trip will be long or the wait protracted, an appropriate fluid, if allowed, may be taken along in the case of an infant. The child's chart should be placed in a bag for protection. The chart itself should be handled only by people with clean hands.

Gown techniques

Gowning. When a clean gown is required, the nurse should put it on before entering the patient's unit or room. Since the gown and the nurse are "clean," any part of the gown may be touched by the nurse as she puts it on. It should be tied at the back of the neck and then the back of the gown should be adjusted in such a way that no part of the nurse's uniform is exposed. Following are two ways in which a gown may be closed:

1. Pull the left-hand side of the back of the gown as far to the right as possi-

ble and lap the right-hand side over the left. Pull the belt around, cross it at the back, and tie it in the front. Push the sleeves up above the wrists (Fig. 33-1, *A*).

2. Hold the right and left inner edges of the back of the gown together and fold over until snugly closed against the wearer's back (Fig. 33-1, *B*). Continue as in 1 above.

Note: Reuse of isolation gowns is not recommended if it can be avoided. Many hospitals are now using paper gowns, which are discarded in the trash.

Removing a gown. The steps for removing an isolation gown are basically the same whether the gown is to be discarded or saved for further use. The procedure is as follows:

1. Untie the belt, letting the ends drop to the side.

2. Turn on the running water.
   a. If faucets are used, they are opened

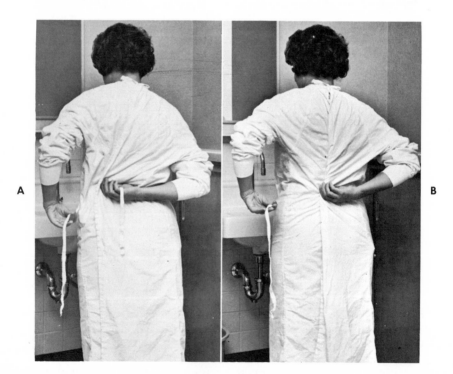

Fig. 33-1. Two methods of gowning. **A,** Right side over left. **B,** Back inside edges together; then roll until snug. (Courtesy Children's Health Center, San Diego, Calif.)

with unwashed hands and closed with clean hands protected by a paper towel.

b. If a knee lever is used, it is turned on and off with a knee covered by the isolation gown.

c. If foot pedals (the most preferable device) are used to control the water flow, one does not need to consider the possibility of contaminating clean hands. Shoes are always considered contaminated.

3. Carefully wash the hands and exposed portion of the arms for 1 minute with an antibacterial detergent, using considerable friction. The use of a brush is overly irritating and unnecessary. The areas are rinsed and patted dry with paper towels. The hands should be kept lower than the elbow when washing, as part of isolation technique, to avoid increasing the area of possible contamination.

4. Untie the neckband with newly washed hands.

5. After discarding the gown, rewash your hands and arms using the same technique described previously, *except,* if a knee lever is used to control the water flow, open it with a hand before washing. If the lever is opened with knee action at this point, the nurse's uniform becomes contaminated. After the hands are washed, close the faucet or knee control with a hand protected by a paper towel.

Leaving the patient's room

The following precautions are taken when leaving the room of an isolation patient:

1. Open the door with the paper towel used to turn off the water. Walk through.

2. Turn around before letting the door close and discard the paper in the wastebasket.

3. All doors to isolation rooms should routinely be kept closed.

Use of masks

There are two drawbacks to the use of face masks. Masks are likely to give a false sense of security to the wearer, and masks, in themselves, may serve as a source of infection unless changed often (approximately every 30 to 60 minutes and always as soon as damp).

However, masks may help filter out some bacteria, thus protecting the wearer or the patient. It is the only practical method we now have, other than good and discreet housekeeping, to protect against airborne organisms. Masks also keep the attendant's hands away from her face!

The following techniques are important in the use of masks:

1. Store masks conveniently outside the patient's unit. Many times they are placed in a paper bag taped on the outside of the patient's room where they are required to be worn.

2. Tie the mask in place before entering the room.

3. Remove a mask after your hands are washed by touching only the supporting ties and dropping it directly into the laundry receptacle.

4. Never leave a patient's room with a mask dangling around your neck!

Use of technique papers

A technique paper enables a nurse to carry out a procedure with greater skill and observance of asepsis by providing a temporary barrier between contaminated and clean objects. A clean paper towel usually serves as a technique paper. Taken directly from the dispenser, it is folded to form at least two layers of paper. It may be placed on a dry contaminated surface with clean hands, serving as a temporary island of cleanliness on which to place articles such as watches, pencils, and perhaps specimen bottles. (The underside of the paper touching the bedside table is contaminated; the upper side is not considered contaminated.)

A watch is not worn in an isolation situation, because hands and arms cannot be properly washed with a watch in place, and a contaminated watch may come into contact with a patient during his care. A watch cannot be sprayed or soaked with Amphyl or other disinfectants—both procedures seem to do something to its insides! However, since a watch is necessary to the nurse, it may be enclosed in a clear, small, waterproof plastic bag or box or placed on a technique paper for a brief period in such a position that the dial may be easily seen.

Neither the chart nor the nursing assignment sheet should be taken into the isolated patient's room. Because of memory problems, some student nurses have found it helpful to initially backfold a border of approximately an inch on a technique paper before placing it on a contaminated surface. This space is used to temporarily write the temperature, pulse, and respiration of the patient with a contaminated pencil, which is left in the unit. When the nurse is ready to leave the unit and has removed her gown, she picks up her watch with clean hands and, using the technique paper, opens the door, reviews the temperature, pulse, and respiration, and throws the paper in the wastebasket. Of course, if parents are in the room, it may not be best to have a slip of paper with the vital statistics of their child's condition in full view.

Service of meals

1. All food prepared for isolation patients in the hospital should be served on disposable dishes. (If special precautions must be taken at home because disposable dishes are not practical, dishes should be scraped in the patient's room and then placed directly in cool water to be boiled at least 10 minutes and then washed or washed in a dishwasher at 180° F.)
2. No serving tray should enter the patient's room. Food in the serving dishes should be lifted from the tray and taken into the room without the tray.
3. Serve the food as soon as possible.

No one enjoys cold meals. Prepare the setting for the children who can feed themselves and then help others who need assistance.

4. Knives, forks, and spoons may be stored in the patient's room. After the meal they are washed and dried at the sink in the room and wrapped in a clean napkin until needed again.
5. Uneaten solid food should be scraped into a paper dish or cup and placed in a refuse sack in the wastebasket. Unfinished liquids may be poured into the toilet.
6. If intake-output records must be kept, the record is posted outside the isolation room, usually on the outside of the patient's door.

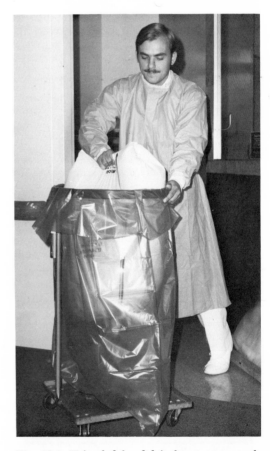

Fig. 33-2. He's glad he didn't forget to properly clear his isolation room of dirty linen. (Courtesy Children's Health Center, San Diego, Calif.)

Care of linen, trash, and diapers

1. Soiled linen, usually with the exception of diapers, should be placed in a laundry hamper in the patient's unit. Handle soiled linen carefully. Do not "wave it in the breeze." Remember, careless handling of linen increases the organism count in the air.
2. At the end of each tour of duty or when the hamper in the room is two-thirds full, close the top of the bag and place it upside down in a clean hamper or a clean bag held by another nurse just outside the door. If the inner bag is made of hot water–soluble plastic, handling of these contaminated linens is reduced. The outer plastic bag ideally should be red or distinctly marked to alert the housekeeping department of potentially infective material.

   Note: A "contaminated nurse" may touch only that part of the outer laundry bag that will be on the inside of the bag when it is closed.
3. Contaminated trash is collected in a plastic bag, which stands in the wastebasket. At the end of a tour of duty or when appropriate, the bag is carefully closed and placed in a clean outer bag just outside the door for disposal.
4. Double-bagged linen or bags of trash should be completely closed as soon as the nurse is able to remove her gown and wash her hands so that contaminated material does not remain unattended in the corridors. Sometimes it is possible for two or more nurses to work together to facilitate the removal of contaminated linen and trash. One will work in the patient's room, and the other(s) will close all the clean outer bags and place them in the approved areas for removal.
5. The handling of contaminated diapers depends on the facilities and services available. Many hospitals use professional diaper services. The in-structions of these companies regarding the pretreatment of diapers (if necessary) and collection should be followed. Any diaper pails used for collections should be closed, ideally with lids that are operated by a foot pedal.

Disposal of urine, feces, emesis, and other body discharges

1. Bedpans and emesis basins are usually emptied directly into the toilet in areas where urban sewage facilities are available. The hospital staff should know the sewage precautions needed in its own community. It is strongly recommended that each isolation unit have its own toilet facilities. In certain situations special precautions may have to be taken in the event of the occurrence of typhoid-related illnesses.
2. Any patient with nasal discharge should have a small paper sack attached to his bedside in which to put used cellulose wipes. When this bag is almost full, it is closed and added to the trash in the large paper bag in the wastebasket.

Disinfection of equipment

1. Disposable equipment is used in an isolation unit as much as possible.
2. Only essential equipment should be taken into an isolation room.
3. Nondisposable, washable items (such as basins, bedpans, spoons, and hemostats) may be washed in the patient's room, sprayed with a disinfectant, and preferably transported directly to a dishwasher that disinfects the utensils. If this is impossible, they may be boiled in water or soaked in disinfectant.
4. Stethoscopes, percussion hammers, and flashlights are usually sprayed with disinfectant. Sphygmomanometers are wiped off with disinfectant. Blood pressure cuffs should have plasticized washable surfaces.

5. If at all possible, disposable needles and syringes should be used. These should be destroyed after use to prevent reuse. The needles should be covered with their protective hoods, placed in a rigid pierce-proof container, and double bagged.

SUGGESTIONS FOR NURSING ORGANIZATION

Suggestions for organizing and completing your daily work in isolation are as follows:

1. Try to have *everything* you need in the room or just outside the room before gowning, including the following:
   a. Linen for the bed
   b. Clean clothes for the patient
   c. Hygienic supplies
   d. Supplies for early morning treatments
   e. Liquids to encourage fluid intake, if appropriate
   f. Plastic sacks, to replace those you will remove when emptying trash or removing diapers or laundry
2. Before ungowning, always ask your patient (if he talks!) if there is anything more he wishes.
3. Use the intercom for assistance, if one is available.
4. Remember, charting and clearing your unit of contaminated linen and waste takes time. Plan your working schedule with this in mind. Be sure you have taken any unnecessary equipment, such as bottles, from the room before you report off duty. At the completion of your morning care, the table tops, bed, and counters in the isolation room should be wiped down with a paper towel moistened with disinfectant.

TERMINATION OF ISOLATION

If isolation precautions are discontinued before the patient is discharged from the hospital, a "termination of isolation" bath is given. If the child's condition is satisfactory and the physician is agreeable, a shampoo followed by a tub bath is ideal. After the tub bath, the child is dressed in clean clothes and returned to a new bed and unit, or he is kept on a clean gurney in another room until his old room can be wiped down and aired or otherwise disinfected. However, if the tub room is used, it too must be disinfected, which is a disadvantage.

If the child's condition or the physical setup of the isolation area precludes a tub bath, another type of bath must be given in his bed. The child is placed on top and under a clean bath blanket. He is given a bed bath, using a fresh clean washcloth, basin, and towel. The nurse giving the bath is dressed in a fresh clean gown. The child is then lifted to a draped uncontaminated gurney, dressed in fresh bedclothes, and covered with a fresh bath blanket. The nurse removes her gown, washes her hands, and takes the child to a new "clean" unit.

Everything transferred from the patient's old isolation unit to his new uncontaminated unit must undergo some type of disinfection. The former isolation room is stripped of everything easily moveable that can be best disinfected in the utility room (including any wall oxygen and suction equipment). The linen is double bagged. All paper goods are discarded in the trash (special papers may be exposed to the sun if it is very important to save them and the disease was not serious). Potted plants may be sprinkled with water and exposed to the sun and air outside for several hours. The stripped room is then either wiped down with a disinfectant (or exposed to ultraviolet light if the organism involved was the tuberculosis bacillus), and the room is completely cleaned.

When a child is discharged from the hospital before termination of isolation is officially completed, the child is placed in a draped wheelchair for the trip to his parents' car. His belongings that are saved are washed or sprayed and placed in a clean bag. His room is then stripped.

Text continued on p. 524.

Table 33-1. Communicable childhood diseases

Disease	Infectious agent and general description	Importance	Mode of transmission	Communicable period	Incubation period	Symptoms	Treatment and nursing care	Prevention
Bacillary dysentery (shigellosis)	*Shigella dysenteriae* and *Shigella paradysenteriae* Acute inflammation of colon	Extremely widespread in areas with poor sanitary facilities and hygiene practices Disease often severe in infancy but mild after age 3 yr.	Direct or indirect contact with feces of infected patients or carriers Contaminated food, water, and flies play important role (Enteric precautions needed)*	As long as patients or carriers harbor organisms (as determined by stool or rectal swab cultures) Healthy carriers common; they should not become food handlers In areas where sanitary treatment of sewage is not routine, stools should be disinfected	1-7 days (usually 3-4 days)	Mild to severe diarrhea; in severe cases blood, mucus, and pus may be seen in stool Abdominal pain, fever, and prostration may be present	Treatment depends on severity of infection Ampicillin drug of choice; chloramphenicol; tetracycline (used after age 8 yr.); furazolidone Paregoric and bismuth may help control diarrhea Keep patient warm; oral fluids may be restricted; intravenous therapy may be necessary to prevent dehydration	Attack appears to confer limited immunity No preventive known other than improved individual and community hygiene
Chicken pox (varicella) (VZ infections)	Virus capable of causing varicella or herpes zoster Mild, chiefly cutaneous infectious disease Varicella—response to primary infection Herpes zoster—reactivation (in debilitated per-	Very common, highly contagious, usually mild disease Complications other than secondary infection from scratching rare; however, encephalitis possible Overwhelming se-	Direct or indirect contact with secretions from mouth or moist skin lesions of varicella or herpes zoster (Respiratory isolation)*	Approximately 24 hr. before rash appears until 6 days after its onset; dried crusts not contagious	10-21 days (usually 14 days)	Slight fever; malaise; rapidly progressing papulovesiculopustular skin eruption in all stages of development, first appearing on trunk and scalp	Keep fingernails short and clean to minimize secondary infections caused by scratching Calamine lotion, oral antihistaminics reduce pruritus	None; immune after one attack Immune serum globulin (ISG) for the corticosteroid-treated child or others at increased risk (see p. 320) Zoster immune globulin (ZIG) may prevent or

Continued.

*Department of Health, Education, and Welfare, Public Health Service, Health Services and Mental Health Administration, Center for Disease Control: Isolation techniques for use in hospitals, Public Health Service Publication No. 2054, Washington, D. C., 1970, U. S. Government Printing Office.

Table 33-1. Communicable childhood diseases—cont'd

Disease	Infectious agent and general description	Importance	Mode of transmission	Communicable period	Incubation period	Symptoms	Treatment and nursing care	Prevention
(VZ infections)—cont'd	sons or persons receiving immunosuppressive therapy) *CAUTION: Contact!*	vere infection seen in children receiving immunosuppressive therapy *CAUTION: Contact!*						modify VZ infections if given within 72 hr. of exposure; available on study basis only from Center for Disease Control, Atlanta, Georgia
Diphtheria	*Corynebacterium diphtheriae* (Klebs-Löffler bacillus) Severe, acute infectious disease of upper respiratory tract and perhaps skin Toxins produced may affect nervous system and heart	Rarely seen because of routine childhood immunization, more comprehensive public health regulations, and enforcement of milk standards and carrier control 5%-10% mortality Serious complications include neuritis, paralysis, and myocarditis	Direct or indirect contact with secretions from respiratory tract or skin lesions of patient or carrier (Strict isolation)*	Variable: 2-4 wk. in untreated persons, or 1-2 days after antibiotic therapy Isolation until satisfactory nose and throat cultures obtained; contacts may be isolated	2-6 days (occasionally longer)	Depend on type and part of upper respiratory area inflamed Formation of fibrinous false membrane, which may or may not be visible in throat or nose Nausea, possible muscle paralysis, and heart complications	Administration of antitoxin, analgesics, erythromycin, and penicillin Prednisone lessens incidence of myocarditis in severe disease Absolute bed rest; gentle throat irrigations; bland, soft diet; humidification Possible need for tracheostomy Watch for muscle weakness	Immunity after one attack, but person may be immune without history of disease Immunity determined by Schick test Routine primary schedule—DTP booster injection on exposure
German measles (rubella, 3-day measles)	Virus Acute infectious disease characterized chiefly by rose-colored macular rash and lymph node enlargement	Very common, frequently occurring in epidemic form Complications rare for victim but may cause deformities of fetus	Usually direct contact with secretions from mouth and nose May be acquired in utero (Respiratory isolation for post-	From 1 wk. before rash appears until approximately 5 days after its onset For discussion of congenital rubella syndrome see p.	14-21 days (usually 18 days)	Rose-colored macular rash occurring first on face, then on all body parts; enlargement and tenderness of lymph nodes; mild fever	Supportive nursing care with good personal hygiene	Rubella vaccine Immune after one attack

Continued.

Disease	Causative agent	Description	Source and transmission	Period of communicability	Incubation period	Symptoms	Treatment	Immunity / prevention
		if contracted by pregnant woman during first trimester	natal infections; strict isolation for congenital rubella syndrome)*	136; affected infants may be infectious up to age 1 yr.				Usually immune after first attack Rarely, second attack seen in some individuals
Gonorrhea (see pp. 136 and 523)								
Herpes zoster (shingles) (VZ infections)	Virus Same virus causes both chicken pox (varicella) and herpes zoster	Overwhelming severe infection seen in children receiving immunosuppressive therapy CAUTION: Contact!	Direct or indirect contact with secretions from mouth or moist skin lesions Zoster less contagious, but susceptible children exposed to zoster lesions may develop chicken pox	Approximately 24 hr. before rash appears until 6 days after its onset	10-21 days (usually 14 days)	Zoster lesions confined to skin over sensory nerves and preceded by local pain, itching, and burning Meningismus associated with cranial nerve involvement	Cut fingernails to prevent scratching Analgesics, sedation, thiamine; prednisone in severe cases; wet compresses to lesions	
Hepatitis, viral (2 types identified)	Both types manifest similarities and differences; may vary with age and general condition of victims	Hepatitis of both types represented fifth most commonly reported communicable disease in 1971	Now believed that both types transmitted through oral, fecal, and parenteral routes			Fever more common in Type A Jaundice for both types may be apparent, fleeting, or persistent with or without itching Headache, anorexia, nausea, vomiting, enlarged liver, abdominal pain, dark urine, weight loss Joint pain more characteristic of Type B Children usually have less severe clinical manifestations	No specific therapy available Supportive rest and nourishing diet In fulminating hepatitis—to combat liver failure, protein withdrawn from diet; neomycin given to suppress bacterial flora in GI tract; possible use of corticosteroids; exchange transfusion?	Type A attack confers immunity for Type A Type B attack confers immunity for Type B, but no cross-immunity conferred ISG recommended for Type A contact Results of ISG given to Type B contracts have been inconsistent Effective screening of blood donors Absolute sterilization of equipment used for drawing blood, or use of disposable equipment
Type A, infectious	Hepatitis A virus: usually acute onset	Type A: highest incidence in civilian populations in persons under 15 years, typically mild in childhood	In addition, urine of patients with Type A hepatitis found to be infectious on the first day of jaundice Ingestion of raw shellfish from polluted waters has caused Type A	Type A: unknown; potentially infectious at least 1 wk. after onset of jaundice and indeterminate period before symptoms	Type A: 15 to 50 days			
Type B, serum	Hepatitis B virus characterized by presence of Australia antigen (hepatitis B	Type B: more common in adults; more often complicated by relapse and pro-	Type B reported more frequently; transmitted through inoculation of contami-	Type B: potentially infectious for indeterminate period before and after active	Type B: 50 to 180 days	Occasionally a rapid, severe (fulminating) type seen characterized by mental confusion, emo-		

Table 33-1. Communicable childhood diseases—cont'd

Disease	Infectious agent and general description	Importance	Mode of transmission	Communicable period	Incubation period	Symptoms	Treatment and nursing care	Prevention
Type B, serum—cont'd	antigen); usually insidious onset	longed liver dysfunction; typically more severe in infants and debilitated patients	nated blood products, needles, and syringes; close and intimate contact Meticulous handwashing technique, enteric isolation,* and blood precautions	symptoms; carrier state possible		tional instability, restlessness, coma, internal bleeding, and possible death		
Measles (rubeola, or 2-week, or red, measles)	Virus Acute infection characterized by moderately high fever, inflammation of mucous membranes of respiratory tract, and macular rash	Very common, highly infectious disease frequently occurring in epidemic form Possible serious complications include pneumonia, otitis media, conjunctivitis, and encephalitis	Direct or indirect contact with secretions from nose and throat, perhaps airborne May be acquired in utero (Respiratory isolation)*	From time of "cold symptoms" until about 3 days after rash appears	About 10 days	Catarrhal symptoms, like a common cold; conjunctivitis; photophobia Fever followed by macular, blotchy rash involving entire body Koplik's spots (eruption on mucous membrane of mouth) diagnostic	Antibiotics (for treatment of secondary bacterial infections) Aspirin and tepid sponge baths for severe cases; various soothing lotions Boric acid eye irrigations; protection from bright lights—eyeshade Observation for onset of pneumonia or ear infection	Live measles vaccine; immune serum globulin (ISG) lessens disease Usually immune after first attack
Meningococcal meningitis (cerebrospinal fever)	Neisseria meningitidis (N. intracellularis) Meningococcus Serious, acute disease caused by	Occurs fairly often where concentrations of people are found (army bases, schools) because of healthy	Direct contact with patient or carrier by droplet spread Organism may be found in	As long as meningococci are found in nose and mouth Usually not infectious after 24 hr.	1-7 days (usually 4 days)	Sudden onset of fever, chills, headache, and vomiting (convulsions fairly common in chil-	Spinal tap and culture needed to confirm diagnosis Temperature control; penicillin G, ampicillin, anal-	Extent of immunity after attack unknown Sulfonamides have been used prophylactically

Continued.

Disease	Description / Cause	Mode of spread (Isolation)	Period of communicability	Incubation period	Symptoms	Treatment / Nursing care	Immunization
	bacteria that invade bloodstream and eventually meninges, causing fever and central nervous system inflammation — carriers — Very severe or relatively mild — Mortality depends on early diagnosis and treatment — Complications include hydrocephalus, arthritis, blindness, deafness, impairment of intellect, and cerebral palsy	urine (Respiratory isolation)*	of appropriate therapy		dren) Cutaneous petechial hemorrhages; stiffness of neck; opisthotonus; joint pain; possibly delirium; convulsions	gesics, and sedatives — Watch for clinical signs of increasing intracranial pressure or meningeal irritation and eye and ear involvement — Maintain dim, quiet atmosphere; turn gently; watch for constipation and urinary retention; attention to fluid balance	during epidemics
Mononucleosis, infectious (glandular fever)	Epstein-Barr (EB) virus — Mildly contagious disease characterized by increase in monocyte-type white cell in blood, lymph node enlargement, fever, and fatigue — Heterophil agglutinin studies positive fairly late in course of disease — Isolation not recommended† — Typically, disease of teen-agers or young adults — Trauma may rarely cause ruptured spleen; hepatitis in 8%-10% of cases — May involve prolonged convalescence	Probably droplets from nose and throat, saliva, or intimate contact (No isolation or precautions recommended)*	Not known — Probably only during acute stage	Unknown (probably 2-6 wk.)	Sore throat, malaise, depression, enlarged spleen, liver, and lymph nodes — Possible jaundice with liver damage	Symptomatic, no specific therapy known — Bed rest, high carbohydrate, protein intake — Possible use of corticosteroids with severe throat involvement and airway obstruction	No immunization available
Mumps (infectious parotitis)	Virus — Acute infectious disease causing inflammation of salivary glands — Possible serious consequences for male after puberty, when an attack is more	Direct or indirect contact with patient by droplet spread (Respiratory	From several days before apparent infection until swelling disappears	14-21 days (usually 18 days)	Tender swelling chiefly of parotid glands in front of and below ear — Headache; mod-	Bed rest; bland, soft diet; analgesics; warm or cold applications to swollen glands	Mumps vaccine — Usually immune after first attack — Mumps immune globulin (human)

†Report of the Committee on Infectious Diseases, Evanston, Ill., 1974, American Academy of Pediatrics.

Table 33-1. Communicable childhood diseases—cont'd

Disease	Infectious agent and general description	Importance	Mode of transmission	Communicable period	Incubation period	Symptoms	Treatment and nursing care	Prevention
Mumps—cont'd	and, at times, testes and ovaries	severe; sterility can be complication Meningitis or encephalitis occur infrequently Mild pancreatitis may be encountered	isolation)*			erate fever; pain on swallowing	Watch for tenderness of testes—scrotal support may be necessary	may help those exposed to have milder cases or avoid symptoms
Poliomyelitis (infantile paralysis)	Virus Acute infectious disease, may occur in many forms and degrees of severity Attacks primarily gastrointestinal and nervous systems; may cause muscular paralysis	New cases uncommon since vaccine When paralysis takes place, many complications may occur involving respiratory, musculoskeletal, urinary, and digestive systems	Direct or indirect contact with pharyngeal secretions and feces of infected persons (many infected persons have no symptoms) (Excretion or enteric precautions)*	Unknown, probably greatest shortly before and after onset of symptoms Usually isolated for 7 days after onset or until fever subsides Virus may persist in stool for weeks; local sewage facilities should be evaluated	7-14 days?	Variable; may include diarrhea, constipation, emesis, painful stiff neck, rigid back, tender skeletal muscles, and respiratory distress Cranial nerve involvement Three main types 1. Inapparent infection, 2. Nonparalytic, and 3. Paralytic a. Spinal, affecting skeletal muscles and diaphragm, b. Bulbar, affecting swallowing, facial	No specific treatment known Supportive treatment depends on patient needs; bed rest, hot packs to relieve muscle spasms, observation for respiratory or bulbar involvement Possible tracheostomy and artificial ventilation if respiratory paralysis occurs; observation for constipation and urinary retention Gentle positioning; physical and occupational therapy	Routine primary schedule and boosters; OPV (Sabin-oral) optimum immunization schedule

518

muscles, and respiration. c. Mixed

Disease								
✱ Rabies (hydrophobia)	Virus Only one nonfatal case reported, acute infectious encephalitis, causing convulsions and muscle paralysis	Exceedingly dangerous Household pets may acquire rabies through bite of rabid wild animals All dogs should be immunized periodically; cats may also be carriers, but impractical to insist on immunization	Bite of rabid animals or entry of infected saliva through previous break in skin or mucous membrane (Strict isolation)*	During clinical course of disease plus 3-5 days before appearance of symptoms (as demonstrated in dogs and cats)	Usually 2-6 wk.	Mental depression, headaches, restlessness, and fever Progresses to painful spasms of throat muscles, especially when attempting to drink Delirium, convulsions, and coma	No effective treatment known Supportive nursing care to help prevent convulsions; analgesics Death usually occurs in about 7 days	Vaccination of dogs; 10-day confinement of any dog who has bitten human Laboratory investigation of brain of dog that dies during this period; if rabies is diagnosed, person bitten must receive rabies vaccine
Staphylococcal infections	Coagulase-positive staphylococci (*Micrococcus pyogenes*, var. *aureus*) pus-producing coccus Descriptions variable	Found almost everywhere; causes many hospital infections; does not respond well to usual antibiotic therapy; extremely difficult to control; anyone may be carrier at intervals Complications include skin lesions, pneumonia, wound infections, arthritis, osteomyelitis, meningitis, and food poisoning	Depends on body area infected Via hands of hospital personnel Asymptomatic nasal carriers common Open suppurative lesions May be airborne Direct or indirect contact with infected secretions Type of isolation depends on area infected	As long as lesions drain or carrier state persists	Variable; 1-10 days to several weeks	Depend on area infected Fever and characteristic signs of inflammation typical	Antibiotics according to drug sensitivity pattern of organism; methicillin, oxacillin Topical antibiotics: bacitracin, neomycin, polymyxin	Good hygiene and aseptic technique best preventive
Streptococcal infections	Strains of beta hemolytic streptococci, usually group A	Interrelated group of infections; septic sore throat probably most	In septic sore throat and scarlet fever, direct or indirect	Variable	2-5 days	Depends on manifestations Septic sore throat, severe pharyngi-	Depends on manifestation Penicillin for at least 10 days	No artificial immunization available Penicillin pro-

Continued.

519

Table 33-1. Communicable childhood diseases—cont'd

Disease	Infectious agent and general description	Importance	Mode of transmission	Communicable period	Incubation period	Symptoms	Treatment and nursing care	Prevention
Strepto-coccal in-fections—cont'd	Diseases include septic sore throat, scarlet fever (scarla-tina), erysipelas, impetigo, puer-peral fever	common Early complica-tions include otitis media May cause serious complications not contagious in themselves—nephritis and rheumatic fever, with possible arthritis and carditis	contact with nasopharyngeal secretions from infected patient; probably air-borne In erysipelas, impetigo, and puerperal fever, direct or in-direct contact with discharges from skin or reproductive tract (type of isolation de-pends on area infected)			tis and fever Scarlet fever, pharyngitis, fever, and fine reddish rash and straw-berry tongue Erysipelas, tender, red skin lesions, and fever often recurrent Puerperal fever, refer to pp. 4 and 170		phylaxis may be used with special groups Good asepsis important
Syphilis (see pp. 134 and 523)								
Tetanus (lockjaw)	Bacillus *Clos-tridium tetani* Acute infectious disease attack-ing chiefly nerv-ous system Wounds deprived of good oxygen supply especially vulnerable	Always considered in event of burns, automobile acci-dents, or punc-ture wounds Mortality of about 35%	Entrance of spores into wounds through contaminated soil Direct or indirect contamination of wounds (No isolation recommended except possibly gloves for wound care)*	None	3-21 days (usually 8 days)	Irritability, rigidity, painful muscle spasms, and in-ability to open mouth Exhaustion and respiratory diffi-culty	Specific—tetanus immune globulin (human); TIG preferred over tetanus antitoxin Sedation plus mus-cle relaxant Quiet, dim room Possible suction and tracheotomy Observation of fluid balance; watch for constipation and respiratory distress; protect from self-injury during	Routine primary immunization; booster at school age and Td every 10 yr.

Disease	Organism and characteristics	Importance and complications	Mode of transmission	Period of communicability	Symptoms and diagnosis	Incubation period	Treatment and nursing care	Prevention and immunity
✱ Tuberculosis	*Mycobacterium tuberculosis* (tubercle bacillus) Typically chronic infection that may affect many body organs Human type most often causes pulmonary infection Bovine type causes much of tuberculosis affecting areas outside lungs	Serious world health problem, particularly in economically deprived areas Infants and young children very susceptible Pulmonary complications, hemoptysis, spontaneous pneumothorax, or spread to other organs with varied symptoms; possible orthopedic problems	Direct or indirect contact with infected patients; body excretions or droplet spread (depending on type) Respiratory tuberculosis often airborne; bovine type may result from drinking milk from infected cows (now rare in U.S.) (Respiratory isolation for pulmonary tuberculosis; secretion precautions for draining lesions)*	Children with uncomplicated primary TB are usually noninfectious because of minimal pulmonary lesions; in chronic TB as long as organism is discharged in sputum or other body excretions Communicability may be reduced by medication, therapy, and teaching cough control and asepsis to patients Body often walls off a primary infection, controlling spread and preventing active disease	Active pulmonary tuberculosis: anorexia, weight loss, night sweats, afternoon fever, cough and dyspnea, fatigue, and hemoptysis; in children dyspnea and cough often absent Diagnosis based on symptoms and microscopic studies of sputum, gastric washings, and chest x-ray examination	From infection to primary lesion, 2-10 wk. Time of appearance of active symptoms variable	Specific—isoniazid (INH); para-aminosalicylic acid (PAS) enhances effect of INH; streptomycin used in addition to INH and PAS in severe cases Nursing care includes provision for mental and physical rest; nutritious diet; observation for toxic drug reactions and increasing respiratory distress; provision for and instructions in personal hygiene; moral support	BCG vaccine to build up immunity in high-risk populations advised by some Early detection and control of known cases through periodic x-ray examination, possible skin tests, and close medical supervision
✱ Typhoid fever (enteric fever)	*Salmonella typhosa,* a bacillus (many types have been identified) Relatively severe febrile systemic infection with symptoms involving lymphoid tissues, intestine, and spleen, which may be accompanied by complete prostration	Always of potential public health importance when community hygiene breaks down Carrier states may persist Complications include intestinal hemorrhage and perforation, thrombosis, cardiac failure, and cholecystitis	Direct or indirect contact with urine and feces of infected patients and carriers Food and water supplies may be infected by contaminated *flies* or unsuspected *carriers;* community sewage facilities should be evaluated; excreta may	As long as typhoid organism appears in feces or urine 2%-5% of those affected become permanent carriers	In children symptoms may be atypical, may at first resemble upper respiratory tract infection; intestinal tract becomes inflamed and even ulcerated; spleen enlarges; fever mounts; pulse relatively slow: rash, "rose spots" may be present	1-3 wk. (usually 2 wk.)	Usually self-limiting; ampicillin or chloramphenicol for chronic disturbances Supportive nursing care; liquid to bland, soft diet as tolerated; bed rest Watch for abdominal distention and hemorrhage; small enemas may be ordered; observation of fluid balance	Immunity usually acquired after one attack Vaccine available

Continued.

521

Table 33-1. Communicable childhood diseases—cont'd

Disease	Infectious agent and general description	Importance	Mode of transmission	Communicable period	Incubation period	Symptoms	Treatment and nursing care	Prevention
Typhoid fever— cont'd	and delirium Condition has prolonged course and convalescence		have to be disinfected before being added to local system (Enteric precautions)*					
✳ Whooping cough (pertussis)	*Bordetella pertussis* (pertussis bacillus) Acute infection of respiratory tract, characterized by paroxysmal cough ending in "whoop," often accompanied by vomiting	Severe disease in infants, may terminate fatally Complications include bronchopneumonia and convulsions, widespread hemorrhages, hernia, and possible activation of pulmonary tuberculosis	Direct or indirect contact with nasopharyngeal secretions of infected patients (droplet infection) (Respiratory isolation)*	From 7 days after exposure to 4 wk. after onset of typical cough Greatest in catarrhal stage before onset of paroxysms	5-21 days (usually within 10 days)	Early symptoms resemble typical common cold Cough worsens and may become violent and paroxysmal Vomiting may be caused by coughing or nervous system irritation; cough may linger after convalescence	Diagnosis confirmed with bacterial studies of exposed cough plates and presence of leukocytosis Immune pertussis globulin (human); erythromycin antibiotic of choice; provision for rest and quiet; sedatives Light nutritious diet; judicious fluid intake to prevent dehydration; weight determinations Observation for onset of respiratory distress or other complications	Immunity usually produced after one attack Routine primary schedule plus boosters

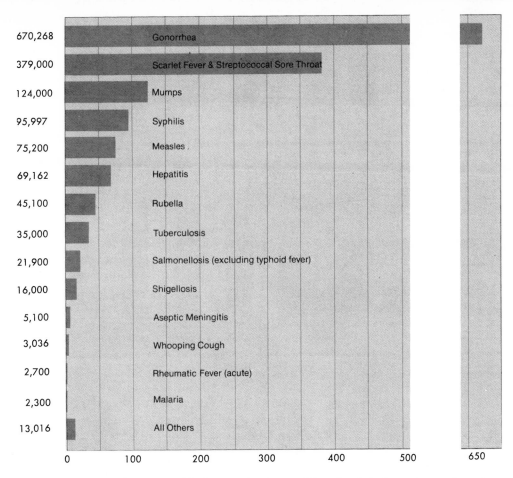

670,268	Gonorrhea
379,000	Scarlet Fever & Streptococcal Sore Throat
124,000	Mumps
95,997	Syphilis
75,200	Measles
69,162	Hepatitis
45,100	Rubella
35,000	Tuberculosis
21,900	Salmonellosis (excluding typhoid fever)
16,000	Shigellosis
5,100	Aseptic Meningitis
3,036	Whooping Cough
2,700	Rheumatic Fever (acute)
2,300	Malaria
13,016	All Others

0   100   200   300   400   500   650

Fig. 33-3. Cases of communicable diseases (in thousands) in the U. S. for 1971. Total number of reported cases of specified notifiable diseases, 1,557,779. Source: Center for Disease Control. (From Maternal and Child Health Service reports on: Promoting the health of mothers and children, FY 1973, Washington, D. C., p. 15. Reprinted with permission, Bureau of Community Health Services, Health Service Administration, U. S. Department of Health, Education, and Welfare.)

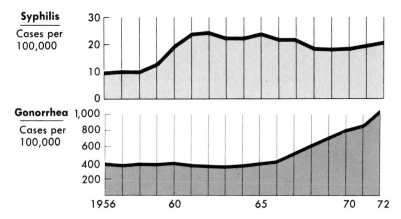

Fig. 33-4. Reported incidence of primary and secondary syphilis and gonorrhea in the U. S. for ages 15 to 19 in 1956-1972. Center for Disease Control. (From Maternal and Child Health Service reports on: Promoting the health of mothers and children, Washington, D. C., FY 1973, p. 22. Reprinted with permission, Bureau of Community Health Services, Health Service Administration, U. S. Department of Health, Education, and Welfare.)

Parents should be told of the precautions, if any, that must be observed at home. If isolation precautions are still necessary, details of ways these precautions may be observed should be discussed so that the parents will feel confident regarding their use. These procedures must be simple and effective. It is better to have a few rules understood and followed wisely than many rules confused and finally disregarded.

SIGNIFICANT COMMUNICABLE DISEASES OF CHILDHOOD AND THEIR NURSING CARE

Descriptions of some of the communicable diseases seen or mentioned most often in pediatrics are included in Table 33-1. Also summarized are nursing points to remember in each case. Fortunately, not all the diseases described will be encountered by nurses today. However, all those described, and some not included, pose a potential threat to our communities (Figs. 33-3 and 33-4). Diseases such as diphtheria, typhoid, and polio, for which we have proved preventives, could again ravage our population if public health standards decline and public education and support for immunization programs are not constantly maintained.

34

Conditions involving the neuromuscular and skeletal systems

All the systems of the body are intimately related. If a difficulty in one part of the body is severe enough or sufficiently prolonged, many body systems—in fact, the entire person—will react. The interdependence of the neuromuscular and skeletal systems is especially noteworthy.

Traumatic, infectious, or toxic injury to the nerve centers or nerve fibers that control the skeletal muscles often leads to wasting of those muscles and an inability to control or perhaps even initiate motion in related parts of the body. Poorly developed, abnormal, or damaged muscles may cause orthopedic deformities. Broken bones frequently cause muscle spasm and pain.

This chapter will attempt to present or review some of the more common neuromuscular and skeletal problems found in children, the methods of treatment, and, of course, the nursing care involved. A number of the problems affecting these interrelated systems are present at birth, or congenital in nature. The more common of these congenital defects were discussed in the chapter treating abnormalities of the newborn infant. For a brief description of hydrocephalus, cranial stenosis (craniosynostosis), microcephaly, spina bifida, clubfoot, congenital dislocated hip, syndactyly, and polydactylism, refer to Chapter 16.

FRACTURES

A very common problem in childhood is a broken bone, or fracture. Roller skates, skate boards, bicycles, and the rather rough-and-tumble life of youngsters (especially boys) contribute to the high incidence of fractures. Probably even more broken bones would occur in childhood if it were not for the relatively plastic condition of the child's skeletal system. The bones of children tend to bend rather than break. Frequently, if a bone does break, it is not completely severed. A portion of the bone remains intact. This type of fracture is called an incomplete, or a *greenstick*, fracture (Fig. 34-1).

Classifications

Other common types of fractures described according to the course of the break sustained include *transverse, spiral,* and *oblique.* A *comminuted* fracture is especially difficult to repair because the bone is typically broken into several pieces. A *depressed* fracture is particularly important when the fractured bony area is the skull and abnormal pressure is exerted on sensitive brain tissue.

Fractures may result from excessive or sudden direct pressure, exaggerated muscular contractions, or a basically unsound bony structure. If an unsound bony structure is the cause, the fracture is termed "pathological." Some of the causes of pathological fractures are osteomyelitis (inflammation of the bone marrow and surrounding bone cells), primary bone tumors or metastases, and osteogenesis imperfecta congenita (congenital brittle bones, a disease of unknown origin in which bones may fracture even before birth, causing characteristic skeletal malformations occasionally accompanied by deafness). If a patient has an underlying bone disease, great care and gentleness must be practiced when turning and positioning him (Fig. 34-2).

A careful note must be made of the general condition of a child who enters the hospital with a fracture of unknown origin, multiple fractures, or a repeated fracture. Sometimes these little patients are the victims of abuse from their own parents, who are unable to meet the daily frustrations of parenthood in a mature manner or who have deep-seated psychological problems. Such children usually exhibit multiple bruises and suffer from malnutrition (battered child syndrome). (See Fig. 34-3 and p. 332.)

Every fracture, irrespective of the course or extent of the break or its basic cause, may be placed in one of two main categories. If a bone is broken but the skin overlying the fracture has not been pierced by the end of the broken bone and there is no opening in the skin that may serve to introduce organisms from the exterior to the bone, the result is called a *simple,* or *closed,* fracture. If, however, the skin has been broken, exposing the bone to

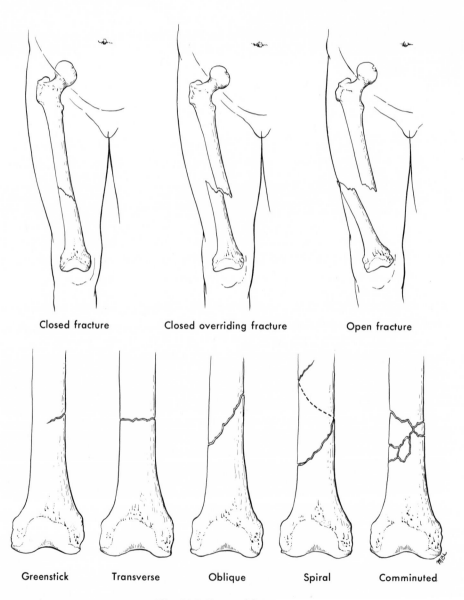

Closed fracture   Closed overriding fracture   Open fracture

Greenstick   Transverse   Oblique   Spiral   Comminuted

Fig. 34-1. Types of fractures.

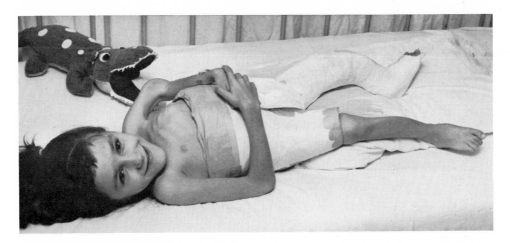

Fig. 34-2. This alert young lady is a victim of osteogenesis imperfecta congenita. She was hospitalized for corrective surgery involving previous fractures. (Courtesy Children's Health Center, San Diego, Calif.)

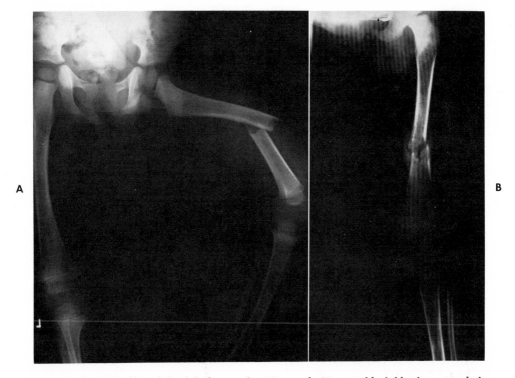

Fig. 34-3. **A,** X-ray film of the left femur of a 19-pound, 2½-year-old child who entered the hospital with multiple body bruises. Provisional diagnosis was "battered child syndrome." **B,** X-ray film showing the same leg after reduction of the fractured femur. The shadowy outline around the break is callus. (Courtesy Naval Regional Medical Center, San Diego, Calif.)

infection, the resulting trauma is called a *compound,* or *open,* fracture. Compound fractures are surgical emergencies because of the increased danger of infection and extensive soft tissue damage usually involved.

First-aid considerations

A nurse encountering an accident victim with unknown injuries should take the following action:

1. Evaluate the safety of the immediate environment. (Turn off ignition of car, set out warning flares if on the highway, etc.) Send someone for help, if possible.
2. Establish an airway if respirations are not present.
3. Control hemorrhage, if present.
4. Restore and maintain breathing, if necessary.
5. Evaluate for spinal injury and fracture. Do not move victim until proper help is available.
6. Keep the patient warm and quiet to prevent and treat shock.

If a victim with spinal injury is moved improperly, the injury may be increased and permanent paralysis or even death may occur. If the victim is conscious but cannot move any extremity, the nurse must consider the possibility of a *broken neck* or cervical fracture. A patient with a possible broken neck should be moved by a team so that no twisting or injurious movement of the spine will take place. He should be transported on a rigid support on his back, *chin up.* The victim with a suspected *broken back* may be unable to move his legs (lower extremity paralysis). He should be moved, log fashion, with considerable help, to a *prone* position and also carried on a rigid support. The prone, or abdominal, position is maintained to prevent flexion of the middle and lower portions of the spine. Persons with suspected spinal injuries should be moved as little as possible. They should be frequently observed to detect the onset of respiratory difficulty and abdominal distention. The higher the in-

jury on the spinal cord, the more body functions will be affected. Nonspinal fractures are less serious but still necessitate careful attention and first aid.

Indications of fracture. Fracture of an extremity may reveal itself early through the presence of the following:

1. Deformity in alignment and swelling
2. Pain or tenderness at the fracture site
3. Loss of function or abnormal mobility of the part
4. A "grating sensation" heard or felt at the suspected point of fracture (crepitus)
5. Black-and-blue areas caused by subcutaneous hemorrhage

However, the real proof of the presence of fracture must be detected by x-ray examination. Sometimes clinical symptoms are virtually lacking or very inconclusive, but the x-ray film reveals a break. Every suspected skeletal injury should be treated as a fracture until proved otherwise.

Use of splints. First-aid treatment of a possible fracture includes limitation of the movement of the injured part by stabilizing the part and the joint above and below the break to relieve muscle spasm and pain and prevent further injury. Splint the arm or leg without attempting to correct any deformity. Do not attempt to straighten it because this may cause still further damage. Do not attempt to push back a broken bone protruding from the skin in the case of a compound, or open, fracture. Just cover the area. If bleeding is present, use direct manual pressure to obtain control. A tourniquet is a potential hazard because it can cause gangrene and loss of a limb. It should be used only as a last resort. If a tourniquet is used, its presence should be clearly indicated by obvious signs or skin markings. Splints may be made from rolled magazines, blankets, or pillows. They should be applied in a position comfortable for the patient. Rings and bracelets on a fractured arm should be removed to avoid difficulty in the event of swelling. The application of ice bags may decrease the possibility of swelling. Do not apply heat. In case of bleeding from an arm or leg, elevate the part if possible.

When a fracture involving the bones of an extremity occurs, usually the muscles attached to the broken bone, which have been under a certain amount of tension, contract as a result of loss of proper skeletal support. The pain associated with the fracture causes the muscles to go into spasm in an effort to splint the injured part. If this spasm is exaggerated, the severed ends of the broken bone may be pulled further out of alignment or may override, causing abnormal shortening of the limb.

Hospital care

Observation. When a patient with a possible bone fracture is first admitted to the hospital, his general condition is evaluated in detail. Vital signs (temperature, pulse, respiration, and blood pressure recordings) are obtained. Elevated blood pressure is important to report because of the possibility of skull fracture. Low blood pressure is equally important because of the possibility of shock. The patient's level of consciousness should be evaluated and the pupils of the eyes checked for abnormal pupil dilatation or inequality of pupil size (other signs of possible skull fracture and brain injury). Depending on the patient's condition, he may be given intravenous solutions or blood. He should not be given any food or fluid by mouth because corrective surgery may be indicated. An x-ray examination of possible fracture sites should be made.

Reduction and casting. If overriding or angulation of a fractured bone has occurred, the displaced bone will be pulled into alignment through some form of traction until the broken fragments are in proper position. The process of bringing the fragments into proper relationship is termed "reducing," or "setting," the fracture. If the fractured bone can be set without performing a surgical operation that actually exposes the involved bone, the procedure is called a *closed* reduction. If it is necessary to expose the site of the fracture

to direct view to secure proper alignment and optimum healing or use some method of internal immobilization such as the installation of a nail, pin, or screws, the procedure is called an *open* reduction. Most children's fractures may be treated by closed reduction.

At times alignment may not be disturbed. The x-ray examination reveals a break, but the bony segments are still in proper relationship. If this is happily the case, no mechanical traction apparatus is needed. A plaster cast or protective splint is applied to maintain correct positioning to assure proper healing. Occasionally there is only a relatively minor disturbance in alignment that can be reduced easily at the time the patient is first seen or may not even require reduction. In children a fracture often stimulates the formation of bone, and, curiously enough, at times the physician may desire a certain amount of overriding to avoid excessive growth of the fractured extremity.

If sufficient initial alignment is difficult or impossible to achieve and maintain, some form of constant pull, or traction, must be exerted to reduce the fracture and bring the ends of the broken bone into proper apposition. The position of the bone and the progress of healing are intermittently checked by x-ray studies. When a sufficient amount of new bone (callus) is formed at the fracture site to help hold the broken segment in position, traction is discontinued and a protective cast is applied, allowing the patient more mobility. For a discussion of the basic nursing care involved in the care of a patient in traction or a cast, refer to Chapter 30.

Fractures involving the legs of infants and young children are often treated by suspending both legs, wrapped in bandages from a frame hanging directly above the bed. The infant's trunk almost entirely rests on the crib mattress, and only the pelvis is raised slightly from the surface of the bed. His legs are suspended at right angles to the mattress. Such an arrangement is called *Bryant's*, or *vertical*, traction (see

529

Fig. 30-3). It is useful in treating lower extremity fractures of children weighing under 25 pounds in the infant or toddler age groups. Even though only one leg may be fractured, both are customarily placed in traction to help stabilize the position and prevent undue twisting on the part of the child. Older children will usually be placed in types of traction similar to but smaller than those used for adults.

The healing of a broken bone, or *union* of a fracture, is accomplished through the deposit of new bone cells. In children, union is usually achieved in a relatively short time. Union is seldom delayed, and it is rare indeed to see a case in which union never takes place.

Rehabilitation. After the bone has united, the weakened muscles attached to the bone may have to be gradually strengthened through a program of exercise as prescribed by the physician. This part of therapy is not so necessary with young children, however, since they start using the part immediately and often do not need the encouragement required by many adults. The resources of the physical therapy department may be used on an inpatient or outpatient basis. The aims of treatment are a return of function, freedom from pain, and a normal appearance.

JOINT AND EXTREMITY PROBLEMS

The skeletal system may become distorted for reasons other than fracture. Some congenital deformities and intervening paralytic or inflammatory diseases of the skeletal system may cause muscular weakness or bone destruction, producing joint instability, which prevents normal weight bearing. Some disorders reduce joint mobility so that the usefulness of a body part is greatly reduced. Other conditions may affect the growth patterns of individual extremities. Various surgical procedures have been devised to increase the effectiveness of various body joints either by increasing their ability to bear weight (increasing joint stability) or by permitting greater motion. If a choice between motion and

stability must be made, the decision is made in favor of stability.

The following are a few of the basic procedures used in some cases to promote healing of or gain greater usefulness for a body part or increase its contribution to the individual's total welfare.

1. *Arthrodesis* is the fusion of a joint to gain stability for weight bearing. It may be accomplished by removing the cartilage from the opposing ends of the bones that form a joint or by grafting bone into the area and then immobilizing it in a cast for a prolonged period to promote fusion. A *triple-arthrodesis* is occasionally performed on a foot; as the name implies, it involves fusion of three joints. It prohibits some lateral movements of the foot itself but preserves ankle motion. Considerable bleeding may be expected after this type of surgery, and considerable pain may be involved. Application of weight to the newly fused part is delayed until fusion is secure, in approximately 2 to 3 months.

2. *Arthroplasty* is the reconstruction of a joint to provide greater movement. The joints usually involved in the procedure are the hip and knee. Recently new procedures that involve the total replacement of those joints have largely supplanted arthroplasty.

3. *Osteotomy* is an opening into or a controlled fracture of a bone to correct a congenital or acquired skeletal deformity. In a *rotational osteotomy* the distal fragment of the bone is turned to secure the desired correction.

4. *Bone block* is an operative procedure that incorporates a piece of bone into a joint to limit motion and help produce increased joint stability. It may precede an arthrodesis.

5. *Tendon transplant* is a procedure in which a tendon from one part of the body is transplanted to another. It may be performed for various reasons—to substitute the action of neighboring strong muscles for paralyzed or weak muscles, to replace badly damaged tendons, or to decrease a deformity caused by exaggerated muscle pull.

6. *Epiphyseal arrest* may be performed to slow up the growth of one extremity in the case of inequality in length. Properly handled, it may also aid in the correction of such deformities as knock-knees or bowlegs. It may be accomplished by the placement of stainless steel staples into the epiphyseal area where bone growth takes place. This procedure stops normal growth. The staples are removed when the desired results are obtained.

CONDITIONS INVOLVING THE BONES AND MUSCLES

Because many pediatric nursing courses are organized according to developmental sequence, the following conditions are presented according to the age group primarily affected. It will readily be seen that such an approach is not without inconsistencies. Some conditions extend to children of all ages; moreover, many problems present in infancy are not diagnosed until later in childhood. In spite of these difficulties, we hope our arrangement meets the needs of nursing teachers and students.

THE INFANT
Torticollis (Fig. 34-4)

Torticollis, or wryneck, is a congenital muscular abnormality possibly associated with birth trauma. Although the defect is minimal at birth, within 2 weeks a palpable fibrous tumor appears in the sternocleidomastoid muscle. The cause of the tumor is

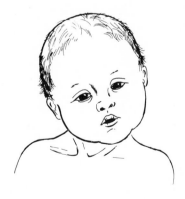

Fig. 34-4. Torticollis, or wryneck; in this case a shortening of the right sternocleidomastoid muscle.

unknown. Within a few months the fibrous tumor gradually disappears, leaving behind a contracture (shortening) of the muscle. The head of the infant is tilted toward the side of the affected muscle, and the chin is rotated to the opposite side. When the condition is recognized, early treatment consists of passive stretching of the involved muscle. Parents are instructed in the exact maneuvers to be done four or five times daily. The reward for faithful treatment is complete and permanent correction in at least 90% of the cases. When torticollis does not respond to conservative measures or when treatment is not consistent, surgery is indicated. The affected muscle is divided or partially excised. The head is immobilized in the corrected position for a period of time. If surgery is delayed until the child is older, postoperative exercises are necessary to prevent a recurrence.

Childhood rickets

One disease resulting from nutritional disturbance is common childhood rickets. The name is misleading, however, because nowadays a classic example of this disease is sometimes difficult to find in the United States. Rickets is always a potential health hazard in communities where there is little sunshine or little exposure of the children to outdoors and a diet deficient in vitamin D and/or calcium or phosphorus. Vitamin D is crucial because it regulates the absorption and deposit of calcium and phosphorus. Most formulas are now specially irradiated or fortified to provide adequate levels of vitamin D to infants and children. Other rich sources are the fish-liver oils. Sunshine, if it is not screened by window glass and clothing or rendered unavailable by air pollution, is the most inexpensive source of vitamin D. Of course, vitamin preparations can be purchased. Cases of rickets may be mild and pass undetected or may be very severe and remarkable. Classic manifestations are knock-knees or bowlegs, kyphosis (humpback) or scoliosis (an abnormal lateral spinal curvature), delayed closure of fontanels and protruding forehead (bossing), thickened wrists and ankles, and enlargement of the cartilaginous area of attachment of the ribs to the sternum, forming the famous *rachitic rosary,* pigeon breast, and contracture of the pelvis. Treatment consists of greater intake of vitamin D, calcium, and phosphorus. It is possible, but not probable, to have an excessive vitamin D intake so discretion should be used in the selection and dosage of therapeutic vitamins.

THE TODDLER
Duchenne's muscular dystrophy

There are a number of conditions that are characterized by a progressive weakening of the musculoskeletal system and eventual wasting of muscle tissue. They differ in the main muscles affected, the course of the disability, and the usual age of onset. Duchenne's or pseudohypertrophic, muscular dystrophy is the commonest form of the progressive types of muscle weakness. The onset of this disease usually occurs within the first 3 years of life. In a few cases the onset commences between the third and sixth years. It is a hereditary sex-linked recessive condition that is said to affect males almost exclusively. In this type of dystrophy, a fatty infiltration of the muscle cells may produce a deceptively large muscle lacking strength, hence its title "pseudohypertrophic" muscular dystrophy. This condition is seen especially in the calf muscles. Intramuscular enzymes, creatine phosphokinase (CPK) and serum aldolase, leak into the blood serum as muscle tissue breaks down. Serum values of these enzymes are very high in the early stages of the disease but decline as the disease progresses, and in the final stages they are only slightly above normal (apparently because there is so little muscle tissue left). The affected young child has difficulty in walking and falls easily as the muscular weakness attacks, in sequence, the muscles of the legs, pelvis, and abdomen. A pronounced lordosis develops as he struggles to remain upright. The child displays a characteristic method of supporting himself when attempting to rise to his feet from a seated posture on the floor. He rises to his knees, extends both legs and arm, grasps the lower part of his legs with his hands, and gradually pushes himself upward in a sort of self-climbing procedure. This is one of the most characteristic signs of muscular dystrophy (Gower's sign). The genetic background of the family, the history and examination of the child revealing the progressive nature of the problem, serum enzyme tests, electromyogram, and muscle biopsy confirm the diagnosis. Muscle biopsy is especially valuable in determining the exact type of muscular problem. Preclinical cases can now be diagnosed by determining serum enzyme levels. The CPK test is a valuable aid in identifying muscular dystrophy carriers.

A diagnosis of muscular dystrophy (no matter what type) is difficult for parents to accept. In the case of the Duchenne type, life expectancy is usually limited to the teen-age period. Death often results from respiratory weakness and intervening infection. The course of the disease is downhill, and it is particularly disheartening for parents who first see their child confined to a wheelchair to eventually see him bedridden to the extent that he needs help to turn over. Many times much can be gained if the parents of such victims can meet together to share their common burdens and learn from one another how certain problems can be met. The local muscular dystrophy associations often sponsor such groups.

The nurse sees the child with muscular dystrophy in the hospital setting chiefly at the time of diagnosis, when orthopedic appliances, such as braces and splints, are being evaluated, or when the presence of other health problems makes it especially difficult to nurse the child at home.

Juvenile rheumatoid arthritis
(Still's disease)

Arthritis, or inflammation of the joints, may be caused by a wide variety of factors, including infection, trauma, and the wear and tear of aging. However, the cause of

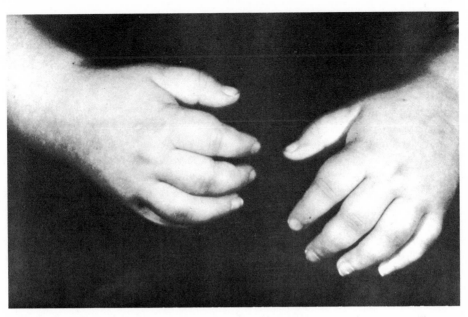

Fig. 34-5. Juvenile rheumatoid arthritis. Spindle-shaped fingers in a 2½-year-old boy. (Courtesy Naval Regional Medical Center, San Diego, Calif.)

the most common form of arthritis encountered in pediatrics, juvenile rheumatoid arthritis (or Still's disease), is unknown.

This disease affects the entire body's health. In studies it is often grouped with the collagen diseases, which affect all the connective tissues of the body. It does not confine itself to symptoms of joint pain, although this is the most remarkable manifestation of the disease. The joints swell and become stiff, slightly warm, and painful with movement. Almost all the joints may eventually become involved, but the knees, ankles, and fingers are most frequently affected. The fingers often assume a spindle shape as a result of the swelling of their middle joints (Fig. 34-5). Unless joint activity is maintained, a joint will become permanently stiffened or immovable, a condition known as *ankylosis* of the joint. For this reason it is important to maintain reasonable joint activity by reducing pain and providing specific tasks or play goals designed to exercise the involved joints.

The rheumatoid patient, unless very careful, is likely to assume positions of comfort, which if maintained for prolonged periods will cause deformities that will interfere with motions necessary to meet the needs of daily living. Mobility should be encouraged as much as tolerated, even during periods of active disease and inflammation. When pain and inflammation are suppressed by salicylates, most children are encouraged to ambulate. The most effective, continuous therapeutic exercise program is provided through the child's own play activities. Play activities should be directed to provide the maximum exercise for the joints most involved. Planned activity and formal exercises will help prevent the stiffness and deformity that result from inactivity. The physical therapist will teach the child and his parents exercises designed to give complete range of motion in each joint.

Fever is a significant manifestation of the disease. It may swing daily as high as 105° F. in the evening and return to normal by morning. The pattern on the temperature chart is usually characteristic and of great value in the differential diagnosis of a patient with acute rheumatoid arthritis.

Other signs and symptoms of rheumatoid

arthritis include enlargement of the liver, spleen, and lymph nodes, anemia, anorexia, pallor, and possibly a salmon-colored, blotchy rash. Infrequently, heart murmurs or carditis is encountered. The relationship (if any) between rheumatoid arthritis and rheumatic heart disease is not clear. The two are usually discussed as separate disorders. Rheumatoid arthritis is aggravated by emotional stress and fatigue.

Kind and understanding parental support, promotion of general health, and physical therapy will achieve most of the therapeutic goals. No specific treatment is known. Although many medications have been tried, aspirin is the drug of choice to relieve pain, reduce swelling, and increase range of motion. It is prescribed four times daily, and the dosage is often increased to toxic levels and then reduced for best results. The children are carefully observed in the clinic and the parents cautioned about early signs of toxicity (p. 328). Indomethacin (Indocin) is a new drug that has been found to be effective in the treatment of rheumatoid arthritis. It is presently being used in the larger clinics, but it is still considered experimental.

Prednisone and other corticosteroid derivatives will help alleviate symptoms of inflammation, but these drugs taken over a prolonged period of time are toxic, and rheumatoid symptoms recur when they are discontinued. So they are prescribed pru-

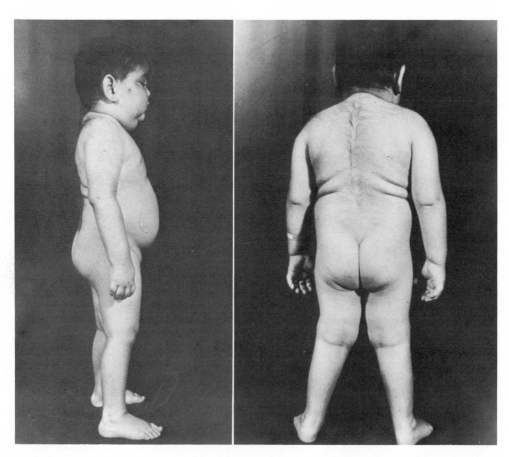

Fig. 34-6. Hypercortisonism in a 2½-year-old boy as a result of intensive steroid therapy. Note moon facies, excessive growth of hair (hirsutism), prominent fat pads, buffalo hump, and marked weight gain. (Courtesy Naval Regional Medical Center, San Diego, Calif.)

dently during periods when joint inflammation does not respond to more conservative therapy. Toxic manifestations of such hormone therapy may include decalcification of the skeleton, altered tissue response to infections and other injuries, personality changes, moon face, abnormal growth of the clitoris in girls, and the appearance of excessive body hair (Fig. 34-6).

Although juvenile rheumatoid arthritis may improve and then worsen over a period of years, usually it gradually subsides as puberty approaches. However, in some cases it may persist actively into adulthood and may leave difficult deformities.

Orthopedic complications of hemophilia

The problem of damaged joints should not be completely closed without at least mentioning another interesting cause of joint difficulty. The child with hemophilia, the classic bleeder, may sustain considerable joint destruction because of "insignificant initiating injuries" followed by hemorrhages into the joints of the knees and elbows. These patients must be placed in traction and protective casts fairly frequently.

The preschool child
Legg-Calvé-Perthes disease (coxa plana)

Legg-Calvé-Perthes disease is a self-limited disease of the hip produced by lack of circulation to the femoral head. The initial degeneration of the femoral head is followed by absorption and regeneration of bone. The entire process takes an average of 4 years.

This developmental disease of the hip is commonly seen in children between 4 and 8 years of age and has a much higher incidence in boys. The initial complaint is usually a limp of several months' duration. Some children have a limp with pain (referred to the knee) that is aggravated by activity and relieved by rest. The primary cause of Legg-Calvé-Perthes disease is unknown. Trauma and synovitis of the hip have preceded some cases. A great variety

of treatment has been used, including 4 years of bed rest. Modern successful treatment of the disease centers around two basic principles: (1) maintaining a full range of motion and (2) keeping the femoral head deep in the socket during its period of healing. In this way the physician seeks to obtain a femoral head that fits well and prevents the development of degenerative arthritis in the later years.

Treatment consists of traction followed by hip bracing in an abducted and slightly internally rotated position to properly align the femoral head and acetabulum. Such bracing removes pressure from the avascular head of the femur. It helps to keep the child ambulatory with the least discomfort and limitation of activity during the years of necessary management. Surgery (Salter procedure) may be indicated where conservative treatment has failed.

The school-age child
Osteomyelitis

Inflammatory bone conditions caused by disease-producing organisms were more common in the past. With increased availability of different types of antibiotics and other helpful medications, osteomyelitis, or inflammation of the bone resulting from infectious agents, has decreased remarkably. If the term "osteomyelitis" is used without a qualifying phrase, it is assumed to mean infection of the bone by either pathogenic staphylococcal or streptococcal organisms. However, broadly speaking, osteomyelitis may also be caused by the tuberculosis bacillus, the gonococcus, or a wide variety of lesser known bacteria. The form of osteomyelitis caused by staphylococci or streptococci may be preceded by some type of local injury to the bone that either introduces the organism directly or weakens the bone so that it is more susceptible to any offending organisms brought to the area by the bloodstream from some distant source of infection.

Blood-borne infections are most common. Boys are more frequently affected than girls. Pain near the end of a long bone and fever are clinically associated with osteomyelitis. The characteristic pain is initially very severe and unremitting because pressure is building up in a closed space. When pus begins to track out under the periosteum, the area is extremely tender, more so than a fracture. Treatment is started on the basis of the clinical examination alone. The child is placed on bed rest, and the affected limb is immobilized. Analgesics are given to lessen the pain. Although blood cultures are positive in only 50% of patients with osteomyelitis, they are taken immediately and during the first few days after examination in the hope of identifying the causative organism. Initially, large doses of broad-spectrum antibiotics are given. X-ray evidence of osteomyelitis is not seen for 10 days following the onset of symptoms. Surgery is considered necessary if improvement is not seen within 36 to 48 hours after antibiotic therapy is instituted. The area of maximum tenderness is drilled to decompress the bone and to allow the pus to drain. The organism responsible for the infection is identified, and a cast is applied to the affected limb. An opening in the cast is made at the surgical site, and the wound is infused with antibiotics for a period of several days before being surgically closed. Intravenous antibiotic therapy is continued for another 3 weeks. During this time the child is kept on bed rest, and the progress of the infection may be monitored by daily sedimentation rates. When the results of this test are near normal, antibiotics can be stopped and, hopefully, the risk of chronic osteomyelitis and extensive bone damage has been minimized.

Bone tumors

Some of the symptoms of infectious osteomyelitis are duplicated when the cause is not pathogenic organisms but the development of abnormal cells, producing a tumor, within the bone. Some of these masses of abnormal tissue are *benign* and of purely local importance. They may cause pain, at times accompanied by fever, and deformity. The tumors may weaken the structure of the bone, but they do not spread (or metastasize) to distant parts of the body. Other types of bone tumors grow rapidly and metastasize early through the bloodstream. These tumors are *malignant*. An osteosarcoma originates in connective tissue (of which bone is one example) and is the most common primarily malignant tumor of bone. School-age boys are affected almost twice as often as girls. The commonest sites are those characterized by active epiphyseal growth (for example, the distal end of the femur and the proximal ends of the tibia and humerus). Initially the child complains of mild pain in the affected part, but in a matter of days to weeks, the pain is constant and severe. As the condition progresses, the tumor mass becomes obvious. Limitation of adjacent joint motion is common. Early diagnosis and immediate treatment are crucial.

X-ray studies are characteristic, but the diagnosis is made only after biopsy and pathological studies of the tissue. Occasionally tumors of the bone in children may be secondary to tumors located elsewhere. When a tissue of bony origin is malignant, aggressive anticancer chemotherapy and radical methods of treatment, including amputation, must be endorsed in an effort to save the patient. The recorded number of 5-year cures is relatively low. Recently, several methods of treating osteosarcoma have been reviewed. The most encouraging results were noted in children who had been treated with supravoltage radiation before biopsy and again 4 to 6 weeks after biopsy. Radical amputation was then carried out if no metastases were found.

Spinal curvature

Spinal deformities such as scoliosis (S-shaped lateral curvature), kyphosis (humpback), and lordosis (exaggerated lumbar curvature) may be the products of many different conditions, including the following:

1. Nutritional deficiencies, such as common childhood rickets (discussed on p. 531)

2. Inflammation of the bony spine (osteomyelitis, tuberculosis, arthritis, or dislocation of the hips)
3. Nerve injury resulting in paralytic conditions and unequal muscle pull (myelomeningocele, poliomyelitis)
4. Primary muscle weakness or dystrophy

Scoliosis

Of the three kinds of abnormal spinal curvatures, scoliosis (or the lateral curvature), is probably the most common spinal deformity encountered in childhood. Lateral curvature of the spine can be divided into two major groups: nonstructural (functional) and structural. The patient can

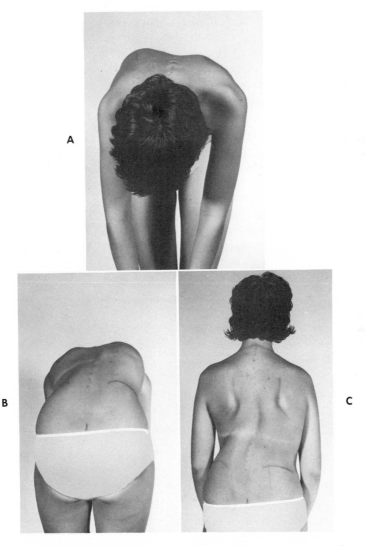

Fig. 34-7. A to C, Idiopathic scoliosis in 14-year-old girl. First visit to orthopedist. Screening positions: standing and forward bend. Observe for: (1) general posture and alignment of the spine: (a) lateral angulation and (b) balance of head, neck, and shoulders over pelvis; and (2) asymmetry: (a) exaggerated flank crease—more prominent on opposite side, (b) high shoulder, (c) position of scapulae, (d) convexity on side of major curve (caused by protruding ribs), (e) prominent hip, and (f) one arm longer than other when hanging free in the forward bend position. (Courtesy Naval Regional Medical Center, San Diego, Calif.)

voluntarily correct a nonstructural curve by altering his position. In functional scoliosis, a condition outside the spine (such as poor posture, pain or muscle spasm, or short leg) has caused a temporary misalignment of the vertebrae. A structural scoliosis is an irreversible lateral curvature that leads to permanent anatomic changes unless early preventive measures are taken.

There are three basic types of structural scoliosis: congenital, paralytic, and idiopathic. Congenital scoliosis results when one side of the vertebral column grows faster than the other. Surgical correction at 1 or 2 years of age may be indicated to prevent greater asymmetrical growth. Paralytic scoliosis may result from polio or other neuromuscular disorders. In order to prevent respiratory complications, some type of stabilization of the spine must be considered, either using an external support or surgery. Idiopathic scoliosis is the most common type, accounting for 80% of the cases classified as structural. It is called idiopathic because the cause is unknown. However, there seems to be a definite familial tendency that suggests a dominant inheritance pattern. The condition is more common in girls and is most apparent during adolescence, although it usually begins much earlier. The pattern of the curve may be cervical, thoracic, lumbar, or a combination of these. The most important aspect of the deformity is its progression with skeletal growth. As the lateral curvature and the rotation of the spine increases, secondary permanent changes develop in the vertebrae and ribs. Misalignment of the spinal joints worsens and eventually leads to painful degenerative spinal joint disease in adult life. In addition to the "crooked back" with a high shoulder, prominent hip, and uneven legs, the deformity of the spine may compromise cardiopulmonary function and shorten the patient's life expectancy. The progression of the curvature is slow and steady, seldom arousing the concern of the parent or child. Poor posture, an uneven hemline and inability to be fitted

for a dress are common complaints that bring the child in for evaluation. Because pain is not associated with the progressive curve, the deformity often reaches 30 degrees before it is detected. The deformity can be clinically evaluated in three positions (Fig. 34-7). Radiological studies confirm the extent of the deformity. The primary (major) curve is greatest in angulation and is the least flexible. It is always more marked than would be expected from the physical appearance (Fig. 34-8).

Screening. The only sure way of preventing the severe curvatures of idiopathic scoliosis, which usually involve major surgical procedures and their inherent risk, is by early recognition. The presence of a mild deformity allows the use of reliable, safe, effective nonsurgical treatment. Most children who demonstrate a curve at 11 or 12 years of age have almost always had it for

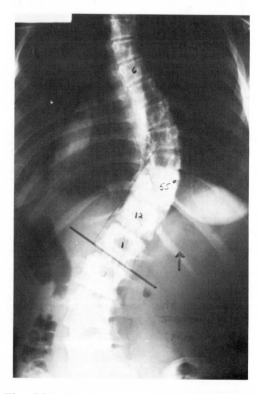

Fig. 34-8. Roentgenogram of 14-year-old girl (same as in Fig. 34-7) shows a 55° right thoracic curve of the spine. (Courtesy Naval Regional Medical Center, San Diego, Calif.)

a number of years. Therefore, screening programs for lateral curvatures should begin before age 10 and should include boys as well as preadolescent girls. Routine inspection of the spine by school nurses can be most rewarding.

Treatment. An orthopedist should determine the need for correction and examine the child with scoliosis at regular intervals to detect any progression of the curve. Curves up to 20 degrees can probably be left alone and watched. Curves that are between 20 to 45 degrees and progressing are stabilized with a brace. The Milwaukee brace (Fig. 34-9) is the standard device used in the nonoperative treatment of mild spinal curvatures. It is designed to provide dynamic correction that incorporates a vertical pushing force between the head and pelvis through adjustable, rigid uprights as well as a lateral corrective force directed toward the convex side of the major curve. The brace is well contoured and cosmetically acceptable. To prevent worsening of

the scoliosis, it is necessary to wear the brace full time, except for brief periods needed for personal hygiene, until complete maturation of the spine has occurred. Correction of the curve is likely when treatment is begun at an early age. Normal activities (such as bike riding and skating) are encouraged while wearing the brace. In fact, an active exercise program is required to maintain good muscle tone. Most children learn to accept the brace, live with it, and have good results.

Surgical correction is usually considered for curves that are over 50 degrees. Surgery offers the best outcome for: (1) curves that are cosmetically objectionable (over 60 degrees) in the preadolescent or postadolescent patient, (2) a growing child in whom conservative measures have failed, and (3) those who experience persistent backache. The operation consists of a spinal fusion that may be supplemented by the insertion and spinal attachment of an internal apparatus. The Harrington rod serves to obtain

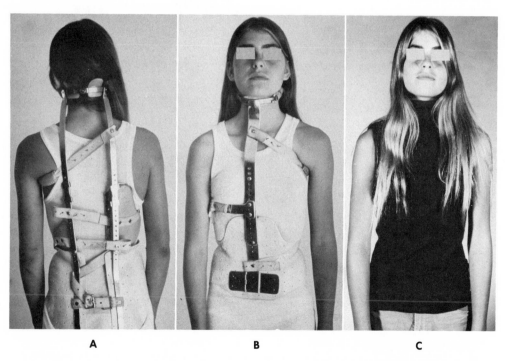

A   B   C

Fig. 34-9. **A,** Thirteen-year-old girl wearing a Milwaukee brace with right thoracic pad, left axillary sling, and left lumbar pad. Overall alignment is good. **B,** Same child front view. Brace is contoured closely to the body. **C,** It can be worn under clothing without being noticed.

539

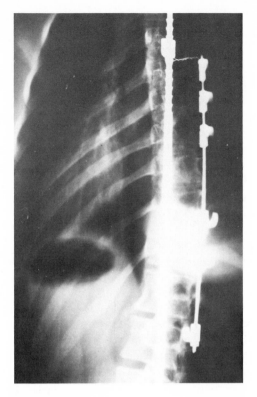

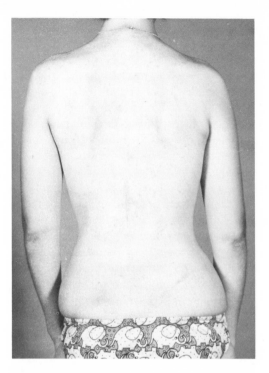

Fig. 34-10. Roentgenogram of back of same patient as in Fig. 34-8 6 months after spinal fusion and Harrington instrumentation. (Courtesy Naval Regional Medical Center, San Diego, Calif.)

Fig. 34-11. Postoperative standing position shows girl's spine reasonably well compensated. (Courtesy Naval Regional Medical Center, San Diego, Calif.)

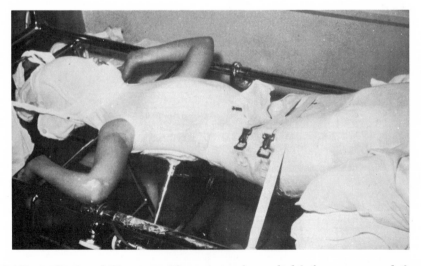

Fig. 34-12. Application of Risser cast. The cast may be applied before surgery and then bivalved for use as a postoperative holding jacket. This photograph shows neck halter, pelvic band, and a positioned localizer helping to maintain the patient's posture on the frame. (Courtesy Paul E. Woodward, M.D., San Diego, Calif.)

correction and to provide an internal type of immobilization (Fig. 34-10). Following spinal fusion, the patient may be placed in a body cast and confined to bed for about 3 months to allow the fused area to become consolidated; then progressive ambulation in the cast is encouraged. The localizer frame devised by Dr. Risser in the early 1950's is commonly used in the application of the jacket cast (Fig. 34-12). Complete union and maturation at the fusion site takes about 1 year.

Halo traction. The halo traction is used in the treatment of a rigid spinal curvature associated with weakness or paralysis of the neck and trunk muscles. It also may be employed in the care of cervical fractures and fusions (Fig. 34-13). The halo consists of a metal ring that is attached to the skull by two posterior pins in the occipital bone and two anterior pins inserted into the temporal bones. It is attached to a weight while countertraction is exerted by weights connected to two Steinmann pins inserted into the distal ends of both femurs. The weights are increased daily as tolerated by the child until maximum correction is obtained.

When maximum correction of the curve is evidenced by x-ray examination, a spinal fusion is usually done. Weighted halo traction may be continued to prevent loss of the correction, or a body cast or jacket is applied, incorporating the halo by means of an extended frame, to maintain the gains accomplished by the original traction and fusion.

NURSING CARE. The procedure should be explained step by step to the child, in words that he can understand. His questions should be answered carefully. He may complain that the pins hurt. This usually indicates that they need to be tightened to make the child more comfortable. The pins are cleaned daily with hydrogen peroxide, and the skin around each pin is painted with an antiseptic.

Proper alignment of all equipment, especially the ropes, is necessary for effective traction. The little patient may prefer to remain in the supine position, but he should be turned at least every 2 hours, from back to side and side to back. The patient is encouraged to breathe deeply for a few minutes each time he is turned. Adequate ventilation of the lungs is extremely important because a respiratory deficit often accompanies advanced scoliosis. Treatment includes promotion of pulmonary function, which is accomplished by specific breathing exercises.

Active and passive range of motion helps maintain muscular strength. Careful attention is given to the skin, especially bony

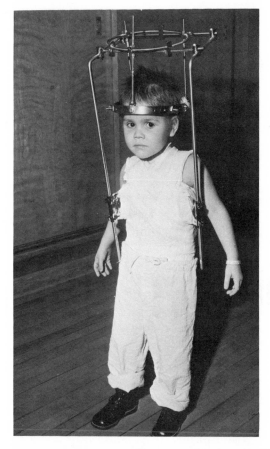

Fig. 34-13. This 4-year-old youngster has congenital deformities of the vertebrae and ribs that caused a severe scoliosis. A spinal fusion was performed. The halo frame and plaster cast combination maintains correction while allowing Ross to move about with relative ease. (Courtesy Children's Health Center, San Diego, Calif.)

prominences and the heels. Neurological and cardiac complications are not uncommon. Appropriate notice should be given to these important considerations without frightening the child. Bowel and bladder difficulties are frequent. They may be lessened by adequate intake of fluids, foods rich in bulk, and occasional laxatives. Remember that immobilization decreases appetite. The child should be given every opportunity to help select his diet when a choice is possible. His psychological growth is just as important as his physical well-being.

Spinal fusion. Casts, which may be worn for an extended period after a spinal fusion make turning the patient much simpler and safer. However, if a cast is not applied after a spinal fusion, care must be exercised so that the spinal column is not twisted during changes in position. The patient's bed should be kept flat unless specific permission has been granted to allow the patient to be on a slight incline while in *supine* position (on his back). A non-casted patient who is allowed to be turned should be gently logrolled from back to side with the use of a turning sheet and at least two nurses (more if the size of the patient indicates that more hands are needed). Such a patient, casted or not, who is turned from his back to a side-lying position should have a pillow between his thighs to prevent the adduction of the top leg and pull on the small of the back. Just how much motion will be allowed a patient will depend on his physician's wishes.

Patients who have had a spinal fusion need the same basic preoperative and postoperative care required for all surgical patients. In addition, they may need the special attention necessary for all casted patients (see Chapter 30). Constipation may be a particular problem; therefore the type of diet, fluid intake, and habit-times need special attention.

Therapy for marked scoliosis is usually long. It characteristically will involve innumerable visits to the physician for evaluation, hospitalization at intervals for cast changes, brace adjustments, or surgical interventions, and physical therapy. The parents and child (young lady or man) need to be constantly encouraged to continue treatment faithfully until optimum, lasting results are achieved.

NERVOUS SYSTEM DISEASES THAT MAY AFFECT THE BONES AND MUSCLES
THE INFANT
Seizure disorders

The term "convulsive seizures" is really not a diagnosis but simply a description of a transient disturbance of the central nervous system. As you have already noted, seizures may be caused by a number of conditions. An elevated body temperature may be the precipitating cause, especially in infancy. Seizures may originate from congenital brain deformities, or increased intracranial pressure caused by tumors, abscess formation, or edema of the brain. Cerebral irritation resulting from toxic or infectious agents may be implicated. A chronic or recurrent convulsive disorder may also be called *epilepsy*. Some writers reserve the term "epilepsy" for recurrent convulsions of the idiopathic variety (cases of unknown cause). There are differences of opinion regarding the role of heredity in cases of idiopathic seizures. Some authorities believe that heredity may be a significant cause; others deny this. Because some states and communities may have laws limiting the activities of those persons who have been diagnosed as epileptic and because the public does not always understand what the word means in a specific case, many physicians hesitate to use this particular term when describing the patient's problem. The nurse would also do well to use the word very discreetly. It has been estimated that approximately 1% of the population has some type of epileptic disorder.

There are many types of seizures; two examples are grand mal (great pain or evil) and petit mal (small pain or evil). Grand mal seizures affect the large muscle groups of the body. Usually the entire body becomes involved in dramatic, involuntary muscular contractions of considerable force. Petit mal seizures, on the other hand, are characterized by minor tremors or brief losses of consciousness revealed perhaps only by a prolonged blank stare or the dropping of an object held in the hand. The frequency of either type of seizure may be extremely variable. A child may experience a seizure rarely or many times during a 24-hour period. Diagnosis is aided by a study of the child's brain waves, or an electroencephalogram.

Children who have grand mal seizures may experience a subjective warning of an impending episode. Such a warning is called an aura. It may occur a few minutes, hours, or, rarely, even days before the attack. It may come in the form of a vague feeling of uneasiness or as some type of sensory cue. For example, the patient may hear, see, or smell things in a particular manner. Such auras are useful to patients because they can seek out places of safety and privacy if they are forewarned of an attack.

The grand mal seizure usually begins with a period of rigidity and temporary respiratory arrest. The first sign of an attack may be involuntary movements of the eyeball (the eyes rolling upward or to the side) and a stiffening of body parts. The patient temporarily suspends respirations and may become cyanotic. Saliva is not swallowed, and the patient may drool. A high-pitched cry may be heard. This first period, called the *tonic* phase, is usually followed by intermittent contractions of the muscles. This secondary period is the so-called *clonic* phase. During this time the tongue and lips may be bitten and saliva, as a result, may be blood tinged.

The nursing care of a patient having a convulsion emphasizes the need to protect the patient from accidental injury and the importance of close observation and report. If possible, a patient should be placed on his side or lie with his face turned to one side to avoid aspiration. He should be placed in an area where the possibility of personal injury as a result of uncontrolled muscular contractions would be minimal: on the floor on a rug, if possible, or in bed. The beds or cribs of patients who experience fairly frequent convulsions of the grand mal type should be equipped with side rails padded with folded blankets or pillows. In the hospital setting nurses are taught to have a well-padded tongue blade readily accessible at the bedside for insertion into the mouth between the back teeth before the onset of the clonic phase of the seizure to prevent mouth injury. If a padded tongue blade is not available, a rolled washcloth may be helpful. In most instances the use of a blade is not required. In some instances it may cause more problems than failure to use anything at all. Nurses should not pry open a patient's mouth to insert a tongue blade. Such a maneuver may cause considerable injury and serves no practical purpose because the damage to the mouth in most cases has already occurred. The Epilepsy Society does not advise the general public to place anything into the victim's mouth. There have been too many incidents of mouth injury or aspiration due, not to the convulsion, but to the insertion of an improper tongue protector.

After first securing a safe position for the convulsing patient, the nurse should focus her powers of observation in order to be able to describe the circumstances and sequence of the attack. She should note the following information:

1. When the seizure began and what type of activity immediately preceded its occurrence
2. What signs of difficulty were first noted, what part of the body was first affected, and how the convulsion progressed
3. How long the attack lasted
4. Whether the patient was incontinent
5. Whether prolonged cyanosis or profuse saliva appeared (may signal the need for the use of oxygen or possible suctioning)

543

In the great majority of cases the seizure subsides, and the child falls into a deep sleep. When finally awake again, he may not remember the seizure but feel tired and sore. He should be reassured regarding the episode and be gently questioned to determine if he had any warning, or aura, of the attack.

Almost all patients who suffer from idiopathic epilepsy and many with organically initiated seizures are receiving some type of anticonvulsant therapy. There are a number of medications available. They are prescribed according to the individual needs of the patient. Some commonly used drugs are diphenylhydantoin (Dilantin) sodium and phenobarbital. The time schedule established for taking anticonvulsants should be faithfully followed to avoid any interruption in treatment and the possible appearance of a seizure. Other methods to help prevent seizures limit fluids and stress a high-fat–low-carbohydrate (ketogenic) diet. Complete or almost complete control can be obtained in approximately half the cases. Many patients can be very well regulated with medical therapy and are able to live fairly normal lives. A few types of epilepsy (for example, petit mal) disappear after puberty; some change their form; others, unfortunately, persist throughout life. The nurse should realize that fatigue, illness, excitement, hyperventilation, blinking lights, or failure to take anticonvulsants may help bring on certain seizures.

The patient and his family need continuous, good medical supervision and counsel. The patient should be encouraged to live life to the fullest within the limits of his disease as imposed by the community and his own sense of responsibility. The intelligence levels of people with epilepsy are very similar to those found in the population as a whole.

The Epilepsy Societies have done considerable work in the area of public education regarding the disorder, attempting to remove false ideas and any legislation that unjustly limits the activities of its victims.

Meningitis

Meningitis, simply stated, is inflammation of the meninges. Not all types of meningitis are infectious, but the infectious types are far more common. The hemophilus influenza bacillus, meningococcus, and pneumococcus are common etiological agents responsible for acute bacterial meningitis in children past 1 month of age. Meningitis usually affects children under 2 years of age, and *Haemophilus influenzae* is by far the most common causative agent. Whatever the cause or age of onset, the treatment of meningitis is always considered a medical emergency! Early recognition and prompt treatment are essential for a favorable recovery. A long and severe infection may result in death or lingering neurological damage.

Typically the child is irritable and restless or drowsy. Previous upper respiratory tract infections, especially ear infections, are associated with *Haemophilus influenzae* meningitis. For this reason, the nurse should impress on parents the importance of continuing medications (for otitis media or other inflammations) and all antibiotics prescribed for as long as ordered. Fever, vomiting, chills, headache, rigidity of the neck and back, and convulsions are common. In more severe cases the child may be in shock or exhibit an involuntary arching of his back known as opisthotonos (Fig. 34-15). A high-pitched cry is characteristic. Meningococcal meningitis is usually accompanied by petechiae, a hemorrhagic skin rash caused by meningococcal invasion of the bloodstream. However, meningococcemia may occur without central nervous system involvement.

A lumbar puncture is done at the slightest suspicion of meningitis, even a convulsion. Parents and children fear a lumbar puncture. Parents should be reassured of the importance and necessity of this procedure. The child, if conscious and old enough to understand, should be mentally prepared just before the procedure. He should be told what is going to happen and why and what he is likely to feel. Re-

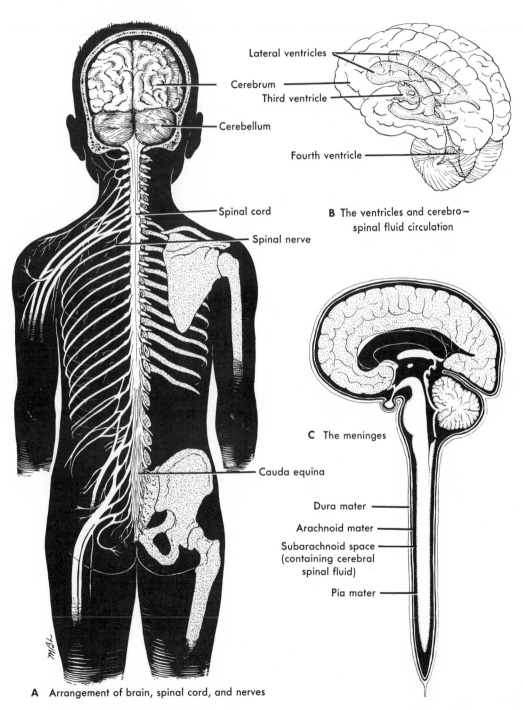

Lateral ventricles

Cerebrum

Third ventricle

Cerebellum

Fourth ventricle

Spinal cord

Spinal nerve

B The ventricles and cerebro—
spinal fluid circulation

C The meninges

Cauda equina

Dura mater

Arachnoid mater

Subarachnoid space
(containing cerebral
spinal fluid)

Pia mater

A Arrangement of brain, spinal cord, and nerves

Fig. 34-14. Simplified central nervous system anatomy and peripheral nerve relationships.

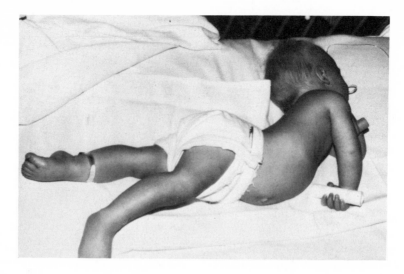

Fig. 34-15. A victim of near drowning showing marked opisthotonos. This posture may be assumed by anyone suffering from severe meningeal irritation. (Courtesy Alan Shumacher, M.D., San Diego, Calif.)

minding him that it is important to lie still during the procedure may provide a sense of control and thereby reduce feelings of helplessness. The assisting nurse must understand the importance of maintaining the position of the child during this procedure. Several holds are possible, depending on the size of the child. A side position is usually preferred. The back of the patient is arched "like a kitten's" to provide greater room for the insertion of the needle between the vertebrae at the level of the iliac crest. The skin is usually prepared with an antiseptic by the gloved physician. At the time of the lumbar puncture the pressure of the fluid within the meninges may be measured by attaching a measuring tube or manometer to the spinal needle. Three specimens of spinal fluid are usually collected consecutively in specially numbered sterile specimen containers. All three containers are sent to the laboratory where they should be immediately examined for cellular and chemical content. A Gram stain or culture is done to identify any organisms that may be present. A Gram stain can often identify an organism at once, before the return of the culture report. At the conclusion of the puncture procedure a

Band-Aid is placed over the site of the needle insertion.

The child is isolated for 24 hours after the start of antibiotic therapy. The meaning of this isolation and why the nurse wears a gown should be explained to parents. If they are not allowed to enter the room, the child's crib should be turned so they might at least see his face.

An intravenous infusion is started as soon as the lumbar puncture is completed. Large doses of ampicillin are given intravenously with fluid and electrolyte replacement. Ampicillin is currently the drug of choice for undiagnosed meningitis. Good supportive care requires that dehydration be corrected promptly, but the alert nurse will guard against overhydration. Symptoms of water intoxication are headache, confusion, sudden weight gain, edema, convulsions, and coma.

Effective restraints must be used to safeguard the infusion. The nurse should carefully position the restrained child on his side during intravenous therapy lest he convulse or aspirate vomitus. Constant nursing care and frequent observation of the child are necessary during the acute phase. Monitoring the vital signs is especially important when increased intracranial pressure is suspected. Slowed pulse, irregular respirations, and elevated blood pressure are signs of increased intracranial pressure and should be called to the physician's attention at once. Cerebral pressure may be lessened either by the infusion of drugs such as mannitol or by surgical intervention. Such methods are often lifesaving.

The infant may be placed in an oxygen-enriched environment in an incubator. The older child may be placed in an oxygen tent. Other nursing responsibilities include control of temperature by sponging and a cool environment. Antipyretics are usually not recommended, because they interfere with monitoring the temperature response, which determines the length of ampicillin therapy. Accurately recording the intravenous intake and the urinary output is important (urinary retention and fecal impactions are real possibilities). As the child progresses favorably, the nurse may safely encourage the parents to hold their infant or toddler during intravenous therapy, allowing for body contact and love, as well as position change. Granting as much freedom from restraint and provision for psychological comforts (such as thumb-sucking) as is consistent with therapy and safety is very important.

The convalescent period should be long enough to permit the child to regain his previous physical status. The young child should be carefully reevaluated at intervals during his convalescence. Residual complications may include hydrocephalus, subdural effusion, incoordination, sensory loss mental deterioration, or behavior problems.

Aseptic meningitis syndrome. This term includes a number of viral disorders that have an acute onset and usually a self-limited course with varying meningeal manifestations. Meningismus, meningeal irritation resulting in complications such as nuchal (neck) or spinal rigidity, is present. Lumbar puncture reveals a sterile culture. To rule out other diseases, hospitalization is necessary for at least 48 hours for obser-

vation. Treatment is supportive and symptomatic.

Neonatal meningitis. Newborns are frequent victims of meningitis. Most often the organisms attacking these babies are *Escherichia coli* and staphylococci. About 1 in every 1,000 to 2,000 newborns is affected. These infections are often associated with low birth weight. Maternal infection, premature rupture of membranes, and complicated deliveries are often part of the obstetrical history. Signs of meningeal irritation are minimal. The infant characteristically is lethargic and irritable and refuses to suck. Vomiting, respiratory distress, and convulsions are common. Penicillin and kanamycin are specific, and medications are given intravenously, usually by scalp vein. The hair should always be shaved in advance. Intensive supportive nursing care is essential. Because of the difficulty in recognizing the disease early and the inability of the debilitated small infant to respond to treatment, prognosis remains very poor, and the children who do survive have a high incidence of cerebral damage.

Subdural hematoma

This condition (really a blood tumor) is most frequently encountered in infants as a result of injury at birth, falls, other trauma, or abnormal bleeding tendencies. (It is also found in cases of "battered children.")

Increased intracranial pressure occurs as a result of bleeding into the potential space just under the dura of the brain, and the brain becomes compressed under the developing collection of bloody fluid. The onset of symptoms may be rapid or slow, depending on the extent of bleeding and the area affected. Diagnosis is made possible through subdural taps, usually performed in infants by insertion of a needle through one side of the anterior fontanel or in the suture line. The area is shaved and cleaned with antiseptic. The child must be carefully restrained (mummy fashion) and the head gently stabilized during the procedure. Withdrawal of abnormal fluid indicates the diagnosis. Successive aspirations and craniotomy may be necessary to relieve pressure and evacuate any membrane that surrounded the hematoma to prevent permanent injury to the brain. Such injury can be manifested by mental retardation and loss of normal motor function. Careful observation and report of vital signs, the tension of the fontanel, eye signs, and any emesis are necessary to prevent such unfortunate complications.

Cerebral palsy (Fig. 34-16)

In reality cerebral palsy is not in itself a disease but a condition that may result from numerous diseases, which may cause damage to those parts of the brain that are responsible for voluntary muscular coordination. Such causes may include pressure on the brain or oxygen deprivation to the brain before or during birth, direct injury,

tumor, embolus or hemorrhage, hydrocephalus, cerebral anoxia and infection or toxicity occurring any time after birth. Cerebral palsy is usually diagnosed in infancy since it is commonly caused by events associated with the prenatal or perinatal period. Treatment may continue throughout the affected person's life. It may be limited and mild or severe and far-reaching involving many body functions. It is said that there are approximately 100 to 600 cases of cerebral palsy per 100,000 persons in the general population.

Since more than the motor areas of the brain may be involved in such injuries and conditions, it is fairly common for children with cerebral palsy to have other symptoms as well. Some are blind; many have disorders in visual perception and may not see objects in the normal way. Since spatial relationships appear distorted, there may be

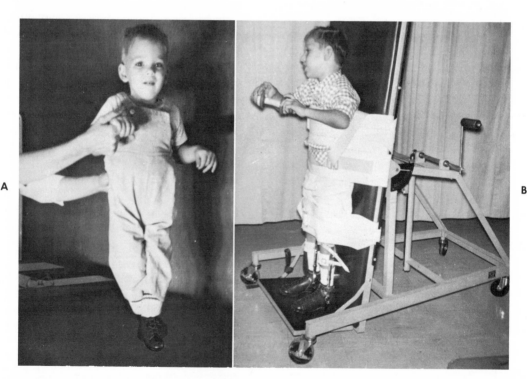

Fig. 34-16. This little fellow cannot walk at all without support. **A,** With support, a scissors gait is present (one foot crossing the other caused by adductor spasticity). **B,** Many hours on the tilt-table and the consistent work and concern of therapists and parents have markedly strengthened this young child's legs. (Courtesy Crippled Children Services, Department of Public Health, San Diego, Calif.)

additional problems in judgment, reading, and writing (words may seem reversed), balance, and coordination. The muscles of the mouth, tongue, and throat may be affected, influencing the ability to receive, chew, and swallow food as well as to speak. A significant percentage of children suffer from hearing loss, a condition that also affects speech. Occasionally the sense of touch may be impaired. Mental retardation is a fairly common complication, although not all children with cerebral palsy are mentally retarded and a few have above average intelligence. The amount of motor difficulty the child experiences is not necessarily indicative of his mental capacity. Some patients are victims of seizures and must receive appropriate medication.

Therapists usually speak of the following three main types of cerebral palsy:

1. *Spastic,* characterized by increased muscle stiffness or tone, exaggerated contraction of affected muscle groups when stimulated (stretch reflex), jerky motions, and a tendency to have contractures. The lower extremities are more often involved. A scissors gait is common.
2. *Athetoid,* characterized by involuntary, uncoordinated purposeless movements involving joint motion rather than single muscle action. The upper extremities are more often involved.
3. *Ataxic,* characterized by loss of a sense of balance and problems in evaluating spatial relationships and the relative positions of body parts.

Subgroupings and combinations of these types of cerebral palsy also occur.

It can readily be appreciated that the care of a cerebral-palsied child and his family cannot be the responsibility of just one practitioner. Their problems are usually too extensive. A team approach is necessary. The team includes the pediatrician, orthopedist, physical therapist, occupational therapist, speech therapist, psychologist, medical-social worker, public health workers, office and hospital nurses, and schoolteachers.

These children and their families often have considerable emotional problems, which may be expressed in the way the parents treat the child and their aspirations for his future. The parents may be overprotective and do too much for the child, making it difficult for him to master the skills of which he is capable. On the other hand, they may expect too much of their child and cause painful frustrations. They may need help in establishing realistic goals and in providing an environment conducive to good mental health as well as good physical health. Parents often have guilt feelings regarding the child's handicap.

Association with other parents with similar problems and psychiatric assistance are often very rewarding. One hopeful aspect of cerebral palsy is that if the initiating cause is not progressive in character, the neuromuscular involvement will not worsen. Cerebral palsy is not a degenerative disease as are, for example, the muscular dystrophies, and considerable improvement can usually be gained. Through physical and occupational therapy, surgical techniques, and medication, youngsters with cerebral palsy are able to meet their daily personal needs and, in some cases, to prepare for self-supporting occupations. Special public school programs may be available in the community that are especially geared to meet the needs of such handicapped children. They may attend some regular public school classes as well as special sessions designed to meet their individual needs during the school day.

When a child with cerebral palsy is hospitalized, it is very important that the hospital staff know his capabilities as an individual. Information regarding successful feeding and dressing techniques, toileting practices, communication aids, and special problems may save hours of frustration and distress. The care of some patients will require little modification, since their total neuromuscular involvement is slight. The care of others will require considerable study and adjustment. A child who has a history of seizures or upper extremity or

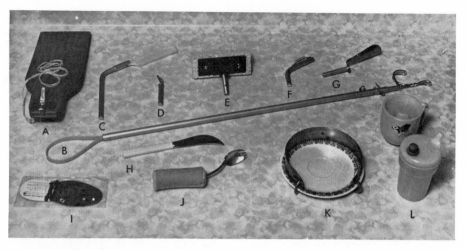

Fig. 34-17. Various aids for everyday activities for the handicapped. *A,* Nail clippers on wooden base, operated by string and foot action; *B,* gadget stick with hook attachment; *C,* comb attachment; *D,* clip attachment; *E,* mop or sponge attachment; *F,* magnet attachment; *G,* shoehorn attachment; *H,* rocker knife; *I,* elastic shoelaces; *J,* built-up handle on swivel fork (Spork); *K,* plate and plate guard; *L,* two types of weighted "trainer cups." (Courtesy Children's Health Center, San Diego, Calif.)

head involvement should not have his temperature taken orally regardless of age.

Each child's diet must be evaluated to make sure that it is appropriate for his age, nutritional needs, and the ability to handle and swallow. Although self-feeding may take considerably more time and cause more disorder, the child should feed himself, as much as possible, using techniques he has been taught. Aids such as swivel spoons, plate guards, training cups, and rocker knives may be invaluable (Fig. 34-17). Occasionally special weights may be attached to the child's arms to help control involuntary motion. Children who because of their condition must be fed should be assisted with patience. Since severely involved children may require the occasional use of suction, an apparatus should be available. When feeding the child, the nurse should hold him in such a way that the child's arm closest to her extends behind her. This often causes the child's head to rotate comfortably to the same side (tonic neck reflex). Gentle support of the chin or stroking of the cheeks may help lip closure and swallowing. Some children who have difficulty swallowing may find

carbonated drinks a problem. Waiting until the carbonation is minimal or serving other types of liquids is helpful.

The child with this condition should receive gentle, deliberate care. Excessive stimulation, sudden jarring movements, and the pressure of "having to hurry" induces greater tenseness and makes performance of relatively simple tasks extremely difficult. These children find it very difficult to relax, and they become fatigued easily. The simplest kind of controlled movement may require a tremendous amount of concentration and energy.

Whenever possible the cerebral-palsied child should have contact with other boys and girls and should not be socially deprived. Contact with other youngsters has frequently been limited. Even those who have moderately severe muscular involvement often enjoy working with Play Dough or modeling clay, finger paints, large blocks, and hand puppets. Music, television, and reading can be enjoyed by many. The occupational therapist may work with the children to perfect certain skills needed to meet everyday needs. These are presented to the young child in the form of games or special projects. His progress, although at times seemingly small, should be recognized and praised. The child responds to this recognition and continues his efforts to improve.

Although it may seem to some critics that a tremendous amount of time, effort, and financial outlay is expended in community programs to help cerebral-palsied youngsters, such programs are rewarding from many points of view. In the long run it is less expensive to educate the individual to achieve his potential than to provide the type of state-supported custodial care offered in the past. It often brings a measure of independence and a feeling of self-respect and personal worth to the individual patient. It brings hope and aid to concerned and burdened parents and inspiration to those who observe and help when they can.

Blindness

Causes of visual loss include hereditary factors, intrauterine or postnatal infections, retrolental fibroplasia (as a result of the use of prolonged high concentrations of oxygen in the care of premature infants), malignant tumors (retinoblastoma), and trauma.

The child who is blind from birth or infancy usually makes a satisfactory adjustment to his lack of visual perception. Special classes or schools may teach him to perform necessary tasks and concentrate on skills that bring special reward—music, reading (through the study of Braille techniques), writing (using Braille typewriters), and learning through the use of tape-recorded instruction.

It is estimated that out of every 100,000 schoolchildren in the United States, more than 34 have been classified legally blind.

The emotional and physical adjustment of the child who becomes blind after having been sighted is more difficult. Both types of blind children need to be treated as much like a sighted child as possible. Parents require special instruction to be able to help their children in the best way

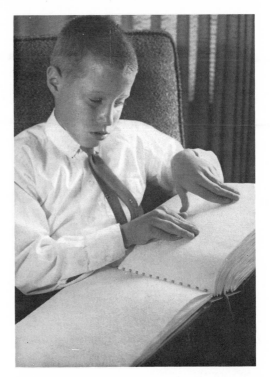

Fig. 34-18. This industrious boy, reading from his Braille Bible, was blinded because of retrolental fibroplasia.

possible and avoid the pitfalls of overprotection or unrealistic demands.

Cataracts

Congenital cataracts are occasionally seen. The student should recall that a cataract is an abnormal opacity of the crystalline lens, located just in back of the pupil. By obstructing the pathway of light to the retina, cataracts can cause partial or total blindness. Congenital cataracts may be caused by infectious agents during the mother's pregnancy (for example, rubella), metabolic disorders in the child, or hereditary factors. Whether corrective surgery is recommended for a child with congenital cataracts will depend on many factors, since surgery may not always produce the desired results.

The amount of movement a child is allowed after the surgical removal of cataracts will depend on the type of procedure performed and the preferences of the attending physician. Some physicians may insist on jacket and elbow restraints as well as sandbags placed at the sides of the head and maintenance of a supine position. Others are more liberal and believe that the agitation that full restraint may cause is more dangerous to the child than most movements he may make. Every effort should be made to reduce crying and prevent vomiting, since they increase intraocular pressure, strain on the sutures, and bleeding. Aspiration is a real danger when the child is maintained on his back, and great care should be taken at feeding time. The child's eyes will be bandaged. His food and surroundings should be described when appropriate. Before touching a child who cannot see, the nurse should speak to be sure that the child is not startled by her care. Again, orientation to the hospital setting, preparation for the postoperative period, and parental support are very important.

Other visual problems

The gift of sight is indeed precious. Proper care of the eyes should be taught to the growing child. It is always better to prevent rather than to treat eye damage. Children should be observed for the following signs of possible visual difficulty:

1. Complaints of poor or blurred vision; inability to see the blackboard well
2. Frequent headaches, dizziness, nausea, or fatigue
3. Burning or "scratchy" eyes
4. Recurrent styes, swollen or red-rimmed eyelids, inflammation and tearing, unequal pupils, or crossed eyes
5. Frequent frowning, squinting, blinking, or grimacing; tilting the head to one side or shutting one eye while inspecting objects; rubbing the eyes often; irritability
6. Difficulty in reading, holding the book too close, or avoiding all "close work."

Myopia and hyperopia. Myopia, or nearsightedness, is hereditary and fairly common in children. Hyperopia, or farsightedness, is less common. Children who must wear glasses to achieve clear vision must be carefully taught to keep their glasses in a case when they are not on their noses. The proper methods of handling and cleaning the lenses should also be demonstrated. When a young patient wearing glasses or contact lenses is admitted to the hospital, a note concerning them should be included in his admission record.

Amblyopia. An eye examination should be routinely made before any child reaches school age (preferably at 3 years of age) to detect problems that may affect normal usage and development of the eyes. If the child has an undetected strabismus (crossed or crooked eyes) or some other visual problem that may cause him to use one eye and not the other, his unused eye may not develop proper vision. This condition has been called *amblyopia.* Its frequency has created considerable concern. It is estimated that 1 in every 20 schoolchildren in the United States suffer from this problem.

Strabismus. Strabismus, or squint, as it is often called, may be treated in several ways, depending on its extent (Fig. 34-20). Some eyes are severely crossed or crooked. Other cases may be difficult to detect. Strabismus is common during early infancy but should not persist. About 1% or 2% of all children continue to have the disorder. It is important because it may eventually cause blindness in the "lazy" eye, and a cosmetic defect may initiate adjustment problems with playmates. For mild conditions, eye exercises may be prescribed. Placing a patch over the unaffected eye to force the use of the weak eye may be all that is necessary. Glasses may be recommended. However, many times a surgical repair of the condition is necessary. This involves the lengthening or shortening of the muscles controlling the position of the eyeball.

The child who has had a squint repair may return to his unit postoperatively with or without eye dressings, according to his physician's preference and his individual

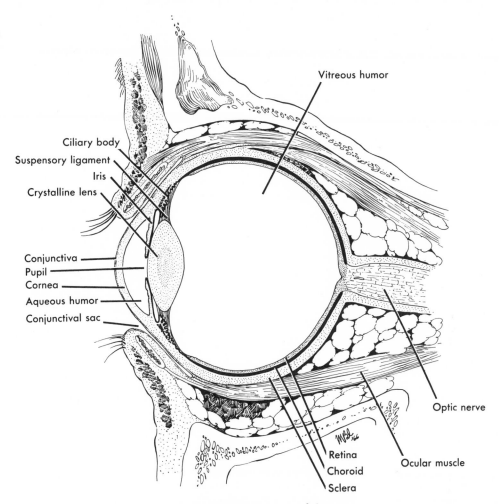

Vitreous humor

Ciliary body
Suspensory ligament
Iris
Crystalline lens

Conjunctiva
Pupil
Cornea
Aqueous humor
Conjunctival sac

Optic nerve

Retina
Choroid
Sclera

Ocular muscle

Fig. 34-19. Basic anatomy of the eye.

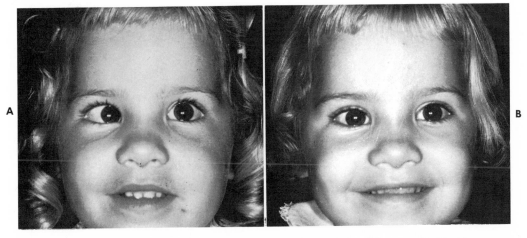

A   B

Fig. 34-20. Repair of squint. **A,** Before surgery. **B,** After surgery. (Courtesy Orville Graves, M.D., La Jolla, Calif.)

needs. He may or may not have restraints, depending on his age, level of consciousness, and ability to cooperate. Many physicians request elbow restraints. If no dressings are in place, the parents should be advised to expect their child to have "bloodshot" eyes. If restraints and dressings are used, it is very important that the child be oriented well to the hospital before his surgery and that he be told that his eyes will be covered after surgery. Some children may benefit from having their eyes bandaged before surgery in order to know what to expect. It is difficult to adequately prepare very young children. Mother's presence at the bedside is the best security. There is usually no postoperative limitation of head movement in the case of squint repair.

Hearing problems

Approximately 5% of preschool-age children have appreciable hearing loss. Almost 3 per 1,000 children are totally or nearly totally deaf. The earlier that hearing loss is detected in the child, the greater the possibility for correcting the hearing loss and reducing speech and personality problems.

It is now advocated that even infants exhibiting hearing loss be fitted with hearing aids so that they may be "tuned in" to the world about them and not suffer from the problems that isolation resulting from deafness creates. Early use of hearing aids may even prevent further hearing loss. Most children can be successfully fitted with one or two aids and learn to talk (Fig. 34-21).

The nurse should be alert for signs of possible deafness. Before 7 to 8 months of age the normal infant attempts to localize sound. At 9 months or more he should be able to localize sources of sound with little difficulty. Older children who have speech that is unclear, problems with consonant formation, or flat or excessively loud voices may be victims of auditory impairment. A child who consistently turns or tips his head or insists that the television be turned up beyond the normal needs of his playmates may also be suffering from hearing loss, as may the child who pulls or pokes at his ears.

Loss of hearing can result from many causes. Either conduction or nerve deafness may occur. Common causes of hearing difficulty are chronic otitis media (middle ear

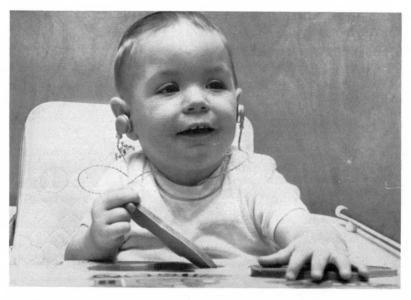

Fig. 34-21. Child with hearing aids during therapy. (Courtesy San Diego Speech and Hearing Center, San Diego, Calif.)

infection), obstruction caused by the presence of a foreign body or excessive wax (cerumen) in the ear canal, congenital malformations involving the external canal or interior of the ear, damage to the auditory nerve caused by prenatal or postnatal infections or toxins, anoxia, or, occasionally, the prolonged use of certain antibiotics such as streptomycin or kanamycin (Kantrex). Many children are left with defective hearing because of the effects of prenatal rubella, or German measles. (Review anatomy of the ear, Fig. 35-4.)

When speaking to a deaf child, one should face him directly, if at all possible, so that he may supplement his limited sound perception with visual cues from your lips. Parents and nurses should take every opportunity to expose the young child to auditory stimulation to help in the improvement of hearing. He cannot hear or learn to listen if there are no sound waves present!

The fact that a child has a hearing defect or wears a hearing aid on admission to the hospital is an important nursing observation. If the child is scheduled for surgery, permission should be sought to allow him to wear the aid until he is anesthetized in the operating room. The aid should be reapplied as soon as he has awakened from surgery. Such permission will greatly reduce the fear of the little patient and facilitate the entire procedure.

THE TODDLER
Encephalitis

Encephalitis is inflammation of the brain, also called the encephalon. Sometimes a disease involves both the meninges and brain tissue; then the condition is labeled meningoencephalitis. One of the meanings of the word element "myelitis" is inflammation of the spinal cord. It is possible to have a widespread inflammation of the central nervous system involving the meninges, brain, and spinal cord, but the terminology that describes the situation is almost as foreboding as the condition itself. Imagine seeing "meningoencephalomyelitis" listed as a tentative diagnosis in a patient's records!

Encephalitis cases may be infectious, postinfectious, or toxic in origin. Some types of encephalitis are caused by viruses that may be carried by infected mosquitoes, ticks, or mites. Encephalitis following rubeola (2-week measles) is relatively common, occurring once in every 600 to 1,000 cases of measles.

Noninfectious forms of encephalitis may be caused by toxins contacted by ingestion or inhalation. Lead poisoning in children, although not as common as formerly, is still reported every year. All furniture and toys used by a young child (who considers tasting at least as important as feeling or smelling) should be protected by nontoxic, lead-free paint.

Encephalitis is often characterized by personality change, headache, drowsiness, convulsion, and fever. Cranial nerves may become paralyzed, affecting speech, muscle strength, and reflex response. Double vision may be reported. Like meningitis, encephalitis may cause mental retardation and residual paralysis.

The nursing care of a child with encephalitis is very much like that of a child with meningitis. Lumbar punctures may be frequently performed to relieve intracranial pressure. The difference between encephalitis and meningitis may not be detected clinically on the basis of demonstrated symptoms. The differentiation is made on the basis of the results from laboratory examinations.

THE PRESCHOOL CHILD
Brain tumors (Fig. 34-22)

Although brain tumors are not found as frequently in children as in adults, they are not uncommon in childhood. Most of these brain tumors are situated rather deeply within the brain structure, making it difficult to assure complete removal of the abnormal cells. About three fourths of the brain tumors occurring in childhood involve the supportive connective tissue of the brain, called *glial* cells. The two most common gliomas are astrocytomas and medulloblastomas. Total resection of an infiltrating cerebral astrocytoma is not usually possible, but a cystic cerebellar astrocytoma is relatively slow growing, usually encapsu-lated, and easier to remove. Symptoms of developing brain tumor may appear very slowly in the case of a slowly progressing lesion. However, some tumors (for example, medulloblastomas) grow rapidly and

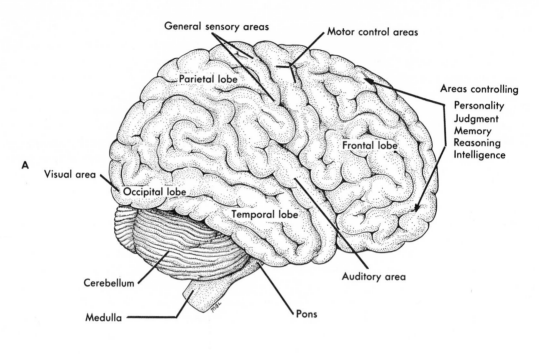

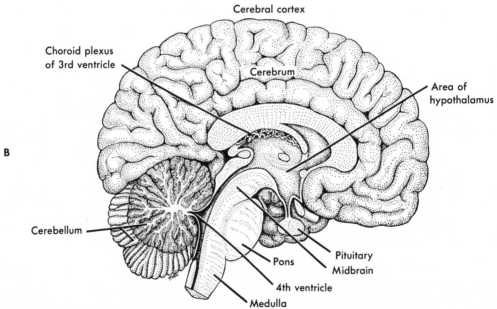

Fig. 34-22. **A,** Surfaces of the brain showing the cerebrum, cerebellum, pons, and medulla with identification of specialized areas of cerebral function. **B,** Simplified sagittal section of the brain showing internal relationships. Brain tumors in children often involve the cerebellum.

cause remarkable signs and symptoms rather soon. The signs and symptoms are those caused by the increased intracranial pressure. They may include headache, dizziness, lethargy, indifference, or irritability. Emesis often occurs (many times unassociated with nausea and not always projectile in character, although projectile vomiting is significant). Double or blurring vision and speech problems are reported fairly often. The pupils may be abnormally or unequally dilated or slow to react to changes in light intensity. Balance and gait may be affected because a large number of childhood brain tumors involve the cerebellum, a part of the brain that plays a significant role in the maintenance of equilibrium. Rigidity, tremors, or convulsions occasionally occur. Local muscle weakness may be present. (Periodic testing of the handgrip is sometimes ordered.) If the child is under 4 years of age, considerable enlargement of the head may still take place because the suture lines are not completely knit, and there may be interference in the ventricular drainage of the cerebrospinal fluid, as well as direct pressure from the enlarging tumor itself. The blood pressure may be elevated and the pulse may be slowed when compared with the normal values for the age group represented by the patient. Respirations may be of the Cheyne-Stokes variety. Fever or wide swings in temperature occasionally occur. Diagnosis may be confirmed through various procedures: spinal taps, skull roentgenograms (x-ray films), brain scans, electroencephalograms, ventriculograms, and arteriograms, as well as clinical observation.

If a nurse is responsible for the care of a child with a possible brain tumor, she must carefully assess his capabilities before attempting to ambulate him and be sure she has sufficient help to avoid falls. Some of these patients have very poor balance. The patient should be observed for any of the signs and symptoms previously described. Observation of vital signs, including blood pressure and eye reactions, should always be part of the nursing care. If intracranial pressure is elevated or mounting, a padded tongue blade should be available at the bedside. Side rails should always be in place.

Surgery and x-ray or cobalt radiation are the treatments currently available. Surgery, of course, is preferred. The complete removal of a well-confined tumor almost always produces a more optimistic prognosis.

Nursing care in the days immediately after a craniotomy, or surgical opening of the skull, is usually a complex affair. The vocational nurse may assist the registered nurse, but she should not have the responsibility of the child's complete bedside care. His condition is too unstable. The patient must be turned slowly and gently to prevent dizziness, nausea, vomiting, and a rise in blood pressure. Since crying elevates the blood pressure, all measures designed to prevent fear or distress are especially important. The head dressings may become damp from cerebrospinal fluid drainage and require reinforcing until they can be changed by the physician. The face, especially the eyes, may be bruised and swollen. Special eye irrigations may be necessary to avoid infection or ulceration resulting from disturbances in tear formation and drainage becaues of trauma. Frequent suctioning may be necessary. Although the child may appear unconscious, he may be able to hear quite well. Conversations at the bedside should be prudent.

As improvement occurs, efforts to rehabilitate the child should be made. Although the patient may eventually die, he may be able to live a relatively satisfying life for many months. Both patient and parents need much physical and emotional support to make the most of this indeterminate and occasionally prolonged period.

• • •

This chapter has covered a great deal of information—perhaps too much! It has treated no subject in depth. However, it is hoped that the student has been challenged to further study the needs of children with neuromuscular and skeletal problems.

35

Conditions involving the respiratory and circulatory systems

If one speaks of the respiratory system without mentioning the circulatory system, only part of an important story is told because these two body systems are intimately related. One might say that the respiratory system begins and ends a story but the circulatory system contributes the bulky middle chapters! For this reason pediatric disorders of the respiratory and circulatory systems are considered here in the same general section, although for convenience they may also be studied as separate units. To put it another way, the respiratory system is responsible for so-called *external respiration,* whereas the circulatory apparatus includes in its duties the responsibility for *internal respiration.*

KEY VOCABULARY

A brief reexamination of basic terminology used in describing respiratory and circulatory action and problems may be helpful:

anemia condition in which there is a reduction of hemoglobin in the blood.
apnea absence of breathing.
atelectasis airless segment of lung.
bronchiectasis abnormal dilatation of the bronchi in response to inflammation, which, if prolonged, will lead to associated structural changes and a chronic productive cough.
Cheyne-Stokes respiration irregular, cyclic-type breathing characterized by a period of increasing respiratory action followed by an interval of apnea.
dyspnea difficult breathing.
edema abnormal, excessive amount of fluid within the body tissues.
emphysema abnormal dilatation and loss of elasticity of the microscopic air sacs, or alveoli, of the lung.

empyema collection of pus in a body cavity, especially the pleural cavity.
eupnea normal breathing.
leukocytosis excessive increase in the number of white blood cells circulating in the blood.
orthopnea condition in which breathing is possible by the patient only when he is in a standing or sitting position.
pneumothorax abnormal collection of air or gas in the pleural cavity between the lung coverings.
remission lessening of severity or abatement of symptoms.
stenosis abnormal narrowing of a passage or opening.

THE RESPIRATORY SYSTEM

In conjunction with the study of disorders of the respiratory system, the student should review Chapter 29, which briefly outlines the basic anatomy and physiology of the respiratory system and discusses methods of aiding respiration and oxygenation.

Respiratory difficulties (such as respiratory distress syndrome, tracheoesophageal fistula, and diaphragmatic hernia) that are particularly associated with the newborn period are discussed in Chapters 17 an 18. In this presentation of respiratory pathology we will begin with a brief anatomical review followed by a consideration of those common problems affecting children in various stages of development.

Anatomical review
The nose

The nose is an extremely interesting structure; although for some people it may not be a cosmetic asset, it performs certain important functions. First of all, it prepares air for entry into the interior of the body.

It filters, warms, and moistens the air. Human beings may also breathe through their open mouths and, except during the period of infancy, do so fairly often. However, large amounts of air that enter the throat through the mouth are not properly warmed to body temperature or 100% humidified. The nose is also involved in the identification of different odors because the olfactory nerve endings are located within the nasal cavity. Many of the finer perceptions of the palate are influenced by the sensitivity of these nerves. Consider how uninteresting food seems when one has a cold and the proper ventilation of the nose is disturbed. A normal nose is also necessary for proper vocal resonance.

The pharynx and trachea

The pharynx is a passageway shared by both the respiratory and digestive systems. It extends from the back of the nasal cavity down past the posteroir portion of the oral cavity to the level of the larynx and esophagus. Consequently, the pharynx is divided descriptively into three parts: nasal, oral, and hypopharyngeal. The larynx and trachea extending from the hypopharynx complete the upper respiratory system.

The lower respiratory tract

The lower respiratory tract is usually considered to include the bronchi, bronchioles, alveoli, which form the tissues of the lungs, and pleurae, or coverings of the lungs. Infectious conditions involving these structures are, for the most part, more difficult to cure and more threatening to general health than those involving the passages of the upper respiratory system.

RESPIRATORY DISORDERS
THE INFANT
Bronchiolitis

Bronchiolitis is a viral respiratory illness with clinical manifestations attributed to inflammatory narrowing of the caliber of the small respiratory passages. The bronchioles are partially or completely obstructed due to mucosal swelling and ex-

udate. The condition is more common in young infants and seldom seen in children over 2 years of age.

Bronchiolitis begins as a simple cold. After several days the infant develops a low-grade fever, shallow, rapid respirations, a harsh exhausting cough, and an expiratory wheeze. Air can usually enter the bronchioles, but expiratory narrowing causes it to be trapped distal to the obstruction. Suprasternal and subcostal retractions are noted on inspiration. The infant is fatigued, irritable, anxious, and unable to eat or sleep. Some infants may even become cyanotic.

The clinical picture of expiratory obstruction with resultant emphysema must be differentiated from bronchial asthma. Epinephrine rarely benefits the infant with bronchiolitis, but striking improvement is seen in the child who has bronchial asthma when it is administered. Often a trial dose of epinephrine is given to the patient in order to rule out the likelihood of bronchial asthma.

Acute bronchiolitis in infants presents a frightening picture. Parents feel helpless, anxious, and actually fear that the life of their child is in jeopardy. Fortunately, mortality is very low, and the most severe aspect of the disease lasts only a day or two. Recovery is almost always complete within 2 weeks. This information is most welcome by the worried parents. Their questions should be answered simply, and they are encouraged to stay at the crib side. The infant should be placed in an atmosphere of cool mist and oxygen. His color, respirations, and pulse need close observation. Rest and hydration are most important. Nasal suctioning is usually necessary before feeding. Fluids should be urged frequently and in small amounts.

Pneumonia

Any inflammation of the lung parenchyma is called pneumonia. All classes of microbiological agents as well as certain noninfectious agents and conditions are known to cause pneumonia. The anatomic pathological changes may involve the lobar, lobular, interstitial, or bronchial areas. Pneumonia is most commonly seen in infants and young children. It is a potentially grave condition, ranking fourth in the cause of mortality in the age group of 1 to 14 years. Early recognition and prompt treatment spare lengthy hospitalization and reduce the incidence of complications. Common pneumonias in infants and children follow:

I. Primary pneumonias (no underlying predisposing condition diagnosed)
  A. Bacterial
    1. Pneumococcal
    2. Staphylococcal
    3. Streptococcal
    4. *Haemophilus influenzae*
  B. Nonbacterial
    1. Viral
    2. *Mycoplasma*
II. Secondary pneumonias (other predisposing conditions diagnosed)
  A. Hypostatic—caused by stasis of respiratory secretions, due to lack of adequate respiration
  B. Asthmatic—due to diminished air exchange
  C. Associated with cystic fibrosis—due to the presence of viscid respiratory secretions that act as excellent culture media
  D. Aspiration pneumonias — involve accidental inhalation of
    1. Hydrocarbons—petroleum distillates such as gasoline and furniture polish
    2. Foreign bodies—popcorn, peanuts, buttons, and other objects

Signs and symptoms

The onset and clinical manifestations of pneumonia vary with the age of the child and the etiological agent. The disease is most frequent in winter and spring. Bacterial pneumonias are often preceded by a viral upper respiratory tract infection, which alters the defense mechanisms of the lower respiratory tract. The classical signs and symptoms are fever, anorexia, listlessness, and cough. At first the cough is wet and loose, but soon it becomes dry and painful. The pain associated with lower lobe pneumonia is frequently referred to the abdomen. For this reason a chest x-ray film should be taken of young children with possible appendicitis to rule out pneumonia before they are sent to surgery. In the young child, fever mounts rapidly and seizures occur frequently. Respirations become rapid and shallow and are accompanied by flaring of the nostrils, grunting, and retractions. The pulse rate is very rapid (it may be doubled). Although meningeal irritation, causing distress such as stiff neck, is often present with upper lobe pneumonia, a spinal tap will rule out coexisting meningitis. Cyanosis coupled with a rapid, weak pulse is always a grave sign. Since proper therapy depends upon knowledge of the causative agents, the common pneumonias will be discussed according to their cause.

Types

Bacterial primary pneumonias. Pneumococcal pneumonia is the most common type encountered in infants and young children. Typically, after symptoms of a mild cold, the infant suddenly refuses his formula and becomes listless. Fever rises rapidly, and respiratory distress is soon apparent. Fortunately, the pneumococcus is very responsive to antibiotic therapy. A dramatic response to penicillin usually takes place within 24 to 48 hours in uncomplicated cases. Response to therapy is delayed in those cases that are complicated by fluid in the pleural space (pleural effusion), empyema, otitis media, or meningitis.

Staphylococcal pneumonia is the most serious of the pneumonias in infancy. It may follow an upper respiratory tract infection, or it may spread to the lungs via the bloodstream from a staphylococcal infection elsewhere in the body. Unless recognized and treated early, the disease characteristically progresses rapidly, causing severe respiratory distress and may be associated with the formation of abscesses and air cysts (pneumatoceles). Antibiotic therapy with methicillin or oxacillin is continued for several weeks. Isolation technique is observed. Pneumothorax is common and treated with continuous closed suction drainage. Hospitalization is long, and mortality ranges from 5% to 50%!

Streptococcal pneumonia is more common in young children than in infants. It is usually preceded by a viral infection such as rubeola, rubella, or varicella. The onset of chills and pleuritic pain may be sudden, or the pneumonia may start with a gradual rise in fever, accompanied by cough. Streptococci cause an interstitial type of pneumonia, with abscesses and pneumatoceles occurring in a number of patients. Empyema usually requires closed-suction drainage. Penicillin G is the antibiotic of choice and is highly effective.

Pneumonia caused by type B *Haemophilus influenzae* is a serious disease. The onset of illness is insidious, and the clinical course may be prolonged over several weeks. Infants and children under 5 years are most often affected and seem prone to bacteremia and empyema. A prolonged, pertussis-like cough sometimes accompanies this type of pneumonia. The *H. influenzae* organism is very sensitive to ampicillin. In order to prevent serious complications, this drug is given in large doses as soon as the disease is diagnosed.

Nonbacterial primary pneumonias. Viral pneumonia can be caused by almost any type of virus. A low-grade fever and coryza precede this interstitial pneumonia, which appears suddenly with the onset of tachypnea and a nonproductive, tight cough. Treatment is symptomatic since antibiotics are of no value unless secondary bacterial complications occur.

Mycoplasma pneumonia is an atypical pneumonia caused by a pathogenic "filterable" microorganism known as *Mycoplasma pneumoniae* (Eaton agent). It is a very small, free-living microorganism that has properties between those of bacteria and viruses. Infection usually results in a self-limited, interstitial pneumonia. Mycoplasma pneumonia occurs most commonly in the adolescent. The onset is abrupt, and symptoms include fever, headache, malaise, chills, and characteristic dry, hacking cough. Later the cough becomes productive, sometimes producing blood-streaked mucus. Treatment is usually symptomatic.

Secondary aspiration pneumonias. Infants and children have been known to aspirate not only their formula but all kinds of food, poisons, and objects. The right upper lobe is frequently involved. Mucosal swelling and obstruction may occur. Symptoms vary depending on the child, the substance, and the amount aspirated. Treatment is supportive and aimed at preventing intercurrent infections. Of course, prevention of these incidents is the best therapy.

Aspiration of petroleum distillates such as kerosene, gasoline, lighter fluid, and furniture polishes causes a very severe chemical pneumonitis, characterized by edema and inflammation. Some petroleum distillates are absorbed from the intestines and then excreted through the lungs. Treatment is symptomatic and may include steroids to reduce inflammatory changes or antibiotics to combat secondary infections.

A number of foreign bodies, including seeds, coins, nuts, popcorn, safety pins, and bones, have been removed from the respiratory passages of young children. (Young children must not eat peanuts or popcorn because of this common problem.) Foreign bodies inhaled into the lungs will occlude the bronchi, causing atelectasis or hyperinflation. The young child will manifest dyspnea, cyanosis, and asymmetric respirations. Incomplete obstruction causes wheezing and, if untreated, fever and cough producing purulent sputum soon develop. Delay in removal of the foreign object by bronchoscopy seriously alters the prognosis. Usually the foreign body becomes embedded, injuring the tissues and causing infection. Permanent damage to the area involved follows prolonged atelectasis.

Diagnosis of the pneumonias

A high white blood cell count (WBC), over 10,000, with increased polymorphonuclear cells and a shift to young forms (bands) is suggestive of bacterial infections. Although a low WBC (5,000 or less) is more typical of viral infections in general, a high WBC usually accompanies viral infections of the lower respiratory tract. Blood cultures obtained prior to antibiotic therapy are very helpful in the identification of specific organisms, especially in those cases in which septicemia is present. Nasopharyngeal cultures are not of great value, since pneumococci, streptococci, *H. influenzae,* and staphylococci can be isolated from healthy children. Tracheal cultures obtained by suction techniques are more helpful in identification of organisms. X-ray films are perhaps the most valuable diagnostic tool in evaluating the extent or type of the pneumonia. Bronchoscopy (visualization of the tracheobronchial tree) may be performed when other procedures have failed to make an adequate diagnosis of the problem. Fluid or tissue may be removed by this method for a culture or cytology studies. Lung biopsy is sometimes necessary when protracted pulmonary disease cannot be explained by other means.

Treatment and supportive nursing care

Specific therapy is important in the treatment of pneumonia. Differentiating viral and bacterial infections is initially difficult. Since pneumococcal pneumonia is the most common pneumonia seen in infants and young children, therapy for all pneumonias is typically begun with penicillin G. Later, when the cause of the pneumonia is established, a more appropriate drug can be given. Supportive care is as important as antibiotic therapy in lessening the severity of the child's illness. Fluids are encouraged and acetaminophen or aspirin is given for fever. Rest in bed is recommended during the febrile stage. Humidification and increased amounts of fluid are necessary for liquefaction of bronchial secretions and excretion of toxic products. Saturated solution of potassium iodide (SSKI) or glyceryl guaiacolate (Robitussin) will help loosen secretions and initiate a productive cough. In general, depressant "cough medicines" are contraindicated in pneumonia because a valuable mechanism used to help clear the bronchial tree would be lost. Physical and inhalation therapies are important in the hospital setting. Bronchial drainage is carried out 3 or 4 times daily (before meals and at bedtime). Viscid secretions will not drain from the bronchi by gravity alone, but deep breathing, reinforced coughing, and physical therapy techniques such as squeezing, cupping, and vibration will assist in their removal. Oxygen administration is frequent.

When the child's appetite improves, he should be offered a nutritious diet of foods that are appealing. Before feeding an infant, one should remove nasal secretions. One or two drops of saline solution may be ordered, followed by gentle suctioning. A restless infant who cannot breathe will not eat.

Nursing care involves careful observation of respiratory patterns, pulse, color, and the general condition of the patient. Observance of the attending physician's positioning orders and frequent modification of body position within the prescribed limits are also important. Patients often breathe better with their heads and chests elevated; babies are often placed in infant seats. Isolation techniques are observed, mainly for staphylococcal pneumonia. Convalescence should not be rushed; adequate time for recuperation is very important to regain strength and weight.

When a child with pneumonia is treated at home or on an outpatient basis, the parents should be carefully instructed about the therapeutic and nursing measures. They should understand that medicines must be taken on time and in the correct amount. In general, young children should be cared for by their parents in the familiar, comforting environment of their own homes. Nevertheless, hospitalization may be advisable during the first 2 or 3 days of illness to confirm diagnosis and to provide inhalation therapy and parenteral administration of drugs and fluid. Infants who are under 6 months of age and have pneumonia are always hospitalized. Other children are hospitalized if they become too sick to take fluids, if they require intense supportive measures (such as IV or oxygen therapy or surgical drainage) because of their diagnosis or condition, or if the family cannot or does not adequately care for them.

Although the diagnosis of pneumonia does not produce the same alarm today that it once did in the hearts and minds of parents, it is still a potential threat to the life and future health of the child. Patients suffering from this disease must be frequently evaluated and expertly nursed.

Cystic fibrosis (mucoviscidosis)

Cystic fibrosis is a hereditary disorder in which there is generalized dysfunction of the exocrine glands, the outward-secreting glands that do not circulate their secretions throughout the bloodstream. Cystic fibrosis especially involves the mucous and sweat glands. When the disease was first described, the pancreatic pathology and digestive difficulties of the patient received much attention. However, cystic fibrosis is usually characterized by the triad of chronic, severe pulmonary disease, pancreatic insufficiency, and abnormally high concentrations of electrolytes in the sweat.

Cystic fibrosis is genetically transmitted as an autosomal recessive trait, but at the present time there is no reliable way to identify individual parents carrying the gene before the disease manifests itself in their offspring. Nor is there any clinically available method to detect the presence of the disease in an unborn child, though researchers are hoping to find such a method of identification. Many attempts have been made to develop a technique that will discover the asymptomatic carriers of the gene, but the metabolic error causing cystic fibrosis remains unknown. A unique substance in the serum of cystic fibrosis patients and their carrier parents has been found to inhibit ciliary movement in oyster gills. The oyster assay in its present stage of development is primarily a research tool that is usually effective in carrier detection and gives promise of the development of a universal test for detection of the cystic fibrosis carrier. If one child has the disease, the risk for each subsequent pregnancy is one in four. That is, each conception has the same 25% chance of producing an affected child (see p. 269 for genetic discussion). The incidence of cystic fibrosis in the United States is 1 per 1,500 live births. Boys and girls appear to be equally involved. Five percent of the white population and less than 1% of the black population are estimated to be genetic carriers of this hidden trait. Cystic fibrosis is a serious disease in terms of numbers inflicted, financial burden, disability and pain involved, and prognosis. Couples who have a child with cystic fibrosis should be made aware of the genetic implications of the disease.

Symptoms. Clinical expression of the disease varies because of differing degrees of involvement of the affected organs and glands. Cystic fibrosis affects the exocrine glands, causing changes in many of the secretions. In a small percentage of cases the disease is diagnosed in the newborn infant nursery because of the detection of meconium ileus. In this condition the meconium, or stool formed by the newborn infant, is even more thick and sticky than normal meconium because of the absence or reduction of normal pancreatic digestive enzymes. The abnormal stool sticks to the walls of the ileum like paste and obstructs the lower digestive tract. The intestine becomes distended, and abdominal distention, or bloating, is noted. No passage of stool occurs. Vomiting and dehydration may ensue. Meconium ileus is a surgical emergency. Any newborn infant who does not pass stool within 24 hours after birth should be especially evaluated and examined for possible obstruction.

Since the pancreatic digestive enzymes may be reduced or absent, foodstuffs (fats and proteins especially) may be poorly digested and assimilated. If much of the food eaten does not leave the digestive tract by the normal processes of assimilation, the child will pass large amounts of feces and develop a protuberant abdomen. During infancy the stools may not be especially bulky or offensive. However, if the child is not treated, the stools may assume these characteristics as he becomes older. The strong odor is caused by the impaired digestion of fats. The diet should provide increased calories and protein with a variable reduction in fat as needed to satisfy the patient's appetite and requirements for growth and development. The child usually has an eager appetite; however, because he is unable to use much of the food he eats (and respiratory complications may interfere with development), his arms and

legs are characteristically spindly, his buttocks are emaciated, and his growth is retarded. Fortunately the digestive problems usually improve with the addition of commercial preparations of pancreatic enzymes given with each meal. The dosage varies with different preparations, the size and content of the meals, and, as indicated, by the character of the stool. Simple carbohydrates are easily digested, and banana products are especially favored. Special formulas reinforced with glucose, skimmed or powdered milk, or banana powder may be utilized. Diets should be supplemented with vitamins prepared in such a way that they can be combined with water (since oil-based vitamins are poorly absorbed). Extra salt intake is necessary because of the large amounts lost in the perspiration. The prescribed amount can be incorpo-

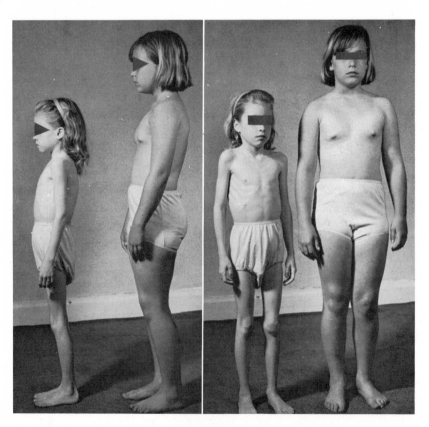

Fig. 35-1. Both these young girls are 10 years old. The youngster on the left demonstrates the effects of severe cystic fibrosis.

rated in the preparation of food and need not be given separately. Heat prostration is a real danger to these children. If excessive sweating is anticipated, NaCl intake should be increased.

The secretions of the mucus-producing glands of the bronchi may become extremely thick and tenacious and block distal bronchioles, causing cough, wheezing, respiratory obstruction, emphysema, and frequently infection (usually by *Staphylococcus aureus* or *Pseudomonas aeruginosa*). The lungs are virtually defenseless against microbes. In severe cases the chronic respiratory disease causes a deformed barrel-type chest, cyanosis, and clubbing of the fingers and toes as a result of secondary hypoxemia (low blood oxygen saturation). Because of the difficulty the heart may encounter in pumping blood through the scarred lung tissue, abnormal dilatation of the right heart and thickening of the right ventricular wall may occur. Death may be the result of heart failure that developed because of the severe respiratory difficulty. Cardiac stress secondary to problems in the action of the lungs is termed "cor pulmonale" (Fig. 35-2).

Diagnosis. A high degree of clinical suspicion is usually the first step in the diagnosis of cystic fibrosis. Infants and children who suffer from recurrent respiratory tract infections or fail to thrive should be especially evaluated. The diagnosis is confirmed by laboratory evidence of abnormally elevated sweat electrolyte levels. Children with cystic fibrosis will have a positive sweat test reaction from birth if enough sweat (100 mg.) can be collected. A positive reaction implies an elevation of

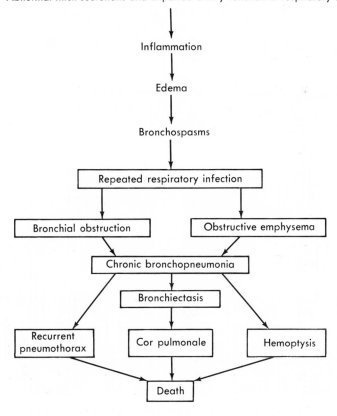

Fig. 35-2. Pathological sequence characteristic of cystic fibrosis.

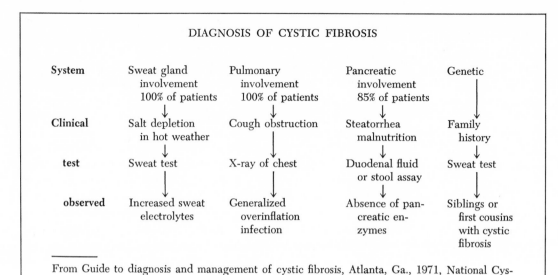

DIAGNOSIS OF CYSTIC FIBROSIS

System	Sweat gland involvement 100% of patients	Pulmonary involvement 100% of patients	Pancreatic involvement 85% of patients	Genetic
Clinical	Salt depletion in hot weather	Cough obstruction	Steatorrhea malnutrition	Family history
test	Sweat test	X-ray of chest	Duodenal fluid or stool assay	Sweat test
observed	Increased sweat electrolytes	Generalized overinflation infection	Absence of pancreatic enzymes	Siblings or first cousins with cystic fibrosis

From Guide to diagnosis and management of cystic fibrosis, Atlanta, Ga., 1971, National Cystic Fibrosis Research Foundation.

the concentration of sodium and chloride above 60 mg./liter. This feature is so pronounced that mothers have noted that their affected children have a "salty taste" when they are kissed.

Although various methods may be used to stimulate the sweat glands, the *pilocarpine iontophoresis* method is the safest and most reliable procedure for including sweat and is the recommended method for making the diagnosis. The sweat stimulation is simple to perform, takes little time (less than 1 hour), and is not painful or inconvenient to the patient.

Another diagnostic finding is the determination of a reduction or absence of the pancreatic enzyme *trypsin* in material aspirated from the duodenum of the patient or in dilutions of fecal material. Still another test involves finding an excessive amount of fat in the child's stool.

Treatment. Treatment is designed to meet the needs of the individual patient. Dietary management and treatment of abnormal salt losses have already been discussed. Pulmonary involvement deserves major emphasis. Control of pulmonary infection requires the use of appropriate antibiotics and effective maintenance of pulmonary hygiene by inhalation therapy together with adequate drainage of bronchial secretions by physical therapy. In some cases the child may sleep and nap in a mist tent. The fine mist particles of ultrasonic nebulizers are thought by some to be especially helpful. Physical therapy includes chest clapping, postural drainage, and breathing exercises. The use of a continuing home pulmonary care program from the time of diagnosis, to prevent progression and complications as much as possible, and long-term antibiotic therapy have improved the life expectancy of children with cystic fibrosis. Children with advanced and steadily increasing pulmonary disease or severe pulmonary infections usually have to be hospitalized for intensive parenteral antibiotic therapy. However, recently, intravenous administration of antibiotics to inpatients and outpatients with acute and chronic infection has been accomplished by use of the Heparin Lock IV. In fact, many hospitalizations can now be avoided by teaching selected children or parents this convenient method of parenteral antibiotic therapy. The Heparin Lock IV consists of a butterfly scalp vein needle attached to a small plastic tube that is sealed by a rubber cap in such a way to protect sterility and patency. It facilitates frequent high intravenous doses of antibiotics without limiting activity. The patient can move about freely with only the lock in place, while the other equipment needed for the intravenous administration of drugs remains at the bedside until the next dose is due. Postural drainage and percussion treatments vital in combating these infections can be more effectively performed. For details of Heparin Lock IV maintenance, see p. 389.

Nursing care. Good nursing care entails a careful observation of the dietary intake and its effect on the child and his elimination. Every effort should be made to offer a variety in the meals within the limitations imposed and to make eating a pleasant experience.

Provision for frequent changes in position to prevent pneumonia and reduce skin problems is an important consideration. Some of these children are very emaciated, and the skin over bony prominences is in special need of care. The rectal area must be meticulously cleaned. Rectal prolapse may occasionally be a complication. A soothing, local ointment may prevent irritation from the bulky stools. Any material soiled by feces should be removed immediately from the child's room. Appropriate air fresheners may be useful. Stools should always be described regarding their size, color, consistency, and odor.

The observation and report of respiratory distress is, of course, of paramount importance. Every effort should be made to protect the child from persons with any type of respiratory tract infection.

Because of the chronic nature of the disease, the severe strain it may place on the family finances, and the psychological needs of the child, home care is recommended except when the child's condition indicates that he or his family need the relief that can be provided through hospitalization. Parents may need much counseling and practical assistance to help meet their child's social and emotional require-

ments, as well as his physical needs. They also must be cautioned against becoming so preoccupied with the sick child that the needs of other family members are continually neglected. Children with diagnosed cystic fibrosis now have a greater than 50% chance of living past 16 years of age. Only rarely will a young man with cystic fibrosis be fertile, since the same mechanisms that typically obstruct other glandular ducts in the body probably interfere with sperm production and transport as well. Female patients have borne children, but their ability to conceive seems to be below normal due to excessive amounts of cervical mucus.

The nurse caring for the child with cystic fibrosis must realize the strain under which the parents may be operating and their feelings of fatigue and frustration. Many families have lost other children because of this disease and have traveled almost the same road to final farewells before. Such a journey is not any easier just because some of the scenery may be familiar.

THE TODDLER

Croup (spasmodic laryngitis, laryngotracheobronchitis)

Acute obstructive subglottic laryngitis, commonly known as spasmodic croup, is part of a viral respiratory disease that involves the larynx, trachea, and bronchi. Mild to severe forms of laryngotracheobronchitis (LTB) typically occur in children between age 6 months and 3 years, during cold weather or after sudden changes in temperature. Acute spasmodic croup is characterized by a sudden onset of inspiratory stridor, hoarseness, and a barklike cough following a 1- to 3-day history of a "cold." These manifestations are due to inflammatory edema and spasm of the vocal cords causing varying degrees of laryngeal obstruction. Most children are awakened without warning in the middle of the night by an acute attack. The child appears extremely anxious and frightened by his respiratory distress. Treatment is

567

symptomatic. High humidity (running hot water in the bathroom) and gentle reassurance are important. Usually the spasms subside in a few hours but often recur for 1 or 2 nights. Certain children seem predisposed to develop this severe laryngospasm and, once they have it, will probably suffer other episodes.

A more severe form of croup results when the inflammatory involvement of the trachea and bronchial tree produces a thick, viscous, purulent exudate. Edema, spasm, and the exudate lead to both inspiratory and expiratory difficulties. As the degree of severity of respiratory distress increases, suprasternal, intercostal, and substernal retractions occur. The child becomes febrile, hypoxic, restless, and desperately anxious. Impending suffocation is a real threat and a terrifying experience for both the child and his parents. This child needs immediate medical management and possible surgical intervention.

During the admission procedure, every effort should be made to avoid aggravation of respiratory distress. The parents should remain at the crib side as the child is gently and calmly placed in an atmosphere of high humidity with oxygen. Maximum humidification is best accomplished with the addition of ultrasonic nebulization to the cool mist of the tent. The moist vapor will help allay irritation of the mucosa and promote liquefaction of the thick secretions. Clear fluids are encouraged and are also extremely important in mobilizing respiratory exudate. Refusal to take fluids orally is serious.

Increased pulse rate, restlessness, stridor, and use of the accessory muscles for breathing must be reported immediately. If the signs and symptoms of acute airway obstruction increase, intubation must be considered before the child is exhausted. Tests of blood gases are most helpful in determining the need for surgical intervention, but unfortunately this procedure may upset the child to such a degree that an emergency tracheostomy is made necessary.

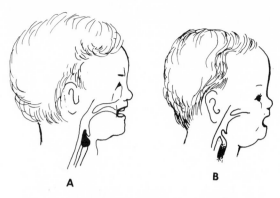

A   **B**

Fig. 35-3. Anatomical difference between acute supraglottic obstruction and acute subglottic obstruction. **A**, Epiglottitis is an acute inflammatory swelling involving the structures above the opening of the trachea (glottis). It most commonly occurs in the preschool child. **B**, Laryngotracheobronchitis is an acute inflammation particularly involving the subglottic area of the larynx, the trachea, and bronchial tree. It most commonly occurs in the toddler.

Recently, intermittent positive pressure breathing (IPPB) and nebulized racemic epinephrine (Vaponefrin) for moderate to severe cases of LTB have been used. At first the child struggles against the face mask, but after a short time he relaxes and his labored breathing subsides. The IPPB procedure is repeated if necessary in 3 to 4 hours. Racemic epinephrine is used for its topical vasoconstrictive effect, resulting in decreased mucosal edema. This treatment has been found to be extremely helpful, and some reports indicate that it prevents the need for tracheostomy.

Acute LTB should not be confused with epiglottitis (acute supraglottic laryngitis), a most serious acute airway problem that may lead to complete respiratory obstruction and death in a few hours (Fig. 35-3).

Foreign bodies in the nose or throat

Children frequently push objects other than their fingers into the nasal cavity. This is probably the result of natural curiosity. If the object does not spontaneously drop out or is not dislodged by sneezing and the episode is not reported by the child, it may be indicated by a bloody or purulent, foul nasal discharge originating from one nostril only. Such a discharge should make one suspect the presence of a foreign body. Removal of such an object should be attempted only by a physician who has the necessary instruments.

If a child is discovered choking, he should be turned upside down. If this simple procedure is not effective alone, a short, controlled blow on the back with the hand, may dislodge the object; however, children who are choking should not be pounded on the back, especially if they are in an upright position, since this may cause a sudden intake of breath and greater aspiration. If respiratory distress continues, the child should be seen immediately by a physician who may have to schedule a chest x-ray examination and perform a bronchoscopy. For discussion of aspiration pneumonia see p. 561.

Bronchitis

Bronchitis is most often caused by the same virus that has invaded other areas of the respiratory tract, or it may be associated with infectious diseases, such as measles. Bronchitis is usually preceded by an upper respiratory tract infection and is a common problem in toddlers. It may remain quite mild or become progressively severe, leading to pneumonia. A disturbing productive cough appears as the disease develops. Paroxysms may occur, particularly when the position of the child is altered, such as in the morning on rising or when first lying in bed after having sat for a period. Vomiting, which is the result of gagging when the secretions are thick, is not uncommon. Since coughing clears the bronchial secretions, cool moisture is preferred until clinical improvement occurs. A generous intake of fluids will thin bronchial secretions, and aspirin or acetaminophen (Tylenol) may be necessary to lessen discomfort or fever. Unless the condition worsens, acute bronchitis is generally a self-limited infection that improves spontaneously in a few days.

THE PRESCHOOL CHILD
Epiglottitis

Acute obstructive supraglottic laryngitis, commonly known as epiglottitis, is usually caused by the *Haemophilus influenzae* type B bacteria. It is characterized by acute respiratory distress, high fever, difficulty in swallowing, drooling, and a "cherry red" epiglottitis. The signs and symptoms of supraglottic obstruction are due to inflammatory edema of the epiglottis. Children between ages 3 and 7 years are most frequently affected. The condition is usually seen in the winter months, and the onset is sudden. The child first complains of a sore throat and difficulty in breathing. Soon he is anxious, unable to eat or drink, prostrated, in a toxic condition, and drooling. Drooling is the most important single sign of impending disaster. One should not be lulled into hopeful, watchful waiting. This child needs to secure his airway, and "emergency" tracheostomies done at the bedside have a 25% mortality. Tracheostomy should not be deferred in the hope that it will not be necessary. Epiglottitis can lead to complete respiratory obstruction and death in just a few hours. It is important not to unduly disturb the child or to separate him from his parents. The diagnosis is confirmed by visualization or by a lateral neck x-ray film, and the child is moved from the emergency room to the operating room where an elective tracheostomy can be performed in an ideal setting. Intravenous antibiotic therapy (ampicillin) and fluids are given.* Arterial blood gases are assessed to assure airway exchange. The child is placed in a mist tent and returned to the pediatric intensive care unit where an experienced staff can give constant care. No child should die from epiglottitis when it is diagnosed and treated promptly.

Epistaxis

Bleeding from the nose is a common disorder of childhood, especially in boys from

---

*Rapkin, R. H.: Tracheostomy in epiglottitis, Pediatrics **52**:426-429, Sept., 1973.

age 4 to 10 years. On the anterior portion of the nasal septum called Kiesselbach's area there is a fragile network of capillaries subject to drying and multiple minor injuries. Picking the nose, forceful blowing, insertion of foreign bodies, and trauma are the usual causes of bleeding.

Placing the child in a sitting position with the head tilted forward while compressing the nares with the thumb and forefinger is often sufficient to facilitate clot formation and stop the bleeding. This posture also prevents blood from dripping down the posterior pharynx, possibly leading to aspiration. Ice packs to the nasal area or to the back of the neck are of little or no value. If bleeding is persistent, an anterior nasal pack consisting of ½ inch of petrolatum-impregnated gauze or an application of agents such as aqueous epinephrine solution (1:1000) or thrombin may be useful.

Any condition that contributes to vascular congestion of the nasal mucosa, such as nasal allergy or sinusitis, increases the frequency of epistaxis. Systemic conditions such as rheumatic, typhoid, or scarlet fever are associated with increased susceptibility to nosebleeds. Bleeding from the posterior region of the nasal cavity is uncommon. At times such nosebleeds may be a symptom of underlying blood dyscrasias such as purpura, leukemia, or conditions associated with a rise in blood pressure. Frequent nosebleeds may or may not be significant. Parental fears can best be allayed by not only stopping the bleeding but also identifying and treating the underlying causes of the disorder.

Deviation of the septum

In some instances the cartilaginous wall, or septum, that divides the nose into two lateral chambers does not occupy the midline. It may deviate toward one side or another as the result of natural development or, more commonly, as an aftermath of trauma. This may indirectly cause occlusion of a nostril and difficult breathing, particularly when the nose is inflamed. This structural anomaly may be corrected surgically by an operation called a submucous resection. To prevent external nasal deformity resulting from the surgery it is usually not performed until adolescence.

Acute nasopharyngitis (acute coryza, common cold)

The so-called common cold has plagued humanity for countless years, and since no specific preventive or treatment has yet been discovered, it will probably be with us to cause consternation for at least several more. Preschool and young school-age children average approximately six colds per year. The common cold is probably caused by several viral organisms that primarily attack the nose and throat. Symptoms include a dry, scratchy, sore, inflamed pharynx and an inflamed nasal mucosa, which produces a clear mucoid nasal discharge that later becomes thick and purulent. These local symptoms are often accompanied by headache, muscular pains, general malaise, and fever. As the viral infection continues, it is often complicated by the intrusion of pathogenic bacteria, which may prolong the congestion and promote the extension of the inflammation to the middle ear, sinuses, larynx, trachea, and even to the bronchi and lungs. It is mainly the possibility of extension that makes the common cold a potentially dangerous condition.

A common cold is probably contagious for a number of hours before symptoms are observed by the patient. It is now believed that the cold sufferer remains contagious for about 8 hours after the onset of visible signs. Contamination by spread of droplets is most common. It is very important to protect infants from exposure to colds because they are affected more seriously than older children. An infant may have a high temperature of 104° F., and febrile convulsions are possible. His ears are almost always affected. His smaller nasal passages are blocked rather easily and difficulties in breathing, nursing, and eating may follow congestion. It is impossible to prevent a child from ever having a cold, but everything possible should be done to protect a baby.

Since nasopharyngitis is due entirely to viruses, there is no specific therapy recommended. Supportive treatment consists of rest, relative isolation, increased fluid intake, and a bland, soft diet as desired. Nasal obstruction in young infants can be partially relieved by humidification or instillation of 1 to 2 drops of normal saline solution in each nostril followed by gentle aspiration with an infant's nasal (or ear) syringe. Phenylephrine (Neo-Synephrine) hydrochloride nose drops (⅛% for infants and ¼% for older children) may also relieve nasal symptoms. Nasal vasoconstrictors should not be used for more than 3 or 4 days because of "rebound phenomena." (When the use of such vasoconstrictors has been prolonged and is suddenly stopped, secretion greatly increases, or "rebounds.")

Mild systemic symptoms and fever may be relieved by proper dosage of aspirin or nonsalicylate acetaminophen (Tylenol or Tempra). Aspirin can be very dangerous to a child whose intake of fluids has declined markedly. Remember, both the amount of aspirin given and the interval and duration of treatment must always be considered. Many children suffer from salicylate poisoning every year! A rule of thumb a nurse may want to remember is that a child of average weight should be given only 1 grain (60 mg.) of aspirin per year of age up to 5 grains and should not be given aspirin more than five times at 4-hour intervals without medical consultation. Dosages for babies under 1 year of age must be very carefully determined. Children over 5 years of age but less than 12 years of age may usually be given 5 grains at a time if administration is not repeated more often than every 4 to 6 hours for a brief period.

To protect the nares or upper lip from excoriation caused by the fairly constant nasal discharge, cold cream or petrolatum may be applied. Antibiotics are indicated in viral infections when secondary bacterial invaders become a problem.

Sinusitis

Nasal obstruction over a period of 3 days is usually followed by an acute sinusitis. Headache and a mucopurulent discharge from one or both nostrils, cough, and a diffusely red pharynx with mucopurulent discharge clinging to the posterior wall are indications that bacteria have invaded the sinuses. Improved ventilation and drainage are primary goals in the treatment. Hot compresses over the painful areas and increased humidification will provide some comfort. Pain and fever are lessened by use of acetaminophen or aspirin. Instillation of nasal vasoconstrictors, preferably by spray, are helpful in shrinking the nasal mucosa and opening the airways. Each nostril should be sprayed once while the child is in a sitting position. About 3 to 5 minutes later, the spraying should be repeated to reach the posterior part of the nose. Oral decongestants such as pseudoephedrine hydrochloride (Sudafed), Triaminic, or Actifed may be useful when local therapy is difficult. Although most acute sinus infections are self-limiting, appropriate antibiotic therapy (culture sensitive) will shorten the course of illness and prevent any further complications.

Otitis media

Otitis media, or inflammation of the middle ear, is a common, difficult problem related to malfunction of the eustachian, or auditory, tube (Fig. 35-4, *A*). Normally this tube protects the middle ear from nasopharyngeal secretions, provides drainage of secretions produced within the middle ear into the nasopharynx, and equalizes the air pressure in the middle ear with that of the atmosphere. Infection, allergy, and enlarged adenoids may commonly disturb any of the above functions.

Acute otitis media is a common complication of upper respiratory tract infection in young children. Respiratory mucosa damaged by viral infection is readily col-

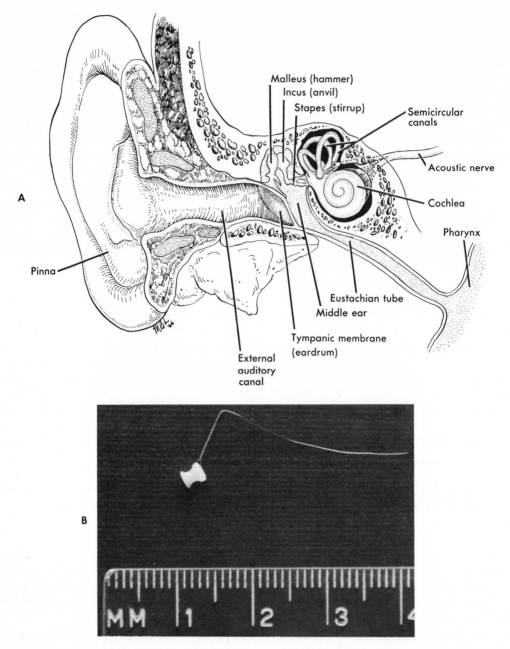

Fig. 35-4. A, Basic anatomy of the ear. B, A typanostomy ventilating tube.

onized by pneumococci, *Haemophilus influenzae,* and group A beta-hemolytic streptococci. Bacteria usually gain access to the middle ear via the eustachian tube. Purulent fluid accumulates in the middle ear, causing severe pain, fever, and irritability. When the eustachian tube becomes in-

flamed, it may swell shut, and the purulent material produced by the infection builds up within the middle ear, causing earache, ringing of the ears, elevated temperature, occasional vomiting, and perhaps spontaneous rupture of the eardrum that may result in a "running ear."

572

Infants are especially susceptible to otitis media and may announce their discomfort by crying, fussy behavior, or pulling at the affected ear. Diagnosis is based on history, symptoms, and the appearance of a bulging eardrum. Antibiotics are the mainstay of therapy. A successful outcome depends in large measure upon early treatment. Parents should be encouraged to notify the pediatrician promptly when the child has an earache. Aspirin, acetaminophen, and Auralgan eardrops may be given for pain, although it usually subsides in 4 to 5 hours after antibiotic therapy has been initiated. Antihistamines and decongestants are often prescribed for the first 5 days in an attempt to clear nasal pharyngitis and inflammation of the eustachian tubes.

Specific antibiotic therapy prevents the dreaded complications of mastoiditis, meningitis, and the incidence of eardrum perforation. Ampicillin, which is effective against both gram-positive and gram-negative bacteria, seems to be the single most useful drug. Widely accepted is combined therapy, such as erythromycin or penicillin with sulfisoxazole. Therapy should be continued for at least 10 days. The nurse must forewarn parents that a follow-up visit to the doctor is essential. The ear must be inspected after 10 days of treatment since the appearance of the drum dictates the duration of therapy. No child is considered cured until there has been resolution of the signs of middle ear disease. Partially treated otitis media is a major cause of meningitis in young children.

In the past, a myringotomy (surgical incision of the eardrum) was commonly done to relieve pressure and evacuate fluid. Since most children respond well to antibiotic therapy, myringotomies are now usually reserved for those few patients whose improvement at follow-up examination has not been satisfactory.

Serous otitis media. Recurrent attacks of acute otitis media characteristically precede serous, or "secretory," otitis media, a nonpurulent middle ear effusion. The fluid varies greatly in its viscosity. When it is very thick the condition is called "glue ear." Serous otitis is relatively common, and since there are no significant symptoms, the development of conductive deafness is a real possibility. Unless definitive measures are instituted to open the eustachian tube, permanent hearing loss may result. Learning difficulties often signal such a hearing loss in school-age children. Children with conductive hearing loss due to serous otitis media should be referred to an otologist. Surgical drainage (myringotomy) is often necessary. The aspirated fluid is cultured, and specific antibiotic therapy may be started. Placement of tiny middle ear ventilating tubes through the eardrum seems to be the best treatment for serous otitis media (see Fig. 35-4, A). The success of tympanostomy tubes is most likely related to improvement of mucous drainage from the middle ear into the nasopharynx. Parents should warn their child not to swim or get water into their ears while the tubes are in place, because the infection may extend.

The most important aspect of long-term management is to relieve the basic cause. Allergies must be investigated and treated, and hypertrophied adenoids must be removed if they truly are obstructing the eustachian tube. A significant advance in the identification of middle ear disease has come with the use of the electroacoustic impedance bridge. A small probe in a rubber cuff is placed in the external canal and attached to the impedance meter. A tympanogram, which reflects the dynamics of the entrie tympanic membrane–middle ear and eustachian tube system, is produced. For detecting otitis media and common conductive defects in children, tympanometry is far more reliable than otoscopic examination. Tympanometry is a simple procedure that can be easily carried out in a short time by nonprofessional personnel.*

Hygiene of the ear. In some instances

---

*Bluestone, C. D., and Shurin, P. A.: Middle ear disease in children, Pediatr. Clin. North Am. **21:** 386, May, 1974.

damage to the ear may follow ill-advised probing of the external auditory canal with such implements as hairpins and match-sticks. It is wise to follow the old saying, "Never put anything in your ear except your elbow." The outer canal should be cleaned only by a washcloth or a tightly rolled piece of cotton. If a collection of hardened wax, or cerumen, is suspected, the ear should be examined, and a physician or nurse trained in the technique of irrigating the ears should carry out the procedure.

Any body opening seems to offer a challenge to some children. Boys and girls will occasionally push foreign bodies into the external ear canal. When foreign bodies are detected, they should be removed by a physician because the general public has neither the knowledge, skill, nor instruments necessary to perform such a task. An irrigation should never be attempted before the child is taken to a physician. If the object is made of vegetable matter, it will swell with the liquid and become more difficult to extract.

THE SCHOOL-AGE CHILD
Adenoids and tonsils

Located on the pharynx are several structures of particular interest to the pediatric nurse. Situated in the nasal pharynx are the pharyngeal tonsils, more often called the adenoids. Farther down on the lateral walls of the oral pharynx are the palatine, or faucial, tonsils, which are the structures indicated when one whispers, "I've just had my tonsils out." These two kinds of tonsils are composed mainly of lymphoid tissue and play a role in the formation of immunoglobulins. In addition they act as a respiratory tract defense mechanism by filtering microbes, thereby helping to prevent microbial invasion of the lower tract. These lymphoid tissues serve a useful purpose and should be preserved unless the problems caused by their continued presence outweigh their possible usefulness. The tonsils and adenoids are present at birth and achieve their major

growth by age 5. It is significant to note that at age 2 the tonsils are normally large, and the adenoids occupy one half of the nasopharyngeal cavity. The peak of adenoid size is reached by puberty, after which they cease to grow and begin to shrink. When adenoids are removed in very young children they usually regrow. In the past, the tonsils and adenoids were thought to be the cause of many ills and were removed without too much hesitation. However, much disillusionment has resulted from the failure of surgery to achieve expected results. Moreover, this often regarded "minor" procedure has taken the lives of many children. In the United States alone there is reliable evidence that over 200 deaths per year result from cardiac arrest, hemorrhage, and infection that follow tonsillectomy.

Indications for removal. Because the adenoids are located close to the opening of the eustachian, or auditory, tube, enlarged adenoids may also be an underlying cause of frequent middle ear infections, or otitis media. The eustachian tube is more horizontal, broader, and shorter in infants and young children than it is in adults; thus, ascending ear infections are fairly common.

Indications for adenoidectomy are: obstructive adenoids with recurrent acute purulent otitis media and chronic serous otitis media with conductive hearing loss. Children with the latter condition require surgical drainage to remove the fluid and placement of tympanostomy tubes in the eardrum to promote ventilation and to prevent reaccumulation of fluid.

Tonsillectomy need not be done with adenoidectomy, since these are two independent procedures with very different indications. The best results from tonsillectomy are obtained when the symptoms have been clearly referable to the tonsils and not to such ills as frequent colds, sore throat, poor appetite, failure to gain weight, postnasal drip, or allergies. Definite indications for tonsillectomy include history of peritonsillar abscess (to prevent a second attack), chronic recurrent group A beta-hemolytic streptococcal tonsillitis (culture proved), and hypertrophied tonsils causing chronic airway obstruction and pulmonary hypertension.

Tonsillectomies and adenoidectomies (T and A surgery) are delayed as long as possible so that children under 4 years of age will not have to be admitted to the hospital and subjected to the psychological stresses that this experience may bring them.

Contraindications and postponements. T and A surgery is contraindicated in those children who have hematologic conditions, such as hemophilia, leukemia, aplastic anemia, or purpura. Routine laboratory screening of candidates for this surgery is particularly important to discover the potential postoperative "bleeder." Bleeding and clotting times and prothrombin levels may indicate need for specific treatment or operative delay. Vitamin K is administered for prothrombin deficiencies. Even when severe systemic disorders such as diabetes and cardiac or renal disease are problems, surgery can usually be safely managed if there is a real need for it. However, T and A surgery is always postponed if any child is beginning to have an upper respiratory tract infection.

Because of the numerous blood vessels in the operative area and the character of the procedure, the most frequent complication of either tonsillectomy or adenoidectomy is hemorrhage. For this reason the nurse should especially watch for symptoms of excessive bleeding and shock. Children who have their tonsils or adenoids removed remain in the hospital for 24 hours after surgery so that close observation can be maintained and any needed emergency measures quickly carried out. If bleeding occurs, it will usually be within the first 24 hours following surgery. The doctor must be called to the bedside, where he can evaluate the seriousness of the situation and try to locate the source of bleeding. Minor bleeding will usually stop when any associated clot, which inadequately obstructs the bleeding yet impedes its constriction, is removed gently by suction and a sponge moistened with lidocaine (Xylocaine) hydrochloride and epinephrine is held firmly against the area for a few minutes. In the event of major hemorrhage from the tonsillar fossae, or bed, reanesthetizing and resuturing may be necessary. Bleeding from the adenoid area is more common. Again, any clot must first be removed, and if the bleeding does not stop, a postnasal pack or Foley-type catheter with inflatable bag can be inserted to remain in place until the next day (Fig. 35-5). Transfusions may be required if bleeeding continues.

Postoperative care. Since the advent and use of recovery rooms, the burden of the immediate postoperative care of the surgical patient carried by the "floor" staff nurse has been lightened. However, it has not been eliminated. After having been gently suctioned and observed for immediate signs of cardiorespiratory distress, the T and A patient returns from the recovery room to his unit. He is best positioned on his side with his anterior chest·at a 45-degree angle with the bed to facilitate oronasal drainage, prevent aspiration, and provide easier observation. His nurse frequently checks his pulse and respirations. She notes the child's level of consciousness and any pronounced restlessness. She observes his skin for color and moisture. She carefully evaluates the amount and kind of oronasal drainage, always asking herself: "Is it profuse? Is it a constant drip or ooze? Is the child swallowing frequently, perhaps swallowing the blood? Does he need suctioning? Approximately how many tissues have been used? What is the color of the discharge?" Persistent, bright red drainage indicates active bleeding. Sometimes it is difficult for a student nurse to evaluate the amount of bleeding considered normal after T and A surgery. She should never feel apologetic for asking a more experienced nurse to help her judge the condition of her patient. Unless special indications develop, blood pressure is not routinely

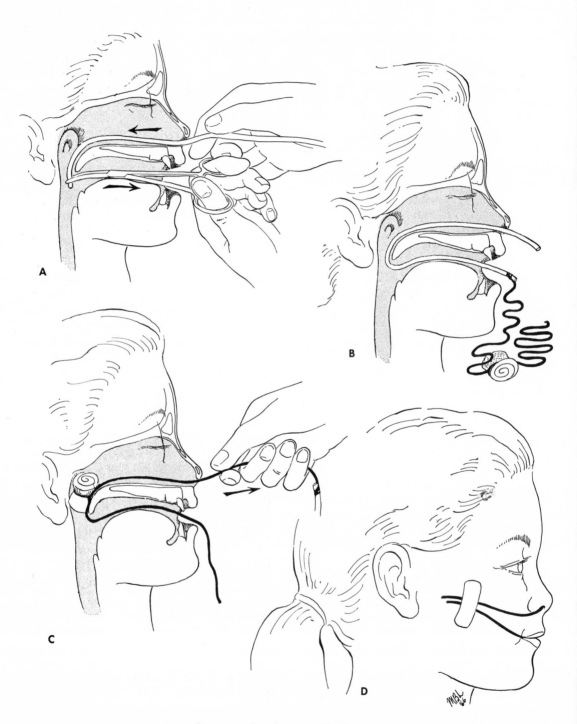

A

B

C

D

Fig. 35-5. Insertion of a postnasal pack to stop bleeding from the adenoid area.

determined on a young child after T and A surgery.

As soon as the child is conscious and responding, he should be given sips of water to ascertain his tolerance of oral fluids. The early introduction of clear, bland fluids helps prevent dehydration and elevated temperature. It also eventually helps to ease the sore throat. By the second day the child is ready for a soft, bland diet. The incidence of postoperative nausea has been greatly reduced through the use of anesthetics other than ether.

Discharge planning should include written instructions for care. Parents and child should be told that his throat will be decreasingly sore for several days. Teaspoon doses of honey may be given as desired to soothe the sore throat or cough. Complaints of earache (referred pain from the throat) are common. Acetaminophen may be prescribed for this discomfort. The child should be told not to blow his nose forcefully. A soft, bland diet should be continued for several days. The child should be encouraged to drink and eat and open his mouth wide. Fluids and food should be given at room temperature. Crisp or hard foods such as popcorn and dry crackers as well as acid foods such as pickles, oranges, grapefruit, and tomatoes should be avoided. About 3 or 4 days after surgery, the child may eat whatever he wishes.

The child should rest and be kept quiet for the first days at home. He may go outside on the third or fourth day, and he may resume his usual activities after 1 week. The school-age child is allowed to return to school at the end of 2 weeks provided there are no infectious diseases among the children in his class.

Signs and symptoms that should be reported promptly by the parents to the physician include fresh bleeding, fever, chest pain, or persistant cough. As already stated, the most common postoperative complication is hemorrhage. Parents should understand that occasional blood-streaked nasal or oral mucus is normal during the first 2 days; but if increased bleeding

should occur, the child must be returned to the hospital promptly (if possible, without causing the child anxiety) for easier and more rapid care. No surgery is without risk. T and A surgery is not a minor operation, nor is it the answer for all ear, nose, and throat problems. It is, however, an effective therapeutic procedure for selected patients.

Streptococcal pharyngitis (strep throat)

Occasionally a severe pharyngitis develops from an infection by the group A beta-hemolytic streptococcus. Such a condition is commonly called a "strep throat." Streptococcal pharyngitis is uncommon before age 2 and almost nonexistent in children less than 1 year of age. Classically, it has a sudden onset, and the child has a high fever, severe sore throat, tender cervical lymph nodes, exudate, a beefy, red pharynx, and petechiae on the soft palate. Unfortunately, strep throat cannot be diagnosed from clinical findings alone, since the same clinical manifestations accompany viral infections. The demonstration of the group A beta-hemolytic streptococcal organism by means of a throat culture is therefore essential for an accurate diagnosis. Since rheumatic fever, heart disease, and glomerulonephritis follow untreated streptococcal infections in a significant number of children, all patients coming to the physician with pharyngeal inflammations should have routine throat cultures taken. The patient's telephone number should be written on the laboratory slip, and those whose culture reveals a beta-hemolytic streptococcus should be notified and treated. While awaiting culture results, patients may be treated symptomatically with saline gargles, lozenges, and aspirin or acetaminophen. The 48-hour delay in starting antibiotic therapy does not increase the incidence of rheumatic fever or glomerulonephritis but is thought to be beneficial in that it gives the patient time to develop an antibody response, which will help prevent future infections by that particular strain of streptococcus. If time is taken to explain this to the patient or his parents, they are most grateful. The patient who is in a toxic state and has physical findings suggesting streptococcal pharyngitis may be given antibiotics immediately, but controlled studies have shown that the speed at which the patient recovers is not appreciably influenced by such treatment. The reason for treating streptococcal pharyngitis with antibiotics is not for a more rapid recovery but for the prevention of complications. Numerous studies have shown that this can be done if the child is treated within 7 days of the onset of his illness. The American Heart Association recommends that streptococcal infections be treated for a period of 10 days with penicillin (or erythromycin if the child is allergic to penicillin). Streptococcal organisms are extremely sensitive to an oral course of penicillin, but since many patients stop their medication prematurely, one intramuscular injection of benzathine penicillin G has been recommended as the treatment of choice. It is also advisable to take throat cultures of asymptomatic family contacts.

Respiratory disease resulting from allergy

About 22 million Americans (1 in 10) suffer from some sort of allergy. Approximately 75% of these have hay fever, asthma, or both. Allergy is the leading chronic disease in children.

The word "allergy" describes an unfavorable reaction in some portion of the body to a normally harmless substance from the outside environment. These substances may be taken into the body through the nose and lungs (pollens, mold spores, animal danders, house dust), through the mouth (foods and drugs), or through the skin (wool, insect bites or stings, and injections). A substance that can produce an allergic reaction is called an *allergen,* but the reaction occurs only in a person sensitive to that substance.

The tendency to become sensitive, or allergic, to some otherwise harmless substance is usually inherited. People vary greatly not only in their susceptibility to allergic diseases, but also in the kind of allergic diseases they have. The organs or tissues in which the allergic reactions occur (lungs, asthma; nose, rhinitis; eyes, conjunctivitis; skin, eczema, urticaria, or hives; gastrointestinal tract, diarrhea) may change during an individual's lifetime. These organs are frequently referred to as target, or shock organs.

The development of allergic sensitivity to a particular substance depends on exposure to that substance as well as the *amount* and *frequency* of such an exposure. An infant who has developed a sensitivity to cow's milk may exhibit this tendency shortly after birth. Throughout his life, he may develop new sensitivities as he undergoes new exposures. The previous sensitivities may remain or may gradually be lost. Although one inherits the tendency to become sensitive to a particular substance, the allergic response develops only *after* exposure to that substance. This exposure can happen in utero. Sensitization may follow the first exposure or may not occur until after repeated exposures. Penicillin allergy is a well-known example of the latter phenomenon.

A general outline of the allergic process follows:

1. A person contacts a substance and produces sensitizing antibodies (such as immunoglobulin E) to that material.
2. These antibodies are then deposited on special cells (mast cells and basophils) in the body.
3. The allergen (substance to which a person is sensitive or allergic) contacts the antibodies attached to these cells in a subsequent exposure.
4. A reaction occurs whereby chemicals, or "allergic mediators" such as histamines, are released from these cells and cause the symptoms of allergy.

Diagnosis of allergy. The best way to find the sources of allergic symptoms is by a careful history of what exposures preceded each attack and what avoidance preceded each attack-free period. Another way in which allergens may be detected is through skin tests. When the test allergen meets antibodies sensitive to that substance in the skin, the chemical mediators are released, resulting in a positive reaction that resembles a mosquito bite. Tests that indicate inhaled allergens are reliable and commonly agree with the patient's symptoms. Although they can be helpful, skin tests for the diagnosis of food allergy are not always reliable. Therefore, different trial diets are sometimes suggested to further evaluate foods as the source of the patient's symptoms.

Treatment of allergy. The best way to treat allergy is to prevent it by separating the patient from the allergen. For example, a fur-bearing pet should not be offered a home with a person having a history of allergic problems. Dust in a patient's bedroom could be minimized by removing cloth draperies, fiber rugs, and using special hypoallergenic pillows and dust-resistant mattresses. The amount of relief from symptoms is in direct proportion to the amount that the exposure is decreased. A second method of treatment consists of immunizing patients to their allergens by injections of these substances in gradually increasing amounts. This regimen is used when allergens (such as pollens) cannot be adequately avoided. The process is called desensitization, hyposensitization, or immunotherapy.

Medications of various types are also employed for relief of symptoms. To be effective for this purpose, medication is often prescribed on a regular daily basis. Regular maintenance doses of medication should be taken as long as there is objective evidence of a symptomatic allergic state. Antihistamines such as tripelennamine hydrochloride (Pyribenzamine) and chlorpheniramine maleate (Chlor-Trimeton Maleate and Teldrin) are often effective for the control of allergic rhinitis. They may be combined with a decongestant such a pseudoephedrine (Drixoral). The xanthine drugs theophylline and aminophylline are most valuable in counteracting bronchospasm in

asthma. The sympathomimetic drugs, such as epinephrine and isoproterenol, are rapid bronchodilators and are the most useful drugs for the relief of anaphylactic shock, acute asthma, hives, or edema. When a regular program is properly planned, the sympathomimetic drugs are less often required. The stimulation threshold can be increased with various combinations of helpful drugs such as Tedral (theophylline 130 mg., ephedrine 24 mg., and phenobarbital 8 mg.). However, such useful combinations often increase the side effects of these drugs. A drug recently approved for use in this country is cromolyn sodium (Intal or Aarane). It is used *prophylactically* and as an adjunct in the treatment and control of the chronic and severely ill asthmatic child. It is administered in powder form by direct inhalation into the bronchial tree. Symptomatic and physical improvements occur without significant side effects. Fewer asthmatic episodes requiring hospitalization and emergency room visits result. Often there is an increase in exercise tolerance. However, there may be a continued need for bronchodilators, although the dose can be decreased. Follow-up care is important.

Rhinitis is one of the most common allergic manifestations in children. It is characterized by sneezing, a profuse, watery nasal discharge, swelling and itching of the nasal mucosa, and often a conjunctivitis. Allergic nasal obstruction is very unpleasant for the child, his parents, and teacher. Frequently it leads to constant sniffling, mouth breathing, snoring, and a nasal voice. Complications such as sinusitis and otitis can result. Allergic rhinitis is commonly classified as seasonal (hay fever) or nonseasonal (perennial). Seasonal allergic rhinitis results most often from plant pollen and mold sensitivity. House dust, animal danders, and foods are the most frequent causes of nonseasonal allergic rhinitis in children. A careful history, physical examination, laboratory aids (such as nasal smears to identify increased eosinophil counts), and skin testing are all important etiological diagnostic measures. Treatment depends upon the results of the diagnostic procedures. When the specific cause can be determined, the allergen is removed if possible. Most nonseasonal allergens, such as animal danders and feathers, can usually be removed to effectively reduce exposure to them.

The antihistaminic drugs are fairly successful in treating some patients with seasonal allergic rhinitis, even though there are innumerable airborne substances that are potentially sensitizing. When it is impossible or impractical to eliminate the causative allergen or control the body's response to its presence, hyposensitization should be considered. Most children with severe allergic rhinitis will require specific treatment. Besides providing symptomatic relief, hyposensitization may lessen the chances of the subsequent development of asthma.

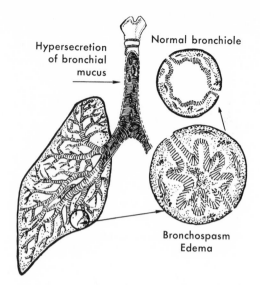

Fig. 35-6. The cardinal anatomical changes in asthma occur at the bronchiole level. Bronchospasm, edema, and hypersecretions of mucus cause severe dyspnea and wheezing.

Asthma

Asthma is the most common major allergic manifestation in childhood. It involves from 1% to 2% of all children. Asthma accounts for 23% of school absenteeism, and in the United States causes over 4,000 deaths annually. It is characterized by difficulty in breathing as the result of spasm of the small bronchi, obstructive edema of the bronchial mucosa, and the production of tenacious secretions, all of which tend to obstruct air exchange (Fig. 35-6). There is more difficulty in exhaling than inhaling. A pronounced expiratory wheeze is usually present. Rapid, shallow inspirations are characteristic. Milder obstruction is frequently manifested by nocturnal or exertional coughing.

Asthma is divided into two major classifications. The first, intrinsic asthma, is commonly seen in the child below age 3 and in older adults. Some allergists think it is caused by sensitivity to infectious agents or their products; this may be called infectious asthma. The second, extrinsic asthma, is caused by specific external allergens such as pollen, house dust, animal danders, and

food. Children with this second type of asthma may develop secondary bacterial or viral infections, which aggravate and prolong symptoms. The clinical course of asthma varies in different children. In addition to the degree of allergic sensitivity and the amount, duration, and frequency of exposure to allergens, a number of nonspecific factors are influential in affecting the response of the patient. Infections, chilling, fatigue, emotional stress, and physical debility all influence the appearance of allergic phenomena.

Treatment of asthma. The treatment of asthma is usually divided into: (1) specific measures, such as elimination of offending allergens and specific desensitization; and (2) nonspecific measures, which include drugs, fluids, and supportive treatment.

Acute attacks of asthma may occur at any time and are related to multiple factors. There may be no single cause. The child exhibits symptoms when he reaches a certain level or threshold of exposure to certain offenders. The cardinal feature is airway obstruction; the patient's shoulders are hunched, his thoracic soft tissues retract as he inspires, and his accessory muscles of respiration bulge with the effort of breathing. His respiratory rate will be rapid and his breathing punctuated by spasms of coughing and audible wheezes. The child is diaphoretic, restless, and fatigued. Difficulty in breathing always produces anxiety, and the patient's anxiety and that of his parents tend to compound his respiratory problems.

Treatment of acute attacks of asthma usually includes the administration of epinephrine (Adrenalin) by injection or isoproterenol by inhalation to produce relatively quick relief. Epinephrine suspension (Sus-Phrine) is a medication often used to achieve more lasting effects. Adequate fluid intake is very important. Following the acute phase, postural drainage after IPPB is very effective in the removal of bronchial secretions or mucous plugs.

A life-threatening situation, *status asthmaticus,* exists when the patient does not clear after 3 consecutive doses of Adrenalin, 1:1,000, given at 20- to 30-minute intervals. These children are critically ill and must be hospitalized.

Children with status asthmaticus need fluids. They may be dehydrated because they have been too ill to eat or drink and have lost fluids by hyperventilating, coughing, and perspiring. Vomiting also adds to the child's dehydrated state. Intravenous administration of fluids is started immediately in order to correct the fluid imbalance, maintain liquified bronchial secretions, and serve as a vehicle for important medications. The nurse should carefully check the amount and time prescribed in order to prevent overhydration. Thereafter, aminophylline, a highly effective bronchodilator, is given intravenously over a 15- to 30-minute period at 4- to 6-hour intervals. Signs of aminophylline intoxication include restlessness, irritability, vomiting, and abdominal pain and should not be confused with increased severity of the asthmatic attack.

Parents should be encouraged to stay at the child's bedside. They need to see what is happening to their child as well as receive explanations of what is being done. Isoproterenol (Isuprel) with IPPB is frequently effective in relieving bronchospasm and dyspnea in children who do not respond to Adrenalin. It is given promptly to all cooperative children 15 minutes after the infusion of aminophylline. This may be followed by chest physical therapy (PT) consisting of vibration, clapping, and coughing in various positions. Chest PT and postural drainage are ordered as soon as the acute phase subsides. It is a significant therapeutic aid for children whose excessive mucus is a problem. It is most effectively performed after bronchodilation is obtained from aminophylline and the aerosol treatment. Hydrocortisone sodium succinate (Solu-Cortef) is given intravenously to children who do not respond to bronchodilators, who have recently had corticosteroids, or who are receiving maintenance doses of steroids. It is important to note that the therapeutic effect of Solu-Cortef is often not seen until 12 hours (and frequently longer) after administration. If the patient improves, corticosteroids may be stopped abruptly after a *short* course. Long-term use of steroids is not recommended because of the serious side effects, which include growth suppression, masking of infection, and osteoporosis. Iodides may be used to raise obstructing mucus, but their effectiveness remains debatable. Antibiotics are indicated in the presence of bacterial infection. However, asthmatic flare-ups are more often associated with viral infections; in these cases antibiotics are not helpful. Oxygen is given to relieve hypoxemia. Since cyanosis is an unreliable sign of hypoxia, arterial blood gas levels should be determined and followed carefully. Oxygen is ordered when the arterial Po_2 is less than 70 mm. Hg. Sodium bicarbonate ($NaHCO_3$) administered intravenously may be needed to correct acidosis.

The nurse who is caring for the child with status asthmaticus must constantly but calmly evaluate the changes and progress that occur. Although most children demonstrate significant improvement after administration of aminophylline, isoproterenol hydrochloride via IPPB, and fluids given intravenously, others do not respond for 12 to 24 hours. During this time, steroids, $NaHCO_3$, antibiotics, and oxygen may be added to their therapeutic regimen. The above measures are usually effective in time. Radiographic studies are most helpful in defining the precise difficulty when management of severe, acute asthma presents a problem. Atelectasis with or without pneumonia, mucus plugs in the bronchi, and spontaneous pneumothorax account for the major complications and must be treated separately. However, sometimes response is not satisfactory, labored breathing persists, and the child becomes exhausted and incoherent. He no longer coughs or wheezes. Inspiratory retractions and cyanosis increase. These are the clinical signs of impending respiratory failure. Blood gases exhibit a decreasing level of oxygen, rising CO_2 retention, and acidosis. This situation might be reversed if the danger is recognized and the child moved to the intensive care unit where adequate equipment and personnel experienced with this grave complication are available. Delivery of 100% humidified oxygen, infusion of isoproterenol and sodium bicarbonate, and mechanical ventilation are necessary measures that must be offered if the child's life is to be saved.

CIRCULATORY DISORDERS

This section introduces the student to some of the more common pediatric problems involving the heart and its vessels and circulating blood. Although some of the frequently encountered congenital heart defects were briefly described in Chapter 16, no mention was made of the surgical possibilities of repair of such defects or the nursing care of the cardiac patient. The following paragraphs will supply these omissions.

Varied abnormalities of the heart and large blood vessels may occur. Some cause little inconvenience. Others are incompatible with life or produce severe problems in their victims.

Diagnostic procedures

To evaluate heart function and detect cardiac abnormalities, an accurate history of the patient's complaints is sought, a complete physical examination is carried out, and various tests and specialized procedures are ordered.

Common noninvasive tests include observation of the shape and action of the heart and great blood vessels by *fluoroscopy*, permanent recording of the size and shape of the heart by *x-ray examination*, external pulse and heart sound recordings by *phonocardiography*, tests of the activity of the heart by *electrocardiography*, and sonar recordings *(echocardiography)*.

Laboratory tests of special significance include a complete blood count and hematocrit and hemoglobin determinations. Patients with cyanotic-type heart disease may have either an excessive amount of circulating red blood cells (polycythemia) manufactured in an attempt to deliver more oxygen to the deprived body cells or may suffer from anemia. If polycythemia is present, the blood thickens and circulation slows down, occasionally causing the development of abnormal clots in the bloodstream, always a dangerous situation.

A special procedure called "angiography" is occasionally arranged. It involves the injection of a contrast medium into the circulation and observation of its flow by x-ray examination or fluoroscopy. When a contrast medium is injected directly into a heart chamber, it is termed "angiocardiography." Such visualization of the aorta is termed "aortography." Special procedures may also include the performance of right or left heart catheterizations, which are concerned with the introduction of a small catheter, seen by x-ray examination, into a vein or artery and its gentle manipulation into various chambers of the heart as well as large associated vessels. This procedure is done on an anesthetized or sedated patient and, although it is not without risk,

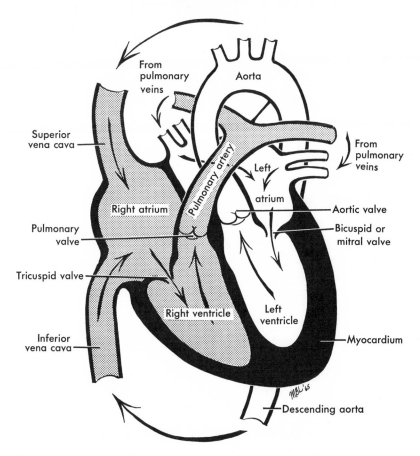

Fig. 35-7. Structure and circulation of the normal heart. The shaded area represents blood with low oxygen content.

yields considerable information. If possible, children are sedated, not anesthetized, so that they may be able to cooperate consciously during the procedure. It reveals the pressure in various areas of the cardio-circulatory system and the percentage of oxygen at different sites. The presence of abnormal openings may be demonstrated by direct passage of the small catheter through the defects or by evaluation of oxygenation patterns.

Children returning to the nursing unit after cardiac catheterization should be treated as postoperative patients. Vital signs—pulse, respirations, and blood pressure—should be noted every 20 minutes until stable. Children should have blood pressure determinations on the arm that is not used for the catheter insertion. A mist tent or oxygen mask should be in readiness as ordered or indicated. Any dressing applied should be noted and observed. It is important to note skin color and temperature and character of the pulse in the extremity catheterized because this may detect arterial occlusion due to thrombus formation.

THE INFANT

Congenital anomalies of the heart and great vessels

About 20,000 infants are born with recognizable heart disease every year in the United States. Formerly, about half of these infants would die within 6 months. Today, early diagnosis and treatment (through palliative or curative surgery) are approximately 90% effective.

Congenital heart disease refers to a structural abnormality or defect present in the heart at birth. These defects may create three problems related to blood flow within the heart and circulatory system. A *volume overload* occurs when more blood than normal enters a ventricle. A *pressure overload* occurs when the outflow of blood is impeded or slowed. Ventricular hypertrophy and finally congestive heart failure may result. *Desaturation,* low oxygen content, of circulating arterial blood, occurs when unoxygenated blood returning from the body mixes with the oxygenated blood returning from the lungs. The result is acidosis due to poor oxygenation of the various organs. Acidosis leads to decreased cardiac performance and still more acidosis. Some congenital anomalies of the heart illustrate all three types of blood flow problems. Early diagnosis and treatment are important.

Signs and symptoms. Infants with serious congenital heart disease often manifest common signs and symptoms that reflect the underlying anomaly. *Cyanosis*—blueness of the lips, nail beds, and mucosal surfaces—may be due to shunting of unoxygenated blood into the left heart, or it may be associated with pulmonary edema. *Tachypnea* is defined as an excessive resting respiratory rate, 45 breaths per minute in the full-term infant or over 60 breaths per minute in the premature infant. Retractions and flaring of the nares occur with each breath. This rapid breathing is a frequent response to low oxygen content in the blood and is often precipitated by mild exercise. *Tachycardia,* an excessively rapid heart rate, may be difficult to evaluate in the infant, particularly if he is moving and crying. A heart rate greater than 200 beats per minute, when infant is at rest, is significant and should be reported at once since infants quickly develop cardiac decompensation (inability to maintain the necessary blood flow). *Effort intolerance* is chiefly manifested by feeding problems. The infant will usually start feedings eagerly but soon becomes fussy and fatigued

and stops feeding. The cycle is often repeated, but the infant seldom finishes his bottle. *Failure to thrive* is also common. Episodes of congestive heart failure and intercurrent pulmonary infection are frequent causes of retarded growth. *Murmurs,* or abnormal heart sounds, occur when the walls of vessels are uneven or when valvular surfaces are irregular. Murmurs represent the most commonly detected physical finding associated with congenital cardiac defects in the infant.

Congestive heart failure (CHF) occurs when the heart can no longer pump blood sufficiently to meet the body's needs. When infants develop CHF in the early months of life, it is usually secondary to structural defects, which produce a pressure or volume overload. In an effort to preserve cardiac output and accommodate the larger volume of residual blood, cardiac dilatation occurs. CHF is typically recognized by a combination of tachypnea and tachycardia associated with hepatomegaly caused by circulatory congestion. The development of CHF warrants prompt cardiac consultation and diagnostic studies. Frequently, surgery offers the only chance of life.

Left-to-right shunts (acyanotic)

Patent ductus arteriosus (PDA). Patent means "open." The condition called patent ductus arteriosus refers to a holdover from the fetal circulation pattern. Review Fig. 5-6. You will remember that the ductus arteriosus is a short blood vessel that connects the pulmonary artery with the aorta, making it unnecessary for the blood circulating through the pulmonary artery to continue on to the nonfunctioning lungs of the fetus. Normally this arterial duct closes soon after birth and within a few weeks becomes a ligament.

If the ductus arteriosus does not close, the higher blood pressure in the aorta, which results after birth, forces well-oxygenated blood from the aorta back into the pulmonary circulation for a return trip to the lungs. This puts an abnormal work load on the left ventricle and may cause a sig-

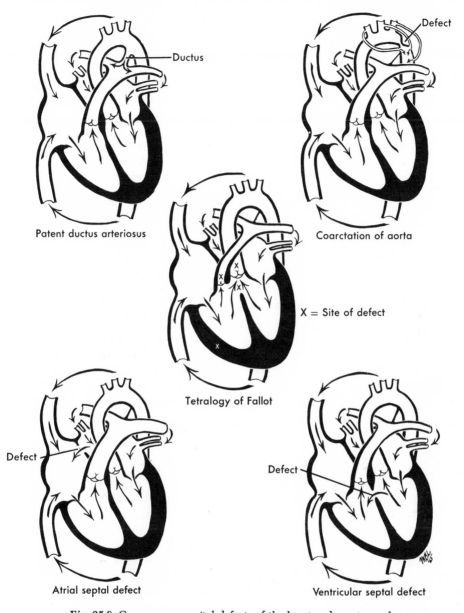

Ductus

Defect

Patent ductus arteriosus

Coarctation of aorta

X = Site of defect

Tetralogy of Fallot

Defect

Defect

Atrial septal defect

Ventricular septal defect

Fig. 35-8. Common congenital defects of the heart and great vessels.

nificant elevation of the blood pressure in the pulmonary circulation. The growth of children suffering from this defect may be impaired if the duct remains large. They may suffer from dyspnea when they are active, and without appropriate treatment their life expectancy is often reduced. The defect does not characteristically produce cyanosis unless pressures in the aorta and pulmonary artery are changed as the result of excessive pulmonary blood flow, which may increase pulmonary vascular resistance. Some premature babies with respiratory distress syndrome may reopen their ductus as a response to poor oxygenation in the lungs. Often this prevents weaning the baby from a mechanical ventilator unless ligation of the ductus is performed.

Diagnosis is usually made on the basis of several findings. The detection of a con-

585

tinuous murmur or an abnormal sound accompanying heart action is only one. A "thrill" may be noted; the word "thrill" in this case refers to a vibration felt over the cardiac area. Blood pressure determinations may reveal a wide range between the systolic and diastolic readings—termed a "wide pulse pressure." The appearance and stamina of the patient are noted. The patent duct may be visualized by aortography or by direct passage of the small catheter through the duct during fluoroscopy.

This condition may be treated surgically, usually with excellent results. The duct is tied off (ligated) or divided.

Atrial septal defect (ASD). An abnormal opening in the wall, or septum, that separates the right and left atria may be the result of the persistence of the foramen ovale, which during fetal life shunts some of the blood from the right to the left side of the heart. It may also be caused by the presence of a septal opening unassociated with normal fetal circulation. Cyanosis does not characteristically occur, since the blood pressure is higher in the left heart and unoxygenated blood does not enter the general circulation. However, if some other abnormality is present (for example, pulmonary artery valve stenosis), right-to-left flow may occur, and cyanosis may result. Children with ASD usually have an overworked right heart and congested pulmonary circulation because of the backflow through the defect to the right atrium. They may demonstrate cardiac enlargement, a systolic murmur, decreased resistance to respiratory tract infections, lowered exercise tolerance, and physical underdevelopment. A decision to attempt surgical correction is based on the condition of the individual child, since some do quite well without operative intervention. Surgery itself presents a small risk. During surgery the defect is either repaired by direct closure with sutures only or by the incorporation of a plastic patch into the repair. The patch is eventually penetrated by growing heart fibers and becomes part of the septum.

Ventricular septal defect (VSD). The presence of an opening between the two ventricles is always an abnormality, whether it occurs in the fetus or newborn infant. How seriously such an opening may disturb normal heart function depends on the position and size of the defect and the presence of other abnormalities in the large vessels of the heart. If a large defect is found in the membranous portion of the septum, symptoms are usually severe. The blood usually travels through the opening from the left to the right ventricle. However, in some cases the shunt may reverse as resistance in the pulmonary capillary bed increases, and the pressure in the right side of the heart mounts. Diagnosis is made on the basis of clinical symptoms, a characteristic heart murmur, and the results of x-ray examination, electrocardiograms, and cardiac catheterization. Specific treatment may be recommended for the individual child and consists of surgical repair by open heart surgery similar to that employed for ASD. Surgical risk is somewhat increased with VSD repair.

Right-to-left shunts (cyanotic)

Tetralogy of Fallot. The word element "tetra" means "four." Tetralogy of Fallot is a heart condition that is characterized by the presence of four heart malformations: an interventricular septal defect, a narrowing of the opening of the pulmonary artery (pulmonary stenosis), an aorta situated very near the septal defect (overriding aorta), and an enlarged, thickened right ventricular wall (right ventricular hypertrophy). Because the narrowed pulmonary artery causes the pressure to rise in the right ventricle, hypertrophy of the right heart wall results, and the shunt of blood through the septal defect goes from right to left, usually causing considerable cyanosis. The infant suffering from tetralogy of Fallot has been called a "blue baby." The moderately to severely affected young child with this diagnosis typically has blue lips and nail beds and a dusky-tinted skin, which becomes more cyanotic on exertion.

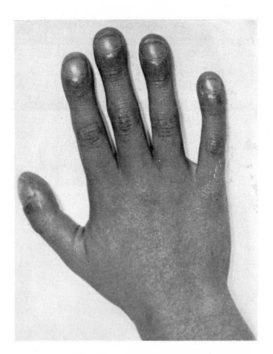

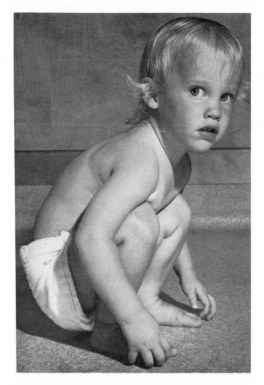

Fig. 35-9. When the ends of the fingers become wide and thick, they are termed "clubbed." These fingers are also very cyanotic. (Courtesy Naval Regional Medical Center, San Diego, Calif.)

Fig. 35-10. The squatting position improves the cardiac output of some children with congenital heart defects.

Clubbing of the fingers and toes is often a feature (Fig. 35-9). Thrill and chest deformity may be noted. The child may have "hypoxic spells" of respiratory distress, deep cyanosis, loss of consciousness, and convulsions. He is small for his age. When the young child with cyanotic heart disease is fatigued, he often squats (Fig. 35-10). This position improves return of blood to the heart, traps desaturated blood in the lower extremities, and improves cardiac output.

Management of "hypoxic spells" may be quite difficult and complex. Initially, when the infant is *excitable,* with respiratory distress, one may use a knee-chest position and administer oxygen. Morphine may be used for sedation. If the infant is flaccid or unconscious, morphine is contraindicated. If metabolic acidosis occurs, sodium bicarbonate may be given intravenously. If these measures fail, propranolol may be

administered intravenously with proper monitoring of vital signs.

Diagnosis depends on clinical manifestations, x-ray examinations, electrocardiograms, angiocardiograms, and cardiac catheterizations. Treatment may be medical or surgical, depending on the condition of the patient. Before open heart surgery was available, surgical techniques were devised to improve the pulmonary circulation by creating an artificial ductus arteriosus, which would recirculate poorly oxygenated blood to the lungs for oxygen enrichment. The Blalock-Taussig operation and the Waterston operation are such techniques. This type of palliative surgery is still useful when the child is considered too small for total correction but is having life-threatening "hypoxic spells." Now open heart surgery with total correction is preferred because the sources of difficulty may be viewed and repaired directly. Without surgical intervention the typical patient with tetralogy of Fallot faces a brief future.

Complete transposition of the great vessels. Transposition of the great vessels is a very serious cyanotic congenital heart defect. In this condition the pulmonary artery originates from the left ventricle, whereas the aorta arises from the right ventricle. Life is possible as long as the foramen ovale or ductus arteriosus remains open or an interventricular septal defect exists. Prominent features are extreme cyanosis and congestive heart failure. Diagnosis is made on the basis of electrocardiogram, x-ray examination, angiocardiogram, and cardiac catheterization. A palliative surgical procedure (Blalock-Hanlen operation) to create or enlarge an ASD may be helpful in prolonging life. A special balloon catheter (balloon septostomy) is often used to create or enlarge an ASD without the high risk of surgery. Total correction is possible by the Mustard procedure. A "baffle," or partition made of pericardium, is placed in such a manner as to redirect the pulmonary venous return within the left atrium to the right ventricle and the systemic return to the left ventricle. Immediate and long-term results have been excellent with an overall mortality of less than 10%.

Obstructive lesions

Pulmonary stenosis. The pulmonary artery carries poorly oxygenated blood from the right ventricle through the pulmonary valve to the lungs where it is reoxygenated. Narrowing of the valve itself or the areas immediately above or below it causes obstruction to the right ventricular outflow. The condition may be so mild that the infant has no symptoms, or it may be so severe that the infant is dyspneic, has effort intolerance, severe cyanosis, and CHF. A loud murmur is heard. The condition is diagnosed by EKG, x-ray film, and cardiac catheterization. Open heart surgical repair is indicated if the right ventricular pressure is high. An incision in the dilated pulmonary artery easily exposes the dome-shaped valvular stenosis, which is then incised (pulmonary valvotomy). If the primary obstruction is below the valve, the obstructing muscle can be resected. The results of this operation are usually excellent, and the risk is low, except in the case of the infant.

Coarctation of the aorta. The aorta is the largest blood vessel in the body. As it leaves the heart it normally arches to the left. Three major vessels sprout from the aortic arch before it starts its descent into the lower thorax and abdomen. These are the innominate, left carotid, and left subclavian arteries, which supply the head and upper extremities with oxygenated blood. The ductus arteriosus joins the aorta in the general area of the left subclavian artery before normal postnatal circulation develops. Sometimes the aorta is abnormally narrowed in the area of the arch, usually involving the segment just past the subclavian artery. Many times smaller "collateral" vessels (usually branches of the subclavian and intercostal arteries) develop and bypass the narrowed portion to help supply circulation to the lower extremities. The narrowing of the aorta is often called "coarctation," since a narrowed figure results when two arcs are drawn side by side, like two C's back to back. The symptoms resulting depend on the location of the coarctation and whether any other blood vessel abnormalities exist.

The presence of coarctation is suspected when there are forceful arterial pulses in the upper extremities but weak or absent pulses in the lower extremities and a systolic murmur is heard. Severe coarctation in the infant, especially if associated with another congenital heart anomaly, may precipitate profound congestive heart failure and require surgical intervention. The older patient may have few complaints, although occasionally headache, leg cramps, excessive fatigue, and frequent nosebleeds may be reported. Diagnosis is confirmed by x-ray examination, electrocardiogram, and aortogram.

Without appropriate treatment the life span is often shortened because of the onset of such complications as cerebral hemorrhage, subacute bacterial endocarditis, or heart failure.

Definitive treatment is surgical. The narrowed portion may be cut out and the adjoining normal-sized segments sewed together. Occasionally the repair involves the insertion of a prosthesis to take the place of a large segment that has to be removed.

Cardiac surgery

Assuming that facilities and skilled physicians are available, surgical treatment of large blood vessel or heart defects depends on the extent of incapacity suffered by the patient, the possibility of a satisfactory repair, and the risk involved. Surgery on the aorta, pulmonary artery, or other associated blood vessels is similar in some respects to heart surgery. However, when the malformations exist in the interior of the heart and cardiac circulation must be interrupted, the difficulty of the procedure and the risk to the patient increase significantly. A heart-lung machine was perfected in 1955. Prior to that time it was impossible to discontinue the beating of the heart long enough to make a lengthly repair without seriously depriving some vital structure (for example, brain or kidneys) of vital carbon dioxide–oxygen exchange and causing tissue damage.

The heart-lung machine receives blood from the patient's venous circulation through tubes inserted into the inferior and superior venae cavae. It removes the carbon dioxide, instills oxygen, regulates blood temperature, and pumps the blood back into the systemic circulation in most cases by way of the femoral artery (called a cardiopulmonary bypass). Needless to say, this is a highly complex procedure, requiring a team of skilled physicians, nurses, and technicians.

A patient with congenital heart defects may undergo surgery as an infant, toddler, or child. To simplify organization, the following discussion will include more than the infant in its scope. Any child who is to have any type of surgery must be carefully prepared for the event. This is especially true in the case of scheduled chest or heart surgery because of the seriousness of the operation and the many procedures that must be carried out that require the trust and cooperation of the child to achieve optimum results.

A prepared child presupposes prepared parents. This does not mean that the parents must feel totally calm and serene or that they and their child must know all the details of the procedure. The former would be unnatural, the latter would be both impossible and undesirable, probably causing many more anxieties than it would ease. How much the child is told will depend on his age, expressed concerns, and intellect. How much the parents are told will depend on their expressed concerns, intellects, and familiarity with the sciences involved. Whatever information is given, however simple, should be truthful.

Children who are scheduled for heart surgery are usually admitted to the hospital several days in advance of the procedure to enable them to learn about the hospital, to become acquainted with some of the nurses who will be caring for them, and to be introduced to some of the equipment and techniques that will be used after surgery. This preliminary period is also used as a period of evaluation of the child. It is a time when his general condition may be observed and nutritional needs noted and, as far as possible, met. His weight is recorded each morning; scheduled blood pressure, respiration, and pulse checks are particularly important. The nurses should be alert for and report any signs of respiratory tract infection or rash, which may indicate the presence of other diseases. Such signs may necessitate a postponement of surgery.

It is usually very helpful to demonstrate some of the equipment that will be used with the child before its use under more stressful conditions is needed. The child may be shown an oxygen tent with humidifier and may get inside to see how the "small house" feels. He may "practice" taking his breathing exercises with the intermittent positive pressure machine or learn how to cough with the nurse holding his chest. Explanations should be calm, factual, and geared to the child's understanding.

Treatment and nursing care of the cardiac patient
Postoperative nursing care

The postoperative nursing care of open heart surgery patients is a nursing specialty in itself. A patient usually remains in the intensive care unit for several days. While the child is in the intensive care unit, his condition is usually monitored by machines that graphically record heart action, arterial and venous blood pressures, respirations, and temperature. In some cases heartbeat may be stimulated by the use of a mechanical pacemaker. The rate and quality of respirations are evaluated; the color and feel of the skin are noted. Chest suction is maintained to prevent a buildup of secretion or gas in the thorax, causing respiratory distress and atelectasis. Humidified oxygen is often administered by an oxygen tent or mask. The urinary catheter is checked often to determine kidney output. Intravenous fluids and blood transfusions are calculated and maintained according to order. Wound drainage and dressings must be checked. Turning and encouraging the patient to cough are extremely important. Intermittent positive pressure may be prescribed. Tracheal as well as nasopharyngeal suctioning may be ordered. Some patients may have temporary tracheostomies. Initially the patient's temperature may be subnormal, but later temperature-reducing procedures may be necessary, including the use of the hypothermia blanket. A relatively high temperature after open heart surgery is fairly common. In some cases it may be caused by a reaction to the massive blood transfusion received. However, the possibility of infection must not be discounted when a patient's temperature rises abnormally.

Continuing care

The patient needs constant, expert nursing observation and care. Many important nursing evaluations must be made during this critical postoperative interval. Caring for this type of patient in the immediate postoperative period is not within the scope of the vocational nurse. However, at times she may be called on to "lend a careful hand," with supervision, during a treatment or to help change the patient's position, depending on his needs and condition. The vocational nurse should know how important it is that the chest tubes remain intact and the drainage bottles and suction machine remain undisturbed. The bottles containing drainage from the chest should always be maintained lower than the lowest level of the child's chest to prevent backflow. To avoid backflow the bottles should be fastened to the floor or to a correctly positioned holder. In the event that a chest bottle should break or the tube should become disconnected, the part of the tube coming from the patient's chest must be immediately clamped off near the chest wall to prevent pneumothorax. Symptoms of pneumothorax include cynanosis, dyspnea, and chest pain.

As the patient's condition improves, his chest suction will be discontinued and the tubes removed. As his condition becomes stable, he may be assigned to the care of a licensed vocational nurse under the supervision of a registered nurse. The nurse should know that the child is usually weighed while undressed each morning before breakfast to determine fluid retention. He may be on a diet that limits sodium and carefully spaces a certain maximum oral fluid intake. The patient's pulse and respirations should be noted and recorded before and after any new activity. During periods of ambulation he should be carefully evaluated for fatigue and given periods of rest as his respirations, pulse, and color dictate. The pulse of these young children and infants is always taken over the heart with a stethoscope, that is, apically, for 1 minute. This technique requires training, since there are normally two sounds to each cardiac cycle. Older children may have radial pulse determinations for 1 minute. The quality as well as the rate should be noted. Occasionally apical-radial pulse determinations will be ordered. These pulse rates are taken simultaneously and then compared; they may be writen 110A/100R. There may be more apical beats than radial beats (pulse deficit), but there is never an excess of radial beats! Blood pressure determinations are routinely made with the patient's pulse and respiration at scheduled intervals. Care must be taken in the selection of the size of cuff—it should cover two thirds of the distance from the shoulder to the elbow, or be 20% wider than the diameter of the patient's arm. Ambulation and activity privileges will be gradually increased. Many times conferences must be arranged with physician-nurse-parent participation to help parents adjust to the new capabilities of their children and avoid the hazards of overprotection. Help regarding school responsibilities to be assumed and even vocational planning may be sought.

Nonsurgical treatment and care

Sometimes a patient's cardiac problem cannot be helped by surgery, or he has to wait until he is in better condition or older before surgery is attempted. In these cases the child is treated by medicines, planned diet, and general health supervision. The nurse should be aware of the types of medications the child is receiving and the expected accomplishments, side effects, and toxic reactions of these medications. Sodium restriction is common. Often patients with cardiac defects must be weighed daily, and accurate intake and output records are maintained. Signs of developing heart failure, cardiac irregularities, or possible respiratory tract infection should be promptly reported. Limitations of activity may be necessary, although many pediatric patients with congenital cardiac defects automatically limit themselves to only the activity they can best tolerate. Quiet play is often more restful than enforced, re-

sented "complete bed rest." The child who must be in an oxygen tent or who demonstrates susceptibility to fatigue should be disturbed as little as possible, and when he is disturbed, several procedures should be carried out at the same time to allow relatively long uninterrupted periods of sleep or rest (for example, TPR and B/P determinations, offering fluids, changing the child's gown or diapers, and shifting his position). Changes of position are important in preventing hypostatic pneumonia and skin breakdown. However, no *vigorous* back rubs should be performed on a patient with a cardiac defect. Proper positioning helps ward off contractures and other deformities and assists proper body function.

Possible complications of congenital cardiac defects
Cardiac decompensation— congestive heart failure (CHF)

Certain complications that may develop in patients with congenital heart prior to, during, or after surgery should be mentioned. Probably the most common is the failure of the heart to continue the circulation of the blood in sufficient volume to meet body needs and prevent abnormal congestion of the blood in certain areas. Sometimes the heart can maintain an adequate blood flow by gradually increasing its size or altering its rate. If this occurs, the heart is said to be in *compensation*. If the heart cannot maintain the necessary blood flow, it is said to be in *decompensation*, or failure. Cardiac failure in infants, whatever the cause, is always a medical emergency.

Pulmonary congestion resulting from the inability of the left ventricle to pump effectively is characterized by pooling of blood in the lung capillaries, causing coughing and dyspnea. Blood-tinged froth may be expectorated. Acute pulmonary edema may necessitate rather drastic measures such as the removal of 5% to 10% of the circulating blood (phlebotomy) or rotating tourniquets on the extremities to reduce the amount of blood returning to the heart at one time.

Congestion of blood in the systemic venous system as the result of inefficient right ventricular contraction may cause nausea and vomiting, enlargement of the liver, and edema. In infants, edema is often best detected by a weight gain. Cyanosis, tachypnea, dyspnea, and tachycardia are major indications for diagnostic studies. But studies are usually undertaken only after CHF is controlled since the baby becomes fatigued by the work of breathing and may have an annoying cough and therefore has difficulty eating and sleeping. Prompt treatment with digoxin, oxygen, and diuretics will decrease heart and respiratory rate and improve color, appetite, and disposition. Digoxin slows and strengthens the heartbeat and induces diuresis. A digitalizing dose (high dose) is given over a period of 12 hours, and a maintenance dose of 10% of the digitalizing dose is usually given every 12 hours. However, digoxin should be withheld and the physician notified if the apical pulse rate in the infant is less than 100. Signs and symptoms of toxicity include anorexia, vomiting, and excessive slowing or irregularity of the pulse rate. Diuretics especially help in relieving the pulmonary congestion that accompanies CHF if response to other forms of treatment is insufficient.

Nursing measures center around making the infant more comfortable and conserving his energy. A sitting position in a cool, humidified oxygen tent is beneficial. Early feeding with soft nipples and allowing for frequent rest periods will reduce fatigue. Uninterrupted sleep should be encouraged by bathing the infant when he is awake and only when absolutely necessary. The recording of accurate, current vital signs, intake and output determinations, and weight is critical. As soon as the child's condition is stable, he is prepared for surgery or discharge until a surgery appointment can be made. The parents should be increasingly involved in his care while he is hospitalized so that they are not unpre-pared when the child goes home. The help of a public health nurse or hospital home visitor can be very valuable in this setting.

Subacute bacterial endocarditis

Any damage to cardiac tissue or a congenital heart or blood vessel anomaly may set the stage for inflammation of the lining of the heart (endocarditis) and arteries (endarteritis). The inflammation usually results from a blood-borne infection, originating at some other body site. It may have its onset after surgical procedures such as dental extraction, tonsillectomy, or adenoidectomy, or it may be spread from an abscess or infection elsewhere in the body. Signs and symptoms include temperature elevation, weight loss, fatigue, anemia, leukocytosis, the presence of petechiae, an enlarged spleen, and perhaps even partial paralysis or other central nervous system symptoms caused by the presence of emboli in the brain that originated in the inflamed heart tissue. Prophylactic antibiotics must be prescribed prior to and during certain procedures that may introduce bacteria into the bloodstream.

Cerebral thrombosis

Cerebral thrombosis may develop when an excess of circulating red blood cells is called into action to increase the oxygen-carrying capacity of the blood. Dehydration may result in a thicker, slower-moving fluid in the blood vessels. Clots, or thrombi, may form, and a cerebral vascular accident may take place. Maintenance of adequate fluid intake, the use of oxygen to relieve episodes of cyanosis, and possibly the cautious use of anticoagulants in patients likely to develop such a complication are suggested means of reducing the risk.

Disorders of the blood and blood-forming organs

The entire cardiovascular apparatus (heart and blood vessels) is designed so that nutrients, hormones, and oxygen reach the individual body tissue cells and waste products from those cells are properly transported for elimination by the kidneys, lungs, or skin. To do this efficiently the circulating fluid within the cardiovascular system—the blood—contains many substances. Of particular interest are the three types of structures called the "formed elements." The red blood cells, or *erythrocytes,* help transport oxygen and carbon dioxide in the blood to and from the lungs. The white blood cells, or *leukocytes,* and antibodies of various types help protect the bloodstream and surrounding body tissues from the intrusion of disease-producing microorganisms and foreign proteins. The platelets, or *thrombocytes* assist in the formation of clots to repair any leak in a damaged blood vessel. However, any lack or defect in the normal makeup of the blood is likely to cause symptoms of disease. It is impossible and of little practical nursing value to describe within the pages of this text all the various problems that may occur when the blood is abnormal. However, four kinds of disorders that are seen with some frequency on the pediatric service will be briefly discussed. They are the *anemias, hemophilias, leukemias,* and *purpuras.*

The anemias

When the term "anemia" is used, it indicates a condition in which the total hemoglobin content of the blood is abnormally reduced, either because of lack of sufficient hemoglobin in the red blood cells or lack of red blood cells. Hemoglobin is the substance in the red blood cells necessary for the normal transport of oxygen to the body cells. The most common cause of anemia in children is iron deficiency. Another anemia that has received much attention lately is sickle cell disease.

Iron deficiency anemia. Pallor, irritability, anorexia, and listlessness usually direct attention to this disorder. The anemia is usually discovered secondarily to the problem that brought the child and his parent to the doctor. Hemoglobin concentrations of less than 11 grams/100 ml. and a hematocrit of less than 33% in a healthy in-

fant strongly suggest iron deficiency. Insufficient iron for synthesis of hemoglobin is the cause of this problem. Children under age 3 and adolescent girls have the highest incidence of this disorder. Causes of anemia other than dietary deficiency include: (1) increased demands during growth (especially of low birth weight and premature infants and adolescents), (2) acute or chronic blood loss, and (3) impaired absorption (severe prolonged diarrhea). Treatment consists of oral administration of iron preparations, preferably ferrous iron, a revision of diet to include iron-rich foods (muscle meats, liver, eggs, wheat, green leafy vegetables), and if the condition is particularly severe or unresponsive due to parental failure to provide the items above, intramuscular injections of iron-dextran complex may be ordered. Packed red cells are rarely given. Since the highest incidence of iron deficiency anemia is in infancy (6 to 18 months), the best and cheapest preventative measure against this form of anemia would be the widespread use of iron-fortified formulas during the entire first year of life. It is possible that the use of such formulas would essentially eliminate all iron deficiency anemia in preschool children. According to some experts this would improve growth, learning, and resistance to disease.

Sickle cell disease. Sickle cell disease is a collective term that embraces several hereditary disorders whose clinical and laboratory features are related to the presence of sickle hemoglobin (Hb S) in red cells. Although a few cases have been reported in the white race, sickle cell disease is found primarily in blacks. About 75,000 black Americans have the disease. Chronic illness of increasing severity and reduction of life span to about 30 years result from hemolytic anemia with its intermittent "crises."

The sickling abnormality is attributed to a mutant gene that is responsible for the synthesis of a type of hemoglobin different from normal. The abnormal change in the shape of the red blood cell from a biconcave disc to a crescent, or sicklelike, shape becomes apparent when hemoglobin is reduced following exposure to low oxygen tensions or changes in pH. The basic defect in sickle hemoglobin is in the alteration of only one amino acid of the 574 that make up normal hemoglobin. This single change is responsible for all the clinical manifestations of sickle cell disease!

Every person possesses a pair of genes that governs the synthesis of hemoglobin. One gene is inherited from each parent. Sickle cell anemia (SCA) is expressed in those persons who receive the mutant sickle cell gene from both parents (homozygous inheritance, SS).

SICKLE CELL TRAIT (SCT). The sickle cell trait is probably the most common defect in hemoglobin found in the United States. It is present in those persons who have re-

ceived Hb S gene from one parent and a normal Hb A gene from the other parent (heterozygous inheritance, AS). The most important consideration in SCT is the genetic risk of SCA for the offspring. Although persons with SCT have as much as 40% Hb S under normal conditions no clinical signs of disease or hemoglobin abnormalities are typically present. Rarely, someone with sickle cell trait will manifest symptoms of stress when exercising strenuously or traveling at high altitudes in nonpressurized airplanes. SCT confers some degree of protection against the lethal effects of malaria, which may account for the major distribution of Hb S in Central Africa and the very fact that SCA exists. The presence of a gene for another abnormal type of hemoglobin, or the gene for thalassemia, should be suspected in a child

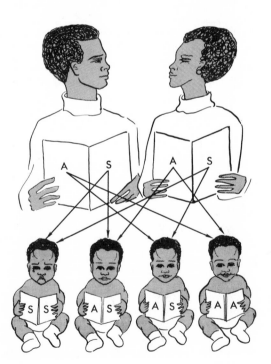

Fig. 35-11. Sickle cell anemia (homozygous inheritance). When both parents carry a sickle cell gene (AS), the possibilities for inheritance in offspring are: one child in four will inherit sickle cell anemia (SS); two children in four will inherit sickle cell trait (AS); one child in four will be normal (AA).

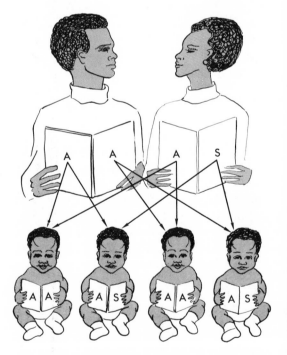

Fig. 35-12. Sickle cell trait (heterozygous inheritance). When only one parent is a carrier of the sickle cell gene (AS), possibilities for inheritance in offspring are: two children in four will be normal (AA); two children in four will carry sickle cell trait (AS).

with SCA when the blood of only one of the parents shows the sickle trait.

Young infants are usually spared the severe symptoms of SCA because of the temporary presence of fetal hemoglobin (Hb F). Hb F is gradually replaced with the Hb S. As the proportion of Hb S increases, the symptoms of anemia appear—usually when the baby is between 6 and 12 months of age.

HEMOLYTIC ANEMIA. This anemia is caused by intravascular sickling that occurs diffusely throughout the body. Sickling red cells often form spontaneously during venous circulation when the red blood cells give up oxygen to the tissues. They also form when there are changes in pH or electrolyte concentration or balance. The body acts quickly to remove these abnormal sickled cells from the bloodstream, and this causes the severe degree of anemia that occurs. In addition, occlusion of blood vessels by sickled cells may interfere with blood supply to vital organs. Damage and death of these organ tissues is the basis of the sickle cell crisis.

The exact events leading to the onset of painful crises are not clearly known. Many of these crises are preceded by infections. Upper respiratory tract infections are often complicated by invasion of the pneumococcus organism. Children with SCA do not handle pneumococcal infections well. Before 2 years of age the "hand-foot" syndrome commonly occurs. The symmetric painful swelling of the hands and feet results from interference with circulation to the metacarpals and metatarsals. If the child's pain is not too severe, increased fluids, application of warmth, and acetaminophen will relieve the pain. In other children the pain may be unbearable and can be relieved only by stronger analgesics. Occlusive episodes after the first or second year of life most frequently occur during the preschool period. Episodes of acute abdominal pain may be severe, accompanied by fever, muscle spasm, nausea, vomiting, and leukocytosis.

A crisis associated with shock is entitled "acute splenic sequestration crisis" (ASSC). The mother notes a rather sudden increase in pallor accompanied by abdominal distention and thirst. By the time the child arrives at the hospital, he has become markedly dyspneic and weak. Left-sided abdominal (splenic) pain is present, and the pulse and respirations are elevated. Prompt diagnosis and treatment are essential to assure survival. Transfusions of packed erythrocytes and plasma expanders should be started immediately on admission. The nurse who recognizes the situation should hasten the admission procedure but be sure to accurately check the child's weight and height. It is imperative to take blood specimens and urine samples immediately and to have special equipment for transfusions ready. Since reduced oxygenation increases sickling, an atmosphere of well-humidified oxygen may be used. The nurse also must keep in mind that parents often fear censure or reproach by those in authority and, in their effort to gain approval, may hide their feelings or hold back information regarding the child. The nurse must give these parents every opportunity to examine their feelings about themselves and the child. She should listen carefully as she works with and encourages the parents, for if she is to really help the child, she must first help them. Because of the rapidity with which a sequestration crisis can occur (and even recur) and its threat of fatality, splenectomy may be performed. The therapy for SCA and its frequent crises remains one of the major clinical problems in pediatric hematology. There is no cure for SCA or even a completely satisfactory treatment for its crises.

DETECTION OF SICKLE HEMOGLOBIN AND COUNSELING. Screening programs for SCA or SCT should not be set up unless genetic counseling service can be provided to those found to carry the trait. Otherwise, the benefits of the screening are largely lost, and anguish may be created over an essentially benign condition. Screening programs must incorporate meaningful education about the nature of SCA and its mode of inheritance as well as individual counseling. In mass screening, Sickledex (sickle-turbidity tube test) or the sickle cell slide test is adequate but positive reactions must be followed by hemoglobin electrophoresis to confirm results. Newborn infants may be screened in the hospital for both the condition and the trait. Such hospital programs facilitate optimal infant care and early diagnosis of crises and provide counseling for the parents.

Nursing care. The nursing care of children with anemia, whatever its basic cause, must take into account the excessive fatigue experienced by most of these boys and girls. Their energy must be conserved. They especially need help and encouragement to build good habits in nutrition. Frequent, small feedings are more successful than large, infrequent meals. The enlarged liver and spleen and tender muscles of some of these patients all demand gentle care. Attention to signs of bleeding (external or internal) is important. Signs of jaundice, increased pallor, increased lethargy, or irritability should be reported. Patients receiving blood transfusions should be carefully observed and protected against possible infiltration of the blood (a potentially serious event). Signs of toxic reactions, complaints of chest or back pain, itching hives, or elevated temperature with or without chills should be noted and reported early. The rate of administration should be closely watched to be sure that the circulatory system is not overloaded.

The hemophilias

Hemophilia A—factor VIII deficiency. Classic hemophilia, antihemophilic globulin (AHG), or factor VIII, deficiency, is a very interesting and disturbing disease involving a defect in the clotting mechanism of the blood. Because of its hereditary feature, it has figured prominently in the history of royal families and has been called the disease of kings. Hemophilia results from a defect in a gene in the X chromosome concerned with blood clotting. It is a sex-linked condition confined almost ex-

clusively to males and may pass from one generation to another from a carrier mother to her son. A male receives only one X, from his mother, which impairs his blood-clotting process. Since the female receives two X chromosomes, one normal gene will ensure normal blood clotting. A girl will only inherit the disease if her father is a hemophiliac and her mother is a carrier.

The defect in clot formation is caused by the lack of antihemophilic globulin, or factor VIII, in the blood plasma. A wide range of factor VIII values (50% to 200%) exists, but in most healthy individuals the average is 100%. A severe hemophiliac has less than 1% of factor VIII. These patients are prone to spontaneous, unprovoked hemorrhage. Mild hemophiliacs have from 2% to 35% of factor VIII and may bleed excessively on minor trauma. Surgical procedures, dental extractions, and even the normal rough-and-tumble existence of young boys are especially hazardous for a hemophilic patient.

Current treatment consists of administration of factor VIII concentrate in any amount necessary to control hemorrhage. However, protection afforded from one infusion rapidly disappears because the concentration of factor VIII falls to half its original level in 8 to 10 hours. Because of this, it is necessary to administer factor VIII as quickly as possible to obtain optimum benefits. The precise level of factor VIII needed to control bleeding is not known exactly, but serious bleeding has been controlled by levels as low as 30%. The combination of immobilization and a level of 10% to 20% is usually adequate to control soft tissue bleeding (provided by 1 to 4 doses of factor VIII plasma concentrate). When desired, a maintenance level is achieved by administering factor VIII at 12-hour intervals. Children with severe hemophilia may be given daily doses in the hope that they might have fewer spontaneous hemorrhages if factor VIII is available. Efforts to control bleeding by using local measures (pressure, cold, or applications of thrombin) should be attempted, if possible. Some cities have hemophilia centers that are prepared to render intravenous therapy to these victims on an outpatient basis. Some patients are being taught to administer the concentrate to themselves.

FACTOR VIII INHIBITORS. A small number (about 5%) of patients with classic hemophilia develop inhibitors (antibodies that destroy factor VIII). The presence of a circulating inhibitor is usually detected by the lack of response to a dose of factor VIII that normally would control the bleeding. Inhibitors may develop in young children after a few exposures to factor VIII, but there is no evidence that the inhibitors are related to the number of transfusions a patient receives. Without exposure to plasma products, the amount of inhibitor gradually decreases, and factor VIII can be given again with full benefit. Effective control of bleeding in patients is very difficult when the inhibitor is circulating.

Hemophilia B—factor IX deficiency (Christmas disease). Factor IX plasma thromboplastic component (PTC) deficiency accounts for about 15% of patients with hemophilia. The causes and symptoms are similar to those of hemophilia A. A factor IX concentrate has recently become available for treatment and is used in the same manner as factor VIII.

Hemophilia C—factor XI deficiency. Factor XI plasma thromboplastin antecedent (PTA) deficiency differs from hemophilias A and B. It is usually a mild disorder and may appear in either boys or girls as the result of an inherited dominant trait. Normal plasma corrects the defect during bleeding episodes. The nursing care of all patients with bleeding problems is similar except that the type of intravenous therapy ordered will differ, depending on the kind of replacement needed.

The parents of a patient with hemophilia are under considerable strain. They must constantly observe the environment of their adventuresome toddler or growing boy. With the help of their attending physician,

they must progressively educate the child to make choices in activity with consideration for the degree of hazard it may entail. They do not want to make their son a psychological cripple, unable to live an interesting, creative life, or a reckless rebel.

Supervision and nursing care. The nursing care of children with hemophilia must emphasize prevention. The sides of infants' cribs should be padded. Toddlers should be denied toys and objects with sharp edges or objects that are easily broken. Rubber toys are very satisfactory for play. Children learning to walk may be fitted with kneepads. Bleeding into the joints may produce considerable pain and deformity. Every effort should be made to prevent stiffening of the joint and loss of function. The nurse must provide her charge with interesting but safe diversion and watch for any signs of increasing bruises or internal or external blood loss. She must observe the child for untoward reaction during transfusion and check whether the intravenous infusion is flowing as ordered. Her care must be gentle and thoughtful.

The home care program. If the factor level could be maintained above 10% in every patient, prevention of all bleeding episodes except those due to trauma could be controlled. This would prevent crippling orthopedic disease due to spontaneous bleeding into the joints.

In an effort to accomplish the goal, selected patients or their parents are being instructed to administer cryoprecipitate and plasma concentrates as necessary at home. Whenever therapy becomes necessary to control minor bleeding episodes, the physician is contacted for advice about the proper dosage. Antihistamines and steroids are kept on hand to be taken by the patient if a transfusion reaction occurs.

Nurses often follow the progress of the patient at home, instructing the family about the importance of accurate records and emphasizing the need for periodic outpatient physical evaluations. The home care program spares patients the expense of frequent hospital visits and the burden of travel and waiting; but most of all, it promotes a more normal life, utilizing the maximum intellectual and social potential of the hemophilic child.

THE TODDLER AND PRESCHOOL CHILD
The leukemias

Leukemia has often been called "cancer of the blood." It is a fatal disease characterized by the overproduction by the body of abnormal, immature, white blood cells (blast forms), which cannot function properly. Since this kind of leukocyte, even when present in tremendous numbers, is incapable of protecting the body from pathogenic microorganisms, intercurrent infections are common. These abnormal white blood cells invade the various tissues of the body, causing pressure symptoms (for example, infiltration of the bone marrow produces severe pain in bones and joints; mediastinal nodes may cause tracheal compression that in turn causes respiratory difficulty and cough). The predominating symptoms depend on the area of the body primarily invaded by the leukemic cells. Diagnosis is suspected on the basis of discovery of immature white blood cell forms in the circulating blood. An unequivocal diagnosis is confirmed by microscopic examination of the bone marrow, usually obtained from the posterior iliac crest. Anemia and a lowered platelet count often complicate the patient's problems. At times the number of circulating white blood cells is extremely elevated. Some cases may demonstrate total white blood cell counts of above 100,000 per mm.[3] In some children the number of white blood cells in the peripheral circulation is relatively low, and proportionately few immature forms are seen; the disease is said to be *aleukemic*. However, at this time the bone marrow may be packed with abnormal cells.

Incidence. Leukemia is the most common form of cancer in children. There is a slightly increased incidence in boys, and the peak age of onset in children is 3 to 4 years of age. Certain children have been

Table 35-1. Incidence of leukemia*

Groups affected	Number affected
Noncaucasian American children under 15 years of age	1 in 5,500
Caucasian American children under 15 years of age	1 in 3,000
Sibling of leukemic child	1 in 720
Children with Down's syndrome	1 in 95
Children exposed to atomic irradiation	1 in 60
Monozygotic twin sibling (with one diagnosed)	1 in 5 (both will get it)

*Peak: white children, 3 to 4 years; nonwhite children, lower.

clearly identified as being at increased risk of developing leukemia (Table 35-1). Although there seems to have been a decline over the last decade in the occurrence of acute leukemia, it accounts for almost 50% of deaths from malignant diseases in children under 15 years of age.

Types. There are a number of different types of leukemia classified according to the kind of white cells principally involved and the relative speed of the disease process. The most common leukemic cell observed in pediatric practice is the undifferentiated form called a "blast," or stem cell, a very immature form of white blood cell, usually of the lymphocytic cell line. Acute lymphoblastic leukemia (ALL) accounts for the majority of cases. Acute granulocytic or myelogenous leukemia (AML) accounts for about 20% of cases. This form, however, does not respond favorably to the antileukemic agents presently available. Acute leukemia is a complex entity, the cause of which remains obscure. Intensive research is now being carried out in an attempt to unravel the origin and development of the disease.

Signs and symptoms. The signs and symptoms of leukemia may be rather slow and insidious in onset or rapid in their development. The child may complain of fatigue and weakness, and lose weight. He may be pale and bruise easily. Fever, with a persistent respiratory tract infection, is a common complaint. Swollen lymph nodes

Table 35-2. Current drugs used in the treatment of leukemia

Agent	Routes of administration	Signs of toxicity
For induction		
Prednisone	Oral	Moon-shaped face, osteoporosis, acne, fluid retention, ulcers, increased susceptibility to infection, personality changes
Vincristine (Oncovin)	IV	Peripheral neuropathy, hair loss
Daunomycin*	IV	Bone marrow depression,† nausea, vomiting, oral ulceration, congestive heart failure
L-Asparaginase*	IV	Chills, fever, nausea, vomiting, hypersensitivity reactions
Adriamycin*	IV	Bone marrow depression,† alopecia, nausea, vomiting, oral ulceration, congestive heart failure
Thioguanine	IV	Bone marrow depression†
For maintenance		
6-Mercaptopurine	Oral	Bone marrow depression,† nausea, vomiting
Amethopterin (methotrexate)	Oral IV Intrathecal	Anorexia, abdominal pain, oral and GI tract ulceration, bone marrow depression,† (hair loss, rare)
Cyclophosphamide (Cytoxan)	Oral IV	Bone marrow depression,† skin rashes, hair loss, hemorrhagic cystitis, oral ulceration, diarrhea
Cytosine arabinoside (Cytosar or ARA-C)	IV Intrathecal	Bone marrow depression,* nausea, vomiting

*Investigational.
†Bone marrow depression is characterized by leukopenia, thrombocytopenia, and anemia.

may be the first symptom that the parent notes. The child's liver and spleen, infiltrated with abnormal cells, may be enlarged. Central nervous system involvement is likely to arise during the course of the disease but is rarely present at the onset. About one out of four children affected suffer leukemic infiltration of the meninges. Increased intracranial pressure occurs and is typically manifested by headache, nausea and vomiting, slowed pulse, and elevated blood pressure. The child is very irritable and tired. Spinal fluid examination confirms the physician's sad suspicions of the nature of the problem. The course of the disease usually involves several hospitalizations and remissions.

Treatment. At this writing no curative treatment for leukemia exists. However, complete remissions of the disease for extended periods have been induced with various drug combinations (research protocols). The major objectives of chemotherapy are the induction of a complete remission and the maintenance of patients in a state of remission for the longest possible time. A complete remission is defined as "restoration to normal health and clinical well-being." Physical and laboratory examinations are negative, blood and bone marrow are considered normal, and all evidence of disease is absent. Best results to date have been achieved with intensive courses of drug combinations and with optimal supportive care, including transfusion of platelets and antibiotic therapy.

Since 1947 when the first brief, temporary remission was induced with aminopterin, antileukemic drug therapy has been greatly improved. Previously the drugs were used singly, with a progression in sequence to another agent as each successive one became ineffective. Then, any one of the drugs was administered coincidently with prednisone. Later the drugs were rotated at regular intervals to avoid development of tolerance while each was still effective. More recently, periodic but intensive parenteral treatment with one drug supplemented by oral administration of another has been advocated.

Dosage schedules as well as the effects of different routes of administration continue to be compared and reevaluated.

Today, modern treatment consists of intermittent administration of high doses of several drugs in combination. The duration of remissions has been increased by the addition of prophylactic therapy to the central nervous system by radiation and/or spinal canal (intrathecal) injections of methotrexate. In an attempt to avoid the immunosuppressive effects of continuous chemotherapy, the maintenance schedules now being used involve intermittent doses of multiple agents in combination, followed by rest periods without therapy, or moderate daily dose schedules periodically reinforced with "induction" agents. Children with acute leukemia should be referred to specialized centers where optimum opportunity for effective therapy is available.

Complete remissions for long periods of time have been induced in almost all patients with ALL. Children in remission must have regular medical supervision, including frequent hematological studies. Relapse is marked by falling hemoglobin levels, thrombocytopenia, severe decreases in the white blood cells called neutrophils, and the reappearance of immature or "blast" cells in the blood and bone marrow.

The length of the first remission is considered to be a prognostic indicator of length of survival. The longer the remission endures, the more optimistic the prognosis. Hopefully all research regimens have been devised to prevent the first relapse, some even at the risk of exposing the patient to the hazards of severe drug toxicity. Intensive research ultimately designed to completely control the growth of leukemic cells continues. In the meantime, a real effort is being made to develop a long-range therapeutic plan for each patient so that treatment can in large part be conducted in cooperation with the patient's physician in his home town.

Supportive care. Platelet transfusions have reduced the number of deaths caused by hemorrhage and increased the opportunity to use effective drugs that depress platelet production. Corticosteroids increase capillary resistance and are useful adjuncts in the control of bleeding. Bleeding from accessible areas is occasionally controlled by the local application of thromboplastin and Gelfoam.

Infection poses the greatest threat to the life of the leukemic child. Drugs used in the control of infection until cultures are available include methicillin or ampicillin for staphylococci, streptococci, and pneumococci. Gentamycin, carbenicillin, or both are used against gram-negative organisms such as *Pseudomonas* and *Proteus*. Oral moniliasis is seen frequently and is treated with nystatin (Mycostatin). Antibiotic therapy administered intravenously with the most up-to-date drugs has diminished effect in the absence of competent white cells. Two methods may be effective in the control of infection: white blood cell transfusions (particularly granulocytes) and germ-free rooms (laminar-flow rooms). These methods of controlling infections are investigational, costly, and not readily available.

Antileukemic drugs may cause a rapid breakdown in the malignant cells, which in turn raises the uric acid load that must be handled by the kidneys. This increased load, especially coupled with a state of dehydration caused by poor fluid intake and vomiting, causes renal injury. Allopurinol helps accelerate the excretion of uric acid and reduces the risk of kidney stone formation. Parenteral fluid therapy also lessens this risk.

Another side effect of some of the antileukemic drugs is that of alopecia, or hair loss, a nondangerous but distressing development. The child and parent can be consoled by the fact that the hair will usually grow back.

The nursing care of the leukemic patient is emotionally taxing. Both the parents and the child need emotional support; a philos-

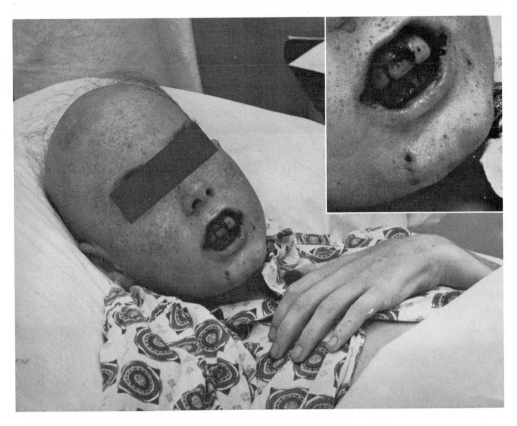

Fig. 35-13. This young boy with leukemia demonstrates the typical mouth lesions. Loss of hair resulted from therapy. (Courtesy Naval Regional Medical Center, San Diego, Calif.)

ophy that recognizes that we can live only one moment at a time and that we are not called on to face all our yesterdays or tomorrows all at once is helpful. For a discussion of the needs of the dying child, his parents, and his nurses, see Chapter 24.

The child with leukemia who is admitted to the hospital because of recurring symptoms is usually very uncomfortable and irritable. Pressure from the large number of white blood cells infiltrating the various body organs makes him sore. He usually does not like to be moved, although changes in position are necessary to avoid respiratory tract infection and skin breakdown. His lowered platelet count leads to easy bruising and spontaneous hemorrhages in many parts of the body. His anemia contributes to his fatigue and pallor. Because of the frequent ulceration of his mucous membranes, oral hygiene must be gentle

(Fig. 35-13). Only soft toothbrushes, gauze, or applicators should be used. Mouthwashes of equal amounts of hydrogen peroxide and saline and the application of viscous lidocaine (Xylocaine) before meals are helpful local measures that often provide comfort.

Fever is often present, and measures to reduce temperature elevation (see Chapter 31) must be frequently employed. Because the rectal mucosa may be bleeding, an axillary temperature may be ordered. The presence of a member of the family at the bedside at frequent intervals is a great help to the patient, and often he will respond by taking fluids offered by the parent when all other overtures are refused. The ability to administer to the needs of their child in these trying days is almost always a source of strength to the parents who feel a need to do something for him.

Table 35-3. Life expectancy of the child with leukemia

Year	Treatment	Survival in months
Acute lymphoblastic		
1937-1953	Supportive	3-5
1954-1962	Prednisone, 6-mercaptopurine, methotrexate	12
1963-1965	Prednisone, 6-mercaptopurine, vincristine, methotrexate, cyclophosphamide	24
1966-1968	Same drugs used in combination	33+
1969-1975	Total therapy	60 (about 5 years)
	Prednisone, vincristine, 6-mercaptopurine, methotrexate, cyclophosphamide, L-asparaginase	
	CNS prophylaxis	
Acute myelogenous		
1975	Daunomycin, thioguanine, vincristine, cytosine, arabinoside, prednisone, cyclophosphamide	6-18

Little routines and special ways of doing things that comfort the child are important to the parent and patient. As much as possible, they should be followed. We the nursing staff should not withdraw from the parents, thinking that there is little we can do. We must continue to provide support throughout the illness.

Prognosis. In childhood, approximately 97% of the leukemias are acute rather than chronic. Before current methods of treatment were available, the survival time for children with acute leukemia from the time of diagnosis until death was sometimes as brief as 3 to 4 weeks and rarely spanned 6 months. Today, almost 50% of children with ALL who get optimal treatment are in uninterrupted remission for at least 4 or 5 years. Until further progress is made, leukemia must still be considered a fatal disease. Death usually comes in the form of massive hemorrhage or infection.

Idiopathic thrombocytopenic purpura

Idiopathic thrombocytopenic purpura (ITP) is a syndrome of unknown cause characterized by bruises, purpura, and petechiae resulting from a marked reduction in the number of platelets (less than 100,000 per mm.[3]). A normal circulating platelet count is 250,000/per mm.[3]. Each normal thrombocyte has a life span of 8 to 10 days. In ITP the platelet may survive only hours. Seepage of blood into the mucous membranes, subcutaneous tissues, and skin occurs. Epistaxis is common. A bone marrow sample reveals impaired thrombocyte formation, which rules out leukemia, the fear of many parents. ITP occurs in all age groups, with a maximum incidence in the preschool group. About half the number of cases are preceded by a febrile upper resipratory tract infection. In most younger patients the disease runs a benign, self-limited course, and most children experience a spontaneous remission within 6 weeks to 4 months.

A large percent of children 10 years of age or over have a more serious chronic type of ITP. In this age group girls are affected more frequently than boys, and the condition is likely to be associated with bleeding and the presence of an antiplatelet factor in the plasma. Steroids have been employed to help prevent bleeding and to suppress the synthesis of antiplatelet antibodies, but to date their use is questionable. Platelet transfusions have been given to control active bleeding, although platelet survival is short. Splenectomy has been followed by a sustained restoration of platelet numbers in some cases.

During the acute phase, activity should be restricted and the child protected from the risk of increased injury. Children with very low platelet counts should be kept in

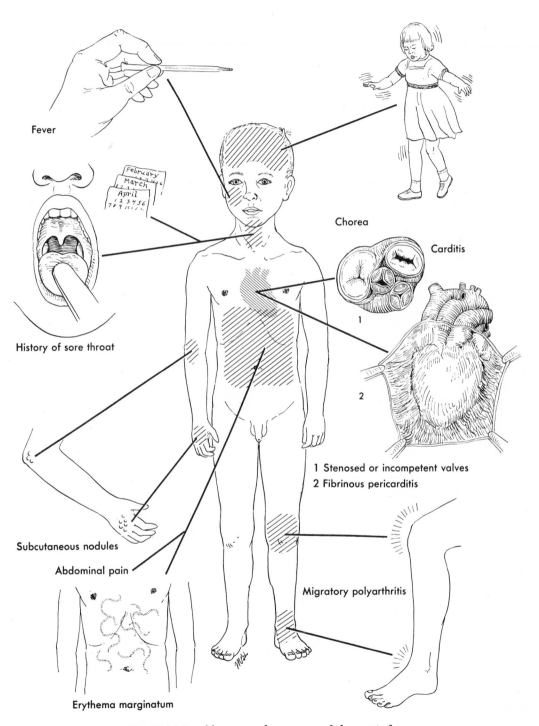

Fever

History of sore throat

Subcutaneous nodules

Abdominal pain

Erythema marginatum

Chorea

Carditis

1 Stenosed or incompetent valves
2 Fibrinous pericarditis

Migratory polyarthritis

Fig. 35-14. Possible signs and symptoms of rheumatic fever.

603

bed if possible. Salicylates and other drugs that foster bleeding should be avoided because they may alter platelet function and trigger spontaneous hemorrhage. Other nursing measures include careful observation of the progress of skin lesions and alertness for any signs of internal bleeding. A major complication, and the most serious risk to the child in the early course of the condition, is intracranial hemorrhage.

THE SCHOOL-AGE CHILD
Rheumatic fever (Fig. 35-14)

Rheumatic fever is properly classed as a collagen disease because it affects the connective tissues in the entire body. However, because its most important complication is extensive cardiac damage, it will be discussed here. Although rheumatic fever may be decreasing in incidence, it is still a chief cause of acquired heart disease.

The mechanism of the disease is not completely known, but it is fairly certain that the symptoms constitute an allergic-type reaction to a prior infection by group A beta-hemolytic streptococcus, which causes the so-called "strep throat," erysipelas, and scarlet fever. However, rheumatic fever itself is not communicable. It is not understood why some people develop rheumatic fever after beta-hemolytic streptococcus infections, whereas others do not. Rheumatic fever is most commonly found in the school-age child.

Signs and symptoms. The symptoms of rheumatic fever vary. It is a rare patient who exhibits all the possible signs and symptoms listed in a textbook. The onset of the condition usually occurs about 2 weeks after the streptococcal infection. However, the infection may have been unapparent at the time. The child may complain of leg aches and joint tenderness, which migrates from joint to joint—one time involving a knee, next an ankle, later a wrist (polyarthralgia). These pains occur during the day as well as the night. When the child begins to have migratory, hot, swollen, tender enlarged joints (polyarthritis), the diagnosis is quickly suggested.

Salicylates relieve the symptoms, and there is no permanent joint damage. The child may fatigue easily and have a fever. The extent of the fever varies considerably, depending on the severity of the disease. He may also report abdominal pain, believed to be caused by lymph node enlargement. Epistaxis (nosebleed) may occur.

Carditis, or inflammation of the heart, happens in about 40% to 50% of cases during the initial attack of rheumatic fever. Constant observation for rapid or irregular pulse, heart murmurs, increased heart size, and signs and symptoms of cardiac failure must be carried out. Small inflammatory nodules or growths may form in the heart. Often they interfere with the action of the mitral or aortic valves, making it difficult for the valves to close properly or open sufficiently. Carditis is the most important feature of rheumatic fever. The prognosis of the patient largely rests on the severity of carditis.

Another sign that may occasionally accompany rheumatic fever is the development of painless *subcutaneous nodules* near the occiput, knuckles, knees, elbows, and spine. These nodules appear late in the course of the attack and are usually associated with severe carditis.

Another feature that may be seen at times, especially in preadolescent girls, is Sydenham's *chorea* (known in earlier times as St. Vitus dance). Chorea may be described as involuntary muscular twitching or movement. It sometimes manifests itself as grimacing. The child may seem exceptionally clumsy and may fail to accomplish muscle tasks involving concentration or fine control. The disorder is characterized by jerky, uncoordinated movements. It may be preceded by a period of emotional instability and behavior problems. It may be so mild as to escape the notice of the casual observer or so severe that it makes normal, daily activities dangerous or impossible. Speech may become slurred and handwriting difficult to decipher.

Still another diagnostic sign of acute rheumatic fever is the appearance of a

JONES CRITERIA (REVISED)
FOR GUIDANCE IN THE DIAGNOSIS OF RHEUMATIC FEVER*

Major manifestations	*Minor manifestations*
Carditis	Clinical
Polyarthritis	Previous rheumatic fever or
	rheumatic heart disease
Chorea	Arthralgia
Erythema marginatum	Fever
Subcutaneous nodules	Laboratory
	Acute-phase reactions:
	erythrocyte sedimentation rate
	C-reactive protein, leukocytosis
	Prolonged P-R interval

Supporting evidence of streptococcal infection

Increased titer of streptococcal antibodies
   ASO (antistreptolysin O)
   Other antibodies

Positive throat culture for group A streptococcus

Recent scarlet fever

---

*The presence of two major criteria, or of one major and two minor criteria, indicates a high probability of the presence of rheumatic fever. Evidence of a preceding streptococcal infection greatly strengths the possibility of acute rheumatic fever. Its absence should make the diagnosis doubtful (except in Syndenham's chorea or long-standing carditis). From Jones criteria (revised) for guidance in the diagnosis of rheumatic fever, New York, © 1967, American Heart Association. Reprinted with permission.

highly distinctive rash known as *erythema marginatum*. This red-line eruption forms irregular patterns on the trunk and extremities but not on the face. However, it is rarely seen.

Diagnosis is made on the evaluation of the signs and symptoms present plus the reports of several laboratory tests. None of the laboratory tests are specific for rheumatic fever, but when made in conjunction with a clinical evaluation of the patient, they are valuable aids. An increased blood *sedimentation rate* and determination of *C-reactive protein* in the blood indicate the presence of an inflammatory process in the body that may be rheumatic fever. It is also possible to detect, with tests such as the *antistreptolysin O titer,* the presence of antibodies in the blood, formed in response to the invasion of streptococci. But as previously stated, not all beta-hemolytic streptococcal infections cause rheumatic fever. Sometimes a nose and throat culture will return a positive result. Other members of the patient's family should be checked for the presence of a streptococcal infection or the carrier state. Rheumatic fever, because of factors not yet completely determined, has a tendency to run in families.

Treatment. Treatment of rheumatic fever includes the prescription of penicillin to eliminate any lingering residual streptococci and prevent a reinfection. Penicillin does not cure the symptoms of rheumatic fever; it only helps prevent further attacks. If the patient is allergic to penicillin, erythromycin may be used to eradicate the streptococcus. Sulfonamides or penicillin is equally useful in preventing reinfections. Aspirin is helpful in controlling the pain of arthritis and lowering the fever. Prednisone is often used in acute cases of carditis, with the hope of decreasing the possibility of permanent heart valve damage. Prednisone is often lifesaving in overwhelming inflammation involving all the structures of the heart.

Nursing care. The nursing care of the child with rheumatic fever depends on the severity of his disease and the symptoms present. When laboratory tests and clinical features indicate that the disease is active and perhaps progressive, every effort should be made to reduce the work load of the heart by providing emotional and physical rest. However, "doing nothing" is not very restful for most children, especially if they do not really feel very sick. The nurse and the patient's family need a great deal of ingenuity to provide rest that is acceptable and therefore therapeutic for the child. Good observation is essential. The pulse rate is taken for a full minute to determine quality and rhythm. Often the determination of the pulse while the patient is sleeping is requested. The nurse should review the signs and symptoms of rheumatic fever and check her charge for indications of these during her care. Possible signs of cardiac failure are extremely important to report (see pp. 591 and 592). Careful positioning and skin care are necessary. The child with symptoms of chorea needs special supportive care; careful explanation of the condition to the parents is a necessity. Chorea may appear as the sole symptom of rheumatic disease. In the event of moderate to severe disability, rest, prolonged warm baths under supervision, and tranquilizers may help. Patient nursing care is a must. The condition usually subsides spontaneously in 2 to 3 months.

When the signs of inflammatory activity subside, the electrocardiogram results are favorable, and the pulse rate is within normal limits, the child may be allowed more freedom. However, he must continue to be carefully evaluated to discover his tolerance for increased exercise. Because recurrences of the disease are fairly common and the possibility of permanent heart damage increases with each attack, it is imperative that the parent understand the importance of continued medical supervision. To prevent recurrences the patient should avoid exposure to infections and receive either daily oral or preferably monthly intramuscular, long-acting penicillin therapy.

• • •

The lungs, heart, blood vessels, and blood are separate anatomical entities. However, if one of these entities is disturbed, the others will invariably respond to meet the physiological needs of the individual. The nurse who recognizes this interdependence is better able to serve the person to whom that deformed heart, inflamed respiratory tract, or abnormal blood belongs.

36

Conditions involving digestion and associated metabolism

A well-behaved digestive system can be a source of great pleasure. The digestive system can also initiate considerable distress, depending on its general condition and the amount of dietary discretion its owner employs. This chapter will briefly present the malformations, infestations, infections, and foreign bodies commonly found in the digestive tracts of children (Fig. 36-1). Also, although it is not considered to be basically a digestive problem, a review of diabetes mellitus will be included, since it influences the metabolism of digested glucose and dietary regulation is required. For the convenience of nursing teachers and students, most of the material will be presented according to the age group primarily affected.

ANATOMY AND PHYSIOLOGY

The digestive system is formed by the mouth, esophagus, gastrointestinal tract, and related organs such as the liver, gallbladder, and pancreas. The adult alimentary canal is an unsterile tract of many shapes and turns, which, if stretched out its entire length, would reach about 30 feet. Although in children the size of the alimentary canal may be greatly abbreviated, its importance is not. Hunger is a primary drive, and appetite, its educated twin, is soon acquired. The child may not know all about his digestive tract, but he knows that it represents a real need. Parents, rather desparingly, have often called it the "bottomless pit." The digestive tract and its accessory organs serve to reduce foodstuffs (carbohydrates, proteins, and fats) to their smallest working chemical units. These

chemical units are then absorbed through the mucous membrane of the intestinal walls and eventually reach the bloodstream to be distributed to the individual cells, providing the body with building materials, heat, and energy. To accomplish this, the digestive system works on food both *mechanically* (through the action of the teeth, tongue, cheeks and muscular contractions of the tract, called *peristalsis*) and *chemically* (through the activity of various enzymes, emulsifiers, acids, and bacteria, which are normally active in different portions of the tract). The student is invited to review Chapter 21 if more details of the digestive process are desired. Substances not absorbed into the rest of the body via the bloodstream or lymphatic system are removed normally by periodic defecation, or bowel movement.

Disorders of the digestive system manifest themselves in several predictable ways. Anorexia, nausea, vomiting, constipation, abdominal distention and pain, diarrhea, and weight loss are common manifestations. The observation of a child's stool is of great importance in pediatrics. The amount, color, consistency, general appearance, and odor of a child's bowel movements can be of real diagnostic significance and aid in evaluating the condition of the digestive tract.

KEY VOCABULARY

digestion process by which food is broken down mechanically and chemically in the gastrointestinal tract and converted into absorbable forms.

endocrine gland structure producing a hormone that is discharged into the bloodstream.

exocrine gland structure that produces a secretion

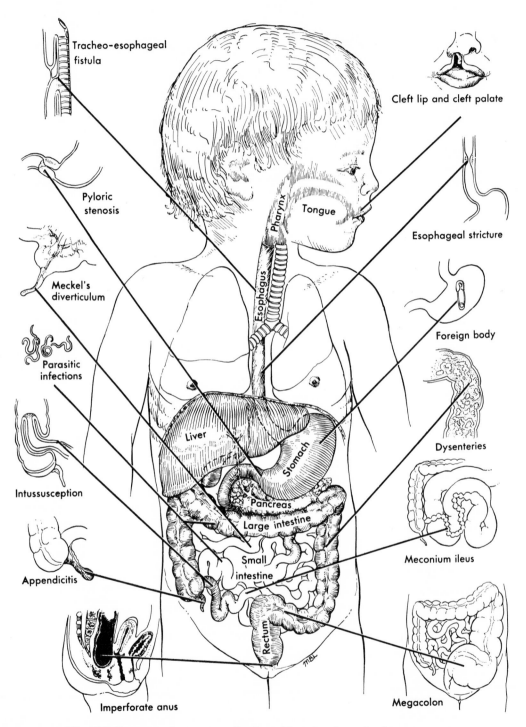

Fig. 36-1. Summary of common pediatric problems involving the digestive system.

that is deposited in a particular area of the body via a duct.

glycosuria presence of glucose in the urine.

hypoglycemia deficiency of glucose in the blood.

ileus obstruction or paralysis of small intestine.

metabolism all energy and material transformations that occur within living cells.

DIGESTIVE AND METABOLIC PROBLEMS

The infant

For a discussion of cleft lip, cleft palate, and esophageal atresia with tracheoesophageal fistula see Chapter 17.

Oral moniliasis

Thrush, or oral moniliasis, mentioned earlier (see p. 191) as a possible complication during the newborn period, results from contamination of the infant's oral cavity with vaginal secretion containing *Candida (Monilia) albicans* at the time of birth or from improper hygiene and feeding techniques after delivery. White, curdlike plaques appear on the tongue and cheeks and adhere to the surface of the mucous membrane (see Fig. 15-4). The mouth may be tender and the desire to eat may be decreased. It may be treated by the oral application of nystatin or even the old standby, gentian violet, 1%. All objects that have entered the infected infant's mouth should be adequately sterilized. The condition usually responds well to therapy. Thrush is also a fairly common condition among children receiving long-term, broad-spectrum antibiotic therapy. The antibiotics destroy the normal flora of the alimentary canal and allow the fungus to multiply without competition. Thrush and other manifestations of *Candida albicans* may be prevented by adding buttermilk or yogurt to the diet. In high-risk patients the regular use of bacterial cultures, such as those found in Lactinex granules or tablets, given at mealtime may be more helpful.

Esophageal stenosis

The narrowing of a child's esophagus, esophageal stenosis, may be congenital in origin; however, more often it is posttrau-matic. The most common cause is probably the ingestion of some corrosive substance such as lye, which burns the tissues and produces scarring, leading to stenosis.

The patient usually must undergo periodic esophageal dilatations by catheters. He may need a gastrostomy, or artificial opening into the stomach, because of difficulty in maintaining nutrition. Surgical excision of the narrowed area and joining together of the remaining parts (anastomosis), replacement of the area by a bowel transplant, or esophageal reconstruction using tissue from the greater curvature of the stomach may be undertaken.

Congenital pyloric stenosis

Abnormal narrowing of the pyloric sphincter, which forms the exit of the stomach, may cause progressive vomiting and malnutrition in the infant (Fig. 36-2). This narrowing is caused by spasm of the sphincter, local edema, and an overgrowth of the circular muscle fibers of the pylorus. The symptoms do not usually begin until the child is approximately 2 to 3 weeks old and rarely have their onset after 2 months of age. This disorder seems to have a slight hereditary tendency and occurs more often in male than female infants.

At first the vomiting is only occasional. However, if the stenosis is unrelieved, it becomes more frequent, forceful, and projectile in character. If this situation persists, the child will lose weight and begin to show signs of dehydration, electrolyte imbalance, and malnutrition. The emesis contains no bile, since the opening to the duodenum is too small to allow such staining. Despite the frequent vomiting, the baby continues to have a good appetite and will take fluids when they are offered. The physician makes his diagnosis on the basis of the history, the clinical examination, and x-ray studies that use a contrast medium. A hard, olive-shaped tumor (the hypertrophied pylorus) may be palpated, and visible, left-to-right peristalsis may be noted as the stomach tries to force the swallowed formula into the duodenum. When this ef-

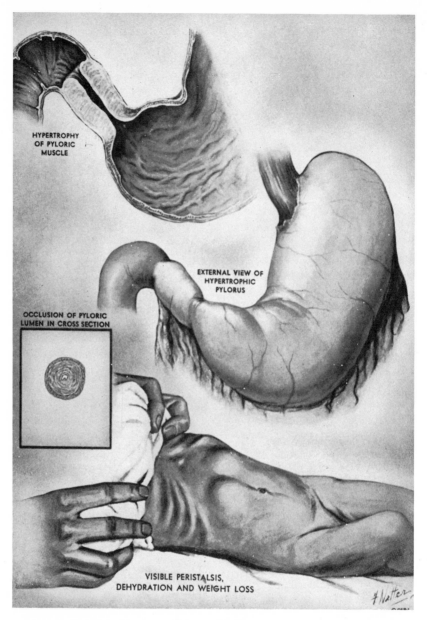

HYPERTROPHY
OF PYLORIC
MUSCLE

EXTERNAL VIEW OF
HYPERTROPHIC
PYLORUS

OCCLUSION OF PYLORIC
LUMEN IN CROSS SECTION

VISIBLE PERISTALSIS,
DEHYDRATION AND WEIGHT LOSS

Fig. 36-2. Congenital hypertrophied pyloric stenosis. (From the CIBA collection of medical illustrations, by Frank H. Netter, M.D., Copyright CIBA.)

fort proves ineffective, the peristaltic waves reverse themselves and emesis results.

In the United States, treatment of pyloric stenosis is usually surgical. A nasogastric tube is inserted prior to surgery to assure that the stomach is empty and to prevent aspiration during the surgery. The procedure is called the Fredet-Ramstedt operation. The surgeon cuts down through the enlarged muscle of the pylorus to the mucous membrane. This relieves the constriction. This operation, when performed on infants well prepared for the procedure, is highly successful in relieving the cause of the persistent vomiting. Postoperative care consists of observation of the surgical site or dressing and careful introduction of glucose water in small amounts as ordered at fairly frequent intervals. The infant should be held at a steep incline while being fed, bubbled well before, during, and after his feeding, and placed in an infant seat or propped on his right side after his feedings. When he is in the infant seat, gravity aids the drainage of the offered fluid. Placing the infant on his right side also aids drainage and helps bubbles come to the top of the stomach where they can be expelled with less formula loss. A side or upright position also helps prevent aspiration. After drinking, the infant should be disturbed as little as possible. It is very important not to overfeed the child. Such a situation leads to possible vomiting and strain on suture lines. If three or four glucose-water feedings are well tolerated, the infant is given progressive amounts of half-strength formula, beginning with 1 ounce. When 2½-ounce feedings are reached, he is started on his usual formula. If the infant retains his formula, he is discharged to the care of his parents. This may be as early as the second postoperative day.

Meckel's diverticulum

A structural leftover from embryonic life is the persistence of a pouch on the ileum called Meckel's diverticulum. At one time a duct joined the umbilicus with the intestine and led to the yolk sac, which gave temporary nourishment to the developing fetus. In the course of normal development this duct closes. However, remnants persist in a small percentage of people. Sometimes they cause difficulty. An open tract, capable of discharging the contents of the small bowel onto the abdominal wall, may endure. More often a blind pouch with no connection or only a cord attachment to the umbilicus remains. Occasionally gastric mucosa is found within the pouch. Meckel's diverticulum may cause ulceration and hemorrhage with symptoms similar to appendicitis or intestinal obstruction. Many times its presence is undiagnosed until exploratory surgery reveals the problem.

Nursing care is similar to that involving any condition that necessitates exploration of the abdominal cavity.

Meconium ileus

Obstruction of the small intestine in the newborn infant caused by the presence of exceptionally thick, sticky meconium is called meconium ileus. The meconium is so gummy that it cannot pass normally through the bowel. Obstruction often occurs near the ileocecal junction. This condition is always indicative of the exocrine disorder, cystic fibrosis of the pancreas, although it is not present in all cases of cystic fibrosis. Meconium ileus results because the pancreas fails to produce the enzymes that normally help liquefy the meconium. See p. 563 for a discussion of cystic fibrosis.

Symptoms include bile-stained emesis, abdominal distention, and absence of the normal meconial stool. This is a difficult pediatric problem because of the type of malfunction, the age of the patient, and other aspects of the total disease process. In mild cases the treatment may be medical, with reliance on special enemas that help dissolve or mechanically clear the impaction and oral administration of pancreatic enzymes. A therapeutic enema of diatrizoate meglumin (Gastrografin) is a promising nonoperative method of relieving the impaction. Intravenous fluid therapy is imperative during this procedure since Gastrografin draws fluid and serum from the intravascular compartment into the lumen of the bowel, hopefully releasing the firm bind of sticky meconium. Many cases, however, require surgery to clear the obstruction. Resection of the intestine and a temporary ileostomy may be necessary. The child is usually very ill, and the prognosis is guarded.

Intussusception

A telescoping of adjacent parts of the bowel is called intussusception (Fig. 36-3). When intussusception occurs, it commonly involves the area of the ileocecal valve. Such an abnormal relationship of parts of

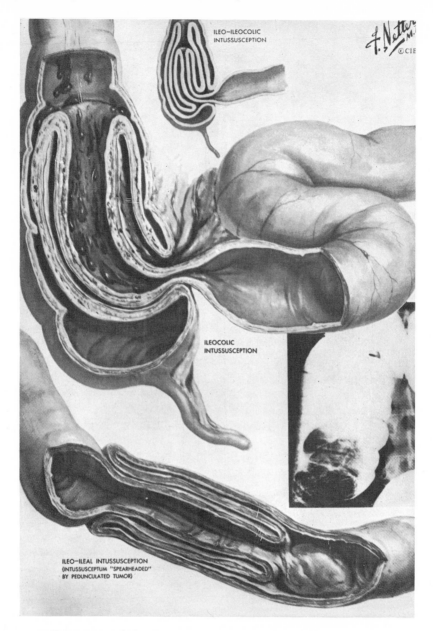

ILEO–ILEOCOLIC
INTUSSUSCEPTION

ILEOCOLIC
INTUSSUSCEPTION

ILEO–ILEAL INTUSSUSCEPTION
(INTUSSUSCEPTUM "SPEARHEADED"
BY PEDUNCULATED TUMOR)

Fig. 36-3. Different types of intussusception. (From the CIBA collection of medical illustrations, by Frank H. Netter, M.D., Copyright CIBA.)

the intestine may disturb circulation to the involved portions and result in gangrene and perforation as well as obstruction of the bowel. This condition most often affects infants and toddlers. The onset is usually sudden. At first the child may draw up his legs and cry out intermittently. Later his discomfort is intensified by progressive vomiting of bile-stained and even fecal emesis. His stools, at first loose, become scanty and characteristically assume the color and consistency of currant jelly because they are formed at this time largely of mucus and blood. If the condition is unrelieved, the child rapidly becomes prostrate. A high temperature develops, and his life is endangered. A favorable prognosis depends on early detection and treatment of the condition.

Diagnosis is made by considering the history, the physical examination, and plain survey films of the abdomen. Treatment of choice in all cases, except those in which peritonitis or frank intestinal obstruction is suspected, is the barium enema. The pressure of the inflowing enema may reduce an intussusception. In some cases reduction comes only after raising the height of the barium or by giving repeated enemas after each evacuation. A small number recur after primary barium enema treatment. When surgery is preferred, the intussusception is identified and usually gently "milked" backward until the telescoping is completely relieved. Resection of a damaged intestine is necessary in other cases.

Congenital megacolon (Hirschsprung's disease)

Classic congenital megacolon, or Hirschsprung's disease, is characterized by lack of normal peristaltic activity in the distal segment of the colon, usually the sigmoid, because of improper nervous control (lack of the necessary nerve ganglia in the musculature of the affected bowel or lack of coordination between the parasympathetic and sympathetic divisions of the nervous system). It is seen more often in males than in females. Signs and symptoms of congenital megacolon appear early in infancy. Constipation, sometimes interrupted by small amounts of stool; progressive abdominal distention, which may be sufficiently marked to cause respiratory embarrassment; anorexia; and occasional vomiting are all indications of the disorder. Pronounced abdominal distention may grossly distort the appearance of the child. Diagnosis is made after a review of the patient's history, palpation and auscultation of the abdomen, rectal examination, x-ray examination, and perhaps a rectal biopsy for microscopic examination of the tissue. Although a rectal biopsy can provide cor-

rect diagnosis of congenital megacolon, it may also initiate the serious complication of enterocolitis.

The condition may be treated medically or surgically, depending on its severity and its response to conservative measures.

Medical management includes almost daily enemas (usually physiological saline solution, 2 teaspoons salt per 1 quart water). Tap water enemas are not given because they are frequently difficult to expel, and therefore, water intoxication is a danger. The amount of fluid given at one time is larger than that given nonaffected children the same age because of the gross distention of the bowel. Digital removal of fecal material from the rectum may be necessary. Stool softeners such as Zymenol or mineral oil may be ordered. The use of drugs that affect the activity of the parasympathetic and sympathetic nervous systems may help obtain more regular bowel movements. A low-residue diet may be helpful in reducing the amount of feces and in keeping the stool soft.

If the condition of the child does not improve sufficiently with medical management, surgical treatment may be elected. The type of procedure done will depend on the age and individual needs of the child. The most satisfactory treatment appears to be an abdominoperineal removal of the abnormal section of bowel with an anastomosis of the remaining normal colon to the anal canal (Swenson's pull-through). A variation of this is the Suavé procedure. Afterward, the child is fed parenterally. Gastric suction and an indwelling urinary catheter are continued for an indefinite period. The anal sphincter may be dilated daily. The presence of bowel sounds and normal stool are eagerly awaited. At times this procedure is inadvisable, and a colostomy is performed.

More common than classic aganglionic megacolon is pseudo-Hirschsprung's disease, which has a psychogenic basis. It does not have an onset in the newborn period; x-ray studies and biopsy studies are negative. Investigation of family living patterns and stresses by qualified personnel is necessary.

Colic

Although colic is often spoken of as a disease entity, it is not a disease but a symptom. In the dictionary it is defined as "acute abdominal pain." However, when parents and nurses speak of "the colic," they are usually referring to the intermittent abdominal distress in the newborn infant that is fairly common in the early months of life. Fortunately, the problem does not always last 3 months, in spite of the frequent use of the phrase "3-month colic." The child and his parents seem to be troubled most in the early evening and night. The baby suddenly draws up his legs on his abdomen, clenches his fists, becomes red in the face, and starts to cry. This goes on intermittently as though he were troubled with periodic intestinal cramping. During these episodes he may pass gas by mouth or rectum.

Various explanations for the abdominal discomfort have been advanced. Probably there are multiple causes. Babies troubled with colic tend to have a low birth weight (5 to 7 pounds). It may be caused basically by an immaturity of the gastrointestinal system. Most explanations of the pain experienced involve the presence of excessive gas in the digestive tract. Excessive air may result from the following:

1. Poor feeding techniques, including failure to tip the bottle sufficiently to assure a full nipple at all times, too rapid feeding, the use of nipples with very small holes, which necessitates considerable suction (and air swallowing) to obtain the formula, and failure to bubble the baby often enough.
2. Excessive use of carbohydrate in the formula, which may cause increased fermentation and gas formation.
3. A tense, nervous baby fostered by a tense, nervous mother.

Attempts to remedy colic consider these possible causes. Various types of bottles and nipples have been marketed as anticolic devices, some of which may merit a try if the baby does not respond to other techniques. Different units using presterilized plastic-bag bottles are available. The physician may recommend a change in formula. Occasionally antispasmodics, tranquilizers, or phenobarbital may be prescribed for both baby and mother! An infant will not be hospitalized because of colic alone, but the nurse may care for colicky babies and must realize why feeding techniques are so important. A baby who is not well bubbled will usually not eat well and is more prone to regurgitation, vomiting, and colic.

The diarrheas

Any diarrheal disease causing profuse fluid loss is a particular threat to the very young person, the very old person, or the debilitated person, regardless of the initiating cause of the diarrhea. Subsequent dehydration and electrolyte imbalance is a very real danger. Fortunately, with the improvement in community sanitation and hygiene, the increased availability of refrigeration, and the adoption of the disinfection techniques used in infant formula preparation, infectious-type diarrheas are not as common in the United States today as they were 50 years ago.

The infant who becomes dehydrated because of diarrhea or diarrhea and vomiting is admitted to the hospital. The infant should be weighed and a stool culture obtained immediately.

Diarrheal disease of early childhood is a syndrome, the course of which varies with age, severity, nutritional status, and cause. Some of the common causes of diarrhea include infection, anatomical abnormalities, malabsorption syndromes, and disease outside the gastrointestinal tract. Most acute diarrheas appear to have a viral cause and frequently accompany acute upper respiratory tract infections. Other causes of infectious diarrheas include staphylococci, pathogenic *Escherichia coli,* and *Salmonella* and *Shigella* microorganisms. Diarrheal disturbances may also be initiated by injudicious diets or emotional upset.

General nursing care. Whatever the cause, acute diarrheal disorders need immediate treatment. The disturbance in intestinal motility and consequent malabsorption causes dehydration and fluid and electrolyte imbalances. Usually diarrhea subsides when fluid and electrolyte therapy is administered intravenously and oral intake is briefly reduced. Oral intake is restricted to rest the gastrointestinal tract and make it less irritable. Antibiotic therapy is indicated for treating diarrheas caused by pathogenic *Escherichia coli* and staphylococci and for severe infections caused by salmonella and shigella-type organisms. Daily calculations of the child's fluid intake and output and his weight must be accurately recorded. Because of the frequency of stools, a special medicated ointment may be prescribed to apply after each cleansing of the perirectal area. A diarrheal stool should be promptly reported, since the physician may have written an order for the administration of a constipating medication after each liquid stool. Of course, the color, consistency, general appearance, and amount of the stool should be faithfully noted and recorded. Rectal temperatures are contraindicated. (See p. 513.)

Abdominal hernias

A hernia is an abnormal protrusion of a portion of the contents of a body cavity through a defect in its surrounding wall, commonly causing abnormal swelling or pressure. The general public calls the condition a "rupture." Common in infancy and childhood are inguinal and umbilical hernias. They are usually congenital.

Inguinal hernia

Hernia repair in the inguinal region is a common surgical procedure. Such hernias are found most often in males. They may be unilateral or bilateral. When the testes originally descend into the scrotum from the abdominal cavity, they are surrounded by a small sac or tube of peritoneum that is continuous with the abdominal lining. Usually this sac soon closes off, making any further communication with the abdominal cavity impossible. However, occasionally the closure is incomplete or does not take place, and the intestine may slip down the open inguinal canal, causing a swelling in the area. This prolapse of the intestine is not important in itself. However, there is a possibility that the misplaced loop of intestine could become trapped (incarcerated) in the inguinal canal or scrotum and the circulation to the trapped segment could become impaired (strangulation), causing intestinal obstruction and gangrene of the bowel.

Inguinal hernia may also develop in girls. The anatomy is different but parallel. The inguinal canals, which are occupied by the round ligaments, may allow loops of intestine to enter the area of the groin. Only 10% of inguinal hernias involve females.

In order to prevent incarceration, all inguinal hernias should be corrected soon after diagnosis. In infants and small children up to 2 years of age, the hernia is repaired in a simple procedure (herniotomy). In older children a slightly more complex procedure is used. A surgical incision is made in a natural skin crease where the scar will not be seen. The hernia sac is carefully tied off. In the case of boys, an abnormal collection of fluid may be found in the scrotal area surrounding the testes (hydrocele). This fluid is aspirated, and the abnormal peritoneal sac is excised. The child usually tolerates the entire procedure very well, and in most cases no postoperative analgesia is required. A protective spray dressing is applied over the new incision. This allows direct observation of the area.

Diapers are usually not applied in a routine fashion until 24 hours after surgery. One approach to the diaper problem is the ues of Stile's dressing (Fig. 36-4). A small bed cradle is placed over the legs of the infant. His diaper is brought upward between his legs and fastened to the frame of the cradle. A long infant gown, securely

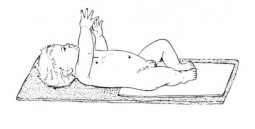

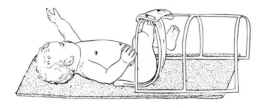

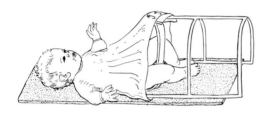

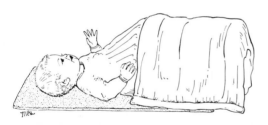

Fig. 36-4. Steps in constructing Stile's dressing. (Be sure that the gown is pulled tightly when attached to the cradle. At times the cradle must be tied to the crib.)

tied in back, is drawn tightly upward over the frame and also fastened with pins. The cradle is then draped with a small blanket. Children are usually discharged on the first postoperative day.

Hospitalization for inguinal hernia repair is not always necessary. A simple herniotomy can be done as an outpatient procedure. Parents are instructed to bring the infant or child to the hospital in a fasting

state about 1 hour before the scheduled procedure. The parents remain with the child until he is taken to the operating room and are present when he awakes. In 2 to 3 hours and when the child is taking fluids, he may be discharged from the hospital. Parents should be reminded to return in 4 days to have the sutures removed from the infant's incision. Older children's sutures are removed on the sixth postoperative day.

Umbilical hernias

Umbilical hernias in infancy are thought to be caused by severe stress to the fresh umbilical wound brought about by crying, coughing, and vomiting. Umbilical hernias often close spontaneously as the child learns to stand and walk and abdominal muscles are strengthened through use. However, umbilical defects greater than 1.5 cm. in diameter in children seldom close spontaneously. (Umbilical hernias are particularly common in black children.) If an umbilical hernia is not closed, the defect often becomes more serious in pregnant women, and the multiparous woman is subject to the dangerous threat of incarceration. In order to prevent this serious problem in adulthood, a more aggressive approach is urged. Prophylactic umbilical hernia repair is recommended for all girls over 2 years and all boys over 4 years of age.

Imperforate anus

The problem of imperforate anus has already been mentioned in Chapter 17. Fig. 17-19 depicts the common types of the malformation encountered. In most cases, surgery for correction must be performed very early to avoid complications and assure a better possibility of success. If a male newborn infant has a rectourethral fistula, surgery must be prompt to avoid intestinal obstruction and ascending urinary tract infection. For infant girls with an associated posterior vaginal anus, corrective surgery may be delayed until the child is 4 to 6 months of age.

Whether an abdominal and/or perineal surgical approach will be necessary depends on the type of defect and the distance of the terminal end of the colon from the perineum. A temporary colostomy may be necessary. After creation or repair of the anorectal area, frequent dilatation of the canal may be ordered.

Galactosemia

One metabolic defect that has dietary significance and has received considerable attention in the literature recently is *galactosemia*. If this congenital error in the metabolism of the sugar galactose is untreated, it may cause physical and mental retardation, cataracts, enlargement of the liver and spleen, and cirrhosis. The body is unable to change galactose to glucose, a chemical reaction that normally takes place primarily in the liver. An enzyme needed to accomplish the task is deficient or missing. Galactose builds up in the bloodstream and spills over into the urine, where it may be identified by appropriate tests.

Early signs of galactosemia in the infant are vomiting, listlessness, and failure to thrive. These signs are not apparent until at least a week or two after birth. Since galactose is present in milk sugar, it is very important that the defect be diagnosed early and that a milk substitute such as Nutramigen or a meat-base formula be used. Like those of children with phenylketonuria (PKU), the diets of galactosemia patients must be very closely supervised to avoid the ingestion of the offending food. Also like the young patient with PKU, the child with galactosemia may be able to gradually expand his dietary horizons after a period of several years on a rigid, restricted regimen.

THE TODDLER AND PRESCHOOL CHILD
Celiac syndrome

The word "celiac" refers to the abdomen. All children with conditions having celiac manifestations have large, protuberant abdomens because of poor absorption of certain foodstuffs from the gastrointesti-

nal tract. The stools are characteristically bulky, pale, greasy, and foul smelling. The arms, legs, and buttocks of these children are emaciated as a result of nutritional deficiency. Although the symptoms may be similar, the underlying causes of the indigestion may be quite varied. The most common pediatric disorders that manifest the celiac syndrome are cystic fibrosis of the pancreas and gluten-induced enteropathy (commonly referred to as *celiac disease,* or chronic intestinal indigestion). Today, celiac disease in its severe, classic form is not as frequent as formerly. However, milder degrees of this difficulty are not rare. The problem usually affects children from 2 to 5 years of age.

Children probably suffer from celiac disease because of an inborn metabolic or enzyme defect or an allergic-type reaction. They are especially sensitive to the ingestion of gluten, a protein commonly found in wheat, rye, and oats. This sensitivity, combined with emotional stress, concurrent infections, and general malnutrition, adds up to a particularly unhappy child. Starches and fats are poorly absorbed. However, simple sugars and nongluten proteins are tolerated. Diagnosis is based on clinical observation, studies of fat content in the stools, and response to a gluten-free diet. These children are often fretful and moody. They frequently have poor appetites. When admitted into the hospital, they may be in *celiac crisis.* A crisis may be precipitated by an upper respiratory tract infection. The child suffers from severe diarrhea, vomiting, dehydration, and weight loss. Immediate and vigorous therapy including fluid, protein, vitamin, and electrolyte replacement is necessary. Recently corticosteroids have been used in treating these children. The effects have been dramatic. Diarrhea and vomiting subside within 2 days, bringing about a striking improvement.

An important part of childhood treatment of celiac disease consists of careful exclusion of the many sources of gluten from the diet. All labels on prepared food must be meticulously read since wheat flour is a frequent additive. The infant or young child is given a high-protein, low-fat, starch-free diet. Simple sugars such as dextrose and sucrose are well received, and banana powder has long been favored. Large amounts of supplementary water-based preparations of vitamins A and D should be given. Long-term diet therapy is recommended for all children. The intolerance of wheat gluten is apparently lifelong.

The child with celiac disease requires patient nursing care to deal with his irritability, regressive behavior, and appetite problems. The nurse should understand the child and why eating has become so burdensome and unrewarding for him. Accurate daily calculation of weight should be made. Detailed charting of the type and amount of intake, as well as accurate stool descriptions, is a necessity.

The patient suffering from celiac disease perspires a great deal and because of his ungainly shape may not move frequently. He should be periodically turned if this is the case. Skin care is a never-ending responsibility.

With good general hygiene and extended dietary management, the tolerance of these children for other types of foods gradually increases, and although upsets may continue irregularly even into adult life, the prognosis as a whole is good. This knowledge usually encourages the parents to continue supervision. A conference with the hospital dietitian before the child's discharge is often very helpful. She has access to special recipes that may make the limited diet prescribed more interesting to the child. She will be able to explain to the mother in more detail the practical implications of the dietary restrictions imposed.

Foreign body ingestion

Children do not limit their experimental tasting and swallowing to articles that are meant to tempt an appetite or even to indigestible items that might appear delicious. All kinds of objects have gone down the "little red lane." Fortunately most complete the entire journey without incident.

One may carefully examine the stool for small round objects that have been ingested. However, sharp or long, angled objects may pose the threat of perforation. If the object is detectable by x-ray examination, it is viewed and periodically watched. If trauma to the tissue seems likely, an operation to retrieve it may be necessary. The abdomen of a child who has swallowed a foreign object should not be palpated. One physician even suggests placing a small sign on the child, cautioning would-be investigators to avoid such maneuvers.

Giving a child large amounts of bread or potato after ingestion of a foreign object is of doubtful value. A laxative should never be given in such circumstances.

Parasitic infestations

All bacteria are parasites; however, when one speaks of *parasitic infestations,* he is usually referring to organisms that are multicellular in their adult form and large enough to be seen with the naked eye. There are many kinds of parasites in this category that trouble mankind. Many of them are found in abundance in tropical areas of the world and represent tremendous public health problems. This text will mention only those found fairly frequently in the United States: pinworms and roundworms.

Oxyuriasis (pinworm, threadworm, or seatworm infestation)

Although the official name of the pinworm is *Enterobius vermicularis,* the name of the disease this small, white, threadlike worm causes is known as oxyuriasis, or enterobiasis, an extremely common infestation. It does not always produce symptoms and often goes undiagnosed.

The pinworm eggs are ingested or possibly inhaled. Most often the child introduces the eggs into his own mouth by his contaminated fingers. His fingers become contaminated by touching objects used by affected children who have not carried out proper toilet hygiene. When the infestation has become established, the child may easily reinfect himself. The eggs are swallowed and hatch in the intestine. They mature in and near the cecum. When the adult female worms are ready to lay their eggs, they migrate down the intestinal tract to the anus. During the night the female worms leave the anus and lay their eggs in the folds of the anal sphincter and the perineum. Occasionally the worms may migrate to the vagina and cause a vaginitis in a little girl. All this activity usually causes considerable local irritation and itching.

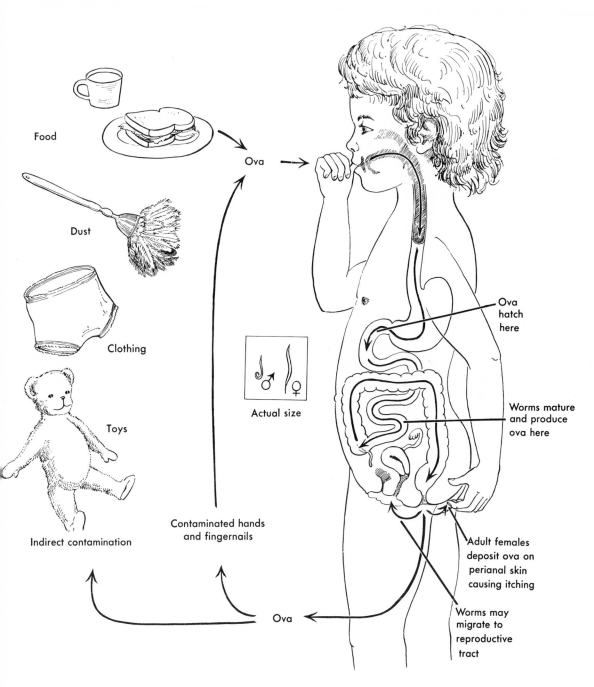

Food

Dust

Clothing

Toys

Indirect contamination

Ova

Actual size

Contaminated hands and fingernails

Ova

Ova hatch here

Worms mature and produce ova here

Adult females deposit ova on perianal skin causing itching

Worms may migrate to reproductive tract

Fig. 36-5. Life cycle of the pinworm *(Enterobius vermicularis).*

The child usually scratches the area, contaminating his fingers with the eggs layed in the region. In the course of time, fingers travel to the mouth again, and the cycle repeats (Fig. 36-5). The interval between the ingestion of an egg and the appearance of the female pinworm at the anus is approximately 6 to 8 weeks.

Usually mild pinworm infestations cause few symptoms other than anal itching and secondary complications caused by scratching. However, in some cases pinworms may cause anorexia, restlessness, and irritability. In cases of large infestations, inflammation of the appendix may occur.

Diagnosis is made on the basis of viewing the worms as they emerge from the anus or are inadvertently expelled on the surface of a stool or by the microscopic detection of the eggs. Since the female lays her eggs in the skin folds outside the body of the child, ova are rarely found in the stool. Usually a so-called Scotch tape test is ordered. The night nurse goes to the bedside of the child before he wakes and shines a light on the rectal region. Sometimes the gravid worms may be seen. She then takes a piece of Scotch tape, which has been fastened "sticky side out" to a tongue blade, and presses it against the rectal area. Some microscopic eggs will adhere to the tape. The tape is then carefully secured to a glass slide "sticky side down" and sent to the laboratory for examination.

In the past when a child was affected, the entire family was treated. Today, only the family members who have symptoms are treated, and a more pleasant form of therapy is available. Doses of piperazine citrate (Antepar), a fruit-flavored syrup, may be ordered for a total of 14 days, or pyrvinium pamoate (Povan) may be given in one or two doses. The nurse and parents should know that pyrvinium pamoate colors the stools red and if the child has an emesis while the medication is still present in the gastrointestinal tract, the emesis may also be reddish.

Other measures must be followed to help assure a cure. Personal toilet hygiene should be stressed. The necessity for hand washing after using the toilet is not grasped by children unless it is taught. Frequent cleansing of the rectogenital area is required. The toilet seat must be cleansed often. Because of the intense itching that may occur at night, an affected child should have very short fingernails, and his hands may be placed in mittens or socks to try to prevent scratching. Snug panties or diapers may also help. Bed linens, towels, underwear, and nightclothes of the infected patient should be washed separately in very hot water, preferably boiled. In the hospital setting the linen is bagged separately and labeled for the benefit of the laundry. Because many children are infested without the nurse's knowledge, it is always good technique to refrain from shaking used bed linen. Instead, it should always be rolled. Waving the child's linens only helps scatter the eggs. Hands must be washed frequently, and a protective cover gown may be worn when intimate care of the patient is required.

Ascariasis (roundworm infestation). Ascaris lumbricoides, the worm that causes ascariasis, looks like a pink or white earthworm. It is usually 6 to 15 inches long. The eggs are found in the soil or on objects contaminated by soil containing involved feces. The disease is perpetuated by poor sanitary facilities and poor hygiene practices.

The microscopic egg is swallowed and hatches in the duodenum. The small intermediate stages of the worm (larvae) pass through the wall of the intestine to penetrate the venules and/or lymphatics. They commonly migrate to the liver, the right side of the heart, and the lungs. The small larvae then penetrate the alveoli and ascend the bronchioles, bronchi, and trachea. On reaching the glottis they are swallowed. These same larvae develop into adult male and female forms in the small intestine. The adult male may be approximately 6 to 10 inches long. The female may be about 8 to 15 inches long and about the diameter of a pencil. The adult worms subsist on the semidigested food in the intestinal canal. Fertilized eggs expelled in feces must undergo a 2- to 3-week period of maturation in the soil before becoming capable of producing disease (Fig. 36-6).

This parasite, because of its migratory habits (even the adult worm may travel up and down the digestive tract, occasionally making an alarming appearance at either end), may cause a variety of symptoms if the infestation is of some intensity. The

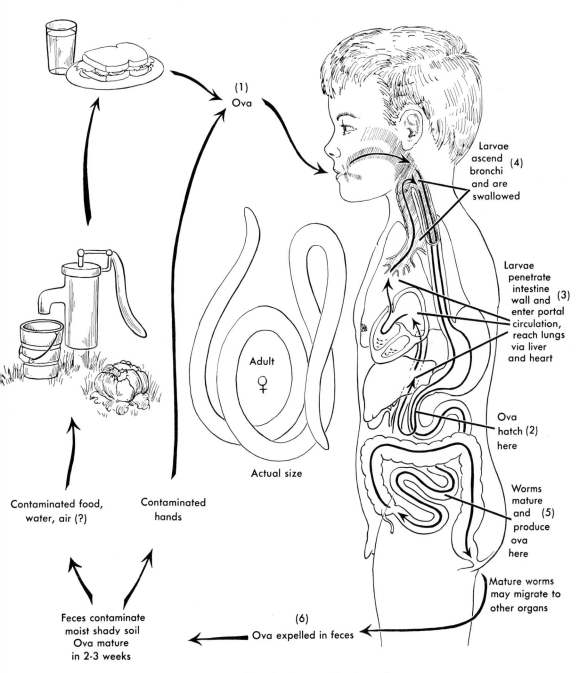

Fig. 36-6. Life cycle of *Ascaris lumbricoides.*

larval migrations may cause nausea and vomiting or initiate symptoms of pneumonitis or intestinal obstruction. They even may produce perforation. Allergic reactions, skin rash, nervousness, and irritability are not uncommon.

Positive diagnosis is made on the basis of finding the ova in the stool or seeing the worms emerge from the gastrointestinal tract. Treatment by piperazine citrate (Antepar) is effective for *Ascaris* infestation, provided that reinfection caused by poor hygiene practices does not occur. All infected persons must be treated to have successful control of the disease. Public education programs teaching general hygiene are a must. Turning infested topsoil under has also been believed helpful. The prognosis is very good unless secondary complications such as pneumonia, intestinal obstruction, or perforation have developed. The outlook then becomes more guarded.

Appendicitis

Inflammation caused by local obstruction or infection of the vermiform appendix, located at the base of the cecum, is a common indication for abdominal surgery. However, it is not always easy to diagnose appendicitis in young children. Other problems may mimic the condition, and the young child is not often very descriptive regarding his general discomfort. Pain may first be felt in the umbilical area. Later it may be localized in the lower right-hand abdominal quadrant. Restlessness, mild constipation or diarrhea, and anorexia followed by nausea and vomiting are often reported. A low-grade fever is characteristic. The white blood cell count is usually elevated. If the inflamed appendix is removed before it has ruptured, recovery is usually prompt and uneventful. However, delay or the use of ill-advised laxatives may result in the rupture of the appendix. Peritonitis may complicate the condition. Recovery in this case is slower, and the risk to the patient is multiplied considerably. The campaign to educate the public not to give laxatives or enemas to persons complaining of abdominal pain has not yet been won.

The patient with a ruptured appendix, related abscess, or peritonitis is very ill. He usually cannot be sent to surgery immediately but must wait until the administration of antibiotics, intravenous fluids, and possible cooling measures are completed in order that he be in the best condition possible for the appendectomy. A nasogastric tube is often passed to relieve flatus and prevent vomiting. At the time of the surgery, a drain is usually placed in the abdominal wound, and drainage may be significant. A high Fowler's position is maintained to prevent the spread of infective material in the abdomen. Intravenous feedings are continued for several days postoperatively, and only ice chips or sips of water are allowed by mouth. Intake and output determinations are important. Today, more and more of these patients are recuperating satisfactorily, and the phrase "ruptured appendix" is no longer as dreaded as it formerly was.

THE SCHOOL-AGE CHILD
Diabetes mellitus

Diabetes mellitus is the most common metabolic disorder of children. It is not a true digestive problem, since carbohydrates are reduced to glucose by the digestive system and the glucose is absorbed into the bloodstream. The difficulty arises because the islands of Langerhans in the pancreas fail to produce the hormone insulin. The glucose in the bloodstream is not subsequently converted and stored or burned properly by the body in the absence of effective insulin.

Diabetes mellitus may manifest itself any time during a person's lifetime. In the United States there are approximately 200,000 known diabetic children under 16 years of age. This group represents about 5% of all known diabetic persons. The earlier the disease appears the more severe it is likely to be. This disorder in glucose metabolism is thought to be hereditary, but the exact pattern of inheritance is unknown.

Mechanism

Glucose is absorbed from the digestive tract, but in diabetes mellitus sufficient functional insulin is not available to convert it to glycogen and store it in the liver and muscles or to burn it properly. It remains at a high level in the bloodstream (hyperglycemia). The large amount of glucose in the blood going to the kidneys cannot be entirely reabsorbed by the tubules of the nephron; therefore glucose spills over into the urine (glycosuria). To excrete the glucose, more water must also be excreted to dilute the glucose. Excessive urine production results.

When the amount of glucose available is insufficient to provide heat and energy to meet the body's needs, protein and fats may be used to help furnish these necessities. However, the metabolism of fat is not complete without the concurrent metabolism of carbohydrate. This incomplete fat metabolism produces ketone bodies (acetone, diacetic acid, and oxybutyric acid) that accumulate abnormally in the blood. Diacetic acid and oxybutyric acid must be neutralized in the body by bases, or alkalies. As the ketones are excreted, the neutralizing bases are also excreted. The body's supply of base is depleted, the sensitive electrolyte balance is upset, and acidosis gradually develops.

Symptoms

In children common symptoms of diabetes mellitus noted may be excessive thirst and fluid intake (polydipsia). This ties in with the increased urinary output (polyuria), which may be so excessive that enuresis; or bedwetting, results. Exceptional appetite (polyphagia) may or may not be present in diabetic children. The affected child demonstrates a slow weight gain or a definite weight loss. He is easily fatigued.

Diabetic ketoacidosis. This is a complex disorder that is the result of untreated diabetes or a disturbance in the glucose-insulin balance of the treated patient. General malaise, nausea, vomiting, and abdominal pain may be present. As acidosis becomes more pronounced, symptoms of dehydration develop. The skin is warm, dry, and often flushed, and the eyeballs are soft and sunken. The body, using every method available to get rid of the abnormal ketones present, expels acetone from the respiratory system as well as the urinary tract. The typical fruity "apple-pie" breath results. Respirations become long, deep, and labored (Kussmaul's respirations). The patient becomes irritable, drowsy, and then unconscious or comatose. His blood pressure is typically low and his pulse rapid and thready.

Treatment of diabetic coma must be intensive. Intravenous therapy to restore the electrolyte balance and provide suitable dosages of insulin is routine. Frequent blood chemistries and urine testing for glucose and acetone levels are mandatory.

Diagnosis

Of course, the primary diagnosis of diabetes mellitus is confirmed with the help of laboratory tests. The presence of glucose in the urine points to the possibility of this disease, but in itself is not conclusive, since some children have a low renal threshold for glucose but no other problem. However, detection of glycosuria coupled with the finding of an elevated blood glucose level (hyperglycemia) is diagnostic, and no further tests are necessary. Children are more likely to have an abrupt onset of the disease than are adults, who tend to develop diabetes gradually.

The oral glucose tolerance test is usually employed to demonstrate carbohydrate intolerance, which confirms the diagnosis of diabetes. After the child has fasted during the night, blood and urine samples are obtained. Then a calculated amount of glucose based on the child's weight is given (1.75 gram of glucose per kilogram of body weight in a specially prepared carbonated beverage). Specimens of blood and urine are secured at intervals for a period of 3 hours. Sometimes continued urine specimens are not ordered because it is not always easy to have a child void on cue.

Diagnosis of diabetes mellitus is made when the blood glucose levels are *greater than* the following normal levels:

110 mg./100 ml. While fasting
170 mg./100 ml. 1 hour ⎫ After ingestion
120 mg./100 ml. 2 hours ⎬ of standard
110 mg./100 ml. 3 hours ⎭ glucose load

Occasionally a physician will order a blood glucose determination 2 hours after a meal to evaluate glucose metabolism. This is termed a "postprandial specimen."

Treatment

The treatment of childhood diabetes mellitus always involves the injection of insulin. The amount and type of insulin prescribed will depend on the patient's caloric requirements (based on his weight, growth rate, and activity) and his individual response to therapy. Some children may be insulin resistant and require exceptionally large doses. In calculating a diabetic diet and the amount of insulin required, one must not only know the total amount of coloric intake derived from carbohydrates, fats, and proteins but also assure the patient an adequate intake of protein and sufficient minerals and vitamins for normal growth.

Basic philosophies. There are basically two different philosophies regarding the diet and management of the child diabetic patient. The traditional, or strict, approach recommends the prescription of a dietary formula based on the child's needs, which is followed closely. Advocates of this type of dietary supervision often believe that the best way for the diabetic patient to avoid complications is to strive toward a sugar-free urine at all times, that is, to be *aglycosuric.*

In recent years a more relaxed system of control has found favor with some physicians. It is usually called the *free,* or *glycosuric,* diet. It allows the patient more freedom of dietary choice and does not strive for sugar-free urine, only ketone-free urine. It counsels moderation in food intake with avoidance of rich carbohydrate or fatty foods. Advocates of this system believe that the frequency of complications is not any greater than when the stricter regimen is followed. It is true that some responsible teen-agers do much better psychologically with the free-type diet.

A middle-of-the-road dietary program is one that follows the American Diabetic Association (ADA) exchange system. A palatable diet should be designed to meet the nutritional needs for growth and physical activity. Calorie sources should be 50% carbohydrate, 15% to 20% protein, and 30% to 35% fat. A common method of calculating the diet assigns 1,000 calories to age 1 year and adds 100 calories per year up to 2,400 calories for girls. After age eleven, boys should add 200 calories rather than 100 calories per year to a total of 2,800 calories. The caloric intake should be divided into three meals and an added after-

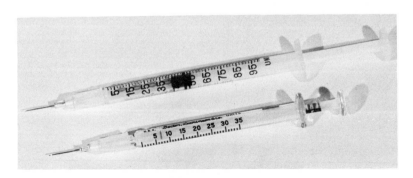

Fig. 36-7. Two types of U100 syringes. The smaller volume syringe that holds 35 units of U100 insulin is preferred in pediatrics.

noon and bedtime snack. A midmorning snack may be necessary for the younger child. Concentrated sweets should be restricted because they require little digestion and are rapidly absorbed into the blood, producing blood glucose levels that may exceed the insulin levels prescribed. This diet provides a fairly constant daily caloric intake, which should balance the same daily insulin regimen and thereby prevent excessive swings in the concentration of glucose in the blood. Effective control can usually be achieved without a strict dietary regimen. With the aid of the dietitian, the diet is adjusted according to the child's needs, family habits, and ethnic customs.

Insulin-food relationships. In the hospital the patient is almost always on a strict type of diet. No food or liquids should be given, with the exception of water or black coffee, without the physician's authorization. The patient should be encouraged to eat all the food served on his tray on time. (Before serving his tray, the nursing staff should determine whether he has received any ordered insulin. The type of insulin he receives will dictate when his meal should be served.) The diabetic patient's tray is returned by his nurse directly to the kitchen. The glucose content of any uneaten portion is calculated, and a replacement (usually a drink) that he must finish is sent to the patient. Any inability to eat or emesis should be promptly reported. The way in which the young patient is adhering to his diet should be carefully reported and recorded. Diet conferences in which the physician and dietitian work along with the older child may be arranged and are often profitable. Sometimes when a youngster feels that he has "made some of the rules," they are easier to keep.

Insulin dosage and administration. One of the essentials in the management of the child with diabetes is to provide a dosage of insulin that can effectively cover a 24-hour period. There are approximately seven types of insulin available on the market. Table 36-1 describes their administration

Table 36-1. Types and action of insulin

Insulin		Onset of action	Strength	Peak† (hours after injection)	Effective duration† (hours)	Time when hypoglycemia most likely occurs
Rapid-acting	Regular Semilente*	½ to 1 hour	U40, U80, U100 U40, U80, U100	2-4	6-8	10 A.M. to lunch
Intermediate-acting	NPH (neutral protamine Hagedorn) Lente* Globin	1 to 2 hours	U40, U80, U100 U40, U80, U100 U40, U80	8-10	12-16	3 P.M. to dinner
Long-acting	PZI (protamine zinc insulin) Ultralente*	4 to 6 hours	U40, U80, U100 U40, U80, U100	14-20	36-72	During night or early morning

*Semilente, Lente, and Ultralente insulins contain no protein.
†Peak and effective duration of action of insulin related to data found in continuous monitoring at the University of Missouri at Columbia. Data from Guthrie, D. W., and Guthrie, R. A.: Juvenile diabetes mellitus, Nurs. Clin. North Am. **8:**594, Dec., 1973.

and activity. They may be grouped as rapid, intermediate, or long acting.

The addition of crystalline zinc to regular insulin aids in preventing reaction at the injection sites but does not alter the basic activity of the medication. Regular or crystalline zinc insulin is used to combat acidosis. It has a rapid but relatively brief action. Many times both rapid-acting and intermediate-acting insulin will be prescribed together.

When a diabetic child is being regulated in the hospital, he is often placed on "regular insulin coverage." The amount of insulin he receives will depend on the amount of glucose found in his urine at specific times during the day. The sites of injection should be changed each day to prevent the atrophy of subcutaneous fat. The child should be taught to keep a record of the daily placement of his insulin. Children 7 and 8 years old often express curiosity about the process of preparing the dosage, and some (who are more dependable and composed) may even be capable of injecting themselves. Children must have considerable practice in preparing dosages with adequate supervision. They should also be taught about the actions of the different insulins in order to understand the relationship between regular, good dietary habits and insulin injections. Children and their parents need to know when the onset, and the peak of the prescribed insulin occur as well as its duration. For example, the onset (the time it takes to be absorbed) of regular insulin occurs ½ to 1 hour after it is injected. If the regular insulin is given at 7:30 A.M., breakfast should be given ½ hour later. The peak action of regular insulin occurs within 2 to 4 hours after injection, and a midmorning snack should be taken during the peak to prevent hypoglycemia. In 5 to 8 hours after the injection, the action of regular insulin has ceased and further injections are needed. The onset of intermediate-acting insulins—NPH (neutral protamine Hagedorn), Lente, and Globin—is 1 to 2 hours after injection. It should be given

early enough so that breakfast can be delayed for at least 1 hour. The peak action of these insulins occurs 8 to 10 hours after injection, and a snack should be given at that time, again to prevent hypoglycemia.

The duration of intermediate-acting insulins is now under study since some investigators feel that it has a shorter duration than previously noted.[*] If this proves to be true, then children will be given a second injection in late afternoon. A two-dose schedule has been used with success. A mixture of one-third regular and two-thirds intermediate-acting insulin is given early in the morning. The second injection consists of intermediate-acting insulin only and is given before supper. The insulin dose can be kept constant when the child and his parents are taught to anticipate his daily activities (exercise) and to vary the nutritional intake to meet his changing needs.

Insulin is a powerful medication, and in most hospitals any nurse giving insulin must show to another nurse the physician's order, the insulin bottle, and the dose drawn up in the syringe before it can be administered.

Insulin shock

Insulin itself may cause problems. Too much insulin may be just as disastrous as too little insulin. A balance between insulin need and insulin available must be maintained to avoid either diabetic acidosis or the other extreme known as insulin shock.

Unlike acidosis, insulin shock may develop quite rapidly, within minutes or hours. The rapidity with which the symptoms appear is greatly influenced by the type of insulin the patient is receiving because peaks of maximum effect differ, depending on the kind of insulin used.

One of the first signs of surplus insulin is a change in personality. This change will take various forms, depending on the patient, but each individual usually reacts in a way that is particularly characteristic for

[*]Guthrie, D. W., and Guthrie, R. A.: Juvenile diabetes mellitus, Nurs. Clin. North Am. **8:**595, Dec., 1973.

him. One may become irritable and edgy. Another may become excited. Some appear sluggish. Fatigue is a common complaint. If the student will recall the way she feels just before a needed lunch, she may be able to remember some of the signs and symptoms of insulin excess more easily. As the reaction increases, sudden, exaggerated hunger pangs, weakness, dizziness, blurred or double vision, dilated pupils, pallor, and rather profuse perspiration are noted. The patient may stagger. Adults suffering from reactions have been falsely accused of being drunk! If the condition is not relieved, the patient will develop deep shock, become unconscious, suffer from possible tremors or convulsions, and, if no treatment becomes available, eventually die.

Nurses and patients should be familiar with the early signs of insulin reaction so that it may be easily counteracted. Children usually learn to recognize their symptoms well. All diabetic persons should carry some rapidly available source of glucose with them in the event that they should feel the beginning of an insulin reaction. Usually a sugar lump or small piece of candy is recommended. In the hospital a small glass of orange juice or crackers are usually given. If no improvement is obtained in 15 minutes, additional food should be given. If it is difficult to get the child to take the necessary oral glucose, an intramuscular or subcutaneous injection of glucagon is ordered. Glucagon activates liver enzymes that break down liver glycogen to produce glucose. It must be remembered that glucagon will not work in the glycogen-depleted child. The family needs to know that glucagon should be given one time only for each episode, and that the child should be fed immediately. Glucagon is available in 1-mg. vials. The usual dose is 0.5 mg. (or ½ vial) for children under 3 years and 1 mg. for children 3 years and over. The intramuscular route is preferred because of more rapid absorption. It usually takes 10 to 20 minutes for glucagon to work. Sometimes intravenous administration by the physician of a 20% to 50% solution of glucose may be required. If the patient has been given a slow-acting, long-duration insulin, response to therapy for hypoglycemia may be slow and treatment more complex. The physician should always be notified of the occurrence of insulin reactions. When a patient complains of symptoms of possible reaction or the nurse is suspicious that such a process is occurring, the nurse should secure and test a current sample of urine if possible. If symptoms of shock are present, the test usually proves negative for glucose and acetone. At times it may be difficult to determine clinically whether the complaints and appearance of the patient are caused by the lack of glucose or too much glucose in the blood. If no laboratory test is feasible, glucagon or intravenous glucose is often ordered. If the difficulty is caused by insulin reaction, the patient responds. If it is not, no real harm will have been done. Insulin shock should be treated promptly. Prolonged, severe hypoglycemia may cause brain damage and subsequent mental deterioration, motor incoordination, and, of course, even death.

As you can see from Fig. 36-8, there are a number of causes of insulin surplus and resulting reaction. Probably the most common cause is uncompensated excessive exercise. Exercise causes sugar to be metabolized more effectively and reduces blood glucose levels. Unless insulin dosage is reduced or glucose intake is increased, insulin reaction is very likely in the presence of unplanned exercise. For this reason it is important for the diabetic child to have periods of regular exercise suitably spaced *after* meals and to recognize the possibility of needed adjustment to compensate for special activities.

Another cause of insulin reaction or shock is failure to eat the planned diet as prescribed (failure to eat enough or to space the food intake conscientiously). Diabetic patients often have ordered interval feedings in the midafternoon and at bedtime. The nurse should be sure that they are given to the patient and that they

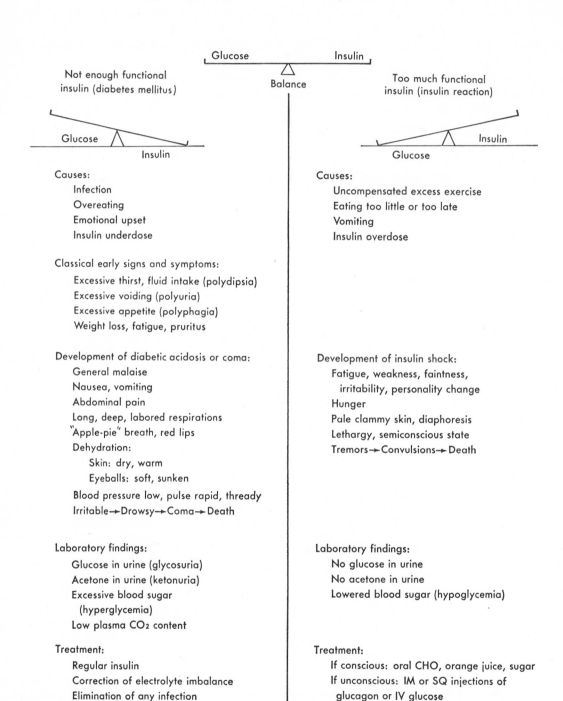

Glucose   Insulin

Balance

Not enough functional
insulin (diabetes mellitus)

Too much functional
insulin (insulin reaction)

Glucose

Insulin

Insulin

Glucose

Causes:
    Infection
    Overeating
    Emotional upset
    Insulin underdose

Classical early signs and symptoms:
    Excessive thirst, fluid intake (polydipsia)
    Excessive voiding (polyuria)
    Excessive appetite (polyphagia)
    Weight loss, fatigue, pruritus

Development of diabetic acidosis or coma:
    General malaise
    Nausea, vomiting
    Abdominal pain
    Long, deep, labored respirations
    "Apple-pie" breath, red lips
    Dehydration:
        Skin: dry, warm
        Eyeballs: soft, sunken
    Blood pressure low, pulse rapid, thready
    Irritable→Drowsy→Coma→Death

Laboratory findings:
    Glucose in urine (glycosuria)
    Acetone in urine (ketonuria)
    Excessive blood sugar
      (hyperglycemia)
    Low plasma CO_2 content

Treatment:
    Regular insulin
    Correction of electrolyte imbalance
    Elimination of any infection

Causes:
    Uncompensated excess exercise
    Eating too little or too late
    Vomiting
    Insulin overdose

Development of insulin shock:
    Fatigue, weakness, faintness,
      irritability, personality change
    Hunger
    Pale clammy skin, diaphoresis
    Lethargy, semiconscious state
    Tremors→Convulsions→Death

Laboratory findings:
    No glucose in urine
    No acetone in urine
    Lowered blood sugar (hypoglycemia)

Treatment:
    If conscious: oral CHO, orange juice, sugar
    If unconscious: IM or SQ injections of
      glucagon or IV glucose

Fig. 36-8. Glucose-insulin balance chart.

are consumed. If the child is nauseated or has an emesis, this should be immediately reported because this condition may also cause an insulin surplus. Meals must be served on time; a long delay after the injection of regular insulin also sets the stage for an episode of hypoglycemia.

Difficulties in determining the regulated doses of insulin may also be a source of glucose-insulin imbalance. The patient may not respond to the dosage as expected. Errors in insulin administration resulting in an overdose are also a real possibility. Great care must be taken in reading the orders and in preparing the injection. One strength (U100) insulin, which is now recommended can be given with much less confusion. If the nurse has been given medical permission to mix two types of insulin in the same syringe, she must be sure of her technique.

1. Inject just enough replacement air into the bottle of cloudy insulin without dipping the injecting needle into the insulin. Remove the needle from the bottle.
2. Withdraw the clear, regular insulin into the syringe, using the proper scale.
3. Withdraw the cloudy insulin into the syringe, using the proper scale.
4. Put an air bubble into the syringe and rock the syringe back and forth to mix the two types.

This technique must be followed in order to prevent the conversion of rapid-acting insulin into a longer-acting type by inadvertent injection of long-acting insulin into a vial of regular insulin.

Because diabetic patients may develop important complications if infection occurs, the technique of preparation and injection should be particularly meticulous.

Acidosis

Acidosis, the opposite body condition from insulin shock, occurs when the insulin available in the blood is insufficient to metabolize the glucose present. We have already discussed the development of acido-

sis in untreated diabetic persons. Treated diabetic patients may occasionally have problems with acidosis.

The most frequent cause for the development of acidosis in a treated diabetic patient is the onset of infection, any infection. Infection greatly intensifies the body's need for insulin, and unless insulin dosage is increased, acidosis may result. Infections of the skin are quite common in diabetic patients. Pruritus is a fairly frequent complaint. At times a vulvitis is the problem that brings the patient to the physician, and diabetes mellitus is subsequently diagnosed. Close attention must be paid to preventing infection and treating vigorously any infection present. Special care of the toenails and feet is encouraged. Nurses do not cut the toenails of diabetic patients.

Failing to follow the prescribed diet or "snitching sweets" may be a possible problem. It takes a great deal of self-understanding and self-discipline to refrain from eating some of the tempting but forbidden foods available, especially if one feels hungry. The development of self-direction and self-control is paramount for the young diabetic person, particularly the young adolescent. Dietary discipline should be encouraged by allowing the youngster to express his frustrations, providing as much variety in the diet as possible, allowing him to participate in its planning, and possibly making provision for a *rare* special treat. With the advent of so many 1-calorie soft drinks, the social life of the teen-ager with diabetes mellitus is a bit less strained. However, he should be cautioned that the label "dietetic foods" does not necessarily mean "foods for the diabetic." The child should be made to believe that ultimately the only person he cheats is himself when he knowingly chooses unwisely or tries to falsify urine tests.

Emotional upset also increases the possibility of acidosis. The insulin requirement rises in periods of stress. The emotionally stable child is much easier to regulate with insulin than a child with many emotional problems.

The difficulty determining the proper dosage of insulin has already been described. Possible errors in the administration of insulin that can result in an underdose as well as an overdose have also been discussed.

Urine tests

Long before the child is ready to give his own insulin injection he will be able to test his urine for the presence of glucose and acetone. Several types of tests for glycosuria are available. They are of varying convenience and expense. In the hospital, Clinitest tablets are usually employed (Fig. 36-9). But any of the commercially available preparations are acceptable, and all simple to use. Urine analysis for the presence of acetone is also routine. The mechanics of these various tests are described on pp. 411 and 412.

Because the type and dosage of insulin must be individualized for each child, all diabetic regimen must utilize some method for monitoring control. Urine glucose tests serve as the most useful guides to assess the level of control. Four kinds of urine specimens may be obtained:

1. The fractional quantitative urine glucose method provides an accurate estimation of diabetic control and pinpoints the time of day when control is poor. When the physician orders fractional specimens, the total urine output between testings is saved. Then at the time of the scheduled urine examination, the entire collected volume is mixed, and tests are made on a specimen from the total volume. For example, Johnny is asked to void at 8:00 A.M. This voiding is added to the urine collection started the previous night for the period from 8:00 P.M. (bedtime) until 8:00 A.M. The collection is mixed and a small amount of the mixture tested. Then the collection is discarded. The next time Johnny voids, the total voiding is placed in the large, empty, clean collection bottle. If he voids again, this voiding, too, is put in the collection bottle. At 12:00 P.M. he is asked to void, and the complete voiding is added to the collection. The urine is mixed and a specimen tested. Four such volumes

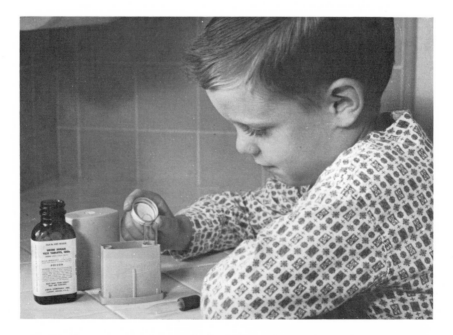

Fig. 36-9. "You're not supposed to touch the tablet with your fingers." Clinitest analysis of urine.

are collected as follows: (1) 8:00 A.M. to noon; (2) noon to 4:00 P.M., (3) 4:00 P.M. to 8:00 P.M., and (4) 8:00 P.M. to 8:00 A.M.

Peak action of the various insulins can be evaluated during these periods. Period 1 reflects rapid-acting insulins; periods 2 and 3 reflect intermediate-acting insulins; and period 4 reflects a 4:30 P.M. second dose of an intermediate- or a long-acting insulin that had been given in the morning. Children in "good control" can tolerate a spill of about 20 to 60 gm. of glucose per day and still maintain normal growth and development. The 24-hour fractional quantitative urine glucose test provides information about the total grams of glucose excreted along with the volume, which helps to accurately assess insulin therapy and enables the physician to make the necessary adjustments.

Periodically, the child's clinical course must be evaluated. Parents (or the child himself) are asked to make several 4-hour urine collections at the same time on different days. Children need not be hospitalized for revaluation because urine should be collected on a "typical" day in terms of nutritional intake, exercise, and emotional stress. When these inherent limitations are considered, the pattern of glucose metabolism and insulin-glucose balance derived from the urine test can be profitably used for adjustments in diabetic therapy.

2. A 24-hour urine collection may be ordered while the child is in the hospital. This is a pooling of the four fractional specimens.

3. The single voided specimen method is a modification of the fractional method. Separate specimens are not collected in a container; rather, the urine is retained in the bladder. If the child is able to retain all his urine during the four intervals, this method of quantitative analysis may be more convenient.

4. The qualitative double-voided specimen method is commonly used. The test reflects the blood glucose level at that moment. Urine specimens are usually secured and tested half an hour before sched-uled meals (that is, at 7:30 A.M., 11:30 A.M., 4:30 P.M., and bedtime). The patient is asked to void (empty his bladder) at 7:00 A.M. Then he is given a glass of water. A portion of the 7:00 A.M. specimen is saved but will be discarded later if it is not needed. At 7:30 A.M. the patient is asked to void again, and a portion of this specimen is tested and reported. The procedure is repeated before lunch, before dinner, and before bedtime. However, practically speaking, it is sometimes difficult for a child to produce the needed urine specimen on schedule. If the second specimen is not forthcoming, the first specimen secured (which had not been thrown away) will be tested, reported, and recorded.

Review of nursing responsibility

The nursing care of the diabetic patient has been discussed throughout this section; however, the following questions should be of assistance in aiding the nurse to organize and evaluate her care:

1. Insulin requirement. Do you know the type of insulin your patient is receiving and when he receives his injections? Do you know how his injections are being rotated?
2. Diet. Do you know what type of diet the physician has prescribed? If a strict diet is ordered (usually the case), have you made sure that your patient has eaten everything or has received a replacement? Do you evaluate his meals for variety and interest? Do you watch for and limit the possibility of the patient obtaining food not calculated in his diet? Does he have a scheduled interval nourishment?
3. Urine testing. Do you know the method to be used? Are you collecting the specimens properly?
4. General hygiene. Is the patient getting as much exercise as possible so that his insulin requirement (because of differences in amounts of exercise taken) will not change greatly on discharge? Is his skin in good condition?

631

Are there any signs of infection anywhere in the body?

5. Glucose-insulin imbalance. Do you know the signs and symptoms of developing insulin shock and acidosis?

6. Patient-parent education and participation. Are you assisting the patient and his parents in learning more about the disease and its treatment and control, depending on their level of understanding? Are you helping the patient to develop attitudes of self-control and feelings of achievement and well-being? Does the child keep records of his insulin intake, urine tests, and general health? How much is he able to participate in his care?

7. What special interests and aspirations does this patient have?

8. What has this patient taught you?

For a diabetic patient to become a contributing citizen in the community and enjoy life to its maximum, he must understand his disease, accept the limitations it imposes, and learn to function in a relatively independent setting. The alert, intelligent, warm-hearted nurse can do much to help him meet these goals.

It is very helpful for patients with diabetes mellitus to be able to room together. They usually are mutually supportive and learn from one another. (Most of the time such learning is positive and beneficial.) Children with this disorder should be encouraged to participate in school, church, and community activities and not look on their metabolic problem as an excuse for difficult behavior or special privileges. The fact that they have diabetes mellitus should not be hidden. Teachers, schoolmates, and employers should be aware of the presence of the condition. In many states there are special summer camping experiences set up for children with this disorder. These 2-week sessions have been of great help to many youngsters.

• • •

A source of much pleasure and occasional pain, the digestive system continually struggles to meet the challenges of unskilled cooks, individual abuse, and emotional stress. Nurses should be able to help prevent or ease some of the difficulties faced by this sensitive body servant. In so doing, they fulfill part of their obligation to the individual whose total well-being is their concern.

37

Conditions involving the genitourinary system

URINARY SYSTEM

The urinary system consists of two kidneys, two ureters, the bladder, and the urethra (Fig. 37-1). The primary function of these organs is to excrete metabolic waste products and other substances not necessary in the blood.

To regulate the composition of blood, the kidneys perform the complex task of secreting urine. The ureters, bladder, and urethra are involved in the transportation, storage, and elimination of the urine.

Kidneys

The kidneys are paired organs located on either side of the vetrebral column, just above the waistline. They lie outside the peritoneal cavity against the posterior abdominal wall.

In the adult the kidneys are about 4½ inches long and 2½ inches wide; they are somewhat bean shaped. On the medial border of each kidney is a concave notch called the *hilus.* The renal artery, renal vein, nerves, and ureter join the kidney at the hilus.

When describing the internal structure of the organ, one may speak of two areas: the functioning portion, the *parenchyma,* and the collecting portion, the *pelvis.* A longitudinal section of the kidney reveals that the parenchyma in turn is composed of two parts: an outer portion called the *cortex* and an inner portion called the *medulla.* The pelvis is formed by the expansion of the upper end of the ureter. The pelvis subdivides to form the major and minor *calyces.*

The physiological structural unit of the kidney is called the *nephron.* The nephron consists of the renal corpuscle plus its tubule. The renal corpuscle consists of the glomerulus (a cluster of connecting capillaries) and Bowman's capsule, into which the capillaries protrude. The proximal and distal convoluted tubules, the loop of Henle, and the renal corpuscle constitute a nephron. The blood supply of the nephron comes from microscopic branches of the renal artery. The renal corpuscle and the convoluting tubules are located in the cortex of the kidney, the loop of Henle and the collecting tubules are located in the medulla. Each kidney contains more than 1 million nephrons.

The kidneys perform the complex task of removing toxic metabolic wastes, such as urea and uric acid, and excessive nontoxic substances, such as water and electrolytes, from the blood. In this way the kidneys regulate the composition and volume of blood. The kidneys also influence blood pressure through complex intermediary mechanisms.

Three processes are involved in the production of urine: filtration, reabsorption, and secretion.

1. *Filtration* takes place under the influence of blood pressure in the renal corpuscle. A single arteriole forms each glomerulus. Water and nonprotein solutes filter out of the glomerulus through Bowman's capsule. Blood cells, platelets, and plasma proteins, due to their large size, are not normally filtered by the glomeruli.

2. *Reabsorption* takes place through the walls of the convoluted tubules and Henle's loop. By means of a highly selective and discriminating process,

633

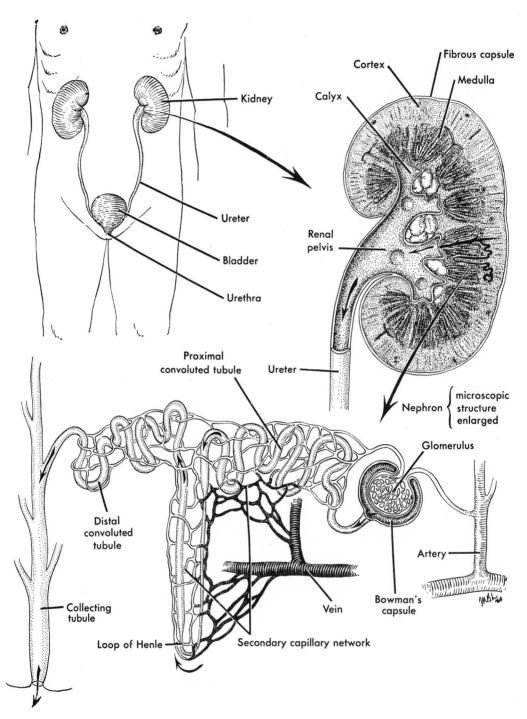

Fig. 37-1. Gross and microscopic structures of the urinary system.

the cells of the tubule efficiently reabsorb certain amounts of water, glucose, and electrolytes. This reclamation process is vital to the maintenance of the fluid and electrolyte balance of the body.

3. *Secretion* takes place in the convoluting tubules. A number of substances are secreted directly into the tubule from the secondary capillary network. In the proximal convoluting tubules, penicillin, iodopyracet (Diodrast), phenolsulfonphthalein, hippuric acid, and creatinine are among the substances secreted and excreted. In the distal convoluting tubule, hydrogen ions and ammonia are secreted in the varying amounts necessary to control and maintain the acid-base balance of the body.

The final filtrate, urine, passes from the distal convoluting tubule into the straight collecting tubule and into the renal pelvis.

In the normal adult approximately 190 liters of blood are filtered through the glomeruli daily. The tubules reclaim about 188.5 liters of filtrate. The remaining filtrate is excreted as urine. The average daily urinary output is about 1,500 ml. In children the daily output of urine varies greatly with the size of the child and his fluid intake.

Ureters

In the adult the ureters are small tubes about ⅕ inch in diameter and 12 inches in length. (The size varies with age.) The expanded upper end of the ureter collects the urine as it forms, and peristaltic waves convey the urine down the ureters and into the bladder. The ureters lie behind the peritoneum and descend from the kidney to the posterior bladder wall. They enter the bladder in an oblique manner, which prevents reflux, or the backflow of urine.

Bladder

The bladder is a dome-shaped, hollow, muscular sac that stores urine. It is located directly behind the symphysis pubis. Three layers of smooth muscle form the bladder wall. These three muscular layers are collectively called the *detrusor muscle*. The outlet of the bladder is surrounded by a band of smooth muscle known as the internal sphincter. The bladder outlet and the two ureteral openings outline a triangular area called the *trigone*.

The detrusor muscle is usually relaxed, allowing the bladder to expand as needed to accommodate urine storage. After a certain volume of urine is collected, the urge to void is felt. In the child this urge is usually recognized when the bladder contains approximately 200 ml. The desire to void is recorded by the sensory parasympathetic endings in the detrusor muscle. If the child decides to void, the detrusor muscle contracts, the internal sphincter opens, and urine enters the posterior urethra. Voiding may be postponed, but when the bladder becomes very full, a point is reached at which even the most desperate efforts can no longer retain the urine.

Urethra

The urethra is a small tube that serves as a passageway for the elimination of urine from the bladder. The external opening of the urethra is called the *urinary meatus*.

The urethra is a comparatively short tube in the adult female; it is about 1½ inches long. In the midportion of the female urethra is a circular striated muscle that forms the external sphincter.

The male urethra is about 8 inches long and also serves as part of the reproductive tract. It is divided into three sections: prostatic, membranous, and penile. The prostatic urethra is about 1 inch long and extends from the internal sphincter of the bladder through the prostate gland to the pelvic floor. The membranous urethra is about ½ inch long and lies between the prostatic and penile sections of the urethra; it is surrounded by the extenal sphincter. The penile urethra is about 6 inches long and extends through the penis, terminating at the urethral meatus.

Urine

Urine is a transparent, amber-colored liquid with a characteristic odor. It is usually acid in reaction. The specific gravity of urine ranges from 1.003 to 1.030. Approximately 95% of urine is water. The remaining 5% consists of wastes from protein metabolism and inorganic components such as sodium and potassium chloride.

The examination of urine is the keystone in diagnosing disorders of the urinary system. A properly collected specimen can yield a wealth of information about renal function and the nature of kidney disorders. Urinalysis also reveals much information about infections and toxic and metabolic disorders.

KEY VOCABULARY

anuria failure of kidney function; lack of urine formation.

albuminuria presence of albumin in the urine.

enuresis bed-wetting at an age when urinary control should be present.

frequency number of repetitions of a periodic process in a unit of time; when speaking of urinary function, the term implies an abnormal increase in the number of voidings.

hematuria presence of blood in the urine.

nocturia excessive urination during the night.

oliguria diminished amount of urine production with subsequent scanty urination.

polyuria abnormally increased urinary output.

proteinuria finding of protein, usually albumin, in the urine.

reflux return or backward flow (e.g., regurgitation of urine from the bladder into the ureter).

uremia toxic condition associated with renal insufficiency and the retention in the blood of nitrogenous substances normally excreted by the kidney.

ANOMALIES OF THE GENITOURINARY TRACT
THE INFANT

The embryological development of the urinary system is closely related to the development of the genital organs in both sexes. Because of this factor, genital and urinary tract deformities will be discussed together. Genitourinary deformities comprise 30% to 40% of all congenital anomalies.

Often a deformity of the genitalia is accompanied by a deformity of the upper urinary tract. Deformities are multiple in approximately 20% of cases and often accompany anomalies in other systems, for example, imperforate anus.

Malformations of the genitourinary tract may lead to death. When the anomaly can be recognized early, surgical correction or treatment is lifesaving. This is true because many anomalies are obstructive and lead to hydronephrosis, which ultimately results in renal failure.

External deformities are obvious and readily detected. However, there is little evidence of internal disease unless it is far advanced. The nurse should be aware of this and know the few signals demanding close observation. It is important to note the number and amount of voidings in the newborn infant. Failure to void within the first 24 hours after birth is a danger sign and should be reported to the physician immediately. Abdominal enlargement or swelling in the area of a kidney also warrants immediate attention.

The signs and symptoms of urinary problems in older children are more easily detected. Crying on urination, urgent and frequent urination, straining to void, and dribbling all may point to genitourinary system difficulties. Unexplained fever, lassitude, weight loss, and failure to thrive are nondescript symptoms but may relate to advanced disease. Serious kidney infections often run a silent course. It is always wise to investigate any of the above signals, since renal failure can be the result of a hidden anomaly.

Renal agenesis

Bilateral renal agenesis is incompatible with life. Autopsy has revealed that it is more common in males than females and not as rare as once believed. *Unilateral renal agenesis* is compatible with life, but the single kidney is more apt to be diseased, since it is often located in the pelvis and associated with other malformations, especially of the ureter.

Double kidney

Duplication of the kidney and ureter is more common in girls than in boys. The ureters from each double kidney may enter the bladder at different points or may unite to enter the bladder as one ureter. Sometimes the ureter from the upper kidney enters the genitourinary tract ectopically, and may cause incontinence. Duplication of the kidney and ureter is clinically significant only when other anomalies causing obstruction or infection exist.

Horseshoe kidney

A horseshoe kidney results when the lower ends of both kidneys fuse, forming a single mass shaped like a horeshoe. The kidneys lie closer to the spine and usually lower than separate kidneys do. Horseshoe kidney may be asymptomatic, but complications, especially infection, are common.

Polycystic kidney

True polycystic disease is always congenital and always bilateral. Polycystic kidneys are larger than the normal kidneys and sometimes are huge, filling the entire abdomen. They contain innumerable cysts, compressing the parenchyma. Such kidneys are constantly prone to infection, obstruction, and stone formation. Treatment can only be palliative. Some children live many years with the condition.

Ureterocele

A ureterocele may be described as a ballooning of the lower end of the ureter because of an abnormally narrow ureteral orifice. Ureteroceles are usually unilateral. Double ureters are commonly associated with the anomaly. When there is an extra ureter, the one that enters the bladder normally is often distorted by the enormous ureterocele. As a result, it becomes obstructed, and kidney infection may ensue. Treatment consists of excising the redundant portion and reconstructing the orifice so that obstruction is eliminated. If an obstruction does not exist, treatment is symptomatic.

Exstrophy of the bladder

Exstrophy of the bladder, fortunately, is a rare condition. It ranks with the most severe anomalies of mankind. Because of a defect in midline closure associated with incomplete development of the pubic arch, the interior of the bladder lies completely exposed through an opening in the lower abdominal wall. A number of genital anomalies may accompany the defect.

The child becomes foul smelling because he is constantly soaked in urine. Often the surrounding skin becomes excoriated, causing great pain. Early in life, the exposed bladder mucosa becomes inflamed, bleeds readily, and is acutely sensitive. Infection is frequent but can usually be controlled by antibiotic therapy.

Treatment is surgical. An anatomical reconstruction of the bladder is the operation of choice. The most desired time for this operation is when the child is between 12 and 18 months old, when he is old enough and strong enough to tolerate a long operative procedure. After this operation, the child is totally incontinent for a period of years; during this time the bladder grows sufficiently to make antireflux operations possible. When the bladder (vesicle) sphincters are made more complete and function somewhat normally, efforts can be directed to make the child continent. Dilatation of the ureter, reflux, and chronic infection often occur when the child is rendered continent too early.

When the ureters are enlarged or the kidney damaged by infection, anatomical reconstruction of the bladder is contraindicated. Other methods of diverting the urine, especially ileal bladder or conduit procedures, are employed.

Exstrophy of the bladder is compatible with life, and the prognosis depends in great measure on the extent of renal damage resulting from defective drainage and infection.

Hypospadias

Hypospadias is a common deformity in which the urethra terminates at some point

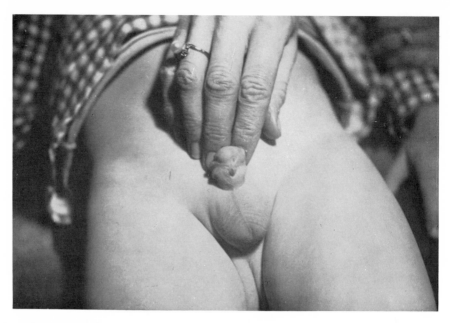

Fig. 37-2. Hypospadias (meatus located on undersurface of penis). (Courtesy Matthew Gleason, M.D., San Diego, Calif.)

on the ventral (under) surface of the penis (Fig. 37-2). The position of the urethra on the penis or perineum will determine the type of treatment. When the urethra terminates near the glans, a high circumcision is performed so that the child can learn to direct his urine stream. Because the prostatic urethra is never involved in hypospadias, the sphincters function normally and the child has good urinary control. Often a meatal stricture is associated with varying degrees of hypospadias. When such a stricture is recognized, it is easily corrected by dilatation or meatotomy.

In the more severe types, a cordlike anomaly may arc the penis downward (chordee). These more extensive deformities all require surgical repair to establish normal control of voiding and make normal reproduction possible later in life. Boys with severe types of hypospadias should not be circumcised, since the foreskin is needed in the repair.

Treatment. Operative repair is usually done in two stages before the child enters school. In this way the child avoids severe ridicule and lasting psychological problems.

The chordee is released early to straighten the penis and allow for normal growth. This is accomplished in the first-stage operation when the child is 2 years of age. When the child is 4 years old or whenever the amount of local tissue permits, a second-stage operation (urethroplasty) is performed. Various plastic techniques have been employed to correct hypospadias, but the Denis Browne technique seems to be most successful.

The difficulties encountered in achieving a successful result in the correction of hypospadias are considerable. The parents should be well aware that more than one operation is usually required. They should also know that after a successful urethroplasty the penis will show scars and that some penile bowing may remain even though the child is able to urinate normally.

Postoperative care. When surgery is completed, the penis is wrapped in petroleum gauze and then covered with a dry gauze bandage. This helps to prevent postoperative swelling, pain, and bleeding. Unless this precaution is taken, necrosis of the glans may occur. A catheter drains the bladder while the incision is healing. The nurse must observe the patient carefully for signs of swelling and bleeding.

After the operations the child is kept on his back. A bed cradle helps to prevent pressure on the operative area. Many times, Stile's dressing will be used (Fig. 36-4).

On the second postoperative day the child may be allowed freedom of movement in his crib, provided the nurse can take time to sit, talk, and play with him. She should attempt to keep his hands busy lest he busy them with his dressing. Parents should be encouraged to stay with their children because they are usually best able to keep them constructively occupied.

Epispadias

When the urethra opens on the dorsal (upper) surface of the penis, the condition is called epispadias. Various degrees of epispadias may occur. However, the deformity is uncommon except when associated with exstrophy of the bladder. Treatment is the same as that for hypospadias or exstrophy.

Intersexual anomalies

A semiemergency exists when simple inspection of the newborn infant's genitalia does not reveal the sex of the child. Chromosome studies are usually helpful in these cases. Exploratory abdominal surgery for gonadal biopsy may also be undertaken to identify the sex of the sexually indeterminate child.

Pseudohermaphroditism

When an individual possesses external genitalia resembling those of one sex and the gonads of the opposing sex, the condition resulting is termed "pseudohermaphroditism." Sometimes a severe hypospadias with undescended testicles or a hypertrophied clitoris and malformed labia cause problems in sex identification. Female pseudohermaphrodites possess ovaries but their external genitalia mimic those of the male. Such masculinization of the female infant is due to an overdeveloped adrenal cortex

(congenital adrenal hyperplasia) and subsequent increased production of male sex hormones (androgens) by the adrenal glands. Male pseudohermaphrodites are chromosomal males, but due to testicular dysfunction and/or other problems, sexual ambiguity is present.

Whatever the condition, it should be corrected but only after the true sex has been determined. Treatment usually consists of corrective plastic procedures on the external genitalia and/or the administration of appropriate missing hormones.

Hermaphroditism

An extremely rare condition exists when a child possesses gonads and genitalia of both sexes. Prompt attention to this problem lessens the possibilities of serious emotional sequelae. Treatment consists of removing the gonads of one sex. Acceptable female genitalia may often be formed by relatively simple procedures. For this practical reason, when a choice can be made, the male gonad tissues are removed and the child is made female. Conversion of sex should be done as soon as possible so that the individual may have an opportunity for a normal, happy, and successful life.

Undescended testicle (cryptorchidism)

Failure of the testes to descend into the scrotum affects about 1% of the male population. The condition is usually unilateral. Frequently an inguinal hernia is present.

There are usually no symptoms associated with undescended testicles except for some tenderness in the inguinal canal. Injury to the testicle is more likely to occur if it is confined to the inguinal canal than if it is in normal scrotal position. Torsion of the undescended testicle may take place, necessitating prompt surgical relief (see p. 469). Development of testicular malignancy is more common in cases of cryptorchidism. Lack of correction may also lead to severe psychological difficulties.

Spontaneous descent, if forthcoming, is usually completed by the first year. If spontaneous descent does not occur, treatment consists of injections of human chorionic gonadotropin (HCG). HCG is believed to lengthen the spermatic cord, allowing the testicle to descend. If this fails, then surgical means are employed to bring the testicle into the scrotum. The optimum age for this procedure (orchiopexy) is disputed. Most physicians agree that after age 10 the testicle will begin to degenerate if not brought down. However, the child with an undescended testicle is often the subject of ridicule and may develop feelings of inferiority. Since normal location of the testicle assures fewer possible complications, it is best that orchiopexy be done before school age. Results of treatment are usually good in unilateral cryptorchidism.

THE TODDLER
Infections of the urinary tract

Whenever a significant number of bacteria (colony counts above 100,000 per milliliter) are found in a urine specimen, one knows that a significant infection of the urinary tract is present. Urinary tract infections are always considered serious and are often difficult to eradicate. Such infections are thought to rank second in frequency only to infections of the respiratory tract.

Ascending infection via the urethra and lower urinary tract is by far the most common way in which urinary tract infections occur. Other routes of infection are the bloodstream and lymphatics. A wide variety of organisms may produce urinary tract infection, but the colon bacilli are responsible for the majority of infections. Repeated infections necessitate a complete evaluation of the urinary tract. An intravenous urogram and a voiding cystourethrogram are necessary to assess renal impairment and the presence of reflux.

Reflux

The incidence of reflux (regurgitation of urine from the bladder into the ureter) detected by cystourethrography during investigation of persistent lower urinary tract infection is significant. It is thought that inflammatory changes in the bladder caused by infection may render the junction of the ureters and bladder temporarily incompetent. Most of these children do well when they receive intensive and specific antimicrobial therapy. There is no progression of renal damage, and reflux frequently disappears.

The diagnosis of primary reflux is considered if infection and reflux persists with renal impairment. Primary reflux seems to be most common in girls with congenitally deficient ureterobladder junction mechanisms. An extensive evaluation of the lower urinary tract reveals an increased reflux but a normal urethra and no significant residual urine or bladder abnormalities. If children with primary reflux continually harbor infection while receiving medication, have persistent recurrence of infection after adequate medical management, and show evidence of continuous renal impairment, surgical intervention is usually required to eliminate reflux and prevent progressive renal damage. The defect is then corrected by reimplanting the ureter into the bladder.

Nursing care. The general postoperative care of this patient is much the same as any surgical patient. The nurse should recognize the importance of changing surgical dressings that have become saturated with urine. Urine is an excellent medium for the growth of bacteria. However, she should be aware that some surgical drains may be purposely attached to the dressings, and special care is therefore required. Some physicians wish to change the dressings themselves for this reason. Drainage tubes must be carefully checked for patency. These postoperative patients may return to the nursing area with as many as five urinary catheters, depending on the extent of the surgery (two nephrostomy tubes inserted into the left and right flanks, draining each kidney pelvis, one suprapubic cystotomy tube that empties the bladder of any urine not drained via the nephrostomy tubes, and two ureteral catheters acting as splints for the newly implanted ureters). Drainage from each of the tubes present should be closely observed and recorded separately. These catheters are never clamped. When the patient is able to be up in a wheelchair, the catheters should be arranged so that they do not kink. The collection bottles must hang below the level of the kidneys, draining freely. Water intake is always encouraged and recorded, particularly in young children who quickly dehydrate. Dehydration promotes the growth of bacteria.

Pain is commonly associated with this type of surgery. Narcotics should be given as ordered on time! Antispasmodic drugs such as propantheline bromide (Pro-Banthine) or methantheline bromide (Banthine bromide) are also ordered. These drugs usually relieve the immediate postoperative colicky pain.

Reflux associated with renal involvement may also be caused by lower tract congenital obstructions. Unless the obstruction is corrected by reconstructive surgery when indicated, pyelonephritis may progress, leading to severe renal impairment.

Pyelonephritis

Pyelonephritis is an infectious process involving the renal pelvis and the working units of the kidney, the nephrons. Infections of the ureter and bladder often coexist. Pyelonephritis is recurrent in nature and is often characterized by repetitive exacerbations of one underlying and continuous infection.

Etiology. Ascending infection is the usual cause of pyelonephritis. Some type of obstructive process may be the causative factor. Infection itself frequently causes inflammation, which leads to scarring and obstruction. Obstruction leads to urinary stasis and persistent infection. Thus both infection and obstruction may assist in perpetuating a chronic infection that proceeds to progressive renal destruction.

Incidence. Pyelonephritis is a common renal disease of childhood. Because of the relatively short female urethra and the ease with which fecal contamination of the urethral orifice may occur, girls' urine is infected at least ten times more frequently

than that of boys. In the cases characterized by obstruction, boys are affected two times more frequently than girls and usually have symptoms before 3 years of age.

Clinical symptoms. Symptoms vary considerably in pyelonephritis. In children under 3 years of age the onset is likely to be abrupt and severe, accompanied by a high temperature, which may reach 104° F. Pallor, anorexia, vomiting, diarrhea, and convulsions may occur. These *acute* symptoms usually disappear in a few days with appropriate treatment.

Older children complain of localized discomfort. Sharp or dull pain in the flank or abdominal tenderness is described. Bladder symptoms such as frequent, urgent, and burning urination are also common complaints. In addition to these problems, chills and fever may be present. Some children demonstrate little or no fever, and symptoms suggestive of pyelonephritis may be almost totally lacking.

In either case, failure to recognize that infection persists allows the slow, but ultimate, destruction of renal substance.

Chronic pyelonephritis occurs over a long period and progresses slowly over many years. As the result of continuous low-grade infection, the patient with pyelonephritis characteristically has a history of recurrent bouts of nonspecific symptoms such as nausea, vomiting, diarrhea, fever, irritability, headache, and transitory urinary abnormalities. Poor general health, anemia, failure to grow, or failure to thrive are typical findings. The child may appear very pale or pasty looking. This condition suggests the late stages of renal damage and the development of uremia. Hypertension frequently appears as the end result of advanced renal scarring and vascular impairment and often accounts for subsequent cerebral hemorrhage or cardiac failure.

Treatment. Urinalysis of a properly collected specimen is the key to successful treatment. Therapy depends primarily on identification of the causative organism and detection and correction of any urinary ab-

641

normality. A carefully collected specimen is essential. The genitalia should be washed, rinsed, and then sponged with a 1:750 benzalkonium chloride (Zephiran) solution, and dried with a sterile pad.

A clean, midstream voided specimen is collected and promptly sent to the laboratory for culture and sensitivity studies. If it is impossible to obtain a specimen by such means, a catheterized specimen may be ordered. Prompt therapy is indicated. Sulfonamides or broad-spectrum antibiotics are administered until the laboratory studies are complete. Specific medications are then ordered and continued for at least 10 days to 2 weeks.

The patient should be placed in bed in a cool, quiet environment until his fever has subsided. A tepid sponge bath may also be ordered. Fluids are encouraged to ensure adequate hydration and a good urine output. An accurate account of the fluid intake and urinary output is essential. Although it is not necessary to insert a catheter for accurate output, a check mark is not sufficient for the information needed. An estimation of the amount of diaper saturation is far more valuable. After removing the diaper, the nurse should carefully wash and dry the child's genitalia before applying the clean diaper. This will prevent further contamination and also protect the skin from becoming irritated and excoriated.

An adequate diet is very important, and every attempt should be made to give the child food that he is able to eat and will eat. A good milk intake will supply the needed protein, carbohydrate, fat, and, most of all, water. Encourage the parents to visit during feeding time. Parents are best able to understand the sick child's desires, and usually the child is more likely to eat for Mom. A daily check of weight, blood pressure, and vital signs offers valuable clues in the early detection of complications.

Prognosis. When the disease is recognized early and treated properly (long-term antibiotic therapy for infection or sur-

gical removal of obstructions), the prognosis is excellent. Chronic infections present a much more serious and difficult problem because severe renal damage is the ultimate result.

Wilms' tumor

Wilms' tumor is one of the most common abdominal neoplasms of childhood. It is a congenital, mixed renal tumor, which develops from abnormal embryonic tissue; it rarely occurs bilaterally. Composed of connective tissue, muscle, blood vessels, glands, and lymphatics, the tumor grows within the renal capsule. Although it distorts the kidney in a bizarre manner, the tumor usually does not invade the renal substance until late in the disease. It grows forward and downward and may occupy as much as half the abdominal cavity. Unfortunately, the tumor often invades the renal veins and metastasizes through the bloodstream to vital organs, especially to the lungs.

Etiology. Like other forms of cancer, the exact cause of Wilms' tumor is unknown.

Incidence. Wilms' tumor accounts for approximately 10% of all cancer in children. Boys and girls are equally affected. About two thirds of all children with Wilms' tumor are diagnosed before 3 years of age. The tumor may be present at birth and is rare after 7 years of age.

Clinical features. The initial manifestation of Wilms' tumor is a mass in the region of the kidney that is often discovered accidently during a routine examination or in the course of daily care. As the tumor grows, the child's abdomen becomes very large, and pressure symptoms soon arise. Constipation, vomiting, abdominal distention, and even dyspnea may occur. Weight loss, pallor, and anemia are common in the late stages. Pain, hematuria, and hypertension are not common but, if present, usually indicate an advanced stage with a grave prognosis.

Treatment and nursing care. When Wilms' tumor is suspected, both the mother and nurse must be careful not to feel or touch the child's abdomen because handling might cause metastasis. Diagnosis is usually confirmed by intravenous pyelography. Occasionally retrograde pyelography and renal arteriography are necessary for differential diagnosis. Treatment consists of prompt surgical removal of the involved kidney. Dissemination of tumor cells sometimes occurs during the operation. Dactinomycin and x-ray therapy are effective against the malignant cells. They may be used preoperatively to reduce the size of the kidney and tumor, rendering removal of the mass easier. Both are administered postoperatively to prevent metastasis. Dactinomycin is given intravenously during surgery, and x-ray therapy may be started before the child awakens from anesthesia. Dactinomycin sensitizes the child to x-ray therapy; therefore, the dosage of radiation is decreased considerably when combined with systemic administration of dactinomycin. This course of treatment is continued intermittently over a 2-year period.

The kidney and perirenal fat are removed through a transabdominal approach. Blood transfusions are often given to replace blood lost during the surgical procedure and to correct preexisting anemia. Intravenous administration of fluids is continued for 24 hours. When the child returns to the ward, he usually assumes a position of comfort. If bleeding occurs, it can easily be detected when pulse rate, respirations, blood pressure, and the child's color are checked often. The dressings should be changed only if necessary, since there is little or no drainage from the incision.

Toxic symptoms from administration of dactinomycin and x-ray therapy may cause more discomfort than does the surgical procedure. Nausea and vomiting, anorexia, malaise, and diarrhea may occur. Dactinomycin is potentially toxic; loss of hair, exfoliation of the skin, and ulceration of the tongue are possible side effects. When side effects occur, the drug is temporarily discontinued. During the interval between medication and x-ray therapy, the child's hair usually grows back.

Complications. The most serious compli-

cation in Wilms' tumor is metastasis. Characteristically, Wilms' tumor metastasizes through the bloodstream to the liver, lungs, brain, and other vital organs. The tumor may also spread by direct extension or by the lymphatics.

Prognosis. The prognosis without treatment is always fatal. When the tumor is discovered early, especially before 2 years of age, the prognosis is very good. Surgical excision plus dactinomycin and x-ray therapy offer a chance of cure even to some children with pulmonary metastases. Follow-up care includes x-ray examination of the lungs monthly for the first 6 months, every 2 months for the next 6 months, and quarterly for the next year in nonmetastatic cases. As the child progresses favorably, an annual examination is sufficient.

THE PRESCHOOL CHILD
Nephrosis

Nephrosis is a chronic, intermittent renal condition characterized by anasarca (marked generalized edema), heavy proteinuria, low serum albumin levels, and high serum cholesterol values. Elevated blood pressure and hematuria are not typical of the disease.

Etiology. The cause of nephrosis is unknown. Remissions are frequent, and the long course of the disease is aggravated by acute infections.

Incidence. Nephrosis seems to be more common in boys than in girls and occurs most frequently between 2 and 6 years of age. The incidence of nephrosis in childhood is 7 per 100,000.

Clinical symptoms. The onset of nephrosis is insidious. Periorbital puffiness may be noted first, and it progresses steadily until the eyes are closed (Fig. 37-3). As the edema increases, the arms, legs, and abdomen reach massive proportions. At the peak of the edema, the child can weigh almost twice as much as usual (Fig. 37-4). Anorexia and varying degrees of diarrhea are commonly found. Discomfort from massive edema causes the child to be irritable and easily fatigued.

643

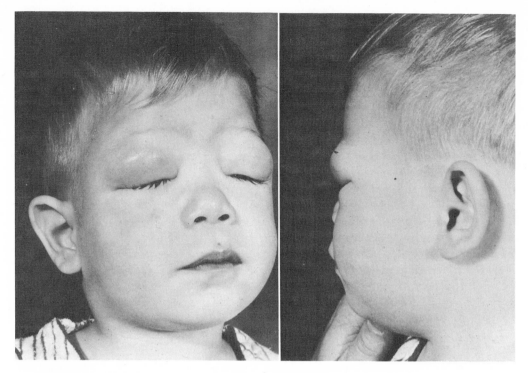

Fig. 37-3. A 2-year-old child with nephrosis. Progressive periorbital edema. (Courtesy Naval Regional Medical Center, San Diego, Calif.)

Complications. The nephrotic child is vulnerable to infections, probably because of loss of gamma globulin in the urine (proteinuria). Bacteremia associated with peritonitis is not uncommon. Upper respiratory tract infections are very dangerous, especially those caused by pneumococci. The severity of these infections should not be underestimated; when a child with nephrosis dies, it is commonly because his condition was complicated by infection.

Treatment and nursing care. The goal of treatment is a child as nearly normal as possible, judged by both clinical well-being and laboratory findings. The aims of nursing care include comforting the patient during the distresses of massive edema, maintaining good nutrition, and preventing intercurrent infections.

The majority of children with nephrosis respond remarkably well to steroid therapy. Large doses of prednisone, given four times daily, usually stimulate diuresis, which occurs from 10 to 14 days after the

initial dose. Recently a maintenance program of prednisone therapy given on alternating days has been found to be extremely useful in minimizing the toxic side effects of the drug. Twice the total daily dose is administered as a single morning dose every other day. Most studies indicate that this schedule appears to sustain desirable antiinflammatory action and diminishes undesirable side effects. When diuresis occurs, other measurable abnormalities usually improve. Proteinuria may disappear, and the serum albumin level appears closer to normal. During remission, steroid therapy is gradually reduced until it can be eliminated completely.

Intermittent steroid therapy, based on proteinuria, is continued during the course of the disease, which sometimes involves several years. Relapses of nephrosis are often associated with intercurrent infections, especially those involving the respiratory and urinary tracts. Immediate intensive antibiotic therapy is mandatory if in-

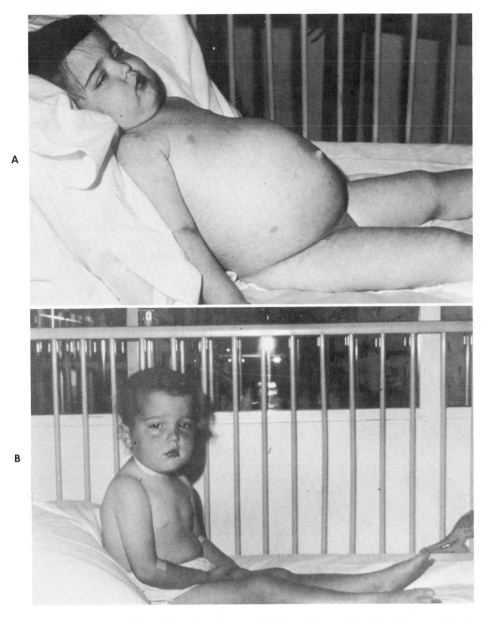

Fig. 37-4. A 2½-year-old child with nephrosis. **A,** Before therapy. **B,** After therapy. (Courtesy Naval Regional Medical Center, San Diego, Calif.)

fection arises. A significant number of upper urinay tract infections have been found in steroid-resistant children. It has been noted that when urinary tract infection is recognized early and treated vigorously, steroid resistance disappears, the nephrosis begins to subside, and the patient rapidly enters remission.

In selecting a hospital room for the nephrotic child, the nurse must remember his increased susceptibility to infection. Placing the child in a double room with another child the same age who has nephrosis is most desirable.

Weighing the child on admission and each morning thereafter is one way of evaluating the amount of edema present. A daily abdominal girth measurement taken in flat position at the level of the umbilicus, just after a breath is exhaled is also helpful. If massive edema is present, the child's self-concept is likely to be greatly distorted. It is important for his parents to be reassured and to be given whatever information is necessary about the condition and its outcome so that they in turn can reassure their child. They should particularly realize the seriousness of the disorder, even though the prognosis is now better than ever before.

Massive edema is most uncomfortable. The skin is stretched thin and easily broken. Keeping the child's body dry and clean will help prevent skin infections. Application of powder between skin surfaces and in skin folds is soothing and protective. If the child is not toilet trained, the nurse must take great care to prevent excoriation of the buttocks and genitalia. Medicines are given orally or intravenously but never by the intramuscular or subcutaneous route. Great care must be taken to protect the edematous skin from injury and subsequent secondary infection. Usually the child is most comfortable in a semi-Fowler's position to reduce respiratory embarrassment. This position may also reduce periorbital edema.

Maintenance of good nutrition is essential because beneath the edema exists a thin, poorly nourished body. Nowadays most physicians have greatly liberalized the diet offered these patients. The child should be given a well-balanced diet, normal for his age. Especially salty foods such as potato chips and pickles should be avoided. High-protein diets do not elevate the low serum protein level, and water restriction is contraindicated because of the child's diminished intravascular volume. Liberalizing the diet and allowing the child some choice will encourage his appetite and help prevent severe nutritional depletion, which readily occurs.

An accurate account of fluid intake is very important when the output is scanty.

Although the nurse may not be able to measure the exact output, she must record approximate amounts each time the child voids.

Bed rest is recommended until diuresis has begun. During the active phase of the disease, the child is usually sluggish and therefore satisfied to be resting most of the time. When massive edema is present, the child is content to rest all the time.

After the child is discharged from the hospital, he is periodically examined until the prednisone has been discontinued without any relapses. Although infection is a common complication in these children while they are receiving prednisone, it is not necessary to interfere with their normal home and school activities. If an outbreak of some infectious disease such as chicken pox (varicella) should occur at school, it is wise to have the child remain at home. Any sign of intercurrent infection must be reported to the physician and treated immediately. Some physicians would rather overtreat than risk the child's life to this most common cause of death.

Prognosis. By controlling infection, antibiotic therapy has greatly reduced the death rate of nephrotic patients. About 80% of the children respond to steroid therapy. Eventually, after many years of intermittent treatment, these children usually fully enjoy healthful living.

THE SCHOOL-AGE CHILD
Glomerulonephritis (nephritis, or Bright's disease)

Acute glomerulonephritis is a bilateral inflammatory disease of the glomeruli. It is characterized by the abrupt appearance of brown or smoky urine 1 to 3 weeks after an acute beta-hemolytic streptococcal infection. The usual clinical manifestations include a mild degree of edema, urinary abnormalities (hematuria, proteinuria, and casts), and varying degrees of hypertension.

Subacute glomerulonephritis sometimes follows the acute condition and is characterized by a progressive downhill course, which may be complicated by the nephrotic syndrome. Death may occur from renal insufficiency or cardiac failure. A few children with very severe cases have been known to recover completely.

Chronic glomerulonephritis is ultimately a fatal disease (unless renal transplants are performed) characterized by a progressive decrease in renal function. This condition usually appears insidiously and may or may not be the sequela to acute glomerulonephritis.

Etiology. Glomerulonephritis is almost always associated with a poststreptococcal infection. It is believed to be the result of an antigen-antibody reaction, secondary to such infections as scarlet fever, tonsillitis and pharyngitis, impetigo, and pneumonia. Isolation of the group A beta-streptococcal organism during the initial infection or a high antistreptolysin O titer in the blood (in response to the previous presence of streptococcal organisms in the body) confirms the diagnosis.

Incidence. Glomerulonephritis is common in children, especially between 5 to 10 years of age. It seems to be more common in boys than girls and is most frequently observed in the late winter months or early spring. This seasonal pattern is related to the peak incidence of streptococcal infections of the upper respiratory tract.

Symptoms. Acute glomerulonephritis is not always recognized because clinical signs and symptoms vary greatly. Microscopic hematuria and proteinuria may be the only signs, or gross hematuria and proteinuria, edema, periorbital puffiness, hypertension, weakness, pallor, anorexia, headache, nausea, and vomiting may be present. Rarely, there is a sudden onset with severe symptoms followed by dysfunction of the brain because of hypertension.

Treatment and nursing care. Necessary bed rest is usually welcomed by the child during the acute phase of the disease. Activities may be resumed as soon as gross hematuria has cleared and signs of edema, hypertension, and other urinary abnormalities have subsided.

The child should be separated from other children who have infections (especially of the upper respiratory tract), but complete isolation is not indicated. He should be observed closely for any recurrences of upper respiratory tract infection, since exacerbations can occur with new strains of streptococcal organisms. However, reinfection by the same nephritogenic strain is generally not possible by virtue of type-specific immunity after infection. Antibiotic therapy is indicated when evidence of infection is present. Prophylactic use of penicillin in the prevention of recurrence is not recommended.

A regular diet without added salt is offered to the child whose case is uncomplicated. If the child is voiding well, fluids are allowed as desired but are not forced. Careful observation of the color and volume of urine serves as a valuable guide in controlling fluid balance. Samples of successive voidings (aliquot urines) may be saved in test tubes, labeled, and placed on a rack for comparison by the physician and nurses. Measurement of fluid intake, urinary output, and daily weight aids in the recognition of early signs of edema.

Temperature and pulse and respiration rates are checked frequently. Blood pressure should be checked often with the proper size sphygmomanometer. The cuff should cover two thirds of the upper arm and should be applied smoothly.

Complications. Changes in mental status such as drowsiness, lethargy, double vision, muscular twitching, and convulsions should be reported at once. Complications can be discovered early when the observant nurse is aware of the clues that indicate that all is not well.

HYPERTENSIVE ENCEPHALOPATHY. Hypertensive encephalopathy is characterized by irritability, headache, vomiting, and blurred or double vision. Convulsions may also occur. The rise in blood pressure is almost always accompanied by a drop in pulse rate. This complication is caused by lack of proper blood supply to the brain, resulting from vasospasm. It usually responds to antihypertensive drug therapy.

CARDIAC DECOMPENSATION. Cardiac decompensation occurs as a result of severe hypertension. Evidences of cardiac involvement include tachycardia, arrhythmia, rapid, difficult breathing, and heart enlargement. When this occurs, salt and fluids are restricted. Treatment is primarily geared to control hypertension and give symptomatic relief of discomfort. Measures include rest in the orthopenic position, administration of oxygen, and sedation. Digitalization is not necessary unless heart failure ensues. Cardiac involvement is greatly decreased when hypertension is adequately controlled.

SEVERE RENAL FAILURE. Severe renal failure is uncommon in children, although urine production may, at times, become scanty or absent. Usually this acute situation is transitory and reversible. When an imbalance of fluids and electrolytes persists, peritoneal dialysis or hemodialysis may be needed to control the uremia.

Prognosis. Acute glomerulonephritis is usually a self-limiting condition, and most children recover completely. A few children present a more complex entity with persistent urinary abnormalities and hypertension, which ultimately results in chronic nephritis and death.

Enuresis

Enuresis may be defined as involuntary voiding of urine, especially at night (nocturnal enuresis), after 4 years of age. However, there appears to be a rather wide age range associated with the neuromuscular maturation of urinary sphincter control. Children with nocturnal enuresis usually have a normal urinary stream and good daytime bladder control. Enuresis may be primary or acquired. When bladder control has never been achieved, enuresis is said to be primary. If enuresis occurs after control has been achieved for at least 1 year, it is said to be acquired.

About 15% of pediatric patients are evaluated because of this disturbance. Enuresis is very common in childhood, and the condition is more prevalent in boys than in girls.

The exact cause of enuresis in most children is unknown. Psychological or developmental disorders are found in many patients, but enuresis may also be caused by an anatomical defect or a systemic disease. The most significant step toward solving the problem is an attempt to find the correct cause. Before a psychological explanation is sought, anatomical abnormalities and organic disease must be ruled out.

Generally, daytime wetting (diurnal enuresis) and other urological symptoms are associated with organic disease. Diabetes mellitus, urinary tract infection, urinary tract anomalies, neurological defects, and obstructions such as meatal stenosis are often responsible for the condition. Psychological problems also account for some cases of enuresis. Improper toilet training, an unhappy environment, a poor mother-child relationship, immaturity associated with other infantile habits, and developmental disturbances, such as jealousy and insecurity, are some psychological causes of enuresis. Whatever the cause, the correction of enuresis is very important to both the child and his parents. For the child it enables him to develop normally and to be like his little friends, and for the parents, correction means peace of mind and a healthy child.

Every enuretic patient should have a careful medical history and physical examination performed to determine if renal enlargements, a distended bladder, a constriction of the external urinary meatus, or a neurological change is present. A very careful urinalysis and urine culture are essential. Intravenous urography, cystography, and cystoscopy are sometimes necessary to diagnose organic causes, since sometimes history and physical examination may be entirely within normal limits.

In the past, medications such as dextroamphetamine sulfate (Dexedrine), anticholinergic drugs, belladonna, and methantheline bromide (to reduce the tone of the detrussor muscle) were widely used without significant success. More recently, imipramine hydrochloride (Tofranil) has been found to completely control the condition in some patients. This drug, however, has some potential toxic manifestations. Thus a physician must carefully evaluate the problem before ordering imipramine hydrochloride and, if he believes it is indicated, the child must be carefully watched for side effects. Facial tics have been reported.

A condition often confused with enuresis is an ectopic ureter in a female in which the ureter empties into the vagina or urethra beyond the sphincter. These children may void normally (from their normal ureters and bladder) but are always wet from constant drainage from the ectopic ureter. Proper surgery will correct this problem.

Enuresis may also diminish through the use of fairly simple techniques. Giving less fluids in the evening may be helpful to some children. Waking the child and taking him to the toilet during the night saves embarrassment to the school-age child. Parents should not threaten or punish their children because they wet the bed. This only increases the child's sense of inferiority and failure and may even deter his will to improve. Instead, every effort should be made to assure the child that he can overcome his condition if he really wants to. Encouragement comes in the form of rewards, for example, being able to go camping or sleep overnight at grandmother's house. Such rewards, together with the child's desire to stay dry, can achieve positive results. Enuretic children without any organic disease or severe psychological problem usually gradually overcome the condition.

Torsion of the testis

Contraction of the cremaster muscle not only elevates the testis but rotates it outward. Depending on the degree of twisting, torsion of the spermatic cord usually causes severe scrotal pain due to an interruption of the blood supply and ensuing necrosis of the testis. Torsion may occur at any age and is not uncommon in the adolescent. It may occur while sleeping, playing games, or jumping into cold water. In order to preserve the fertility and viability of the testis, prompt diagnosis and action must be taken to relieve the condition. Immediate steps, such as manipulative reduction or surgical intervention to untwist the testis, are necessary to save the organ. Surgical exploration must be done within 6 hours to verify the success of any manipulative attempts to reduce the malrotation. Bilateral orchiopexy (fixation of both testes in the scrotum) is usually performed since recurrence occurs frequently.

unit eleven
Suggested selected readings and references

Abrahamson, J.: Repair of inguinal hernias in infants and small children, Clin. Pediatr. 12:617-621, Oct., 1973.

Allue, X., Rubio, T., and Riley, H. D., Jr.: Gonococcal infections in infants and children, Clin. Pediatr. 12:584-588, Oct., 1973.

Altshuler, A.: Complete transposition of the great arteries, Am. J. Nurs. 71:96-98, Jan., 1971.

Balderson, S.: In orthopedic surgery children need extensive nursing care, AORN J. 19:1047-1052, May, 1974.

Barga, J. L.: How to treat nosebleed, Am. Fam. Physician 8:66-73, Aug., 1973.

Beaumont, E.: Portable IPPB machines, Nurs. '73 3:26-31, Jan., 1973.

Beaumont, E.: Product information: urinary drainage systems, Nurs. '74 4:52-60, Jan., 1974.

Beaumont, E., and Wiley, L.: Hearing aids are a nursing responsibility, Nurs. '74 4:67, June, 1974.

Betson, C., Valoon, P., and Soika, C.: Cardiac surgery in neonates: a chance for life, Am. J. Nurs, 69:69-73, Jan., 1969.

Blair, J., and Fitzgerald, J. F.: Treatment of nonspecific diarrhea in infants, Clin. Pediatr. 13:333-337, April, 1974.

Bonine, G. N.: The myelodysplastic child: hospital and home care, Am. J. Nurs. 69:541-544, March, 1969.

Boone, J. E., Baldwin, J., and Levine, C.: Juvenile rheumatoid arthritis, Pediatr. Clin. North Am. 21:871-884, Nov., 1974.

Bowman, B. H.: Genetic counseling in cystic fibrosis, Am. Fam. Physician 8:112-118, Dec., 1973.

Brewer, E. M.: Major problems in clinical pediatrics. Juvenile rheumatoid arthritis, vol. 6, Philadelphia, 1970, W. B. Saunders Co.

Brodie, B., and Von Haam, J.: Children born with adrenogenital syndrome, Am. J. Nurs. **67:** 1018-1021, May, 1967.

Brown, M. R., and Lillibridge, C. B.: When to think of celiac disease, Clin. Pediatr. **14:**76-82, Jan., 1975.

Butler, I., and Johnson, R.: Central nervous system infections, Pediatr. Clin. North Am. **21:** 649-668, Aug., 1974.

Carver, D. H., editor: The Pediatric Clinics of North America. Symposium on infectious diseases, vol. 21, no. 2, Philadelphia, 1974, W. B. Saunders Co.

Chan, J. C. M.: Dietary management of renal failure in infants and children, Clin. Pediatr. **12:**707-713, Dec., 1973.

Chilcote, R. R., and Balhner, R. L.: Infection in childhood cancer: experience in management of infection in acute leukemia, Pediatr. Ann. **3:**71-88, May, 1974.

Clifton, J.: Collecting 24-hour urine specimens from infants, Am. J. Nurs. **69:**1660-1661, Aug., 1969.

Cogen, R.: Cardiac catheterization: preparing the child, Am. J. Nurs. **73:**80-82, Jan., 1973.

A commonsense guide to family dental care, Parents' Magazine and Better Homemaking **49:** 14, March, 1974.

Condon, M. R.: The cardiac child: what his parents need to know, Nurs. '73 **3:**60-61, Oct., 1973.

Connor, G. H., Hughes, D., Mills, M. J., and others: Tracheostomy, Am. J. Nurs. **72:**68-74, Jan., 1972.

Coogan, J. P.: Motivating the unmotivated patient, Nurs. '74 **4:**31-36, Feb., 1974.

Corbary, L. J.: VD: U. S. number one epidemic, J. Pract. Nurs. **24:**20-23, June, 1974.

Cyphert, F. C.: Back to school for the child with cancer, Nurs. Digest **2:**48-53, Jan., 1974. Condensed from J. School Health **43:**215-217, April, 1973.

Daniel, W. A.: The adolescent patient, St. Louis, 1970, The C. V. Mosby Co.

Deney, J.: How you can help the asthmatic patient, Nurs. Care **7:**10-13, Feb., 1974.

Dison, N.: A mother's view of tonsillectomy, Am. J. Nurs. **69:**1024-1027, May, 1969.

Down, J., and others: Acute respiratory failure in infants and children, Pediatr. Clin. North Am. **19:**423-445, May, 1972.

Drachman, R. H.: Acute infections gastroenteritis, Pediatr. Clin. North Am. **21:**711-737, Aug., 1974.

Duckett, C. L.: Caring for children with sickle cell anemia, Children **18:**227-231, Nov.-Dec., 1971.

Elliott, R. A., and Holhn, J. F.: Use of commercial porcine skin wound dressings, Plast. Reconstr. Surg. **52:**401-405, Oct., 1973.

Ellis, E. F.: Symposium on pediatric allergy, vol. 22, Philadelphia, 1975, W. B. Saunders Co.

Erikson, R. A.: Cranial check: a basic neurological assessment, Nurs. '74 **4:**67, Aug., 1974.

Feeney, R.: Preventing rheumatic fever in school children, Am. J. Nurs. **73:**265, Feb., 1973.

Fernbach, D. J., and Starling, K. A.: Acute leukemia in children, Pediatr. Ann. **3:**13-26, May, 1974.

Foley, M. F.: Pulmonary function testing, Am. J. Nurs. **71:**1134-1139, June, 1971.

Forman, B. H., and others: Management of juvenile diabetes mellitus: usefulness of 24-hour fractional quantitative urine glucose, Pediatrics **52:**257-263, Feb., 1974.

Foss, G.: Breaking architectural barriers with crutches, wheelchairs and walkers, Nurs. '73 **3:** 16-31, Oct., 1973.

Frobisher, M., and Fuerst, R.: Microbiology in health and disease, ed. 13, Philadelphia, 1973, W. B. Saunders Co.

Froelich, L.: Care of the infant with exstrophy of the bladder, Nurs. Clin. North Am. **2:**573, Sept., 1967.

Gardner, P.: Antimicrobial drug therapy in pediatric practice, Pediatr. Clin. North Am. **21:** 617-648, Aug., 1974.

Geis, D. P., and Lambertz, S. E.: Acute respiratory infections in young children, Am. J. Nurs. **68:**294-297, Feb., 1968.

Gillon, J. E.: Behavior of newborns with cardiac distress, Am. J. Nurs. **73:**254-257, Feb., 1973.

Goda, S.: Speech development in children, Am. J. Nurs. **70:**276-278, Feb., 1970.

Guide to diagnosis and management of cystic fibrosis, 1971, Atlanta, National Cystic Fibrosis Research Foundation.

Guthrie, D. W., and Guthrie, R. A.: Juvenile diabetes mellitus, Nurs. Clin. North Am. **8:**587-603, Dec., 1973.

Harkness, L.: Bringing epilepsy out of the closet, Am. J. Nurs. **74:**875-876, May, 1974.

Heal, L. W.: Evaluation of an integrated approach to the management of cerebral palsy, Except. Child. **40:** March, 1974.

Herrin, J. T., and Crawford, J. D.: The seriously burned child. In Smith, C. A., editor: The critically ill child, Philadelphia, 1972, W. B. Saunders Co., pp. 46-61.

Hiles, D. A.: Strabismus, Am. J. Nurs. **74:**1082-1089, June, 1974.

Hughes, W. T., and others: Infectious diseases in children with cancer, Pediatr. Clin. North Am. **21:**583-615, Aug., 1974.

Humphrey, N., and others: Parenteral hyperalimentation for children, Am. J. Nurs. **72:**286-288, Feb., 1972.

Hyde, J. S., editor: The Pediatric Clinics of North

America. Pediatric allergy, vol. 16, no. 1, Philadelphia, 1969, W. B. Saunders Co.

Isolation techniques for use in hospitals, Atlanta, 1970, U. S. Department of Health, Education, and Welfare, Center for Disease Control.

Jacoby, F. G.: Nursing care of the patient with burns, St. Louis, 1972, The C. V. Mosby Co.

Johnson, A.: Rheumatic fever: a continuing threat, Nurs. '74 3:57-59, March, 1974.

Keaveny, M. E., moderator: creative nursing care for acute leukemia, Nurs. '73 3:19-23, June, 1973.

Keegan, L. G.: Dispelling the myth of the apical-radial pulse in digitalis therapy, Am. J. Nurs. 72:1434-1435, Aug., 1972.

Kelalis, P. P., Burke, E. C., and Stickler, G. B.: The riddle of vesicoureteral reflux, Clin. Pediatr. 11:495-496, Sept., 1972.

Keush, G.: Bacterial diarrheas, Am. J. Nurs. 73:1028-1032, June, 1973.

Khan, A. J., and Pryles, C. V.: Urinary tract infection in children, Am. J. Nurs. 73:1340-1343, Aug., 1973.

Knox, L. L., and McConnell, F.: Helping parents to help deaf infants, Children 15:183, Sept.-Oct., 1968.

Kravis, L. P.: The complications of acute asthma in children, Clin. Pediatr. 12:538-549, Sept., 1973.

Krugman, S., and Ward, R.: Infectious diseases of children and adults, St. Louis, 1973, The C. V. Mosby Co.

Kunsman, J.: Nursing care after primary excision, RN 37:25-26, Aug., 1974.

Kurth, J. S.: Correct application of the Thomas splint and Pearson attachment, Nurs, '73 3:20-24, July, 1973.

Lane, P. A.: Home care of a toddler in a spica cast: what it's really like, Am. J. Nurs. 71:2141-2143, Nov., 1971.

Lane, S., and Wiley, L., editors: Rheumatic heart disease: a teenager's torment, Nurs. '74 3:51-56, March, 1974.

Lanser, J., and Pancoast, A.: Caring for the asthmatic—at home, in school and on the job, Nurs. '73 3:62-64, Nov., 1973.

Lapides, J., editor: The Urologic Clinics of North America. Symposium on the neurogenic bladder, vols. 1 and 2, Philadelphia, 1974, W. B. Saunders Co.

Larson, C. B., and Gould, M.: Orthopedic nursing, ed. 8, St. Louis, 1974, The C. V. Mosby Co.

Lascari, A. D.: The reactions of families to childhood leukemia, Clin. Pediatr. 12:210-214, April, 1973.

Lawrence, P. A.: U-100 insulin: let's make the transition trouble free, Am. J. Nurs. 73:1539, Sept., 1973.

Lecks, H. I., Kravis, L. P., and Wood, D. W.: Clinical experience with the use of cromolyn sodium in asthmatic children, Clin. Pediatr. 13:420-425, May, 1974.

Lee, R. M.: Day surgery has added benefits for children, AORN J. 19:632-635, March, 1974.

Lee, R. V.: Antimicrobial therapy, Am. J. Nurs. 73:2044-2048, Dec., 1973.

Leventhal, B. G., and Hersh, S.: Modern treatment of childhood leukemia, Child. Today 3:2-6, May-June, 1974.

Lice on the loose, J. Pract. Nurs. 23:34, Dec., 1973.

Lilly, J. R., and Peck, C. A.: Immediate porcine heterografting of burns in children, J. Pediatr. Surg. 9:335-340, June, 1974.

Lindh, K., and Rickerson, G.: Spinal-cord injury: you can make a difference, Nurs. '74 4:41-45, Feb., 1974.

Linshaw, M. A., and Gruskin, A. B.: Management of the nephrotic syndrome, Clin. Pediatr. 13:45-51, Jan., 1974.

Littmann, D.: Stethoscopes and auscultation, Am. J. Nurs. 72:1238-1241, July, 1972.

MacEwen, G. D., and O'Connor, B. J.: The Chiari osteotomy, AORN J. 19:1060-1064, May, 1974.

Magnus, R. A.: Parent involvement in residential treatment programs, Child. Today 3:25-27, Jan.-Feb., 1974.

Mahoney, J. A.: Viewpoints on attitudes and actions toward handicapped children, J. Pract. Nurs. 24:40-41, April, 1974.

Makker, S. P., and Heymann, W.: The idiopathic nephrotic syndrome of childhood, Am. J. Disturbed Child. 127:830-837, June, 1974.

Matheney, N. M., and Snively, W. D.: Fluid balance, ed. 2, Philadelphia, 1974, J. B. Lippincott Co.

May, C. M.: Wheelchair patient for a day, Am. J. Nurs. 73:650-651, April, 1973.

McClure, P. D.: Idiopathic thrombocytopenic purpura in children, Pediatrics 55:68-74, Jan., 1975.

McFarlane, J.: Children with diabetes—special needs during growth years, Am. J. Nurs. 73:1360-1363, Aug., 1973.

McKendry, J. B. J., and Stewart, D. A.: Enuresis, Pediatr. Clin. North Am. 21:1019-1028, Nov., 1974.

Miezio, P.: Care of the child with myelomeningocele, Nurs. Digest 1:45-51, Nov., 1973. Condensed from Highlights in Nursing, vol. 10, April, 1973.

Mira, M., and Hoffman, S.: Educational programming for multihandicapped deaf-blind children, Except. Child. 40:513-514, April, 1974.

Moffenson, H. D., and Greensher, J.: Peritoneal dialysis, Clin. Pediatr. 11:534-537, Sept., 1972.

Morgan, C. V., Jr., and Orcutt, T. W.: The care and feeding of chest tubes, Am. J. Nurs. 72:305-308, Feb., 1972.

Murray, B. S., Elmore, U., and Sawyer, J. R.: The patient has an ileal conduit, Am. J. Nurs. **71**: 1560-1565, Aug., 1971.

Murray, J. D.: The continuing problem of purulent meningitis in infants and children, Pediatr. Clin. North Am. **21**:967-980, Nov., 1974.

Nellhaus, G.: Brain tumors in childhood, Pediatr. Ann. **3**:18-37, June, 1974.

New dental projects for poor children, Health Serv. Rep. **87**:605-608, Aug.-Sept., 1972.

Newburger, E. H.: A conceptual approach to the child with exceptional nutritional requirements: the management of patients with complex nutritional problems as addressed with a simple conceptual model, Clin. Pediatr. **8**:456-467, Aug., 1973.

Pidgeon, V.: The infant with congenital heart disease, Am. J. Nurs. **67**:289-293, Feb., 1967.

Pierce, W. S., and Waldhansen, J. A.: Surgical approaches in congenital heart disease, Pediatr. Clin. North Am. **19**:333-353, May, 1972.

Pinney, M. S.: Postural drainage in infants, Nurs. '72 **2**:45-48, Oct., 1972.

Pochedly, C. E.: Sickle cell anemia: recognition and management, Am. J. Nurs. **71**:1948-1951, Oct., 1971.

Pochedly, C. E.: The child with neuroblastoma, Am. Fam. Physician **5**:74-79, Feb., 1972.

Pochedly, C. E.: The child with leukemia, Springfield, Ill., 1973, Charles C Thomas, Publisher.

Pochedly, C., and Necheles, I. F.: Childhood cancer, Springfield, Ill., 1973, Charles C Thomas, Publisher.

Posey, R. A.: Babies with heart disease, Nurs. '74 **4**:40-45, Oct., 1974.

Rabinowitz, M.: Why didn't anyone tell me about bottle mouth cavities? Child. Today **3**:18-20, March-April, 1974.

Rapkin, R. H.: Tracheostomy in epiglottitis, Pediatrics **52**:426-429, Sept., 1973.

Rapkin, R. H., and Eppley, M. L.: The recognition of streptococcal pharyngitis, Clin. Pediatr. **10**:706-710, Dec., 1971.

Reece, R. M.: Keeping immunizations up to date, Am. Fam. Physician **9**:119-125, March, 1974.

Reeves, K. R.: Acute epiglottitis—pediatric emergency, Am. J. Nurs. **71**:1539-1541, Aug., 1971.

Report of the Committee on Infectious Disease, part I, ed. 17, Evanston, Ill., 1974, American Academy of Pediatrics.

Rice, A. K.: Common skin infections in school children, Am. J. Nurs. **73**:1905-1909, Nov., 1973.

Robbins, S. M., and Finklestein, J.: Reducing the emotional and economic costs of hospitalization of acutely ill asthmatics, Clin. Pediatr. **12**:550-554, Sept., 1973.

Roberts, F. B.: The child with heart disease, Am. J. Nurs. **72**:1080-1084, June, 1972.

Ruben, M.: Balm for burned children, Am. J. Nurs. **66**:297-302, Feb., 1966.

Sanchez, A.: Anesthesia in pediatric orthopedic surgery, AORN J. **19**:1054-1059, May, 1974.

Sato, F. F.: New devices for continuous urine collection in pediatrics, Am. J. Nurs. **69**:804-805, April, 1969.

Schwartz, D. C., and West, T. D.: Cardiac catheterization in infants and children, Heart and Lung **3**:407-414, May-June, 1974.

Schwartz, E.: The treatment of hemophilia, Pediatr. Clin. North Am. **15**:473-481, May, 1968.

Scoliosis: affectionate, yet firm postoperative nursing care, Nurs. '74 **4**:49-55, Aug., 1974.

Sells, C., and Sells, M.: Scoliosis screening in public schools, Am. J. Nurs. **74**:60-62, Jan., 1974.

Seto, D., and Heller, R.: Acute respiratory infections, Pediatr. Clin. North Am. **21**:683-710, Aug., 1974.

Sheehy, E.: Primary excision: innovation in pediatric burn care, RN **57**:21-25, Aug., 1974.

Shumway, C. A.: Iron deficiency anemia, Pediatr. Clin. North Am. **19**:855-864, Nov., 1972.

Simone, J. V.: Childhood leukemia: the changing prognosis, Hosp. Practice **9**:54-68, July, 1974.

Smallpox vaccination in the U. S.: The end of an era, J. Pediatr. **30**:600-608, Sept., 1972.

Sparks, J. P.: Torsion of the testis in adolescents and young adults, Clin. Pediatr. **11**:484-486, Aug., 1972.

Spicher, C.: Nursing care of children hospitalized with infections, Nurs. Clin. North Am. **5**:123-129, March, 1970.

Stadnyk, S., and Bindschadler, N.: A camp for

children with cystic fibrosis, Am. J. Nurs. **70:** 1691-1693, Aug., 1970.

Stamford, P.: Victory over rabies, RN **37:**65-76, May, 1974.

Stern, R. C., and others: Use of a "Heparin Lock" in the intermittent administration of intravenous drugs, Clin. Pediatr. **9:**521-523, Sept., 1972.

Stinson, V.: Porcine skin dressings for burns, Am. J. Nurs. **74:**111-112, Jan., 1974.

Striker, T. W., and Schreiber, M.: Respiratory problems associated with congenital heart disease, Heart and Lung **3:**401-406, May-June, 1974.

Tachdjian, M. O.: Pediatric orthopedics, Philadelphia, 1972, W. B. Saunders Co.

Taranta, A., and Moody, M.: Diagnosis of streptococcal pharyngitis and RF, Pediatr. Clin. North Am. **18:**125-143, Feb., 1971.

Tetrault, S. M., and Scott, R. B.: Recreation and hobbies as developmental supports for a child with sickle cell anemia, Clin. Pediatr. **13:**496-497, June, 1974.

TeWinkle, M. B.: Immunization and communicable diseases, J. Pract. Nurs. **23:**22-25, March, 1974.

Turner, H. G.: The A & P of normal respiration, Nurs. Clin. North Am. **3:**383-401, Sept., 1968.

Van Der Horst, R. L.: On teething in infancy, Clin. Pediatr. **12:**607-610, Oct., 1973.

Webb, K. J.: Early assessment of orthopedic injuries, Am. J. Nurs. **74:**1048-1052, June, 1974.

Whitman, W. F.: Wilms' tumor and neuroblastoma, Am. J. Nurs. **68:**526-535, March, 1968.

Williams, S. R.: Nutrition and diet therapy, ed. 2, St. Louis, 1973, The C. V. Mosby Co.

Wilson, H. D., and Eichenwald, H. F.: Sepsis neonatorum, Pediatr. Clin. North Am. **21:**571-582, Aug., 1974.

Wilson, P.: Iron-deficiency anemia, Am. J. Nurs. **72:**502-504, March, 1972.

Wood, M., Kenny, H. A., and Price, W. R.: Silver nitrate treatment of burns, Am. J. Nurs. **66:** 518, March, 1966.

Zellweger, H., and Antonik, A.: Newborn screening for Duchenne muscular dystrophy, Pediatrics **55:**30-34, Jan., 1975.

General bibliography

Blake, F., Wright, F., and Waechter, E.: Nursing care of children, ed. 8, Philadelphia, 1970, J. B. Lippincott Co.

Broadribb, V.: Foundations of pediatric nursing, Philadelphia, 1973, J. B. Lippincott Co.

Brunner, L. S., and others: The Lippincott manual of nursing practice, Philadelphia, 1974, J. B. Lippincott Co.

Cooke, R. E., editor: The biological basis of pediatric practice, Philadelphia, 1969, W. B. Saunders Co.

Gellis, S. S., and Kagan, B. M.: Current pediatric therapy, ed. 6, Philadelphia, 1973, W. B. Saunders Co.

Green, M., and Haggerty, R. J.: Ambulatory pediatrics, Philadelphia, 1968, W. B. Saunders Co.

Hughes, J. G.: Synopsis of pediatrics, ed. 3, St. Louis, 1971, The C. V. Mosby Co.

Kendig, E. L., editor: Pulmonary disorders, vol. 1, Philadelphia, 1972, W. B. Saunders Co.

Latham, L. C., and Heckel, R. V.: Pediatric nursing, ed. 2, St. Louis, 1972, The C. V. Mosby Co.

Leifer, G.: Principles and techniques in pediatric nursing, ed. 2, Philadelphia, 1973, W. B. Saunders Co.

Marlow, D. R.: Textbook of pediatric nursing, ed. 4, Philadelphia, 1973, W. B. Saunders Co.

Marsh, J. B., and Dickens, M.: Armstrong and Browder's nursing care of children, ed. 4, Philadelphia, 1973, F. A. Davis Co.

Raffensperger, J. G., and Primrose, R. B.: Pediatric surgery for nurses, Boston, 1968, Little, Brown and Co.

Report of the Committee on Infectious Diseases, ed. 17, Evanston, Ill., 1974, American Academy of Pediatrics.

Scipien, G. M.: Comprehensive pediatric nursing, New York, 1975, McGraw-Hill Book Co.

Shirkey, H. C.: Pediatric therapy, ed. 4, St. Louis, 1972, The C. V. Mosby Co.

Slobody, L. B., and Wasserman, E.: Survey of clinical pediatrics, ed. 6, New York, 1974, McGraw-Hill Book Co.

Smith, C. A., editor: The critically ill child, Philadelphia, 1972, W. B. Saunders Co.

Smith, C. H.: Blood diseases of infancy and childhood, ed. 3, St. Louis, 1972, The C. V. Mosby Co.

Vaughan, V. C., and McKay, R. J.: Textbook of pediatrics, ed. 10, Philadelphia, 1975, W. B. Saunders Co.

Wallace, H. M., and others, editors: Maternal and child health practices, Springfield, Ill., 1973, Charles C Thomas, Publisher.

Glossary

abduction (ăb-dŭk'shŭn) movement away from the midline.

abortion (à-bŏr'shŭn) termination of a pregnancy before viability; may be spontaneous or induced; definitions of viability may vary.

abrasion (ă-brā'zhŭn) loss of superficial tissue, skin, or mucous membrane because of friction.

abruptio (ăb-rŭp'shē-ō) a tearing away from.

abruptio placentae (plá-sĕn'tē) premature separation of a normally implanted placenta.

abscess (ăb'sĕs) a focus of suppuration within a tissue; pocket of pus.

abstinence (ab'stĭ-nents) going without voluntarily; refraining from sexual intercourse.

acetabulum (ăs-ĕ-tăb'ū-lŭm) rounded cavity on the external surface of the innominate bone that receives the head of the femur.

acidosis (as-ĭ-dō'sis) abnormal increase in acidity of the blood and tissues.

acinus (ăs'ĭ-nŭs) (pl. acini) smallest division of a gland, often referring to the mammary glands.

adenoids (ăd'ĕ-noyds) grouping of lymphoid tissue located on the posterior wall of the nasopharynx (the pharyngeal tonsils).

adnexa (ăd-nĕx'à) accessory parts of a structure; uterine adnexa—oviducts and ovaries.

afebrile (ā-fĕb'rĭl) without fever.

afibrinogenemia (ā-fī"brĭn-ō-jĕ-nē'mĭ-à) lack of the protein fibrinogen in the blood, causing problems in coagulation.

aggregate (ăg'grĕ-gāt) total substances making up a mass.

airway normal passageway for respired air or a device used to prevent or correct respiratory obstruction.

albinism (ăl'bĭn-ĭsm) abnormal but nonpathogenic absence of pigment in skin, hair, and eyes.

albumin (ăl-bū'mĭn) one kind of protein.

albuminuria (ăl-bū'-mĭ-nū'rĭ-à) presence of albumin in the urine.

alignment (ă-līn'ment) arranging in a line.

alimentation (ăl-ĭ-mĕn-tā'shŭn) the general process of nourishing the body.

alkalosis (ăl"kà-lō'sĭs) abnormal increase of alkalinity of the blood and tissues.

allergen (ăl'er-jĕn) any substance that produces an allergic response.

alveolus (ăl-vē'ō-lŭs) (pl. alve'oli) a little hollow or cavity; the air sac or cell of the lung tissue.

ambivalence (ăm-bĭv'à-lĕnts) simultaneous feelings of attraction and repulsion, love and hate for a person, object, or action.

amblyopia (ăm-blĭ-ō'pē-à) reduction or dimness of vision in one eye without apparent associated organic abnormality.

amenorrhea (ā-mĕn-ō-rē'à) absence of menstruation.

amnesic (ăm-nē'sĭk) capable of producing amnesia, or loss of memory.

amniocentesis (ăm'nē-ō-sĕn-tē'sĭs) puncture of the intrauterine amniotic sac usually through the abdominal wall to obtain sample of amniotic fluid.

amniotic (ăm-nē-ŏt'ĭk) pertaining to the amnion, the innermost of the fetal membranes that secretes the fluid inside the bag of waters.

analgesic (ăn'ăl-jē'sĭk) capable of producing analgesia, or relief from pain.

anaphylactic shock (ăn"à-fī-lăk'tĭk) a syndrome that occasionally occurs after the reintroduction of a substance (antigen) into a person or animal previously sensitized to it; characterized by circulatory collapse and shock.

anasarca (ăn-à-sär'kà) a marked generalized edema.

anastomosis (ă-năs'tō-mō'sĭs) a natural or surgical joining of blood or lymph vessels, or a surgically created communication between different hollow organs or parts of the same organs.

ancillary (ăn'sĭ-ler-ē) subordinate or auxiliary.

android (ăn'droyd) manlike; adjective used to describe a male-type pelvis.

anemia (ăn-ē'mē-à) condition in which there is a reduction of hemoglobin in the blood.

anencephalus (ăn-ĕn-sĕf'à-lŭs) monstrosity lacking a cerebrum, cerebellum, and part of the cranium.

Glossary

anesthetic (ăn'ĕs-thĕt'ĭk) capable of producing anesthesia, that is, complete or partial loss of feeling.

angiocardiography (ăn″jē-ō-cär-dē-ŏg'rä-fē) injection of contrast material into the circulation and observation of its flow by x-ray or fluoroscope.

anion (ăn'ī-ăn) particle of matter (ion) carrying a negative electrical charge.

ankylosis (ăn-kĭ-lō'sĭs) abnormal immobility and consolidation of a joint.

anorexia (ăn-á-rĕk'sē-á) loss of appetite.

anoxia (ăn-ŏk'sē-á) lack of oxygen.

antagonistic (ăn-tăg-á-nĭs'tĭk) acting with antagonism, that is, in opposition to an agent or principle; counteracting; hostile.

antenatal (ăn-tē-nā'tál) before birth; prenatal.

antepartal (ăn-tē-pär'tál) before delivery.

anteroposterior (ăn'tĕr-ō-pŏs-tĭr'ē-ur) from front to back.

antiarrhythmic (ăn″tē-á-rĭth'mĭk) preventing (or effective against) arrhythmia, or irregular cardiac contractions.

antibody (ăn'tĭ-bŏd-ē) protective protein substance formed by the body in the presence of pathogenic organisms or foreign materials.

antisepsis (ăn″tĭ-sĕp'sĭs) literally "against infection or decay"; the use of procedures usually involving chemicals (antiseptics) that hinder the growth of microorganisms without necessarily destroying them.

antitoxin (ăn-tĭ-tŏk'sĭn) protective protein formed by the body in response to the presence of a toxin; a preparation containing antibodies designed to produce passive immunization.

anuria (á-nyur'ē-á) failure of kidney function; lack of urine formation.

apnea (ăp'nē-á) absence of respiration, temporary or permanent.

areola (á-rē'ō-lá) (pl. areolae) ring of pigment on the breast surrounding the nipple.

arteriogram (är-tĭr'ē-ō-grăm) x-ray procedure that reveals aterial pathways injected with special contrast materials.

artery (är'ter-ē) blood vessel that carries blood away from the heart.

arthritis (är-thrī'tis) inflammation of a joint, usually accompanied by pain and frequently by changes in structure.

arthrodesis (är″thrŏd-ē'sĭs) surgical fusion of a joint performed to gain stability for weight bearing.

arthroplasty (är'thrō-plăs-tē) surgical formation or reconstruction of a joint.

asepsis (á-sĕp'sĭs) literally "without infection or decay"; refers to the absence of living ·disease-producing microorganisms or to procedures that produce such an absence.

asphyxia (ăs-fĭk'sē-á) lack of oxygen and excessive carbon dioxide build-up in the body resulting

from an abnormal gaseous environment or disease.

aspiration (ăs-pĭ-rā'shun) process of drawing in or out as by suction.

assimilation (á-sĭm-ĕ-lā'shun) processes whereby the products of digestion change to resemble the chemical substances of the body tissues, first passing through the lacteals and blood vessels.

astrocytoma (ăs-trō-sī-tō'má) tumor of the brain tissue.

ataxic (á-tăk'sĭk) pertaining to ataxia, or the incoordination of the voluntary muscles; one possible result of brain damage.

atelectasis (ăt-ĕ-lĕk'tá-sĭs) lack of proper lung expansion. A collapsed or airless segment of lung.

athetoid (ăth'ĕ-toyd) pertaining to athetosis, or the presence of involuntary, purposeless weaving motions of the body, or its extremities; one possible result of brain damage.

atopic (á-tŏp'ĭk) pertaining to allergic responses, particularly those of a hereditary nature.

atresia (á-trē'zhuh) lack of a normal opening or canal.

atrium (ā'trē-ŭm) (pl. atria) a cavity or sinus; one of two upper chambers of the heart.

atrophy (ăt'rá-fē) lack of nourishment; wasting or reduction in size of cells, tissues, organs, or regions of the body.

attenuated (á-tĕn'ye-wātd) to make thin; to weaken or reduce in force.

attitude (ăt'ĭ-tüd) in speaking of fetal position, refers to the degree of flexion of the baby's head and extremities in the uterus.

aura (är'á) subjective warning of an impending epileptic seizure.

auscultation (aws-kŭl-tā'shŭn) process of listening for sounds produced in some body cavity.

autoclave (aw'tō-clāv) appliance used to sterilize objects by steam under pressure.

autonomy (aw-tŏn'á-mē) state of self-government or self-direction.

autosomes (äw'tō-sōhm) all chromosomes except sex determining X and Y.

bacillus (bá-sĭl'ŭs) (pl. bacilli) a rod-shaped bacterium.

barrier techniques various forms of isolation.

basophil (bā'sō-fĭl) one type of white blood cell.

bilirubin (bĭl-ĭ-rū'bĭn) orange or yellow pigment in bile; a product of red blood cell destruction; elevated levels in the blood may cause jaundice.

biopsy (bī'ŏp-sē) procurement of a specimen of tissue for microscopic examination.

booster injection substance or dose used to renew or increase the effect of a drug or immunizing agent.

bossing rounded protuberance, particularly on the skull, in the area of the forehead; one possible manifestation of rickets.

656

bradycardia (brăd″ē-kär′dē-à) slowness of the heartbeat; in adults, usually a rate of less than 60 beats per minute.

Braxton Hicks (brăx′ton hĭks) *contractions* contractions of the uterus that occur throughout pregnancy that help enlarge the uterus to accommodate the growing fetus; during the last weeks of pregnancy they may become very noticeable; false labor contractions.

breech (brēch) *birth* delivery of the child feet or buttocks first.

bronchiectasis (brŏn-kē-ĕk′tà-sĭs) abnormal dilatation of the bronchi in response to inflammation, which may lead to structural changes and chronic cough.

buffer apparatus or substance serving to neutralize the shock of opposing forces.

bulbar (bŭl′bär) pertaining to the "bulb" or medulla of the brain and the cranial nerves.

calcaneus (kăl-kā′nē-ŭs) heel bone or os calcis; type of clubfoot in which only the heel touches the ground; patient may walk on inner side of heel.

callus (kăl′ŭs) new bone formation at the site of a healing fracture.

calyx (kā′lĭks) (pl. calyces) small subdivision of the pelvis of the kidney.

Candida albicans (kăn′dĭ-dà ăl′bĭ-kănz) formerly called *Monilia albicans;* a yeastlike fungus that may infect various portions of the body, causing a variety of symptoms (e.g., leukorrhea, dermatitis, stomatitis).

cannula (kăn′ū-là) (pl. cannulae) small tube; large needle sheath used for the removal of fluid from body cavities.

canthus (kăn-thŭs) (pl. canthi) corner at each side of the eye where the eyelids meet.

caput succedaneum (kă′pŭt sŭk-sē-dā′nē-ŭm) abnormal collection of fluid under the scalp.

cardiovascular (kär-dē-ō-văs′kūl-är) pertaining to the heart and blood vessels.

caries (kăr′ēz) dental decay.

carrier person or animal capable of transmitting a contagious or hereditary disease but showing no outward sign of the disease.

cast solid mold usually made of plaster to help protect, position, or immobilize a part; microscopic sediment that has been partially shaped by the kidney tubules; any other body discharge or excretion retaining the shape of a body part that held it.

catalyst (kăt′à-lĭst) substance that speeds the rate of a chemical reaction without itself being permanently altered by the reaction.

catamenia (kăt-à-mē′nē-à) menses or menstruation.

cataract (kăt′à-răkt) abnormal opacity of the crystalline lens of the eye.

catheter (kăth′ĕ-ter) a hollow tube for insertion into a cavity or a canal for the purpose of discharging its fluid contents or introducing other substances into it.

cation (kăt′ĭ-àn) particle of matter (ion) carrying a positive electrical charge.

cecum (sē′kŭm) blind pouch that forms the first portion of the large intestine or colon; the attachment for the appendix.

celiac (sē′lē-ăk) *disease* chronic intestinal indigestion.

cellulitis (sĕl-ū-lī′tĭs) inflammation of the cellular or connective tissues.

cephalhematoma (sĕf-ăl-hē-mà-tō′mà) swelling on the head due to a collection of bloody fluid under the periosteum of the skull as the result of trauma.

cephalic (sĕ-făl′ĭk) pertaining to the head.

cephalocaudal (sĕf-à-lō-cawd′àl) moving from the head toward the base of the spine.

cerumen (sĕ-rü′mĕn) ear wax.

cervical (sĕr′vĭ-kàl) pertaining to the neck or cervix.

cesarean (sĕz-ăr′ē-àn) *section* an abdominal delivery made possible by incising the uterine and abdominal walls.

Chadwick's (chăd′wĭks) *sign* violet tinge of the cervical and vaginal mucous membranes; a probable sign of pregnancy.

chancre (shăng′ker) craterlike lesion seen in first-stage syphilis.

Cheyne-Stokes (chān′ stōks) *respiration* irregular, cyclic-type breathing characterized by a period of increasing respiratory action followed by an interval of apnea.

chloasma gravidarum (klō-ăz′mà grăv-ĭ-dā′rŭm) deepening pigmentation of skin during pregnancy, especially of the face; "mask of pregnancy."

chordee (kŏr-dē′) abnormal downward curvature of the penis.

chorea (kō-rē′à) involuntary muscular twitching or movement.

choriocarcinoma (kō-rĭ-ō-kär-sĭ-nō′mà) rare malignancy associated with hydatid mole or pregnancy.

chorion (kō′rĭ-ŏn) outermost membrane of the growing fertilized egg; one of two membranes that later form the "bag of waters."

chorionic gonadotropin (kō′rē-ŏn-ĭk gŏ-năd′ō-trō′pĭn) a gonad-regulating hormone produced by the outermost tissue covering the fetus in early pregnancy.

chorionic villi (vĭl′ī) fingerlike tissue projections of chorion on the outer wall of the fertilized egg.

chromosomes (krō′mà-sōmz) microscopic structures seen fairly easily in the nucleus of a cell during its reproduction, which contain the genes or determiners of heredity.

cisternal (sĭs-tĕr′nàl) *puncture* puncture with a hollow needle between the cervical vertebrae, through the dura mater, into the cisterna at the base of the brain.

clavicle (klăv′ĭ-kàl) collarbone.

clitoris (klī′tà-rĭs) the small, sensitive erectile structure located at the anterior junction of the labia minora.

coagulation (ko-ăg-ye-lā′shun) process of clotting.

coccus (kŏk′ŭs) (pl. cocci) spherical-shaped bacterium.

coitus (kō′ĭ-tŭs) sexual intercourse.

colic (kŏl′ĭk) intermittent pain caused by spasm of any hollow or tubular soft organ; abdominal cramping fairly common in first three months of infancy.

collagen (kŏl′à-jĕn) substance existing in many of the body's connective tissues.

collateral (kà-lăt′er-àl) situated at the sides; supplementary, reinforcing.

colostrum (kŏl-ŏs′trŭm) breast secretion produced by the mother the first few days after delivery.

colporrhaphy (kŏl-pōr′à-fē) surgical repair of the walls of the vagina.

comatose (kō′mà-tōs) in a coma or abnormally deep sleep caused by illness or injury.

comedo (kŏm′ē-dō) (pl. comedones) discolored, dried, oily secretion plugging the pores of the skin; blackhead.

comminuted (kŏm′ĭ-nŭt-ĕd) broken into many pieces; comminuted fracture, a crushed bone.

compatible able to work together; not in opposition; able to be mixed without destructive changes.

compression (kom-presh′un) a squeezing together; state of being pressed together.

conception (kon-sĕp′shŭn) union of the male sex cell, spermatozoon, and the female sex cell, ovum; fertilization; beginning of a new being.

conduit (kŏn′dü-ĭt) a tube or other device conveying water on other fluid from one region to another.

condyloma (kŏn-dĭ-lō′mà) wartlike growth usually found near the anus or vulva; the broad, flat form (c. latum) is characteristic of syphilis in its secondary stage.

congenital (kon-jĕn′ĭ-tàl) existing at birth.

conjugate (kŏn′jū-gāt) an anteroposterior diameter of the pelvis.

conjunctiva (kŏn-jŭnk-tī′và) mucous membrane that lines the inner surface of the eyelid and covers the anterior portion of the eye.

contaminated soiled, stained, touched or exposed in such a manner that the article in question becomes unsafe to use as intended or without barrier techniques.

continence (kŏnt′ĭ-nĕnts) control of bladder or bowel function, or self-restraint, especially in regard to sexual intercourse.

contraception (kŏn-trà-sĕp′shun) prevention of the fertilization of an egg or ovum.

contracture (kon-trăk′chur) permanent contraction of a muscle resulting from spasm or paralysis causing limitation of motion; high resistance to the passive stretch of a muscle.

contusion (kŏn-tū′zhŭn) injury that does not result in breaking the skin; a black and blue area; a bruise.

convulsion (kon-vŭl′shŭn) violent, involuntary contraction or series of contractions of the muscles.

corium (kō′rĭ-ŭm) dermis layer of the skin; "true skin."

cor pulmonale (kōr pŭl-mŏn-ăl′ē) cardiac enlargement or failure secondary to respiratory disease.

cortex (kōr′tĕks) outer or more superficial part of an organ.

coryza (kō-rī′zà) "common" head cold.

crepitus (krĕp′ĭ-tŭs) grating sensation sometimes heard or felt at the site of a fracture; crackling sound heard in certain diseases.

cretinism (krē′tĭn-ĭzm) infantile hypothyroidism characterized by mental retardation and other disturbances in mental and physical development.

crust an external protective layer; scab.

cryptorchidism (krĭpt-or′kĭd-ĭzm) failure of the testicles to descend into the scrotum.

cul-de-sac of Douglas blind pouch formed by the peritoneal lining of the abdominal cavity located between the uterus and rectum.

curettage (kü-ret′àj) (uterine) scraping with a curette to remove contents of uterus (as in inevitable, incomplete, or early therapeutic abortion), to obtain specimens for use in diagnosis, or to remove growths (e.g., polyps).

CVA cardiovascular accident.

cyanosis (sī-ăn-ō′sĭs) bluish or grayish coloration of the skin caused by poor oxygenation of the blood.

cystitis (sĭs-tī′tĭs) inflammation of the urinary bladder.

cystocele (sĭs′tō-sēl) prolapse of the urinary bladder caused by the weakened tissue wall between the bladder and vagina.

cystourethrogram (sĭs″tō-ū-rĕth′rō-gram) x-ray film of the bladder and urethra.

cytoplasm (sī′tō-plăz-ŭm) portion of a cell inside the cell membrane but outside the nucleus.

debilitate (dē-bĭl′ĭ-tāt) to produce weakness; enfeeble.

debridement (dā-brēd-mŏn′) surgical removal of dead, damaged, or contaminated tissue.

debris (dà-brē) rubbish; ruins.

decalcification (dē-kăl-sĭ-fī-kā′shŭn) removal of or withdrawal of lime salts from bone.

deciduous (dē-sĭd′ū-ŭs) *teeth* baby or milk teeth.

decubitus (dē-kū′bĭ-tŭs) bedsore.

dehydration (dē-hī-drā′shŭn) condition in which the body tissues lack normal fluid content.

dentition (děn-tĭsh'ŭn) process or time of teething.

dermatitis (děr-mà-tī'tĭs) *venenata* skin disturbance caused by external irritants.

detrusor (dē-trü'sor) *muscle* smooth muscle of the bladder wall.

diaphoresis (dī-ă-fō-rē'sĭs) profuse sweating.

diaphragmatic (dī-à-frăg-măt'ĭk) *hernia* protrusion of abdominal contents through an abnormal opening in the diaphragm.

diaphysis (dī-ăf'ĭ-sĭs) shaft or middle part of a long bone.

diastolic (dī-ăs-tŏl'ĭk) pertaining to diastole—the blood pressure at the time of greatest cardiac relaxation.

digestion (dī'jěs'chěn) process by which food is broken down mechanically and chemically in the gastrointestinal tract and converted into absorbable forms.

digital (dĭj'ĭ-tàl) pertaining to the digits, that is, the fingers or toes.

digitalization (dĭj-ĭ-tăl-ĭ-zā'shŭn) administration of digitalis to slow and strengthen the heartbeat (particularly the initial administration of the drug).

dilatation (dĭl-à-tā'shŭn) expansion of an organ or orifice; dilation.

diploid (dĭp'loyd) having double the number of chromosomes found in the ova or sperm, the normal chromosome number for body cells.

disorientation (dĭs-ō-rē-ĕn-tā'shŭn) inability to evaluate properly direction, location, time surroundings, or personal role.

distal (dĭs'tàl) farthest from the trunk of the body or from a specific point of reference.

distention (dĭs-tĕn'shŭn) (also distension) inflation, stretch, ballooning.

diuresis (dī″ū-rē'sĭs) increased urine output.

diuretic (dī-ū-rĕt'ĭk) agent that increases the secretion of urine.

diverticulum (dī-ver-tĭk'ū-lŭm) (pl. diverticula) sac or pouch in the walls of a canal or organ, especially the colon.

ductus arteriosus (dŭk'tŭs är-tēr-ē-ō'sŭs) short blood vessel located between the pulmonary artery and aorta in the fetus.

ductus deferens (dŭk'tŭs děf'ěr-ěnz) excretory duct of the testicle; vas deferens.

dyscrasia (dĭs-krā'zhē-à) undefined disease, malfunction, or abnormal condition, often used when speaking of abnormalities of the blood.

dysentery (dĭs'ĕn-tĕr-ē) inflammation of the intestines, especially of the colon, usually characterized by mild to severe diarrhea.

dysmenorrhea (dĭs-mĕn-ō-rē'à) painful or difficult menstruation.

dyspnea (dĭsp-nē'à) difficult breathing.

dystocia (dĭs-tō'shà) difficult labor, particularly difficulty in the mechanics of childbirth.

ecchymosis (ĕk-ĭ-mō'sĭs) black-and-blue mark caused by hemorrhage into the skin, usually a relatively large area.

eclampsia (ě-klămp'sē-à) major toxemia of pregnancy characterized by convulsion of a pregnant or newly delivered patient who classically displays signs of albuminuria, hypertension, and edema; if the patient has these symptoms but has not convulsed, she is termed "preeclamptic."

ecology (ĭ-kŏl'à-jĭ) interrelationships of organisms and their environment as manifested by natural cycles and rhythms.

ectopic (ĕk-tŏp-ĭk) *pregnancy* pregnancy that develops in an abnormal place (e.g., in the uterine tube, abdomen, or ovary).

edema (ē-dē'ma) abnormal, excessive amount of fluid within the body tissues.

edematous (ě-dĕm'ăt-ŭs) characterized by the presence of edema; that is, an abnormal amount of fluid in the tissues.

effacement (ĕf-ās'měnt) (of the cervix) shortening and thinning of the cervix or neck of the uterus.

effleurage (ĕf'lü-rahzh) the stroking movement used in massage.

effusion (ē-fu'-shun) escape of fluid into an area.

ejaculation (ē-jăk-ū-lā'shŭn) ejection of the seminal fluid from the male urethra.

electroencephalogram (ē-lĕk-trō-ĕn-sĕf'à-lō-grăm) tracing made by an apparatus designed to detect and record brain waves.

electrolyte (ē-lĕk'trō-līt) substance that, in solution, conducts electric current.

embolus (ĕm'bō-lŭs) (pl. emboli) foreign substance traveling in the circulatory system; e.g., a blood clot or air.

embryo (ĕm'brē-ō) unborn young of any creature in an early stage of development when specific identification is difficult with the naked eye.

emesis (ĕm'ě-sĭs) referring to vomiting or the substance vomited.

emission (ē-mĭsh'ŭn) discharge (e.g., discharge of semen), especially involuntary.

emphysema (ĕm-fĭ-sē'mà) abnormal dilatation and loss of elasticity of the alveoli or air sacs of the lungs.

empyema (ĕm-pī-ē'mà) collection of pus in a body cavity, especially the pleural cavity.

encephalitis (ě-sĕf-à-lī'tĭs) inflammation of the encephalon, that is, the brain.

encephalopathy (ĕn-sĕf″à-lŏp'à-thē) any dysfunction of the brain.

endarteritis (ĕnd-är-tĕr-ī'tĭs) inflammation of the lining of the arteries.

endocarditis (ĕn-dō-kär-dī'tĭs) inflammation of the lining of the heart.

endocrine (ĕn'dō-krĭn) pertaining to ductless glands that discharge their secretions (hormones) directly into the bloodstream.

endometritis (ĕn-dō-mē-trī'tĭs) inflammation of the endometrium, or lining of the uterus.

endotracheal (ĕn'dō-trā'kē-ȧl) within the trachea.

engagement (ĕn-gāj'mĕnt) in obstetrics, refers to the entrance of the presenting part of the fetus into the true pelvis; the passage of the largest diameter of the presenting part into the true pelvis.

engorgement (ĕn-gōrj'mĕnt) in obstetrics, refers to the swelling of the breasts because of local congestion of the veins and lymphatics associated with lactation.

enterobiasis (ĕn"tĕr-ō-bī'ȧ-sĭs) disease caused by pinworm infestation.

enterostomy (ĕn-tĕr-ŏs'to-mĭ) surgical opening into the intestine through the abdominal wall.

enuresis (ĕn-ū-rē'sĭs) bed-wetting at an age when urinary control should be present.

epicanthus (ĕ-pĭ-kǎn'thŭs) fold of skin extending from the nose to the median end of the eyebrow, characteristic of the Mongolian race.

epidemiological (ep'ĭ-dē"mē-o-loj'ĭ-kȧl) pertaining to the study of epidemics, their origin and prevention or, more broadly, the origins of any condition.

epididymis (ĕp-ĭ-dĭd'ĭ-mĭs) (pl. epididymides) small oblong organ, situated on the testis, containing a coiled extension of the tubules of the testis, which eventually joins the vas deferens.

epiphysis (ĕ-pĭf'ĭ-sĭs) (pl. epiphyses) end of a long bone.

episiotomy (ĭ-pĭz-ē-ŏt'ȧ-mē) surgical incision extending from the soft tissue of the vaginal opening into the true perineum performed to protect the perineum from laceration or help hasten the delivery of an infant.

epispadias (ĕp-ĭ-spā'dē-ȧs) abnormal condition in which the urethral opening is located on the upper (dorsal) surface of the penis.

epistaxis (ĕp-ĭ-stăk'sĭs) nosebleed.

epithelial (ĕp"ĭ-thē'lē-ȧl) pertaining to the outermost layer of the skin and/or the lining tissue of hollow organs and inner passages of the body.

equilibrium (ē-kwĭ-lĭb'rē-um) equal balance, between powers; mental balance; equality of effect.

equinus (ē-kwī'nŭs) condition characterized by a tiptoe walk affecting one or both feet, often associated with clubfoot.

Erbs' palsy (erbz pawl'zē) injury to the brachial plexus causing partial paralysis of the arm.

erectile (ē-rĕk'tĭl) capable of becoming erect.

erysipelas (ĕr-ĭ-sĭp'ĕ-lŭs) acute febrile disease, with localized inflammation and swelling of the skin and subcutaneous tissue accompanied by systemic disturbance of variable degree, caused by a streptococcus.

erythema (ăr-ĭ-thē'mȧ) redness of the skin; characteristic red blotches on the skin of the newborn infant.

erythema marginatum (märj-ĭ-nå'tŭm) rash occasionally seen in cases of rheumatic fever.

erythroblast (ĕ-rĭth'rō-blăst) immature, inadequate form of red blood cell normally found only in the bone marrow.

erythroblastosis fetalis (ĕ-rĭth"rō-blăst-ō'sĭs fē-tă'lĭs) hemolytic disease of the newborn characterized by anemia, jaundice, enlarged liver and spleen, and the presence of erythroblasts circulating in the bloodstream.

erythrocyte (ĕ-rĭth'rō-sīt) red blood corpuscle or cell.

eschar (ĕs'kär) thick crusts that may form over burned areas on the body, composed of hardened drainage.

esophageal (ĕ-sŏf"ȧ-jē-ȧl) pertaining to the esophagus, or food tube, leading from the throat to the stomach.

estrogen (ĕs'trō-jĕn) class name for a female sex hormone; more particularly, the hormonal secretion of the ovary that builds up the lining of the uterus and promotes feminine characteristics.

eupnea (ūp-nē'ȧ) normal breathing.

excoriation (ĕks-kō-rĭ-ā'shŭn) scraping of the skin's surface through injury.

excrete (ek-skrēt) separate and eliminate from an organic body.

exocrine (ĕks'ō-krĭn) term applied to glands whose secretion reaches an epithelial surface either directly or through a duct.

exstrophy (ĕks'trō-fē) eversion or the turning inside out of a part with or without the abnormal exposure of the part.

exudate (ĕks'ū-dāt) accumulation of a fluid in a cavity; drainage flowing from one body area to another; drainage from wounds.

fallopian (fȧ-lō'pē-on) *tubes* uterine tubes, or oviducts, leading from the uterine cavity toward each ovary.

familial (fȧ-mĭl'ē-ȧl) pertaining to or characteristic of a family.

fascia (fǎsh'ē-ȧ) fibrous connective tissue found under the skin or covering, supporting, and separating muscles and other organs.

febrile (fēb'rĭl or fĕb'rĭl) state of being feverish.

fertilization (fĕr-tĭ-lĭ-zā'shŭn) union of male and female sex cells; conception.

fetus (fē'tŭs) later stages of the developing young of an animal within the uterus or egg when the species is distinguishable by the naked eye.

FHR fetal heart rate.

fibrinogen (fī-brĭn'ō-jĕn) protein in the blood plasma necessary to coagulation.

fistula (fĭs'tū-lȧ) (pl. fistulae) abnormal tubelike passageway from a normal body cavity or canal to another body cavity or to the outside of the body.

flaccid (flǎ'sĭd) soft, flabby, relaxed; lacking normal tension or tone.

flexion (flĕk'shŭn) act of being bent.

follicle (fŏl'ĭ-kȧl) small secretory sac or cavity; protective tissue envelope of the female sex cell, or ovum.

fontanel (fŏn'tȧ-nĕl) soft spot found between the cranial bones of the skull of an infant, formed where sutures meet or cross.

foramen (fō-rā'mĕn) small opening.

foramen ovale (ō-vā'lē) normal opening between the atria in the heart of the fetus.

foreskin (fōr'skĭn) prepuce, or fold of skin covering the glans penis.

fornix (fōr'nĭx) (pl. fornices) arch or fold.

fourchet (für-shĕt') tense band of mucous membrane connecting the posterior ends of the labia minora.

frenulum (frĕn'ū-lŭm) (pl. frenula) fold of mucous membrane extending from the underside of the tongue to the floor of the mouth at the midline.

frequency (frē'kwĕn-sē) number of repetitions of a periodic process in a unit of time; when speaking of urinary function, the term implies an abnormal increase in the number of voidings.

FSH follicle-stimulating hormone.

fundus (fŭn'dŭs) (pl. fundi) part of an organ opposite its opening; top of the uterus.

funic souffle (fū'nĭk sü-fȧl) sound sometimes heard over the pregnant uterus having same rate as fetal heartbeat; it may be related to compression of the umbilical cord.

furuncle (fū'rŭng-kȧl) infected hair follicle; a boil.

fusion (fū'shŭn) process of uniting.

galactosemia (gȧ-lăk″tō-sē'mē-ȧ) metabolic condition involving the metabolism of galactose, which may produce mental retardation and other symptoms.

gamete (găm'ēt) male or female reproductive cell capable of entering into union with each other in the process of fertilization.

gamma globulin (găm'mȧ glŏb'ū-lĭn) blood protein fraction containing most of the protective immune antibodies.

gastroenteritis (găs″trō-ĕn-ter-ī'tĭs) inflammation of the mucosa of the stomach and intestines.

gastrostomy (găs-trŏ'stȧ-mē) intentional establishment of an opening into the stomach through the abdominal wall, usually for artificial feeding.

gavage (gȧ-vȧzh') feeding through a stomach tube passed either nasally or orally.

gene (jēn) hereditary determiner located on the chromosomes.

genetics (jĕ-nĕt'ĭks) study of inheritance or genes.

genitalia (jĕn-ĭ-tāl'ē-ȧ) organs of generation or reproduction.

gestation (jĕs-tā'shŭn) period of intrauterine fetal development; pregnancy.

gingivitis (jĭn″jĭ-vī'tĭs) inflammation of the gums.

glans penis (glănz pē'nĭs) sensitive portion (tip) of the penis.

glioma (glī-ō'mȧ) tumor involving the supportive tissue of the brain or glial cells.

glomerulus (glō-măr'ū-lŭs) (pl. glomeruli) cluster or coil of connecting capillaries located at the top of the expanded end (Bowman's capsule) of the urinary tubules in the kidney.

glottis (glŏt'ĭs) opening of the larynx including the associated vocal cords.

gluten (glü'tĕn) protein found in wheat, rye, and oats.

gluteus (glü-tē'us) any of the three muscles that form the buttocks.

glycosuria (glī-kō-sü'rē-ȧ) presence of glucose in the urine.

gonadotropic (gō-năd-ō-trō'pĭk) relating to stimulation of the gonads, that is, the ovaries or testes.

gravida (grăv'ĭ-dȧ) pertaining to the number of pregnancies a woman has had; a pregnant woman.

gumma (gŭm'mȧ) soft gummy tumor that may develop during third stage of syphilis.

gynecoid (gī'nĕ-coyd or jĭn'ĕ-coyd) womanlike; typical female pelvis.

gynecomastia (gī-nĕ-kō-măs'tĭ-ȧ or jĭn-ĕ-kō-măs'tĭ'ȧ) swelling of the newborn or adult male breast tissue.

habilitate (hȧ-bĭl'ĭ-tāt) equip for working and for everyday tasks or activities.

hallucination (hȧ-lū-sĭ-nā'shŭn) false perception having no relation to reality and not accounted for by any external stimuli; may be visual, auditory, olfactory, etc.

Hegar's (hā'gärz) *sign* softening of the uterine isthmus, the area between the cervix and body of the uterus; a probable sign of pregnancy.

hemangioma (hē-măn-jē-ō'mȧ) blood vessel tumor.

hematocrit (hē-măt'ȧ-krĭt) *reading* the percentage of whole blood volume occupied by red blood cells after they have been separated through use of a centrifuge.

hematoma (hē-mȧ-tō'mȧ) tumor composed of blood cells, resulting from tissue injury.

hematuria (hē-mȧ-tü'rĭ-ȧ) presence of blood in the urine.

hemoglobin (hē-mō-glō'bĭn) oxygen-carrying protein pigment found in the red blood cells.

hemolytic (hē-mō-lĭt'ĭk) pertaining to or causing the breakdown of red blood cells.

hemoptysis (hē-mŏp'tĭ-sĭs) presence of blood-stained sputum.

hemorrhoid (hĕm'ō-royd) rectal varicosity; "pile."

heparinized (hĕp'er-rĭn-īzed) containing heparin employed as an anticoagulant.

hermaphroditism (her-măf'rō-dīt-ĭsm) possession by one individual of the gonads and external genitalia of both sexes.

hernia (hĕr'nĭ-à) rupture; an abnormal protrusion of a portion of the contents of a body cavity because of a defect in its surrounding walls, frequently causing swelling, pressure symptoms, or other complications.

herpes (hĕr'pēz) *simplex* viral infection characteristically causing an eruption of small, clustered blisters on the skin or mucous membranes.

heterozygous (hĕt"er-ō-zī'gŭs) having the two members of one or more pairs of genes dissimilar.

homozygous (hō"mō-zī'gŭs) having both of a given pair of genes alike.

hordeolum (hŏr-dē'ō-lŭm) sty or infection involving the eyelash follicle.

hormone (hŏr'mōn) internal secretions of thyroid gland, pancreas, etc. Chemical substance originating in an organ, gland, or part that is conveyed through the blood to another part of the body, helping to regulate body processes.

Hutchinson's (hŭch'ĭn-sŭnz) *teeth* notched teeth characteristic of congenital syphilis.

hydatidiform (hī"dà-tĭd'ĭ-fōrm) *mole* condition in which the fertilized ovum becomes altered and an abnormal tissue develops instead of a baby and normal placenta.

hydrocele (hī'drō-sēl) abnormal collection of fluid in the lining tissue of the testis.

hydrocephalus (hī-drō-sĕf'à-lŭs) collection of abnormal amounts of cerebrospinal fluid within the cranium, causing enlargement of the immature skull.

hydrophobia (hī-drō-fō'bē-à) rabies; fear of water.

hymen (hī'mĕn) membrane partially covering the vaginal opening; "the maindenhead."

hyperalimentation (hī"per-ăl'ĭ-mĕn-tā'shŭn) overfeeding or giving nourishment in great amounts per vein.

hypercalcemia (hī-per-kăl-sē'mē-à) excessive amount of calcium in the blood.

hypercapnia (hī"per-kăp'nē-à) (increased P_{CO_2}) excessive amount of carbon dioxide in the blood.

hyperemesis gravidarum (hī-pĕr-ĕm'ē-sĭs grăv-ĭ-dā'rŭm) persistent, exaggerated nausea and vomiting during pregnancy.

hyperglycemia (hī-pĕr-glī-sē'mē-à) excessive amount of glucose in the bloodstream.

hyperkalemia (hī-per-kà-lē'mē-à) excessive amount of potassium in the blood.

hypernatremia (hī-per-nà-trē'mē-à) excessive amount of sodium in the blood.

hypertension (hī-per-tĕn'shŭn) abnormal elevation of the blood pressure, especially the diastolic pressure.

hypertonic (hī"per-tŏn'ĭk) excessive or above normal in tone or tension; containing excessive amounts of salts.

hypertrophy (hī-per'trō-fē) increase in size or bulk; excessive development.

hyperventilation (hī-per-vĕn-tĭl-ā'shŭn) overbreathing accompanied by a carbon dioxide deficit commonly causing dizziness as well as tingling and numbness in the hands.

hypnotic (hĭp-nŏt'ĭk) medication that causes sleep.

hypocalcemia (hī-pō-kăl-sē'mē-à) abnormally low blood calcium level.

hypodermoclysis (hī-pō-dĕr-mŏk'lĭ-sĭs) infusion of fluids into the tissue spaces below the skin and above the muscle layer by means of a needle placed in the subcutaneous tissue.

hypogastric (hī-pō-găs'trĭk) pertaining to lower middle area of the abdomen.

hypoglycemia (hī-pō-glī-sē'mē-à) deficiency of glucose in the blood.

hypokalemia (hī-pō-kà-lē'mē-à) deficiency of potassium in the blood.

hyponatremia (hī-pō-nā-trē'mē-à) deficiency of sodium in the blood.

hypospadias (hī-pō-spā'dē-às) condition characterized by the abnormal opening of the urethra on the undersurface of the penis.

hypostatic (hī-pō-stăt'ĭk) pertaining to the settling of a deposit or congestion in an area, caused by lack of proper activity.

hypotension (hī-pō-tĕn'shun) abnormal decrease of systolic and diastolic blood pressure.

hypothalamus (hī-pō-thăl'à-mŭs) area of heat control and other body regulation located near the base of the brain.

hypothermia (hī"pō-thur'mē-à) pertaining to subnormal temperature of the body.

hypoxia (hī-pŏks'ē-ă) lack of adequate amount of oxygen.

hysterotomy (hĭs-tĕr-ŏt'ō-mē) opening of the uterus; cesarean section.

icterus (ĭk'tĕr-ŭs) jaundice; a yellow tint to the skin.

idiopathic (ĭd-ē-ō-păth'ĭk) adjective meaning that the cause of the condition is unknown.

ileostomy (ĭl"ē-ŏs'tà-mē) surgical formation of a fistula or artificial anus through the abdominal wall into the ileum, or an ileal pouch created as a part of the Bricker procedure.

ileum (ĭl'ē-ŭm) lower portion of small intestine.

ileus (il'ē-ŭs) obstruction or paralysis of small intestine.

iliopectineal (ĭl"ē-ō-pĕk-tĭnē-al) *line* imaginary line dividing the upper or false pelvis from the lower or true pelvis; the linea terminalis forming the brim or inlet of the pelvis.

immunity (ĭ-mū'nĭ-tē) ability to protect oneself against the development of infectious disease.

impaction (ĭm-păk'shŭn) state of being lodged and retained abnormally in a part or strait; a large accumulation of relatively hard stool in the rectum or colon, difficult to move.

imperforate (ĭm-pĕr'fōr-āt) without an opening.

impetigo (ĭm-pĕ-tī'gō) contagious skin infection

662

caused by coagulase-positive staphylococci or beta-hemolytic streptococci.

implantation (ĭm-plăn-tā′shŭn) nesting of the fertilized ovum in the wall of the uterus; artificial placement of a substance in the body.

incarcerated (ĭn-kär′sĕr-ā-tĕd) trapped; confined.

incest (ĭn′sĕst) sexual intercourse between those of near relationship.

incontinence (ĭn-kŏn′tĭ-nĕnts) inability to retain urine or feces because of loss of sphincter control.

incubation (ĭn-kū-bā′shŭn) *period* period of time that must elapse between the infection of an individual at the time of exposure until the appearance of signs and symptoms of the disease.

inertia (ĭn-ĕr′shà) sluggishness; absence of activity; resistance to movement or change.

infanticide (ĭn-făn′tĭs-īd) killing of an infant.

infectious (ĭn-fĕk′shŭs) *disease* disorders caused by organisms that invade tissue and cause symptoms of illness.

infecund (ĭn′fĕk-ŭnd) unfruitful; infertile; inability to conceive.

infertile (ĭn-fer′til) inability of a man or woman to conceive.

infusion (ĭn-fū′zhun) introduction of a solution into a vein.

inguinal (ĭn-gwĭ-nàl) pertaining to the region of the groin.

inhibitor (ĭn-hĭb′ĭt-er) agent that curtails or stops certain activity.

insemination (ĭn′sĕm-ĭ-nā-shŭn) (artificial) injection of semen into the uterine canal by a process unrelated to intercourse.

integumentary (ĭn-tĕg-ū-mĕn′tà-rē) referring to the integument, that is, the skin, including the hair, nails, oil and sweat glands, and superficial sensory nerve endings.

interstitial (ĭn-tĕr-stĭsh′àl) *fluid* body fluid found outside the bloodstream in the spaces between the tissue cells.

intertrigo (ĭn″ter-trē′gō) a reddened skin eruption produced by friction of adjacent parts; chafing.

intubation (ĭn″tü-bā′shŭn) introduction of a tube into a hollow organ or passageway to keep it open.

intussusception (ĭn-tŭs-sŭs-sĕp′shŭn) telescoping of adjacent parts of the bowel, usually in the ileocecal region.

in utero (ū′tĕr-ō) inside the uterus.

inversion (ĭn-vĕr′shŭn or ĭn-vĕr′zhŭn) a turning upside down, inside out, or end to end.

involution (ĭn-vō-lū′shŭn) a turning or rolling inward; the reverse of evolution, a term especially used to describe the return of the uterus to approximately its prepregnant size and position after childbirth.

iodophor (ĭ-ō′dà-fōr) an antiseptic containing iodine combined with detergent or an agent or carrier that enhances its solubility.

ion (ĭ′àn) one or more atoms carrying an electrical charge.

IPPB intermittent positive pressure breathing device used to help expand the lungs.

ischial (ĭs′kē-àl) *spines* the two relatively sharp bony projections protruding into the pelvic outlet from the ischial bones that form the lower lateral border of the pelvis, used in determining the progress of the fetus down the birth canal.

isolation (ĭ-sō-lā′shŭn) prevention of direct or indirect contact with a person with a contagious disease during its period of communicability by the observance of certain barrier techniques designed to prevent the spread of illness.

jaundice (jawn′dĭs) yellow tinge to the skin or sclerae; icterus.

karyotype (kăr′ē-ō-tīp) the total characteristics of the chromosomes of a cell nucleus including number, form, size, and grouping, usually photographed, cut out and arranged on a card for study.

kernicterus (ker-nĭk′ter-ŭs) yellow staining of the basal ganglia of the brain in the jaundiced newborn infant; a complication of Rh factor incompatibility.

ketogenic (kē-tō-jĕn′ĭk) *diet* high-fat, low-carbohydrate diet.

ketone (kē′tōn) *bodies* group of compounds produced during the oxidation of fatty acids; one example is acetone.

kwashiorkor (kwash-ĭ-ōr′kōr) disease resulting from protein deprivation in infancy and childhood, common in certain parts of Africa.

kyphosis (kī-fō′sĭs) humpback.

labia majora (lā′bē-à mà-jō-rà) (sing. labium) (two fleshy, hair-covered folds located on both sides of the perineal midline, extending from the mons veneris almost to the anus in women.

labia minora (mĭ-nō′rà) two small folds of tissue covering the vestibule located just under the labia majora in women.

laceration (lăs-er-ā′shŭn) jagged cut or tear.

lacrimal (lăk′rĭm-àl) *glands* tear glands.

lactation (lăk-tā′shŭn) process of milk production or the period of breast feeding in mammals.

lactogenic (lăk-tō-jĕn′ĭk) inducing the secretion of milk (e.g., the lactogenic hormone *prolactin* or LTH).

lanugo (là-nü′gō) soft, fine hair on the body of the fetus or newborn.

laparotomy (lăp-à-rŏt′ō-mē) abdominal operation; surgical opening of the abdomen.

laryngospasm (lär-ĭng′gō-spă-zŭm) spasm of the muscles of the larynx.

larynx (lär′ĭnks) voice box.

lesion (lē′zhŭn) any change or irregularity in tissue resulting from disease or injury.

lethargic (lĕth-är′jĭk) drowsy; sluggish.

leukemia (lū-kē′mē-a) disease characterized by overproduction of abnormal, immature, white blood cells; "cancer of the blood."

leukocyte (lü′kō-sīt) white blood cell.

leukocytosis (lü-kō-sī-tō′sĭs) excessive increase in the number of white blood cells circulating in the blood.

leukopenia (lü-kō-pē′nē-à) abnormal decrease of circulating white blood cells.

leukorrhea (lü-kō-rē′à) abnormal white or yellowish cervical or vaginal discharge.

levator ani (lĕ-vā′tŏr ā′nē) major muscle that helps form the pelvic diaphragm or floor.

ligament (lĭg′à-mĕnt) strong, fibrous tissue that serves to connect bone to bone or to support an organ.

ligation (lī-gā′shŭn) closing off by tying, especially arteries, veins, tubes, or ducts.

lightening (līt′ĕn-ĭng) descent of the fetus into the true pelvis, which lessens pressure on the maternal thorax and abdomen.

linea nigra (lĭn′ē-à nī′grà) dark line that develops during pregnancy extending from the pubis to the umbilicus.

lipoids (lĭp′oydz) fatty-type substances.

lipoprotein (lĭp″ō-prō′tēn) simple protein combined with a lipid or fatlike substance.

lithotomy (lĭth-ŏt′à-mē) removal of a calculus, usually a urinary tract stone.

lochia (lō′kē-à) vaginal drainage after childbirth.

lordosis (lŏr-dō′sĭs) exaggerated lumbar curvature; swayback.

lues (lū′ēz) syphilis.

lumbar puncture needle insertion into the subarachnoid space of the spinal cord between the lumbar vertebrae for diagnosis or therapy.

luteal (lü′tē-àl) *hormone* progesterone.

lymphocyte (lĭm′fō-sīt) one kind of white blood cell.

macule (măk′ūl) flat spot or stain.

malaise (mà-lāz′) discomfort, uneasiness.

mandible (măn′dĭ-bŭl) jawbone.

mastitis (măs-tī′tĭs) inflammation of the breast.

maturation (măt-ū-rā′shŭn) process of developing, ripening, or becoming more adult.

meatotomy (mē-à-tŏt′ō-mē) incision of the urinary meatus or opening to enlarge the passage.

meatus (mē-ā′tŭs) passage or opening.

meconium (mē-kō′nē-ŭm) first feces of the fetus or newborn.

medulla (mē-dŭl′à) inner portion of an organ (e.g., the medulla of the kidney or adrenal gland).

megacolon (mĕg-à-kō′lŏn) abnormally large colon.

megaloblast (mĕg′à-lō-blăst) a large, early form of red blood cell with a characteristic nuclear pattern, found in the blood where there is vitamin B₁₂ or folic acid deficiency.

menarche (mĕ-när′kē) first menses or menstruation experienced by a girl.

meningitis (mĕn-ĭn-jī′tĭs) inflammation of the meninges covering the spinal cord or brain.

meningococcemia (mĕ-nĭn-gō-kŏk-sē′mĭ-à) presence of meningococci in the blood.

meningococcic (mĕ-nĭn-gō-kŏk′sĭk) *meningitis* cerebrospinal fever.

menopause (mĕn′ō-pawz) period that marks the permanent cessation of menstrual activity.

menorrhagia (mĕn-ō-rā′jē-à) abnormal, excessive bleeding at time of the menstrual period.

menses (mĕn′sēz) menstruation.

menstruation (mĕn-strū-ā′shŭn) monthly elimination of a bloody vaginal discharge, the portion of the lining of the uterus that had been prepared for the fertilized egg in the event of pregnancy.

mentum (mĕn′tŭm) chin.

metabolic (mĕt-à-bŏl′ĭk) pertaining to the physical and chemical changes that take place within a living organism.

metabolism (mē-tăb′à-lĭz-ĕm) all energy and material transformations that occur within living cells.

metacarpal (mĕt″à-kär′pàl) pertaining to one of the five bones of the hand.

metastasis (mē-tăs′tà-sĭs) spread of a disease (e.g., cancer) from its primary location to secondary locations; the colonizing element.

metrorrhagia (mē-trō-rā′jē-à) presence of bloody vaginal discharge between menstrual periods.

microcephaly (mī-krō-sĕf′à-lē) failure of the brain to develop to a normal size.

milia (mĭl′ē-à) (sing. milium) pinpoint white or yellow dots commonly found on the nose, forehead, and cheeks of newborn babies resulting from nonfunctioning or clogged sebaceous glands.

miliaria rubra (mĭl-ē-ā′rĭ-à rü′brà) heat rash; prickly heat.

milk leg phlebitis of the femoral vein, occasionally found in women after delivery.

miscarriage spontaneous abortion.

mohel (moy′ĭl) an ordained Jewish circumciser.

molding shaping of the baby's head as it travels through the birth canal.

Monilia (mō-nĭl′ē-à) see moniliasis.

moniliasis (mō-nĭ-lī′à-sĭs) yeast infection of the skin or mucous membranes caused by *Candida albicans*, formerly called *Monilia albicans*; commonly found in the vagina; infection of the mouth is termed thrush.

monocyte (mŏn′ō-sīt) type of white blood cell.

mortality (mŏr-tăl′ĭ-tē) state of being mortal, subject to death or destined to die; the death rate.

morula (mŏr′ü-là) mass of dividing cells resembling a mulberry, resulting from the fertilization of an ovum; an early stage of life.

mosaicism (mō-zā′ĭ-cĭzm) the presence of body

cells with differing genetic contents in the same individual.

motile (mō'tĭl) capability of spontaneous movement.

mucosa (mū-kō'sȧ) mucous membrane.

mucous (mū'kŭs) (adj.) secreting or containing mucus; slimy.

mucoviscidosis (mū-cō-vĭs-ĭd-ō'sĭs) cystic fibrosis of the pancreas; a disease affecting the exocrine glands involving primarily the respiratory and digestive systems.

mucus (mū'kŭs) (n.) slippery secretion produced by the mucous membranes.

multifactorial caused by many factors; involving many genes or combinations of genes.

multiform (mŭl'tĭ-form) having many forms or shapes.

multigravida (mŭl-tĭ-grăv'ĭ-dȧ) woman who has had two or more pregnancies.

multipara (mŭl-tĭp'ȧ-rȧ) strictly speaking, a woman who has been delivered of two or more infants of 500 Gm. or more; however, in the delivery room, a woman in the process of labor with her second child is called a multipara.

musculature (mŭs'kū-lȧ-tūr) arrangement and condition of the muscles in the body or its parts.

myelitis (mī-ĕl-ī'tĭs) inflammation of the spinal cord or bone marrow.

myelomeningocele (mī''ĕl-ō-mĕ-nĭng'ō-sēl) herniation of elements of the spinal cord and the meninges through an abnormal opening in the spine.

myocarditis (mī''ō-kär-dī'tĭs) inflammation of the muscular tissue of the heart.

myomectomy (mī-ō-mĕk'tō-mē) removal of a portion of muscle or muscular tissue.

myometrium (mī''ō-mē'trē-ŭm) the muscular layer of the uterus.

myopia (mī-ō'pē-ȧ) nearsightedness.

myringotomy (mĭr-ĭn-gŏt'ō-mē) incision into the eardrum.

necrosis (nĕk-rō'sĭs) death of tissue.

neonatal (nē-ō-nā'tȧl) concerning the newborn infant or the first 4 weeks of life.

neoplasm (nē'ō-plă-zŭm) tumor.

nephron (nĕf'rŏn) working unit of the kidney; the renal corpuscle and its tubule.

nephrosis (nĕf-rō'sĭs) renal disease of unknown cause seen in children, characterized by massive edema and albuminuria.

neutrophil (nū'trō-fĭl) one kind of white blood cell.

nevus (nē'vŭs) (pl. nevi) mole, pigmented area, or vascular tumor on the skin.

nitrous oxide (nī'trŭs ŏk'sīd) laughing gas (N_2O).

nocturia (nŏk-tū'rĭ-a) excessive urination during the night.

nodule (nŏd'ūl) small aggregate of cells.

nuchal (nū'kȧl) pertaining to the neck.

nucleus (nū'klē-ŭs) central point about which matter is gathered; controlling portion of a cell regulating metabolism and reproduction of the cell.

nulligravida (nŭl-ĭ-grăv'ĭ-dȧ) woman who has never been pregnant.

nullipara (nŭl-ĭp'ȧ-rȧ) woman who has never delivered an infant of 500 Gm. or more.

nurture (ner'cher) to feed, rear, foster, care for; nourishment, care, and training of growing children or things.

nystagmus (nĭs-tăg'mŭs) constant, involuntary movement of the eyeballs.

oblique (ō-blēk') slanting; inclined.

obturator (ŏb'tū-rā''tŏr) small, curved rod with an olive-shaped tip that fits inside a tracheostomy tube to aid in its insertion.

occiput (ŏk'sĭ-pŭt) occipital bone or back part of the skull.

occlude (ŏ-klūd') to close or plug.

occult (ŏ-kŭlt') obscure, hidden.

oliguria (ŏl-ĭ-gū'rē-ȧ) diminished amount of urine production with subsequent scanty urination.

omphalocele (ŏm'făl-ō-sēl) absence of the normal abdominal wall in the region of the umbilicus creating defects of varying sizes.

opaque (ō-pāk') lacking transparency.

ophthalmia neonatorum (ŏf-thăl'mē-ȧ nē-ō-nă-tōr'-ŭm) inflammation of the eyes of the newborn infant, particularly that caused by gonorrheal organisms.

opisthotonos (ŏ-pĭs-thŏt'ō-nŏs) involuntary arching of the back because of irritation of the brain or spinal cord.

orchiopexy (or''kē-ō-pĕk'sē) surgical fixation of a testis or testicle in the scrotum to correct undescent.

orthopnea (ŏr-thŏp-nē'ȧ) condition in which breathing is possible only when the patient is in a standing or sitting position.

orthostatic (ŏr-thō-stăt'ĭk) concerning an erect position or related to a standing position.

osmosis (ŏs-mō'sĭs) passage of a liquid (solvent), usually water, through a semipermeable partition separating solutions of different concentrations to equalize the concentration of any substance dissolved in the solutions.

ossification (ŏs-ĭ-fĭ-kā'shŭn) process of bone formation.

osteomalacia (ŏs''tē-ō-mȧ-lā'shē-ȧ) adult rickets or softening of the bone.

osteomyelitis (ŏs''tē-ō-mī-ĕ-lī'tĭs) inflammation of the bone marrow and surrounding cells.

osteoporosis (ŏs''tē-ō-po-rō'sĭs) deossification with decrease in bone tissue resulting in structural weakness.

otitis media (ō-tī'tĭs mē'dē-ȧ) middle ear infection.

ovary (ō'vȧ-rē) paired, almond-shaped gland that produces female hormones and female sex cells, or ova.

oviduct (ō′vĭ-dŭkt) fallopian, or uterine, tube.

ovulation (ŏ-vŭ-lā′shŭn) rupture of an ovarian follicle and the expulsion of the ovum.

oxytocic (ŏk-sē-tō′sĭk) medication that stimulates the uterus to contract.

palliative (păl′ē-ā-tĭv) alleviate without curing.

palpation (păl-pā′shŭn) examination by touch or feel.

papule (păp′ūl) small, solid elevation on the skin; the typical early stage of a pimple.

paracentesis (păr-ă-sĕn-tē′sĭs) artificial withdrawal of fluid by puncture of a body cavity, especially the abdominal cavity.

paralytic (păr-ă-lĭt′ĭk) person suffering from loss of the ability to move a part or parts of his body.

parametrium (păr″ă-mē′trē-ŭm) the outermost covering of the uterus formed in part by a portion of the peritoneum.

parenchyma (pà-reng′kĭ-mà) functioning portion of an organ as distinguished from supportive cells forming its framework.

parenteral (pà-rĕn′ter-ăl) pertaining to methods of drug or food administration other than through the use of the gastrointestinal tract (e.g., intravenous or subcutaneous routes).

paresis (pà-rē′sĭs) organic mental illness; partial or incomplete paralysis.

paroxysmal (păr″ŏk-sĭz′măl) of the nature of a sudden attack.

parturient (păr-tū′rē-ĕnt) laboring or newly delivered mother.

parturition (păr-tū-rĭsh′ŭn) childbirth; delivery.

patency (pā′tĕn-sē) state of being freely open.

pathogen (păth′ō-jĕn) microorganism or substance capable of producing a disease.

pathological (păth′à-lŏj′ĭ-kàl) caused by or involving disease; concerning disease.

pediculosis (pĕ-dik-ū-lō′sĭs) infestation of an individual by head, body, or pubic lice.

pelvimeter (pĕl-vĭm′ĕ-ter) device used to measure the pelvis.

pendulous (pĕn′dū-lŭs) hanging; lacking proper support.

percussion (per-kush′ŭn) tapping the body lightly but sharply for diagnosis or therapy.

perinatal (pĕr-ĭ-nāt′ăl) associated with the period before or after birth.

perineum (per-ĭ-nē′ŭm) area of the external genitalia in both male and female; specifically, the area between the vagina and the anus or the scrotum and the anus.

periorbital (pĕr′ē-or′bĭt′ăl) the periosteum or outermost tissues covering the bone within the orbit of the eye.

periosteum (pĕr-ĭ-ŏs′tē-ŭm) fibrous membrane that forms the covering of bones except at their articular surfaces.

peripheral (per-ĭf′er-ăl) located at the surface or away from the center of the body.

peristalsis (pĕr-ĭs-tăl′sĭs) progressive, wavelike movement that occurs involuntarily in hollow tubes of the body, especially the alimentary canal.

peritoneum (pĕr″ĭt-o-nē′ŭm) the serous membrane lining the interior of the abdominal cavity and surrounding the contained internal organs.

peritonitis (pĕr-ĭ-tō-nī′tĭs) inflammation of the peritoneum.

permeable (pur′mē-à-bàl) capable of being penetrated.

per se (per sā) essentially; by itself; of itself.

pertussis (per-tŭs′ĭs) whooping cough.

petechiae (pà-tē′kē-ī) small, bluish purple dots on the skin resulting from capillary hemorrhages.

petrification (pĕt″rĭ-fĭ-kā′shŭn) process of turning into stone.

phagocytosis (făg″ō-sī-tō′sĭs) ingestion and digestion of bacteria and microscopic particles by phagocytes, certain white blood cells.

pharynx (făr′ĭnks) musculomembranous passageway at the back of the nose and mouth partially shared by both the respiratory and digestive systems.

phlebitis (flĕ-bī′tĭs) inflammation of a vein.

phlebotomy (flĕ-bŏt′ō-mē) purposeful opening of a vein, usually to let out a considerable amount of blood for therapy.

photophobia (fō-tō-fō′bē-à) unusual intolerance to light.

pica (pī′kà) an abnormal craving for substances not meant for consumption.

pigmentation (pĭg-mĕn-tā′shŭn) coloration resulting from the deposit of certain substances in the skin.

pipette (pī-pĕt′) narrow calibrated glass tube with both ends open, used to measure and transfer liquids from one container to another by application of oral suction.

pituitary gland (pĭ-tū′ĭ-tăr-ē) endocrine gland located at the base of the brain involved in many body functions; the "master gland."

placenta (plà-sĕn′tà) flattened, circular mass of spongy vascular tissue attached to the inside of the uterine wall that serves as the metabolic link between the fetus and the mother; from its surface protrudes the umbilical cord that carries food and oxygen to the fetus and waste away from the fetus; also serves as a point of attachment for the bag of waters that encloses the fetus.

placenta previa (prē′vē-à) low implantation of the placenta near or over the cervix within the uterine cavity causing hemorrhage late in pregnancy.

plantar (plăn′tär) concerning the sole of the foot.

platelet (plāt′lĕt) (blood platelet) thrombocyte, a necessary element for blood clot formation.

platypelloid (plăt″ē-pĕl′oyd) abnormal type of female pelvis, flattened from front to back.

pneumatocele (nü-mă′ō-sēl) a herniation of lung tissue; a sac or tumor containing gas.

pneumomediastinum (nü″mō-mē-dē-ăs-tī′nŭm) air or gas in the mediastinal tissues located between the lungs.

pneumonia (nü-mō′nē-á) inflammation of the lung tissue.

pneumothorax (nü-mō-thō′răks) collection of air or gas in the pleural cavity (the potential space between the two coverings of the lungs).

polyarthritis (pŏl″ē-är-thrī′tĭs) inflammation that involves more than one joint, often migratory in character.

polycystic (pŏl-ē-sĭs′tĭk) composed of many cysts, that is, little sacs usually containing fluid.

polycythemia (pŏl″ē-sī-thē′mē-á) abnormal condition characterized by an excess of red blood cells.

polydactylism (pŏl-ē-dăk′tĭl-ĭzm) presence of extra fingers or toes.

polydipsia (pŏl-ē-dĭp′sē-á) excessive thirst and fluid intake.

polyhydramnios (pŏl″ē-hī-drăm′nē-ōs) an excessive volume of amniotic fluid.

polymorphonuclear (pŏl″ē-mor-fō-nü′klē-er) leukocyte having a lobated or segmented nucleus.

polyphagia (pŏl-ē-fā′jē-á) excessive appetite.

polyuria (pŏl-ē-ū′rē-á) excessive urinary output.

portal of entry avenue by which an infectious agent gains entrance into the body.

precipitate (prē-sĭp′ĭ-tāt) *delivery* delivery that occurs with such rapidity that proper preparation and medical supervision are lacking.

preeclampsia (prē-ĕk-lămp′sē-á) toxemia of pregnancy uncomplicated by convulsion or coma (see eclampsia).

prehension (prē-hĕn′shŭn) use of the hands to pick up small objects; grasping.

prepuce (prē′pŭs) foreskin of penis.

presentation in obstetrics, relationship of the length of the fetus to the length of the uterus.

presenting part part of the baby that comes through or attempts to come through the pelvic canal first; often synonymous with "obstetrical presentation."

primigravida (prī-mĭ-grăv′ĭ-dà) woman who is having or has had one pregnancy.

primipara (prī-mĭp′á-rá) strictly speaking, a woman who has been delivered of one infant over 500 Gm.; however, in the delivery room, a woman in the process of labor with her first viable child is called a primipara.

progesterone (prō-jĕs′tĕr-ōn) female sex hormone manufactured by the corpus luteum of the ovary and, during pregnancy, by the placenta; aids in preparing the lining of the uterus for pregnancy and maintaining a pregnancy once established.

prolapse (prō-lăps′) a falling out of place (e.g., a rectocele).

prophylactic (prō-fĭ-lăk′tĭk) that which prevents disease.

prophylaxis (prō-fĭ-lăk′sĭs) preventive treatment.

prostate (prŏs′tāt) exocrine gland found at the base of the male bladder that secretes an alkaline fluid stimulating sperm motility.

prosthesis (prŏ-thē′sĭs) artificial body part.

proteinuria (prō-tē-ĭn-ū′rē-á) finding of protein usually albumin, in the urine.

prothrombin (prō-thrŏm′bĭn) chemical substance found in the blood, necessary to coagulation.

protozoa (prō-tō-zō′á) (sing. protozoon) simple microscopic animals, usually single celled.

protrusion (prō-trü′zhŭn) state or condition of being forward or projecting.

pruritus (prü-rī′tŭs) itching.

pseudohermaphroditism (sū″dō-hĕr-măf′rō-dĭt-ĭzm) condition in which an individual possesses external genitalia resembling those of one sex and the internal sex organs or gonads of the opposing sex.

psychosis (sī-kō′sĭs) serious mental disturbance involving personality disintegration and loss of contact with reality.

ptyalism (tī′á-lĭzm) excessive salivation.

puberty (pū′ber-tē) period in life when one becomes capable of reproduction.

puerperium (pū-er-pĭr′ē-ŭm) six-week period following delivery.

purpura (pur′pū-rá) purple discoloration that occurs as a result of spontaneous bleeding into the skin or mucous membranes.

pustule (pŭs′tūl) pus-filled papule; a superficial cutaneous abscess.

pyelogram (pī′ĕl-ō-grăm) roentgenogram of the ureters and renal pelves.

pyelonephritis (pī″ĕl-ō-nĕf-rī′tĭs) infection of the renal pelvis and the working units of the kidney, the nephrons.

pyogenic (pī-ō-jĕn′ĭk) producing pus.

pyrosis (pī-rō′sĭs) heartburn.

quarantine (kwär′ăn-tēn) confinement of a person or group of persons who have been exposed to a contagious disease to a specific place without outside contacts for the duration of the longest usual incubation period of the disease in question.

quickening (kwĭk′ĕn-ĭng) maternal identification of fetal motion; felt by multiparas at about the sixteenth week of pregnancy and by primiparas 2 weeks later.

rectocele (rĕk′tō-sēl) prolapse or displacement of the rectum because of the weakening of the rectovaginal wall.

reduction (rē-dŭk′shŭn) in orthopedics, refers to

realignment of a broken bone or the correct placement of a dislocation.

reflux (rē′flŭks) return or backward flow (e.g., regurgitation of urine from the bladder into the ureter).

regurgitation (rē-gŭr-jĭ-tā′shŭn) return of solids or fluids to the mouth from the stomach; any abnormal backflow of fluid within the body.

remission (rē-mĭsh′ŭn) lessening of severity or abatement of symptoms.

reservoir (rĕz′er-vwâr) chamber or receptacle for holding fluid; store; reserve.

retinoblastoma (rĕt-ĭn-ō-blăs-tō′må) malignant tumor of the eye.

retraction (rē-trăk′shŭn) state of being drawn back.

retroflexion (rĕt-rō-flĕk′shŭn) bending or flexing backward; an abnormal position of the uterus bent backward toward the rectum, forming an angle between the cervix and the body of the organ.

retrograde (rĕt′rō-grād) moving backward; degenerating from better to worse.

retrolental fibroplasia (rĕ″tro-lĕn′tål fĭ″brō-plā′zē-å) an oxygen-induced separation of the retina of the eye behind the lens; characteristic of premature infants.

retroversion (rĕt-rō-ver′shŭn) turning or state of being turned back; backward displacement of the body of the uterus so that the cervix points toward the symphysis pubis instead of toward the sacrum.

Rh blood factor blood protein found in approximately 85% of the American population; those persons who possess it are termed Rh positive.

rheumatism (rü′må-tĭzm) any of numerous conditions characterized by inflammation or pain in muscles, joints, or fibrous tissue.

rhinitis (rī-nī′tĭs) inflammation of the nasal mucosa.

rickets (rĭk′ĕts) disturbance in skeletal development because of poor nutritional intake or absorption of vitamin D and/or calcium or phosphorus; characterized by abnormal softening of the bones.

roentgenogram (rĕnt-gĕn′ō-gram) x-ray film.

rubella (rü-bĕl′å) German, or 3-day, measles.

rubeola (rü-bē′ō-lå) red, or 2-week, measles.

sacrum (sā′krŭm) fused bone that with the coccyx forms the lower portion of the spine and posterior surface of the pelvis.

salmonellosis (săl″mō-nĕl-ō′sĭs) infection (including typhoid) caused by ingesting foods containing species of the genus *Salmonella*.

sarcoma (sär-kō′må) malignant tumor originating in connective tissue.

scabies (skā′bēz) infestation of the skin by the itch mite *Sarcoptes scabiei;* "7-year itch."

sclera (sklĕ′rå) (pl. sclerae) white outercoating of the eyeball extending from the optic nerve to include the cornea.

scoliosis (skō-lĭ-ō′sĭs) abnormal lateral spinal curvature.

scrotum (skrō′tŭm) pouch forming part of the male external genitalia containing the testicles and part of the spermatic cord.

scultetus (skŭl-tē′tŭs) *binder* many-tailed abdominal binder.

seborrhea (sĕb-ōr-ē′å) functional disorder of the sebaceous (oil) glands of the skin and/or scalp causing crusting and scaling; on the scalp it may be called dandruff, milk crust, or cradle cap, depending on the location and density of the scaling.

sedative (sĕd′å-tĭv) medication that quiets and reduces tension.

semen (sē′mĕn) fluid discharge from the male reproductive organs that contains the sperm destined to fertilize the female ovum.

sensitization (sĕn-sĭ-tĭ-zā′shŭn) process of making a person reactive to a substance such as a drug, plant, fiber, or serum.

sepsis (sĕp′sĭs) presence or state of contamination, putrefaction, or infection.

septicemia (sĕp-tĭ-sē′mē-å) disease condition resulting from the absorption of pathogenic microorganisms and/or the poisons resulting from infectious processes into the blood.

sequestrum (sē-kwĕs′trŭm) (pl. sequestra) fragment of a diseased, decaying bone that has become separated from surrounding tissue.

serology (ser-ōl′ō-jĭ) study of blood serum.

show as used in obstetrics, the blood-tinged mucoid vaginal discharge that becomes more pronounced and red as cervical dilatation increases during labor.

shunt (shŭnt) to turn away from; to divert; a normal or artificially constructed passage that diverts a flow from one main route to another.

sibling (sĭb′lĭng) one of two or more children of the same parents.

smegma (smĕg′må) cheesy secretion of the sebaceous glands found in the area of the labia minora and the clitoris of the female or the prepuce in the male.

spastic (spăs′tĭk) type of muscular action characterized by stiff, uncoordinated movement.

spasticity (spăs-tĭs′ĭ-tē) stiff, awkward, uncoordinated movements caused by hypertension of the muscles, usually caused by brain damage.

sperm male sex cell, spermatozoon, carrying the male hereditary potential.

spermatozoon (sper″må-tō-zō′on) (pl. spermatozoa) male sex cell.

sphincter (sfĭngk′ter) circular muscle constricting or closing an opening.

spore (spōr) protective form assumed by some bacilli (usage in bacteriology).

stasis (stā'sĭs) a cessation of flow in blood or other body fluids.

station (stā'shŭn) depth of the presenting part in the pelvic canal as measured by the relationship of the presenting part to the ischial spines of the pelvis.

status asthmaticus (stăt'ŭs ăz-măt'ĭ-kŭs) a severe asthmatic condition that does not respond to usual treatment.

steatorrhea (stē-ăt-ōr-rē'á) presence of excessive fat in the stool; increased secretion of the oil glands.

stenosis (stĕn-ō'sĭs) abnormal narrowing of a passage or opening.

sterile (stĕr'ĭl) free of living microorganisms, including spore forms.

stoma (stō'má) a mouth or opening of a pore; a body opening, natural or artificial; term usually applied to a colostomy, ileostomy, or ileobladder opening.

strabismus (strá-bĭz'mŭs) crossed or crooked eyes; squint.

streptococcus (strĕp-tō-kŏk'ŭs) (pl. streptococci) spherical microorganism that forms a pattern like beads on a string.

striae (strī'ē) stretch marks often seen on the skin of pregnant women where weight gain has been marked.

stridor (strī'dōr) harsh-sounding respirations.

subcostal (sŭb-kŏs'tál) lying beneath a rib or ribs or just below the last rib adjacent to the abdomen.

subinvolution (sub-ĭn-vō-lū'shŭn) incomplete return of a part to its normal position or dimensions; term usually applied to an abnormal, incomplete return of the uterus to its prepregnant state after childbirth.

subluxation (sŭb"lŭk-sā'shŭn) incomplete dislocation of a bone.

supine (sü-pīn') positioned on the back or palm up.

suprapubic (sü"prá-pū'bĭk) above the pubis.

suprasternal (sü"prá-stur'nál) above the sternum adjacent to the neck.

syndactylism (sĭn-dăk'tĭl-ĭzm) fusion or webbing of two or more fingers or toes.

syndrome (sĭn'drōm) complete picture of a disease; all the symptoms of a disease considered as a whole.

systolic (sĭs-tŏl'ĭk) *pressure* pertaining to systole; blood pressure at the time of greatest cardiac contraction.

tachycardia (tăk"ē-kär'dē-á) excessive rapidity of the heart's action.

tachypnea (tăk"ĭp-nē'á) rapid rate of breathing.

talipes (tăl'ĭ-pēz) any of a number of deformities of the ankle or foot, usually congenital; clubfoot.

talipes valgus (văl'gŭs) the toes are turned out.

talipes varus (vā'rŭs) the toes are turned in.

telangiectasia (tel-ăn"jē-ĕk-tā'zē-á) small reddened areas often found on the eyelids, midforehead, and nape of the neck on newborn infants, caused by superficial dilatation of capillaries.

tendon (tĕn'dŭn) fibrous tissue that connects muscle to bone or other structures.

teratogenic (tĕr"á-tō-gĕn'ĭk) capable of causing congenital malformation.

testis (tĕs'tĭs) (pl. testes) paired, oval, male sex gland that produces a male sex hormone and spermatozoa.

testosterone (tĕs-tŏs'tĕr-ōn) male hormone produced by the testes.

tetanus (tĕt'á-nŭs) lockjaw; a state of sustained muscular contraction.

tetany (tĕt'á-nē) nervous affection characterized by intermittent tonic spasms of the muscles that may be caused by inadequate calcium levels in the bloodstream.

therapeutic (thĕr-á-pū'tĭk) having medicinal or healing properties; a healing agent.

thermal (ther'măl) pertaining to heat.

thoracentesis (thō-răs-ĕn-tē'sĭs) removal of fluids through the chest wall by the insertion of a special needle.

thrombocyte (thrŏm'bō-sīt) blood platelet necessary to coagulation.

thrombocytopenic (thrŏm"bō-sī"tō-pēn'ĭk) pertaining to abnormal decrease in the number of platelets in the blood.

thrombophlebitis (thrŏm"bō-flē-bī'tĭs) inflammation of a vein in conjunction with the development of a blood clot.

thrombosis (thrŏm-bō'sĭs) formation of a blood clot.

thrombus (thrŏm'bŭs) blood clot formed in a blood vessel or cavity of the heart.

thrush (thrŭsh) fungous infection caused by *Candida albicans* in the mouth or throat, especially in infants; characterized by white patches that adhere to the mucous membranes.

tincture (tĭngk'tūr) substance that, in solution, is diluted with alcohol.

tinea capitis (tĭn'ē-á kăp'ĭ-tĭs) ringworm of the scalp.

tinea corporis (kōr'por-ĭs) any fungous skin disease, especially ringworm of the body.

tinea pedis (pēd'ĭs) fungous skin disease or ringworm of the foot; commonly called athlete's foot.

torsion (tōr'shŭn) act of or condition of being twisted.

torticollis (tŏr-tĭ-kŏl'ĭs) wryneck or tilting of the head caused by the abnormal shortening of either sternocleidomastoid muscle.

toxemia (tŏk-sē'mē-á) presence of poisonous products in the blood and body; disease of unknown mechanism suffered by some pregnant women, characterized by high blood pressure, albumin in the urine, and edema (see eclampsia and preeclampsia).

toxoid (tŏks'oyd) preparation that contains a toxin or poison produced by pathogenic organisms capable of producing active immunity against a disease but too weak to produce the disease itself.

tracheostomy (trā-kē-ŏst'ō-mē) surgical opening of the trachea through the neck to help assure an airway; a planned intervention usually of some duration or permanence.

traction (trăk'shŭn) process of pulling.

translocation (trănz"lō-kā'shŭn) displacement of part or all of one chromosome onto another.

transverse (trăns-vĕrs') *presentation* presentation in which the fetus lies crosswise in the pelvis and cannot be delivered vaginally unless turned.

trauma (träw'mȧ) injury or wound; a painful emotional experience.

trichomonas vaginitis (trī-kŏm'ō'nȧs vȧ-jī-nī'tīs) inflammation of the vagina caused by the parasitic protozoa *Trichomonas vaginalis* that results in itching and a profuse, bubbly, yellow discharge.

trigone (trī'gōn) triangular space; triangular area in the urinary bladder formed by the urethral outlet and the two ureteral openings.

trimester (trī-mĕs'tĕr) three-month period of time.

trisomy (trī'sō-mē) occurrence of three of a given chromosome in a cell rather than the normal diploid number of two.

trophozoite (trŏf-ō-zō'īt) animal spore during its developmental stage; motile form of the ameba.

turgor (tur'gur) normal tension in living cells; distention or swelling.

ulcer (ŭl'ser) raw area often depressed or forming a cavity caused by loss of normal covering tissue.

ultrasonography (ŭl"trȧ-sō-nŏg'rȧ-fē) pulse echo diagnosis or technique using high-frequency, inaudible sound waves.

umbilicus (ŭm-bĭl'ĭkŭs or ŭm-bĭ-lī'kŭs) site of the umbilical cord attachment; the navel.

uremia (ū-rē'mē-ȧ) toxic condition associated with renal insufficiency and the retention in the blood of nitrogenous substances normally excreted by the kidney.

ureter (ū-rē'tur/ūr'ĕ-ter) long tubes conveying the urine from the kidneys to the urinary bladder.

ureterocele (ū-rē'ter-ō-sēl) ballooning of the lower end of the ureter.

urethra (ū-rē'thrȧ) the canal through which the urine is discharged.

urethroplasty (ū-rē'thrō-plăs-tē) operation to correct hypospadias; surgical repair of the urethra.

urogram (ū'rō-gram) x-ray photograph of any part of the urinary tract.

urticaria (ur-tĭ-kā'rē-ȧ) wheals; hives; large, slightly raised, reddened or blanched areas often accompanied by intense itching.

uterine inertia (ū'ter-ĭn ĭn-er'shȧ) abnormal relaxation of the uterus either during labor, causing lack of obstetrical progress, or after delivery, causing uterine hemorrhage.

uterus (ū'ter-ŭs) hollow, muscular organ that serves as a protector and nourisher of the developing fetus and aids in its expulsion from the body; the womb.

vaccine (văk'sēn) preparation containing killed or weakened living microorganisms that, when introduced into the body, cause the formation of antibodies against that type of organism, thereby protecting the individual from the disease.

vaccinia (văk-sĭn'ē-ȧ) (generalized) numerous vaccination sites resulting from the spread of the vaccine to open lesions after a routine smallpox vaccination.

vagina (vȧ-jī'nȧ) canal opening between the urethra and anus in the female that extends back to the cervix of the uterus.

valgus (văl'gŭs) term denoting position meaning "turned outward" or "twisted"; applied to a clubfoot with the toes turned outward.

varicella (văr-ĭ-sĕl'ȧ) chicken pox; acute contagious disease, commonly of childhood, characterized by a body rash seen simultaneously in all stages of development.

varicosity (văr-ĭ-kŏs'ĭ-tē) abnormal swollen vein, the walls of which are thinned and weakened.

variola (vȧ-rī'ō-lȧ) smallpox; severe contagious disease characterized by the formation of a typical rash and pronounced prostration; may cause death.

varus (vā′rŭs) term denoting position meaning "turned inward"; applied to a clubfoot with the toes turned inward.

vas deferens (văs dĕf′er-ĕnz) excretory duct of the testis.

vasodilator (văs-ō-dī-lā′tŏr) drug that dilates the blood vessels.

vein (vān) blood vessel that carries blood to the heart.

ventricle (vĕn′-trĭk-ŭl) small cavity or chamber; one of two lower chambers of the heart; one of several cavities in the brain where cerebrospinal fluid is formed or drains.

ventriculogram (vĕn-trĭk′ū-lō-grăm) diagnostic test in which air is introduced into the ventricles of the brain through surgical openings in the scalp.

vernix caseosa (vĕr′nĭks cāz-ē-ō′sà) yellowish, creamy substance on the fetus caused by the secretion of the oil glands of the skin.

version (ver′shŭn) in obstetrics, the changing of the fetal presentation by internal or external manual maneuvers.

vertigo (ver′tĭ-gō) dizziness.

vesicle (vĕs′ĭ-kŭl) elevation of the skin, obviously containing fluid; a blister.

vesicular (vĕs-ĭk′ū-lar) blisterlike.

vestibule (vĕs′tĭ-būl) triangular space between the labia minora in which the openings of the urethra, vagina, and Bartholin's glands are located.

viable (vī′à-bŭl) capable of life; capable of living outside the uterus; subject to legal definition.

virulent (vĭr′ū-lĕnt) very poisonous; infectious.

virus (vī′rŭs) submicroscopic infective agent.

viscosity (vĭs-kŏs′ĭ-tē) state of being thick, gummy, or sticky.

vulnerable susceptible to being wounded; in an unfavorable condition.

vulva (vŭl′và) external female genitalia.

wheal (wēl) large, slightly raised, reddened or blanched area, often accompanied by intense itching.

zygote (zī′gōt) fertilized egg.

Index